Macleod's
Clinical Examination

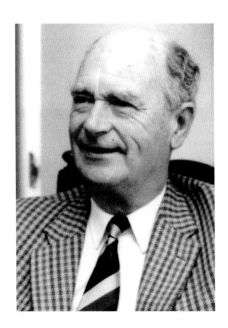

John Macleod (1915–2006)

John Macleod was appointed consultant physician at the Western General Hospital, Edinburgh, in 1950. He had major interests in rheumatology and medical education. Medical students who attended his clinical teaching sessions remember him as an inspirational teacher with the ability to present complex problems with great clarity. He was invariably courteous to his patients and students alike. He had an uncanny knack of involving all students equally in clinical discussions and used praise rather than criticism. He paid great attention to the value of history taking and, from this, expected students to identify what particular aspects of the physical examination should help to narrow the diagnostic options.

His consultant colleagues at the Western welcomed the opportunity of contributing when he suggested writing a textbook on clinical examination. The book was first published in 1964 and John Macleod edited seven editions. With characteristic modesty he was very embarrassed when the eighth edition was renamed *Macleod's Clinical Examination*. This, however, was a small way of recognising his enormous contribution to medical education.

He possessed the essential quality of a successful editor – the skill of changing disparate contributions from individual contributors into a uniform style and format without causing offence; everybody accepted his authority. He avoided being dogmatic or condescending. He was generous in teaching others his editorial skills and these attributes were recognised when he was invited to edit *Davidson's Principles and Practice of Medicine*.

Content Strategist: Laurence Hunter
Content Development Specialist: Helen Leng
Project Manager: Anne Collett
Designer: Miles Hitchen
Illustration Manager: Karen Giacomucci

Macleod's

Clinical Examination

14th Edition

Edited by

J Alastair Innes
BSc PhD FRCP(Ed)

Consultant Physician, Respiratory Unit, Western General
Hospital, Edinburgh; Honorary Reader in Respiratory Medicine,
University of Edinburgh, UK

Anna R Dover
PhD FRCP(Ed)

Consultant in Diabetes, Endocrinology and General Medicine,
Edinburgh Centre for Endocrinology and Diabetes, Royal
Infirmary of Edinburgh; Honorary Clinical Senior Lecturer,
University of Edinburgh, UK

Karen Fairhurst
PhD FRCGP

General Practitioner, Mackenzie Medical Centre, Edinburgh;
Clinical Senior Lecturer, Centre for Population Health Sciences,
University of Edinburgh, UK

Illustrations by Robert Britton and Ethan Danielson

ELSEVIER   Edinburgh   London   New York   Oxford   Philadelphia   St Louis   Sydney   2018

ELSEVIER

First edition 1964
Second edition 1967
Third edition 1973
Fourth edition 1976
Fifth edition 1979

Sixth edition 1983
Seventh edition 1986
Eighth edition 1990
Ninth edition 1995
Tenth edition 2000

Eleventh edition 2005
Twelfth edition 2009
Thirteenth edition 2013
Fourteenth edition 2018

ISBN   978-0-7020-6993-2
International ISBN   978-0-7020-6992-5

Notices

ELSEVIER your source for books, journals and multimedia in the health sciences

www.elsevierhealth.com

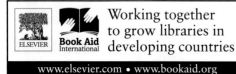

Working together to grow libraries in developing countries

www.elsevier.com • www.bookaid.org

The publisher's policy is to use **paper manufactured from sustainable forests**

Printed in Europe
Last digit is the print number: 9   8   7   6   5   4   3   2

Contents

Preface

Despite the wealth of diagnostic tools available to the modern physician, the acquisition of information by direct interaction with the patient through history taking and clinical examination remains the bedrock of the physician's art. These time-honoured skills can often allow clinicians to reach a clear diagnosis without recourse to expensive and potentially harmful tests.

This book aims to assist clinicians in developing the consultation skills required to elicit a clear history, and the practical skills needed to detect clinical signs of disease. Where possible, the physical basis of clinical signs is explained to aid understanding. Formulation of a differential diagnosis from the information gained is introduced, and the logical initial investigations are included for each system. *Macleod's Clinical Examination* is designed to be used in conjunction with more detailed texts on pathophysiology, differential diagnosis and clinical medicine, illustrating specifically how the history and examination can inform the diagnostic process.

In this edition the contents have been restructured and the text comprehensively updated by a team of existing and new authors, with the aim of creating an accessible and user-friendly text relevant to the practice of medicine in the 21st century.

Section 1 addresses the general principles of good interaction with patients, from the basics of taking a history and examining, to the use of pattern recognition to identify spot diagnoses. Section 2 deals with symptoms and signs in specific systems and Section 3 illustrates the application of these skills to specific clinical situations. Section 4 covers preparation for assessments of clinical skills and for the use of these skills in everyday practice.

An expertly performed history and examination of a patient allows the doctor to detect disease and predict prognosis, and is crucial to the principle of making the patient and their concerns central to the care process, and also to the avoidance of harm from unnecessary or unjustified tests.

We hope that if young clinicians are encouraged to adopt and adapt these skills, they not only will serve their patients as diagnosticians but also will themselves continue to develop clinical examination techniques and a better understanding of their mechanisms and diagnostic use.

The 14th edition of *Macleod's Clinical Examination* has an accompanying set of videos available in the online *Student Consult* electronic library. This book is closely integrated with *Davidson's Principles and Practice of Medicine* and is best read in conjunction with that text.

JAI, ARD, KF
Edinburgh, 2018

Acknowledgements

The editors would like acknowledge the immense contribution made by Graham Douglas, Fiona Nicol and Colin Robertson who edited the three previous editions of Macleod's Clinical Examination. Together they re-shaped the format of this textbook and their efforts were rewarded by a substantial growth in both its sales and international reputation.

The editors would like to acknowledge and offer grateful thanks for the input of all previous editions' contributors, without whom this new edition would not have been possible. In particular, we are indebted to those former authors who step down with the arrival of this new edition. They include: Elaine Anderson, John Bevan, Andrew Bradbury, Nicki Colledge, Allan Cumming, Graham Devereux, Jamie Douglas, Rebecca Ford, David Gawkrodger, Neil Grubb, James Huntley, John Iredale, Robert Laing, Andrew Longmate, Alastair MacGilchrist, Dilip Nathwani, Jane Norman, John Olson, Paul O'Neill, Stephen Payne, Laura Robertson, David Snadden, James C Spratt, Kum-Ying Tham, Steve Turner and Janet Wilson.

We are particularly grateful to the following medical students, who undertook detailed reviews of the book and gave us a wealth of ideas to implement in this latest edition. We trust we have listed all those who contributed, and apologise if any names have been accidentally omitted: Layla Raad Abd Al-Majeed, Ali Adel Ne'ma Abdullah, Aanchal Agarwal, Hend Almazroa, Alhan Alqinai, Amjed Alyasseen, Chidatma Arampady, Christian Børde Arkteg, Maha Arnaout, Rashmi Arora, Daniel Ashrafi, Herry Asnawi, Hemant Atri, Ahmed Ayyad, Kainath N Azad, Sadaf Azam, Arghya Bandhu, Jamie Barclay, Prithiv Siddarth Saravana Bavan, Rajarshi Bera, Craig Betton, Apoorva Bhagat, Prachi Bhageria, Geethanjali Bhas, Navin Bhatt, Shahzadi Nisar Bhutto, Abhishek Ghosh Biswas, Tamoghna Biswas, Debbie Bolton, Claude Borg, Daniel Buxton, Anup Chalise, Amitesh Kumar Chatterjee, Subhankar Chatterjee, Farhan Ashraf Chaudhary, Aalia Chaudhry, Jessalynn Chia, Bhaswati Chowdhury, Robin Chowdhury, Marshall Colin, Michael Collins, Margaret Cooper, Barbara Corke, Andrea Culmer, Gowtham Varma Dantuluri, Abhishek Das, Sonali Das, Aziz Dauti, Mark Davies, Adam Denton, Muinul Islam Dewan, Greg Dickman, Hengameh Ahmad Dokhtjavaherian, Amy Edwards, Muhammad Eimaduddin, Laith Al Ejeilat, Divya G Eluru, Emmanuel Ernest, El Bushra El Fadil, Fathima Ashfa Mohamed Faleel, Malcolm Falzon, Emma Farrington, Noor Fazal, Sultana Ferdous, Matthew Formosa, Brian Forsyth, David Fotheringham, Bhargav Gajula, Dariimaa Ganbat, Lauren Gault, Michaela Goodson, Mounika Gopalam, Ciaran Grafton-Clarke, Anthony Gunawan, Aditya Gupta, Digvijay Gupta, Kshitij Gupta, Sonakshi Gupta, Md. Habibullah, Kareem Haloub, Akar Jamal Hamasalih, James Harper, Bruce Harper-McDonald, Jon Harvey, Alexandra Hawker, Raja K Haynes, Emma Hendry, Malik Hina, Bianca Honnekeri, Justina Igwe, Chisom Ikeji, Sushrut Ingawale, Mohammad Yousuf ul Islam, Sneha Jain, Maria Javed, Ravin Jegathnathan, Helge Leander B Jensen, Li Jie, Ali Al Joboory, Asia Joseph, Christopher Teow Kang Jun, Janpreet Kainth, Ayush Karmacharya, JS Karthik, Aneesh Karwande, Adhishesh Kaul, Alper Kaymak, Ali Kenawi, Abdullah Al Arefin Khadem, Haania Khan, Muhammad Hassan Khan, Sehrish Khan, Shrayash Khare, Laith Khweir, Ankit Kumar, Vinay Kumar, Ibrahim Lafi, Armeen Lakhani, Christopher Lee, David Lee, Benjamin Leeves, Soo Ting Joyce Lim, Chun Hin Lo, Lai Hing Loi, Chathura Mihiran Maddumabandara, Joana Sousa Magalhães, Aditya Mahajan, Mahabubul Islam Majumder, Aaditya Mallik, Mithilesh Chandra Malviya, Santosh Banadahally Manjegowda, Jill Marshall, Balanuj Mazumdar, Alan David McCrorie, Paras Mehmood, Kartik Mittal, Mahmood Kazi Mohammed, Amber Moorcroft, Jayne Murphy, Sana Mustafa, Arvi Nahar, Akshay Prakash Narad, Shehzina Nawal, Namia Nazir, Viswanathan Neelakantan, Albero Nieto, Angelina Choong Kin Ning, Faizul Nordin, Mairead O'Donoghue, Joey O'Halloran, Amit Kumar Ojha, Ifeolu James Oyedele, Anik Pal, Vidit Panchal, Asha Pandu, Bishal Panthi, Jacob Parker, Ujjawal Paudel, Tanmoy Kumar Paul, Kate Perry, Daniel Pisaru, David Potter, Dipesh Poudel, Arijalu Syaram Putra, Janine Qasim, Muhammad Qaunayn Qays, Mohammad Qudah, Jacqueline Quinn, Varun MS Venkat Raghavan, Md. Rahmatullah, Ankit Raj, Jerin Joseph Raju, Prasanna A Ramana, Ashwini Dhanraj Rangari, Anurag Ramesh Rathi, Anam Raza, Rakesh Reddy, Sudip Regmi, Amgad Riad, Patel Riya, Emily Robins, Grace Robinson, Muhammad'Azam Paku Rozi, Cosmin Rusneac, Ahmed Sabra, Anupama Sahu, Mohammad Saleh, Manjiri Saoji, Saumyadip Sarkar, Rakesh Kumar Shah, Basil Al Shammaa, Sazzad Sharhiar, Anmol Sharma, Homdutt Sharma, Shivani Sharma, Shobhit Sharma, Johannes Iikuyu Shilongo, Dhan Bahadur Shrestha, Pratima Shrestha, Anurag Singh, Kareshma Kaur Ranjit Singh, Nishansh Singh, Aparna Sinha, Liam Skoda, Ethan-Dean Smith, Prithviraj Solanki, Meenakshi Sonnilal, Soundarya Soundararajan, Morshedul Islam Sowrav, Kayleigh Spellar, Siddharth Srinivasan, Pradeep Srivastava, Anthony Starr, Michael Suryadisastra, Louisa Sutton, Komal Ashok Tapadiya, Areeba Tariq, Imran Tariq, Jia Chyi Tay, Javaria Tehzeeb, Daniel Theron, Michele Tosi, Pagavathbharathi Sri Balaji Vidyapeeth, Amarjit Singh Vij, Cathrine Vincent, Ghassan Wadi, Amirah Abdul Wahab, James Warrington, Luke Watson, Federico Ivan Weckesser, Ben Williamson, Kevin Winston, Kyi Phyu Wint, Harsh Yadav, Saroj Kumar Yadav, Amelia Yong, Awais Zaka and Nuzhat Zehra.

How to make the most of this book

The purpose of this book is to document and explain how to:

- interact with a patient as their doctor
- take a history from a patient
- examine a patient
- formulate your findings into differential diagnoses
- rank these in order of probability
- use investigations to support or refute your differential diagnosis.

Initially, when you approach a section, we suggest that you glance through it quickly, looking at the headings and how it is laid out. This will help you to see in your mind's eye the framework to use.

Learn to speed-read. It is invaluable in medicine and in life generally. Most probably, the last lesson you had on reading was at primary school. Most people can dramatically improve their speed of reading and increase their comprehension by using and practising simple techniques.

Try making mind maps of the details to help you recall and retain the information as you progress through the chapter. Each of the systems chapters is laid out in the same order:

- Introduction: anatomy and physiology.
- The history: common presenting symptoms, what questions to ask and how to follow them up.
- The physical examination: what and how to examine.
- Investigations: how to select the most relevant and informative initial tests, and how these clarify the diagnosis.
- Objective Structured Clinical Examination (OSCE) examples: a couple of short clinical scenarios included to illustrate the type of problems students may meet in an OSCE assessment of this system.

- Integrated examination sequence: a structured list of steps to be followed when examining the system, intended as a prompt and revision aid.

Return to this book to refresh your technique if you have been away from a particular field for some time. It is surprising how quickly your technique deteriorates if you do not use it regularly. Practise at every available opportunity so that you become proficient at examination techniques and gain a full understanding of the range of normality.

Ask a senior colleague to review your examination technique regularly; there is no substitute for this and for regular practice. Listen also to what patients say – not only about themselves but also about other health professionals – and learn from these comments. You will pick up good and bad points that you will want to emulate or avoid.

Finally, enjoy your skills. After all, you are learning to be able to understand, diagnose and help people. For most of us, this is the reason we became doctors.

Examination sequences

Throughout the book there are outlines of techniques that you should follow when examining a patient. These are identified with a red 'Examination sequence' heading. The bullet-point list provides the exact order in which to undertake the examination. To help your understanding of how to perform these techniques many of the examination sequences have been filmed and these are marked with an arrowhead.

▶ Clinical skills videos

Included with your purchase are clinical examination videos, custom-made for this textbook. Filmed using qualified doctors, with hands-on guidance from the author team, and narrated by former Editor Professor Colin Robertson, these videos offer you the chance to watch trained professionals performing many of the examination routines described in the book. By helping you to memorise the essential examination steps required for each major system and by demonstrating the proper clinical technique, these videos should act as an important bridge between textbook learning and bedside teaching. The videos will be available for you to view again and again as your clinical skills develop and will prove invaluable as you prepare for your clinical OSCE examinations.

Each examination routine has a detailed explanatory narrative but for maximum benefit view the videos in conjunction with the book. See the inside front cover for your access instructions.

Key points in examinations: photo galleries

Many of the examination sequences are included as photo galleries, illustrating with captions the key stages of the examination routine. These will act as a useful reminder of the main points of each sequence. See the inside front cover for your access instructions.

Video contents

- Examination of the cardiovascular system.
- Examination of the respiratory system.
- Examination of the gastrointestinal system.
- Examination of the neurological system.
- Examination of the ear.
- Examination of the thyroid gland.
- Examination of the musculoskeletal system.

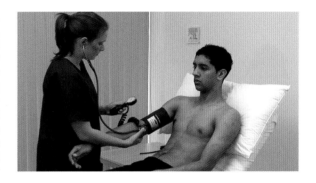

Video production team

Director and editor
Dr Iain Hennessey

Producer
Dr Alan G Japp

Sound and narrators
Professor Colin Robertson
Dr Nick Morley

Clinical examiners
Dr Amy Robb
Dr Ben Waterson

Patients
Abby Cooke
Omar Ali

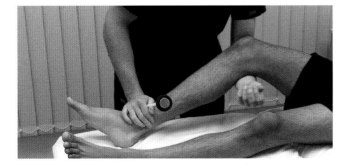

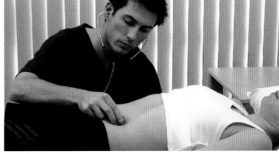

Contributors

Anthony Bateman MD MRCP FRCA FFICM
Consultant in Critical Care and Long Term Ventilation, Critical Care NHS Lothian, Edinburgh, UK

Shyamanga Borooah MRCP(UK) MRCS(Ed) FRCOphth PhD
Fulbright Fight for Sight Scholar, Shiley Eye Institute, University of California, San Diego, USA

Kirsty Boyd PhD FRCP MMedSci
Consultant in Palliative Medicine, Royal Infirmary of Edinburgh; Honorary Clinical Senior Lecturer, Primary Palliative Care Research Group, University of Edinburgh, UK

Ivan Brenkel FRCS(Ed)
Consultant Orthopaedic Surgeon, Orthopaedics, NHS Fife, Kirkcaldy, UK

Gareth Clegg PhD MRCP FRCEM
Senior Clinical Lecturer, University of Edinburgh; Honorary Consultant in Emergency Medicine, Royal Infirmary of Edinburgh, UK

Steve Cunningham PhD
Consultant and Honorary Professor in Paediatric Respiratory Medicine, Royal Hospital for Sick Children, Edinburgh, UK

Richard Davenport DM FRCP(Ed)
Consultant Neurologist, Western General Hospital and Royal Infirmary of Edinburgh; Honorary Senior Lecturer, University of Edinburgh, UK

Neeraj Dhaun PhD
Senior Lecturer and Honorary Consultant Nephrologist, University of Edinburgh, UK

Anna R Dover PhD FRCP(Ed)
Consultant in Diabetes, Endocrinology and General Medicine, Edinburgh Centre for Endocrinology and Diabetes, Royal Infirmary of Edinburgh; Honorary Clinical Senior Lecturer, University of Edinburgh, UK

Colin Duncan MD FRCOG
Professor of Reproductive Medicine and Science, University of Edinburgh; Honorary Consultant Gynaecologist, Royal Infirmary of Edinburgh, UK

Kirsty Dundas DCH FRCOG
Consultant Obstetrician, Royal Infirmary of Edinburgh; Honorary Senior Lecturer and Associate Senior Tutor, University of Edinburgh, UK

Andrew Elder FRCP(Ed) FRCPSG FRCP FACP FICP(Hon)
Consultant in Acute Medicine for the Elderly, Western General Hospital, Edinburgh; Honorary Professor, University of Edinburgh, UK

Karen Fairhurst PhD FRCGP
General Practitioner, Mackenzie Medical Centre, Edinburgh; Clinical Senior Lecturer, Centre for Population Health Sciences, University of Edinburgh, UK

Jane Gibson MD FRCP(Ed) FSCP(Hon)
Consultant Rheumatologist, Fife Rheumatic Diseases Unit, NHS Fife, Kirkcaldy, Fife; Honorary Senior Lecturer, University of St Andrews, UK

Iain Hathorn DOHNS PGCME FRCS(Ed) (ORL-HNS)
Consultant ENT Surgeon, NHS Lothian, Edinburgh, UK; Honorary Clinical Senior Lecturer, University of Edinburgh, UK

Iain Hennessey FRCS MMIS
Clinical Director of Innovation, Consultant Paediatric and Neonatal Surgeon, Alder Hey Children's Hospital, Liverpool, UK

J Alastair Innes BSc PhD FRCP(Ed)
Consultant Physician, Respiratory Unit, Western General Hospital, Edinburgh; Honorary Reader in Respiratory Medicine, University of Edinburgh, UK

Alan G Japp PhD MRCP
Consultant Cardiologist, Royal Infirmary of Edinburgh; Honorary Senior Lecturer, University of Edinburgh, UK

David Kluth PhD FRCP
Reader in Nephrology, University of Edinburgh, UK

Alexander Laird PhD FRCS(Ed) (Urol)
Consultant Urological Surgeon, Western General Hospital, Edinburgh, UK

Elizabeth MacDonald FRCP(Ed) DMCC
Consultant Physician in Medicine of the Elderly, Western
General Hospital, Edinburgh, UK

Hadi Manji MA MD FRCP
Consultant Neurologist and Honorary Senior Lecturer,
National Hospital for Neurology and Neurosurgery,
London, UK

Nicholas L Mills PhD FRCP(Ed) FESC
Chair of Cardiology and British Heart Foundation Senior
Clinical Research Fellow, University of Edinburgh; Consultant
Cardiologist, Royal Infirmary of Edinburgh, UK

Nick Morley MRCS(Ed) FRCR FEBNM
Consultant Radiologist, University Hospital of Wales,
Cardiff, UK

Rowan Parks MD FRCSI FRCS(Ed)
Professor of Surgical Sciences, Clinical Surgery, University of
Edinburgh; Honorary Consultant Hepatobiliary and Pancreatic
Surgeon, Royal Infirmary of Edinburgh, UK

Ross Paterson FRCA DICM FFICM
Consultant in Critical Care, Western General Hospital,
Edinburgh, UK

John Plevris DM PhD FRCP(Ed) FEBGH
Professor and Consultant in Gastroenterology, Royal Infirmary
of Edinburgh, University of Edinburgh, UK

Stephen Potts FRCPsych FRCP(Ed)
Consultant in Transplant Psychiatry, Royal Infirmary of
Edinburgh; Honorary Senior Clinical Lecturer, University of
Edinburgh, UK

Colin Robertson FRCP(Ed) FRCS(Ed) FSAScot
Honorary Professor of Accident and Emergency Medicine,
University of Edinburgh, UK

Jennifer Robson PhD FRCS
Clinical Lecturer in Surgery, University of Edinburgh, UK

Janet Skinner FRCS MMedEd FCEM
Director of Clinical Skills, University of Edinburgh; Emergency
Medicine Consultant, Royal Infirmary of Edinburgh, UK

Ben Stenson FRCPCH FRCP(Ed)
Consultant Neonatologist, Royal Infirmary of Edinburgh;
Honorary Professor of Neonatology, University of
Edinburgh, UK

Michael J Tidman MD FRCP(Ed) FRCP (Lond)
Consultant Dermatologist, Royal Infirmary of Edinburgh, UK

James Tiernan MSc(Clin Ed) MRCP(UK)
Consultant Respiratory Physician, Royal Infirmary of
Edinburgh; Honorary Senior Clinical Lecturer, University of
Edinburgh, UK

Naing Latt Tint FRCOphth PhD
Consultant Ophthalmic Surgeon, Ophthalmology, Princess
Alexandra Eye Pavilion, Edinburgh, UK

Oliver Young FRCS(Ed)
Clinical Director, Edinburgh Breast Unit, Western General
Hospital, Edinburgh, UK

Nicola Zammitt MD FRCP(Ed)
Consultant in Diabetes, Endocrinology and General Medicine,
Edinburgh Centre for Endocrinology and Diabetes, Royal
Infirmary of Edinburgh; Honorary Clinical Senior Lecturer,
University of Edinburgh, UK

Section 1

Principles of clinical history and examination

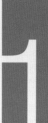

Karen Fairhurst
Anna R Dover
J Alastair Innes

Managing clinical encounters with patients

The clinical encounter

The clinical encounter between a patient and doctor lies at the heart of most medical practice. At its simplest, it is the means by which people who are ill, or believe themselves to be ill, seek the advice of a doctor whom they trust. Traditionally, and still most often, the clinical encounter is conducted face to face, although non-face-to-face or remote consultation using the telephone or digital technology is possible and increasingly common. This chapter describes the general principles that underpin interactions with patients in a clinical environment.

Reasons for the encounter

The majority of people who experience symptoms of ill health do not seek professional advice. For the minority who do seek help, the decision to consult is usually based on a complex interplay of physical, psychological and social factors (Box 1.1). The perceived seriousness of the symptoms and the severity of the illness experience are very important influences on whether patients seek help. The anticipated severity of symptoms is determined by their intensity, the patient's familiarity with them, and their duration and frequency. Beyond this, patients try to make sense of their symptoms within the context of their lives. They observe and evaluate their symptoms based on evidence from their own experience and from information they have gathered from a range of sources, including family and friends, print and broadcast media, and the internet. Patients who present with a symptom are significantly more likely to believe or worry that their symptom indicates a serious or fatal condition than non-consulters with similar symptoms; for example, a family history of sudden death from heart disease may affect how a person interprets an episode of chest pain. Patients also weigh up the relative costs (financial or other, such as inconvenience) and benefits of consulting a doctor. The expectation of benefit from a consultation – for example, in terms of symptom relief or legitimisation of time off work – is a powerful predictor of consultation. There may also be times when other priorities in patients' lives are more important than their symptoms of ill health and deter or delay consultation. It is important to consider the timing of the consultation. Why has the patient presented now? Sometimes it is not the experience of symptoms themselves that provokes consultation but something else in the patients' lives that triggers them to seek help (Box 1.2).

1.1 Deciding to consult a doctor
• Perceived susceptibility or vulnerability to illness • Perceived severity of symptoms • Perceived costs of consulting • Perceived benefits of consulting

1.2 Triggers to consultation
• Interpersonal crisis • Interference with social or personal relations • Sanctioning or pressure from family or friends • Interference with work or physical activity • Reaching the limit of tolerance of symptoms

A range of cultural factors may also influence help-seeking behaviour. Examples of person-specific factors that reduce the propensity to consult include stoicism, self-reliance, guilt, unwillingness to acknowledge psychological distress, and embarrassment about lifestyle factors such as addictions. These factors may vary between patients and also in the same person in different circumstances, and may be influenced by gender, education, social class and ethnicity.

The clinical environment

You should take all reasonable steps to ensure that the consultation is conducted in a calm, private environment. The layout of the consulting room is important and furniture should be arranged to put the patient at ease (Fig. 1.1A) by avoiding face-to-face, confrontational positioning across a table and the incursion of computer screens between patient and doctor (Fig. 1.1B). Personal mobile devices can also be intrusive if not used judiciously.

For hospital inpatients the environment is a challenge, yet privacy and dignity are always important. There may only be curtains around the bed space, which afford very little by way of privacy for a conversation. If your patient is mobile, try to use a side room or interview room. If there is no alternative to speaking to patients at their bedside, let them know that you understand your conversation may be overheard and give them permission not to answer sensitive questions about which they feel uncomfortable.

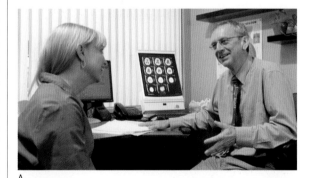

A

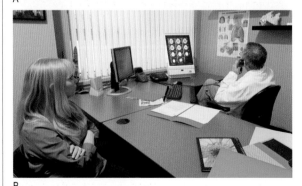

B

Fig. 1.1 **Seating arrangements.** A In this friendly seating arrangement the doctor sits next to the patient, at an angle. B Barriers to communication are set up by an oppositional/confrontational seating arrangement. The desk acts as a barrier, and the doctor is distracted by looking at a computer screen that is not easily viewable by the patient.

Opening the encounter

At the beginning of any encounter it is important to start to establish a rapport with the patient. Rapport helps to relax and engage the person in a useful dialogue. This involves greeting the patient and introducing yourself and describing your role clearly. A good reminder is to start any encounter with 'Hello, my name is … .' You should wear a name badge that can be read easily. A friendly smile helps to put your patient at ease. The way you dress is important; your dress style and demeanour should never make your patients uncomfortable or distract them. Smart, sensitive and modest dress is appropriate. Wear short sleeves or roll long sleeves up, away from your wrists and forearms, particularly before examining patients or carrying out procedures. Avoid hand jewellery to allow effective hand washing and reduce the risk of cross-infection (see Fig. 3.1). Tie back long hair. You should ensure that the patient is physically comfortable and at ease.

How you address and speak to a patient depends on the person's age, background and cultural environment. Some older people prefer not to be called by their first name and it is best to ask patients how they would prefer to be addressed. Go on to establish the reason for the encounter: in particular, the problems or issues the patient wishes to address or be addressed. Ask an open question to start with to encourage the patient to talk, such as 'How can I help you today?' or 'What has brought you along to see me today?'

Gathering information

The next task of the doctor in the clinical encounter is to understand what is causing the patient to be ill: that is, to reach a diagnosis. To do this you need to establish whether or not the patient is suffering from an identifiable disease or condition, and this requires further evaluation of the patient by history taking, physical examination and investigation where appropriate. Chapters 2 and 3 will help you develop a general approach to history taking and physical examination; detailed guidance on history taking and physical examination in specific systems and circumstances is offered in Sections 2 and 3.

Fear of the unknown, and of potentially serious illness, accompanies many patients as they enter the consulting room. Reactions to this vary widely but it can certainly impede clear recall and description. Plain language is essential for all encounters. The use of medical jargon is rarely appropriate because the risk of the doctor and the patient having a different understanding of the same words is simply too great. This also applies to words the patient may use that have multiple possible meanings (such as 'indigestion' or 'dizziness'); these terms must always be defined precisely in the course of the discussion.

Active listening is a key strategy in clinical encounters, as it encourages patients to tell their story. Doctors who fill every pause with another specific question will miss the patient's revealing calm reflection, or the hesitant question that reveals an inner concern. Instead, encourage the patient to talk freely by making encouraging comments or noises, such as 'Tell me a bit more' or 'Uhuh'. Clarify that you understand the meaning of what patients have articulated by reflecting back statements and summarising what you think they have said.

Non-verbal communication is equally important. Look for non-verbal cues indicating the patient's level of distress and mood. Changes in your patients' demeanour and body language during the consultation can be clues to difficulties that they cannot express verbally. If the their body language becomes 'closed' – for example, if they cross their arms and legs, turn away or avoid eye contact – this may indicate discomfort.

Handling sensitive information and third parties

Confidentiality is your top priority. Ask your patient's permission if you need to obtain information from someone else: usually a relative but sometimes a friend or a carer. If the patient cannot communicate, you may have to rely on family and carers to understand what has happened to the patient. Third parties may approach you without your patient's knowledge. Find out who they are, their relationship to the patient, and whether your patient knows the third party is talking to you. Tell third parties that you can listen to them but cannot divulge any clinical information without the patient's explicit permission. They may tell you about sensitive matters, such as mental illness, sexual abuse or drug or alcohol addiction. This information needs to be sensitively explored with your patient to confirm the truth.

Managing patient concerns

Patients are not simply the embodiment of disease but individuals who experience illness in their own unique way. Identifying their disease alone is rarely sufficient to permit full understanding of an individual patient's problems. In each encounter you should therefore also seek a clear understanding of the patient's personal experience of illness. This involves exploring the patients' feelings and ideas about their illness, its impact on their lifestyle and functioning, and their expectations of its treatment and course.

Patients may even be so fearful of a serious diagnosis that they conceal their concerns; the only sign that a patient fears cancer may be sitting with crossed fingers while the history is taken, hoping inwardly that cancer is not mentioned. Conversely, do not assume that the medical diagnosis is always a patient's main concern; anxiety about an inability to continue to work or to care for a dependent relative may be equally distressing.

The ideas, concerns and expectations that patients have about their illness often derive from their personal belief system, as well as from more widespread social and cultural understandings of illness. These beliefs can influence which symptoms patients choose to present to doctors and when. In some cultures, people derive much of their prior knowledge about health, illness and disease from the media and the internet. Indeed, patients have often sought explanations for their symptoms from the internet (or from other trusted sources) prior to consulting a doctor, and may return to these for a second opinion once they have seen a doctor. It is therefore important to establish what a patient already understands about the problem. This allows you and the patient to move towards a mutual understanding of the illness.

Showing empathy

Being empathic is a powerful way to build your relationship with patients. Empathy is the ability to identify with and understand patients' experiences, thoughts and feelings and to see the world as they do. Being empathic also involves being able to convey that understanding to the patient by making statements such as 'I can understand you must be feeling quite worried about what this might mean.' Empathy is not the same as sympathy, which is about the doctor's own feelings of compassion for or sorrow about the difficulties that the patient is experiencing.

Showing cultural sensitivity

Patients from a culture that is not your own may have different social rules regarding eye contact, touch and personal space. In some cultures, it is normal to maintain eye contact for long periods; in most of the world, however, this is seen as confrontational or rude. Shaking hands with the opposite sex is strictly forbidden in certain cultures. Death may be dealt with differently in terms of what the family expectations of physicians may be, which family members will expect information to be shared with them and what rites will be followed. Appreciate and accept differences in your patients' cultures and beliefs. When in doubt, ask them. This lets them know that you are aware of, and sensitive to, these issues.

Addressing the problem

Communicating your understanding of the patient's problem to them is crucial. It is good practice to ensure privacy for this, particularly if imparting bad news. Ask the patient who else they would like to be present – this may be a relative or partner – and offer a nurse. Check patients' current level of understanding and try to establish what further information they would like. Information should be provided in small chunks and be tailored to the patient's needs. Try to acknowledge and address the patient's ideas, concerns and expectations. Check the patient's understanding and recall of what you have said and encourage questions. After this, you should agree a management plan together. This might involve discussing and exploring the patient's understanding of the options for their treatment, including the evidence of benefit and risk for particular treatments and the uncertainties around it, or offering recommendations for treatment.

Concluding the encounter

Closing the consultation usually involves summarising the important points that have been discussed during the consultation. This aids patient recall and facilitates adherence to treatment. Any remaining questions that the patient may have should be addressed, and finally you should check that you have agreed a plan of action together with the patient and confirmed arrangements for follow-up.

Alternatives to face-to-face encounters

The use of telephone consultation as an alternative to face-to-face consultation has become accepted practice in parts of some healthcare systems, such as general practice in the UK. However, research suggests that, compared to face-to-face consultations, telephone consultations are shorter, cover fewer problems and include less data gathering, counselling/advice and rapport building. They are therefore considered to be most suitable for uncomplicated presentations. Telephone consultation with patients increases the chance of miscommunication, as there are no visual cues regarding body language or demeanour. The telephone should not be used to communicate bad news or sensitive results, as there is no opportunity to gauge reaction

or to offer additional support. When using the telephone, it is even more important to listen actively and to check your mutual understanding frequently.

Similarly, asynchronous communication with patients, using email or web-based applications, has been adopted by some doctors. This is not yet widely seen as a viable alternative to face-to-face consultation, or as a secure way to transmit confidential information. Despite the communication challenges that it can bring, telemedicine (using telecommunication and other information technologies) may be the only means of healthcare provision for patients living in remote and rural areas and its use is likely to increase, as it has the advantage of having the facility to incorporate the digital collection and transmission of medical data.

Professional responsibilities

Clinical encounters take place within a very specific context configured by the healthcare system within which they occur, the legal, ethical and professional frameworks by which we are bound, and by society as a whole.

From your first day as a student, you have professional obligations placed on you by the public, the law and your colleagues, which continue throughout your working life. Patients must be able to trust you with their lives and health, and you will be expected to demonstrate that your practice meets the expected standards (Box 1.3). Furthermore, patients want more from you than merely intellectual and technical proficiency; they will value highly your ability to demonstrate kindness, empathy and compassion.

1.3 The duties of a registered doctor

Knowledge, skills and performance

- Make the care of your patient your first concern
- Provide a good standard of practice and care:
  - Keep your professional knowledge and skills up to date
  - Recognise and work within the limits of your competence

Safety and quality

- Take prompt action if you think that patient safety, dignity or comfort is being compromised
- Protect and promote the health of patients and the public

Communication, partnership and teamwork

- Treat patients as individuals and respect their dignity:
  - Treat patients politely and considerately
  - Respect patients' right to confidentiality
- Work in partnership with patients:
  - Listen to, and respond to, their concerns and preferences
  - Give patients the information they want or need in a way they can understand
  - Respect patients' right to reach decisions with you about their treatment and care
  - Support patients in caring for themselves to improve and maintain their health
- Work with colleagues in the ways that best serve patients' interests

Maintenance of trust

- Be honest and open, and act with integrity
- Never discriminate unfairly against patients or colleagues
- Never abuse your patients' trust in you or the public's trust in the profession

Courtesy General Medical Council (UK).

Fundamentally, patients want doctors who:

- are knowledgeable
- respect people, healthy or ill, regardless of who they are
- support patients and their loved ones when and where needed
- always ask courteous questions, let people talk and listen to them carefully
- promote health, as well as treat disease
- give unbiased advice and assess each situation carefully
- use evidence as a tool, not as a determinant of practice
- let people participate actively in all decisions related to their health and healthcare
- humbly accept death as an important part of life, and help people make the best possible choices when death is close
- work cooperatively with other members of the healthcare team
- are advocates for their patients, as well as mentors for other health professionals, and are ready to learn from others, regardless of their age, role or status.

One way to reconcile these expectations with your inexperience and incomplete knowledge or skills is to put yourself in the situation of the patient and/or relatives. Consider how you would wish to be cared for in the patient's situation, acknowledging that you are different and your preferences may not be the same. Most clinicians approach and care for patients differently once they have had personal experience as a patient or as a relative of a patient. Doctors, nurses and everyone involved in caring for patients can have profound influences on how patients experience illness and their sense of dignity. When you are dealing with patients, always consider your:

- A: attitude – How would I feel in this patient's situation?
- B: behaviour – Always treat patients with kindness and respect.
- C: compassion – Recognise the human story that accompanies each illness.
- D: dialogue – Listen to and acknowledge the patient.

Confidentiality and consent

As a student and as a healthcare professional, you will be given private and intimate information about patients and their families. This information is confidential, even after a patient's death. This is a general rule, although its legal application varies between countries. In the UK, follow the guidelines issued by the General Medical Council. There are exceptions to the general rules governing patient confidentiality, where failure to disclose information would put the patient or someone else at risk of death or serious harm, or where disclosure might assist in the prevention, detection or prosecution of a serious crime. If you find yourself in this situation, contact the senior doctor in charge of the patient's care immediately and inform them of the situation.

Always obtain consent before undertaking any examination or investigation, or when providing treatment or involving patients in teaching or research.

Social media

Through social media, we are able to create and share web-based information. As such, social media has the potential to be a valuable tool in communicating with patients, particularly by facilitating access to information about health and services, and by providing invaluable peer support for patients. However, they also have the potential to expose doctors to risks, especially when there is a blurring of the boundaries between their professional and personal lives. The obligations on doctors do not change because they are communicating through social media rather than face to face or through other conventional media. Indeed, using social media creates new circumstances in which the established principles apply. If patients contact you about their care or other professional matters through your private profile, you should indicate that you cannot mix social and professional relationships and, where appropriate, direct them to your professional profile.

Personal responsibilities

You should always be aware that you are in a privileged professional position that you must not abuse. Do not pursue an improper relationship with a patient, and do not give medical care to anyone with whom you have a close personal relationship.

Finally, remember that, to be fit to take care of patients, you must first take care of yourself. If you think you have a medical condition that you could pass on to patients, or if your judgement or performance could be affected by a condition or its treatment, consult your general practitioner. Examples might include serious communicable disease, significant psychiatric disease, or drug or alcohol addiction.

J Alastair Innes
Karen Fairhurst
Anna R Dover

General aspects of history taking

The importance of a clear history

Understanding the patient's experience of illness by taking a history is central to the practice of all branches of medicine. The process requires patience, care and understanding to yield the key information leading to correct diagnosis and treatment.

In a perfect situation a calm, articulate patient would clearly describe the sequence and nature of their symptoms in the order of their occurrence, understanding and answering supplementary questions where required to add detail and certainty. In reality a multitude of factors may complicate this encounter and confound the clear communication of information. This chapter is a guide to facilitating the taking of a clear history. Information on specific symptoms and presentations is covered in the relevant system chapters.

Gathering information

Beginning the history

Preparation

Read your patient's past records, if they are available, along with any referral or transfer correspondence before starting.

Allowing sufficient time

Consultation length varies. In UK general practice the average time available is 12 minutes. This is usually adequate, provided the doctor knows the patient and the family and social background. In hospital, around 10 minutes is commonly allowed for returning outpatients, although this is challenging for new or temporary staff unfamiliar with the patient. For new and complex problems a full consultation may take 30 minutes or more. For students, time spent with patients learning and practising history taking is highly valuable, but patients appreciate advance discussion of the time students need.

Starting your consultation

Introduce yourself and anyone who is with you, shaking hands if appropriate. Confirm the patient's name and how they prefer to be addressed. If you are a student, inform patients; they are usually eager to help. Write down facts that are easily forgotten, such as blood pressure or family tree, but remember that writing notes must not interfere with the consultation.

Using different styles of question

Begin with open questions such as 'How can I help you today?' or 'What has brought you along to see me today?' Listen actively and encourage the patient to talk by looking interested and making encouraging comments, such as 'Tell me a bit more.' Always give the impression that you have plenty of time. Allow patients to tell their story in their own words, ideally without interruption. You may occasionally need to interject to guide the patient gently back to describing the symptoms, as anxious patients commonly focus on relating the events or the reactions and opinions of others surrounding an episode of illness rather than what they were feeling. While avoiding unnecessary repetition, it may be helpful occasionally to tell patients what you think they have said and ask if your interpretation is correct (reflection).

The way you ask a question is important:

- Open questions are general invitations to talk that avoid anticipating particular answers: for example, 'What was the first thing you noticed when you became ill?' or 'Can you tell me more about that?'
- Closed questions seek specific information and are used for clarification: for example, 'Have you had a cough today?' or 'Did you notice any blood in your bowel motions?'

Both types of question have their place, and normally clinicians move gradually from open to closed questions as the interview progresses.

The following history illustrates the mix of question styles needed to elucidate a clear story:

When did you first feel unwell, and what did you feel? (Open questioning)

Well, I've been getting this funny feeling in my chest over the last few months. It's been getting worse and worse but it was really awful this morning. My husband called 999. The ambulance came and the nurse said I was having a heart attack. It was really scary.

When you say a 'funny feeling', can you tell me more about what it felt like? (Open questioning, steering away from events and opinions back to symptoms)

Well, it was here, across my chest. It was sort of tight, like something heavy sitting on my chest.

And did it go anywhere else? (Open but clarifying)

Well, maybe up here in my neck.

What were you doing when it came on? (Clarifying precipitating event)

Just sitting in the kitchen, finishing my breakfast.

How long was the tightness there? (Closed)

About an hour altogether.

So, you felt a tightness in your chest this morning that went on for about an hour and you also felt it in your neck? (Reflection)

Yes that's right.

Did you feel anything else at the same time? (Open, not overlooking secondary symptoms)

I felt a bit sick and sweaty.

Showing empathy when taking a history

Being empathic helps your relationship with patients and improves their health outcomes (p. 5). Try to see the problem from their point of view and convey that to them in your questions.

Consider a young teacher who has recently had disfiguring facial surgery to remove a benign tumour from her upper jaw. Her wound has healed but she has a drooping lower eyelid and facial swelling. She returns to work. Imagine how you would feel in this situation. Express empathy through questions that show you can relate to your patient's experience.

So, it's 3 weeks since your operation. How is your recovery going?

OK, but I still have to put drops in my eye.

And what about the swelling under your eye?

That gets worse during the day, and sometimes by the afternoon I can't see that well.

And how does that feel at work?

Well, it's really difficult. You know, with the kids and everything. It's all a bit awkward.

I can understand that that must feel pretty uncomfortable and awkward. How do you cope? Are there are any other areas that are awkward for you, maybe in other aspects of your life, like the social side?

The history of the presenting symptoms

Using these questioning tools and an empathic approach, you are now ready to move to the substance of the history.

Ask the patient to think back to the start of their illness and describe what they felt and how it progressed. Begin with some open questions to get your patient talking about the symptoms, gently steering them back to this topic if they stray into describing events or the reactions or opinions of others. As they talk, pick out the two or three main symptoms they are describing (such as pain, cough and shivers); these are the essence of the history of the presenting symptoms. It may help to jot these down as single words, leaving space for associated clarifications by closed questioning as the history progresses.

Experienced clinicians make a diagnosis by recognising patterns of symptoms (p. 362). With experience, you will refine your questions according to the presenting symptoms, using a mental list of possible diagnoses (a differential diagnosis) to guide you. Clarify exactly what patients mean by any specific term they use (such as catarrh, fits or blackouts); common terms can mean different things to different patients and professionals (Box 2.1). Each answer increases or decreases the probability of a particular diagnosis and excludes others.

In the following example, the patient is a 65-year-old male smoker. His age and smoking status increase the probability of certain diagnoses related to smoking. A cough for 2 months increases the likelihood of lung cancer and chronic obstructive pulmonary disease (COPD). Chest pain does not exclude COPD since he could have pulled a muscle on coughing, but the pain may also be pleuritic from infection or thromboembolism. In turn, infection could be caused by obstruction of an airway by lung cancer. Haemoptysis lasting 2 months greatly increases the chance of lung cancer. If the patient also has weight loss, the positive predictive value of all these answers is very high for lung cancer. This will focus your examination and investigation plan.

What was the first thing you noticed wrong when you became ill? (Open question)

I've had a cough that I just can't get rid of. It started after I'd had flu about 2 months ago. I thought it would get better but it hasn't and it's driving me mad.

Could you please tell me more about the cough? (Open question)

Well, it's bad all the time. I cough and cough, and bring up some phlegm. It keeps waking me at night so I feel rough the next day. Sometimes I get pains in my chest because I've been coughing so much.

Already you have noted 'Cough', 'Phlegm' and 'Chest pain' as headings for your history. Follow up with key questions to clarify each.

Cough: *Are you coughing to try to clear something from your chest or does it come without warning?* (Closed question, clarifying)

Oh, I can't stop it, even when I'm asleep it comes.

Does it feel as if it starts in your throat or your chest? Can you point to where you feel it first?

It's like a tickle here (points to upper sternum).

Phlegm: *What colour is the phlegm?* (Closed question, focusing on the symptom)

Clear.

2.1 Examples of terms used by patients that should be clarified

Patient's term	Common underlying problems	Useful distinguishing features
Allergy	True allergy (immunoglobulin E-mediated reaction) Intolerance of food or drug, often with nausea or other gastrointestinal upset	Visible rash or swelling, rapid onset Predominantly gastrointestinal symptoms

Indigestion	Acid reflux with oesophagitis
	Abdominal pain due to:
	  Peptic ulcer
	  Gastritis
	  Cholecystitis
	  Pancreatitis
		Retrosternal burning, acid taste
		Site and nature of discomfort:
		  Epigastric, relieved by eating
		  Epigastric, with vomiting
		  Right upper quadrant, tender
		  Epigastric, severe, tender

Arthritis	Joint pain Muscle pain Immobility due to prior skeletal injury	Redness or swelling of joints Muscle tenderness Deformity at site
Catarrh	Purulent sputum from bronchitis Infected sinonasal discharge Nasal blockage	Cough, yellow or green sputum Yellow or green nasal discharge Anosmia, prior nasal injury/polyps
Fits	Transient syncope from cardiac disease Epilepsy Abnormal involuntary movement	Witnessed pallor during syncope Witnessed tonic/clonic movements No loss of consciousness
Dizziness	Labyrinthitis Syncope from hypotension Cerebrovascular event	Nystagmus, feeling of room spinning, with no other neurological deficit History of palpitation or cardiac disease, postural element Sudden onset, with other neurological deficit

Have you ever coughed up any blood? (Closed question)

Yes, sometimes.

When did it first appear and how often does it come? (Closed questions)

Oh, most days. I've noticed it for over a month.

How much? (Closed question, clarifying the symptom)

Just streaks.

Is it pure blood or mixed with yellow or green phlegm?

Just streaks of blood in clear phlegm.

Chest pain: Can you tell me about the chest pains? (Open question)

Well, they're here on my side (points) when I cough.

Does anything else bring on the pains? (Open, clarifying the symptom)

Taking a deep breath, and it really hurts when I cough or sneeze.

Pain is a very important symptom common to many areas of practice. A general scheme for the detailed characterisation of pain is outlined in Box 2.2.

2.2 Characteristics of pain (SOCRATES)

Site
- Somatic pain, often well localised, e.g. sprained ankle
- Visceral pain, more diffuse, e.g. angina pectoris

Onset
- Speed of onset and any associated circumstances

Character
- Described by adjectives, e.g. sharp/dull, burning/tingling, boring/stabbing, crushing/tugging, preferably using the patient's own description rather than offering suggestions

Radiation
- Through local extension
- Referred by a shared neuronal pathway to a distant unaffected site, e.g. diaphragmatic pain at the shoulder tip via the phrenic nerve (C_3, C_4)

Associated symptoms
- Visual aura accompanying migraine with aura
- Numbness in the leg with back pain suggesting nerve root irritation

Timing (duration, course, pattern)
- Since onset
- Episodic or continuous:
  - If episodic, duration and frequency of attacks
  - If continuous, any changes in severity

Exacerbating and relieving factors
- Circumstances in which pain is provoked or exacerbated, e.g. eating
- Specific activities or postures, and any avoidance measures that have been taken to prevent onset
- Effects of specific activities or postures, including effects of medication and alternative medical approaches

Severity
- Difficult to assess, as so subjective
- Sometimes helpful to compare with other common pains, e.g. toothache
- Variation by day or night, during the week or month, e.g. relating to the menstrual cycle

---

Having clarified the presenting symptoms, prompt for any more associated features, using your initial impression of the likely pathology (lung cancer or chronic respiratory infection) to direct relevant questions:

Do you ever feel short of breath with your cough?

A bit.

How has your weight been? (Seeking additional confirmation of serious pathology)

I've lost about a stone since this started.

The questions required at this point will vary according to the system involved. A summary of useful starting questions for each system is shown in Box 2.3. Learn to think, as you listen, about the broad categories of disease that may present and how these relate to the history, particularly in relation to the onset and rate of progression of symptoms (Box 2.4).

To complete the history of presenting symptoms, make an initial assessment of how the illness is impacting on the life of your patient. For example, breathlessness on heavy exertion may prevent a 40-year-old builder from working but would have much less impact on a sedentary retired person. 'Can you tell me how far you can walk on a good day?' is a question that can help to clarify the normal level of functioning, and 'How has this changed since you have been unwell?' can reveal disease impact. Ask if the person undertakes sports or regular exercise, and if they have modified these activities because of illness.

2.3 Questions to ask about common symptoms

System	Question
Cardiovascular	Do you ever have chest pain or tightness? Do you ever wake up during the night feeling short of breath? Have you ever noticed your heart racing or thumping?
Respiratory	Are you ever short of breath? Have you had a cough? If so, do you cough anything up? What colour is your phlegm? Have you ever coughed up blood?
Gastrointestinal	Are you troubled by indigestion or heartburn? Have you noticed any change in your bowel habit recently? Have you ever seen any blood or slime in your stools?
Genitourinary	Do you ever have pain or difficulty passing urine? Do you have to get up at night to pass urine? If so, how often? Have you noticed any dribbling at the end of passing urine? Have your periods been quite regular?
Musculoskeletal	Do you have any pain, stiffness or swelling in your joints? Do you have any difficulty walking or dressing?
Endocrine	Do you tend to feel the heat or cold more than you used to? Have you been feeling thirstier or drinking more than usual?
Neurological	Have you ever had any fits, faints or blackouts? Have you noticed any numbness, weakness or clumsiness in your arms or legs?

2.4 Typical patterns of symptoms related to disease causation

Disease causation	Onset of symptoms	Progression of symptoms	Associated symptoms/pattern of symptoms
Infection	Usually hours, unheralded	Usually fairly rapid over hours or days	Fevers, rigors, localising symptoms, e.g. pleuritic pain and cough
Inflammation	May appear acutely	Coming and going over weeks to months	Nature may be multifocal, often with local tenderness
Metabolic	Very variable	Hours to months	Steady progression in severity with no remission
Malignant	Gradual, insidious	Steady progression over weeks to months	Weight loss, fatigue
Toxic	Abrupt	Rapid	Dramatic onset of symptoms; vomiting often a feature
Trauma	Abrupt	Little change from onset	Diagnosis usually clear from history
Vascular	Sudden	Stepwise progression with acute episodes	Rapid development of associated physical signs
Degenerative	Gradual	Months to years	Gradual worsening with periods of more acute deterioration

2.5 Example of a drug history

Drug	Dose	Duration	Indication	Side-effects/patient concerns
Aspirin	75 mg daily	5 years	Started after myocardial infarction	Indigestion
Atenolol	50 mg daily	5 years	Started after myocardial infarction	Cold hands (?adherence)
Co-codamol (paracetamol + codeine)	8 mg/500mg, up to 8 tablets daily	4 weeks	Back pain	Constipation
Salbutamol MDI	2 puffs as necessary	6 months	Asthma	Palpitation, agitation

MDI, *metered-dose inhaler.*

Past medical history

Past medical history may be relevant to the presenting symptoms: for example, previous migraine in a patient with headache, or haematemesis and multiple minor injuries in a patient with suspected alcohol abuse. It may reveal predisposing past or underlying illness, such as diabetes in a patient with peripheral vascular disease, or childhood whooping cough in someone presenting with bronchiectasis.

The referral letter and case records often contain useful headlines but the patient is usually the best source. These questions will elicit the key information in most patients:

- What illnesses have you seen a doctor about in the past?
- Have you been in hospital before or attended a clinic?
- Have you had any operations?
- Do you take any medicines regularly?

Drug history

This follows naturally from asking about past illness. Begin by checking any written sources of information, such as the drug list on the referral letter or patient record. It is useful to compare this with the patient's own recollection of what they take. This can be complicated by patients' use of brand names, descriptions of tablet number and colour and so on, which should always be translated to generic pharmaceutical names and quantitative doses for the patient record. Ask about prescribed drugs and other medications, including over-the-counter remedies, herbal and homeopathic remedies, and vitamin or mineral supplements. Do not forget to ask about inhalers and topical medications, as patients may assume that you are asking only about tablets. Note all drug names, dosage regimens and duration of treatment,

along with any significant adverse effects, in a clear format (Box 2.5). When drugs such as methadone are being prescribed for addiction, ask the community pharmacy to confirm dosage and also to stop dispensing for the duration of any hospital admission.

Concordance and adherence

Half of all patients do not take prescribed medicines as directed. Patients who take their medication as prescribed are said to be adherent. Concordance implies that the patient and doctor have negotiated and reached an agreement on management, and adherence to therapy is likely (though not guaranteed) to improve.

Ask patients to describe how and when they take their medication. Give them permission to admit that they do not take all their medicines by saying, for example, 'That must be difficult to remember.'

Drug allergies/reactions

Ask if your patient has ever had an allergic reaction to a medication or vaccine. Clarify exactly what patients mean by allergy, as intolerance (such as nausea) is much more common than true allergy. Drug allergies are over-reported by patients: for example, only 1 in 7 who report a rash with penicillin will have a positive penicillin skin test. Note other allergies, such as foodstuffs or pollen. Record true allergies prominently in the patient's case records, drug chart and computer records. If patients have had a severe or life-threatening allergic reaction, advise them to wear an alert necklace or bracelet.

Non-prescribed drug use

Ask all patients who may be using drugs about non-prescribed drugs. In Britain about 30% of the adult population have used illegal or non-prescribed drugs (mainly cannabis) at some time. Useful questions are summarised in Box 2.6.

Family history

Start with open questions, such as 'Are there any illnesses that run in your family?' Follow up the presenting symptoms with a question like 'Have any of your family had heart trouble?' Single-gene inherited diseases are relatively uncommon in clinical practice. Even when present, autosomal recessive diseases such as cystic fibrosis usually arise in patients with healthy parents who are unaffected carriers. Many other illnesses are associated with a positive family history but are not due to a single-gene

disorder. A further complication is that some illnesses, such as asthma and diseases caused by atheroma, are so common in the UK population that their presence in family members may not greatly influence the risk to the patient.

Document illness in first-degree relatives: that is, parents, siblings and children. If you suspect an inherited disorder such as haemophilia, construct a pedigree chart (Fig. 2.1), noting whether any individuals were adopted. Ask about the health of other household members, since this may suggest environmental risks to the patient.

Social history and lifestyle

No medical assessment is complete without determining the social circumstances of your patient. These may be relevant to the causes of their illness and may also influence the management and outcome. Establish who is there to support the patient by asking 'Who is at home with you, or do you live alone?' For those who live alone, establish who is their next of kin and who visits regularly to support them. Check if your patient is a carer for someone vulnerable who may be at risk due to your patient's illness. Enquire sensitively if the patient is bereaved, as this can have profound effects on a patient's health and wellbeing.

Next establish the type and condition of the patient's housing and how well it suits them, given their symptoms. Patients with severe arthritis may, for example, struggle with stairs. Successful management of the patient in the community requires these issues to be addressed.

Smoking

Among other things, tobacco use increases the risk of obstructive lung disease, cardiac and vascular disease, peptic ulceration,

---

2.6 Non-prescribed drug history

- What drugs are you taking?
- How often and how much?
- How long have you been taking drugs?
- Have you managed to stop at any time? If so, when and why did you start using drugs again?
- What symptoms do you have if you cannot get drugs?
- Do you ever inject? If so, where do you get the needles and syringes?
- Do you ever share needles, syringes or other drug-taking equipment?
- Do you see your drug use as a problem?
- Do you want to make changes in your life or change the way you use drugs?
- Have you been checked for infections spread by drug use?

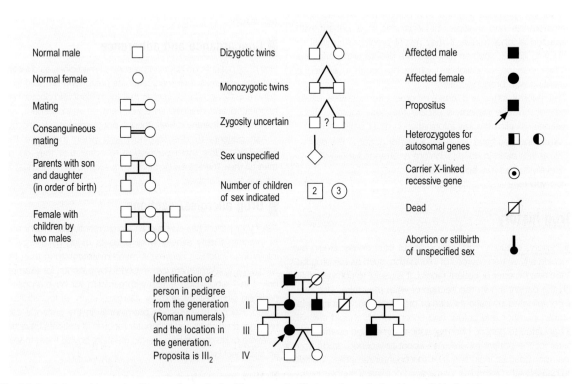

Fig. 2.1 **Symbols used in constructing a pedigree chart, with an example.** The terms 'propositus' and 'proposita' indicate the man or woman identified as the index case, around whom the pedigree chart is constructed.

intrauterine growth restriction, erectile dysfunction and a range of cancers.

Most patients recognise that smoking harms health, so obtaining an accurate history of tobacco use requires sensitivity. Ask if your patient has ever smoked; if so, enquire what age they started at and whether they still smoke now. Patients often play down recent use, so it is usually more helpful to ask about their average number of cigarettes per day over the years, and what form of tobacco they have used (cigarettes, cigars, pipe, chewed). Convert to 'pack-years' (Box 2.7) to estimate the risk of tobacco-related health problems. Ask if they have smoked only tobacco or also cannabis. Never miss the opportunity during history taking to encourage smoking cessation, in a positive and non-judgemental way, as a route to improved health. Do not forget to ask non-smokers about their exposure to environmental tobacco smoke (passive smoking).

Alcohol

Alcohol causes extensive pathology, including not only hepatic cirrhosis, encephalopathy and peripheral neuropathy but also pancreatitis, cardiomyopathy, erectile dysfunction and injury through accidents. Always ask patients if they drink alcohol but try to avoid appearing critical, as this will lead them to underestimate their intake. If they do drink, ask them to describe how much and what type (beer, wine, spirits) they drink in an average week. The quantity of alcohol consumed each week is best estimated in units; 1 unit (10 mL of ethanol) is contained in one small glass of wine, half a pint of beer or lager, or one standard measure (25 mL) of spirits.

Alcohol problems

The UK Department of Health now defines hazardous drinking as anything exceeding 14 units per week for both men and women. Binge drinking, involving a large amount of alcohol causing acute intoxication, is more likely to cause problems than if the same amount is consumed over four or five days. Most authorities recommend at least two alcohol-free days per week.

Alcohol dependence occurs when alcohol use takes priority over other behaviour that previously had greater value. Warning signs in the history are summarised in Box 2.8.

Occupational history and home environment

Work profoundly influences health. Unemployment is associated with increased morbidity and mortality while some occupations are associated with particular illnesses (Box 2.9).

Ask all patients about their occupation. Clarify what the person does at work, especially about any chemical or dust exposure. If the patient has worked with harmful materials (such asbestos or stone dust), a detailed employment record is needed, including

---

2.7 Calculating pack-years of smoking

A 'pack-year' is smoking 20 cigarettes a day (1 pack) for 1 year

$$\frac{\text{Number of cigarettes smoked per day} \times \text{Number of years smoking}}{20}$$

For example, a smoker of 15 cigarettes a day who has smoked for 40 years would have smoked:

$$\frac{15 \times 40}{20} = 30 \text{ pack-years}$$

2.8 Features of alcohol dependence in the history

- A strong, often overpowering, desire to take alcohol
- Inability to control starting or stopping drinking and the amount that is drunk
- Drinking alcohol in the morning
- Tolerance, where increased doses are needed to achieve the effects originally produced by lower doses
- A withdrawal state when drinking is stopped or reduced, including tremor, sweating, rapid heart rate, anxiety, insomnia and occasionally seizures, disorientation or hallucinations (delirium tremens); this is relieved by more alcohol
- Neglect of other pleasures and interests
- Continuing to drink in spite of being aware of the harmful consequences

---

2.9 Examples of occupational disorders

Occupation	Factor	Disorder	Presents
Shipyard workers, marine engineers, plumbers and heating workers, demolition workers, joiners	Asbestos dust	Pleural plaques Asbestosis Mesothelioma Lung cancer	>15 years later
Stonemasons	Silica dust	Silicosis	After years
Farmers	Fungus spores on mouldy hay	Farmer's lung (hypersensitivity pneumonitis)	After 4–18 hours
Divers	Surfacing from depth too quickly	Decompression sickness Central nervous system, skin, bone and joint symptoms	Immediately, up to 1 week
Industrial workers	Chemicals, e.g. chromium Excessive noise Vibrating tools	Dermatitis on hands Sensorineural hearing loss Vibration white finger	Variable Over months Over months
Bakery workers	Flour dust	Occupational asthma	Variable
Healthcare workers	Cuts, needlestick injuries	Human immunodeficiency virus, hepatitis B and C	Incubation period >3 months

employer name, timing and extent of exposure, and any workplace protection offered.

Symptoms that improve over the weekend or during holidays suggest an occupational disorder. In the home environment, hobbies may also be relevant: for example, psittacosis pneumonia or hypersensitivity pneumonitis in those who keep birds, or asthma in cat or rodent owners.

Travel history

Returning travellers commonly present with illness. They risk unusual or tropical infections, and air travel itself can precipitate certain conditions, such as middle-ear problems or deep vein thrombosis. The incubation period may indicate the likelihood of many illnesses but some diseases, such as vivax malaria and human immunodeficiency virus, may present a year or more after travel. List the locations visited and dates. Note any travel vaccination and anti-malaria prophylaxis taken if affected areas were visited.

Sexual history

Take a full sexual history only if the context or pattern of symptoms suggests this is relevant. Ask questions sensitively and objectively (see later). Signal your intentions: 'As part of your medical history, I need to ask you some questions about your relationships. Is this all right?'

Systematic enquiry

Systematic enquiry uncovers symptoms that may have been forgotten. Start with 'Is there anything else you would like to tell me about?'

Box 2.10 lists common symptoms by system. Asking about all of these is inappropriate and takes too long, so judgement and context are used to select areas to explore in detail. For example:

- With a history of repeated infections, ask about nocturia, thirst and weight loss, which may indicate underlying uncontrolled diabetes.
- In a patient with palpitation are there any symptoms to suggest thyrotoxicosis or is there a family history of thyroid disease? Is the patient anxious or drinking too much coffee?
- If a patient smells of alcohol, ask about related symptoms, such as numbness in the feet due to alcoholic neuropathy.

Closing the interview

Using simple language, briefly explain your interpretation of the patient's history and outline the likely possibilities. Be sensitive to their concerns and body language. Ask the patient if they already have ideas and concerns about the diagnosis (p. 5), so these may be addressed directly. Always give the patient a final opportunity to raise additional concerns ('Is there anything else you would like to ask?').

Make sure patients are involved in any decisions by suggesting possible actions and encouraging them to contribute their thoughts. This way, you should be able to negotiate an agreed plan for further investigation and follow-up. Tell them that you will communicate this plan to other professionals involved in their care.

Difficult situations

Patients with communication difficulties

If your patient does not speak your language, arrange to have an interpreter, remembering to address the patient and not the interpreter.

If your patient has hearing or speech difficulties such as dysphasia or dysarthria, consider the following:

- Write things down for your patient if they can read.
- Involve someone who is used to communicating with your patient.
- Seek a sign language interpreter for a deaf patient skilled in sign language.

Patients with cognitive difficulties

Be alert for early signs of dementia. Inconsistent or hesitant responses from the patient should always prompt you to suspect and check for memory difficulties. If you do suspect this, assess the patient using a cognitive rating scale (p. 331). You may have to rely on a history from relatives or carers.

Sensitive situations

Doctors sometimes need to ask personal or sensitive questions and examine intimate parts. If you are talking to a patient who may be suffering from sexual dysfunction, sexual abuse or sexually transmitted disease, broach the subject sensitively. Indicate that you are going to ask questions in this area and make sure the conversation is entirely private. For example:

Because of what you're telling me, I need to ask you some rather personal questions. Is that OK?

Can I ask if you have a regular sexual partner?

Follow this up with:

Is your partner male or female?

If there is no regular partner, ask sensitively:

How many sexual partners have you had in the past year?

Have you had any problems with your relationships or in your sex life that you would like to mention?

If you need to examine intimate areas, ask permission sensitively and always secure the help of a chaperone. This is always required for examination of the breasts, genitals or rectum, but may apply in some circumstances or cultures whenever you need to touch the patient (p. 20).

Emotional or angry patients

Ill people feel vulnerable and may become angry and frustrated about how they feel or about their treatment. Staying calm and exploring the reasons for their emotion often defuses the situation. Although their behaviour may be challenging, never respond with anger or irritation and resist passing comment on a patient's account of prior management. Recognise that your patient is upset, show empathy and understanding, and ask them to explain why: for example, 'You seem angry about something' or 'Is there something that is upsetting you?' If, despite this, their anger escalates, set boundaries on the discussion, calmly withdraw,

2.10 Systematic enquiry: cardinal symptoms

General health

- Wellbeing
- Appetite
- Weight change
- Energy
- Sleep
- Mood

Cardiovascular system

- Chest pain on exertion (angina)
- Breathlessness:
  - Lying flat (orthopnoea)
  - At night (paroxysmal nocturnal dyspnoea)
  - On minimal exertion – record how much
- Palpitation
- Pain in legs on walking (claudication)
- Ankle swelling

Respiratory system

- Shortness of breath (exercise tolerance)
- Cough
- Wheeze
- Sputum production (colour, amount)
- Blood in sputum (haemoptysis)
- Chest pain (due to inspiration or coughing)

Gastrointestinal system

- Mouth (oral ulcers, dental problems)
- Difficulty swallowing (dysphagia – distinguish from pain on swallowing, i.e. odynophagia)
- Nausea and vomiting
- Vomiting blood (haematemesis)
- Indigestion
- Heartburn
- Abdominal pain
- Change in bowel habit
- Change in colour of stools (pale, dark, tarry black, fresh blood)

Genitourinary system

- Pain passing urine (dysuria)
- Frequency passing urine (at night: nocturia)
- Blood in urine (haematuria)
- Libido
- Incontinence (stress and urge)
- Sexual partners – unprotected intercourse

Men

If appropriate:
- Prostatic symptoms, including difficulty starting (hesitancy):
  - Poor stream or flow
  - Terminal dribbling
- Urethral discharge
- Erectile difficulties

Women

- Last menstrual period (consider pregnancy)
- Timing and regularity of periods
- Length of periods
- Abnormal bleeding
- Vaginal discharge
- Contraception

If appropriate:
- Pain during intercourse (dyspareunia)

Nervous system

- Headaches
- Dizziness (vertigo or lightheadedness)
- Faints
- Fits
- Altered sensation
- Weakness
- Visual disturbance
- Hearing problems (deafness, tinnitus)
- Memory and concentration changes

Musculoskeletal system

- Joint pain, stiffness or swelling
- Mobility
- Falls

Endocrine system

- Heat or cold intolerance
- Change in sweating
- Excessive thirst (polydipsia)

Other

- Bleeding or bruising
- Skin rash

---

and seek the assistance and presence of another healthcare worker as a witness for your own protection.

Talkative patients or those who want to deal with many things at once may respond to 'I only have a short time left with you, so what's the most important thing we need to deal with now?' If patients have a long list of symptoms, suggest 'Of the six things you've raised today, I can only deal with two, so tell me which are the most important to you and we'll deal with the rest later.'

Set professional boundaries if your patient becomes overly familiar: 'Well, it would be inappropriate for me to discuss my personal issues with you. I'm here to help you so let's focus on your problem.'

Anna R Dover
J Alastair Innes
Karen Fairhurst

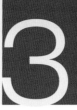

General aspects of examination

General principles of physical examination

The process of taking a history and conducting a physical examination is artificially separated in classical medical teaching, to encourage learners to develop a structured approach to information gathering. However, your physical assessment of patients undoubtedly begins as soon as you see them, and the astute clinician may notice signs of disease, such as subtle abnormalities of demeanour, gait or appearance, even before the formal consultation begins. The clinician can be likened to a detective, gathering clues, and the physical assessment of a patient can then be seen as the investigation itself!

Historically, great importance has been placed on the value of empirical observation of patients in the formulation of a differential diagnosis. Modern technological advances have increased the reliance on radiological and laboratory testing for diagnosis, sometimes even at the bedside (such as portable ultrasound or near-patient capillary blood ketone testing), and this has called into question the utility of systematic physical examination in modern practice. Nevertheless, the importance of performing a methodical and accurate physical examination cannot be overstated. The inconstancy of physical signs and the need to monitor patient progress by repeated bedside assessment, often conducted by different clinicians, mean that a standardised approach to physical examination resulting in reproducible findings is crucial. Additionally, the interpretation of many diagnostic investigations (such as detection of interstitial oedema on a chest X-ray in heart failure) is subject to variation between clinicians, as is the detection of physical signs (such as audible crackles on auscultating the lungs). Furthermore, the utility of many diagnostic investigations relies heavily on the pre-test probability (the likelihood of the disease being present prior to the test being performed; p. 362), which depends on information gathered during the history and examination. Finally, there are a number of conditions, or syndromes, that can be diagnosed only by the detection of a characteristic pattern of physical signs. Thus by mastering structured skills in physical examination, clinicians can improve the reliability and precision of their clinical assessment, which, together with the appropriate diagnostic investigations, lead to accurate diagnosis.

Preparing for physical examination

It is important to prepare both yourself and your patient for the physical examination. As a clinician, you must take reasonable steps to ensure you can give the patient your undivided attention, in an environment free from interruption, noise or distraction. Always introduce yourself to the patient, shake hands (which may provide diagnostic clues; Box 3.1 and see later) and seek permission to conduct the consultation. Make sure you have the relevant equipment available (Box 3.2) and that you have observed local hand hygiene policies (Fig. 3.1). As discussed on page 4, privacy is essential when assessing a patient. At the very least, ensure screens or curtains are fully closed around a ward bed; where possible, use a separate private room to avoid being overheard. Seek permission from the patient to proceed to examination, and offer a chaperone where appropriate to prevent misunderstandings and to provide support and encouragement for the patient. Regardless of whether the patient is the same

3.1 Information gleaned from a handshake

Features	Diagnosis
Cold, sweaty hands	Anxiety
Cold, dry hands	Raynaud's phenomenon
Hot, sweaty hands	Hyperthyroidism
Large, fleshy, sweaty hands	Acromegaly
Dry, coarse skin	Regular water exposure Manual occupation Hypothyroidism
Delayed relaxation of grip	Myotonic dystrophy
Deformed hands/fingers	Trauma Rheumatoid arthritis Dupuytren's contracture

3.2 Equipment required for a full examination

- Stethoscope
- Pen torch
- Measuring tape
- Ophthalmoscope
- Otoscope
- Sphygmomanometer
- Tendon hammer
- Tuning fork
- Cotton wool
- Disposable Neurotips
- Wooden spatula
- Thermometer
- Magnifying glass
- Accurate weighing scales and a height-measuring device (preferably a calibrated, wall-mounted stadiometer)
- Personal protective equipment (disposable gloves and apron)
- Facilities for obtaining blood samples and urinalysis

gender as the doctor or not, chaperones are always appropriate for intimate (breast, genital or rectal) examination. Chaperones are also advised if the patient is especially anxious or vulnerable, if there have been misunderstandings in the past, or if religious or cultural factors require a different approach to physical examination. Record the chaperone's name and presence. If patients decline the offer, respect their wishes and record this in the notes. Tactfully invite relatives to leave the room before physical examination unless the patient is very apprehensive and requests that they stay. A parent or guardian should always be present when you examine children (p. 307).

The room should be warm and well lit; subtle abnormalities of complexion, such as mild jaundice, are easier to detect in natural light. The height of the examination couch or bed should be adjustable, with a step to enable patients to get up easily. An adjustable backrest is essential, particularly for breathless patients who cannot lie flat. It is usual practice to examine a recumbent patient from the right-hand side of the bed. Ensure the patient is comfortably positioned before commencing the physical examination.

Seek permission and sensitively, but adequately, expose the areas to be examined; cover the rest of the patient with a blanket or sheet to ensure that they do not become cold. Avoid unnecessary exposure and embarrassment; a patient may appreciate the opportunity to replace their top after examination of the chest before exposing the abdomen. Remain gentle towards the patient at all times, and be vigilant for aspects of the examination that may cause distress or discomfort. Acknowledge any anxiety or concerns raised by the patient during the consultation.

3

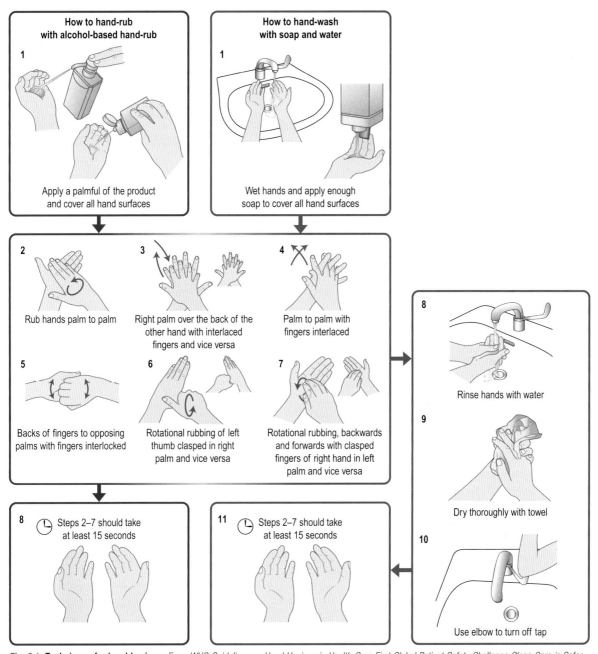

Fig. 3.1 **Techniques for hand hygiene.** *From WHO Guidelines on Hand Hygiene in Health Care First Global Patient Safety Challenge Clean Care is Safer Care; http://www.who.int/gpsc/clean_hands_protection/en/ © World Health Organization 2009. All rights reserved.*

Sequence for performing a physical examination

The purpose of the physical examination is to look for the presence, or absence, of physical signs that confirm or refute the differential diagnoses you have obtained from the history. The extent of the examination will depend on the symptoms that you are investigating and the circumstances of the encounter. Often, in a brief, focused consultation (such as a patient presenting to a general practitioner with headache), a single system (the nervous system in this case) will be examined. In other circumstances, however, a full integrated physical examination will be required and this is described in detail on page 362.

There is no single correct way to perform a physical examination but standardised systematic approaches help to ensure that nothing is omitted. With experience, you will develop your own style and sequence of physical examination. Broadly speaking, any systematic examination involves looking at the patient (for skin changes, scars, abnormal patterns of breathing or pulsation, for example), laying hands on the patient to palpate (feel) and percuss (tapping on the body), and finally using a stethoscope, where appropriate, to listen to the relevant system (auscultate). This structured approach to the examination of the system can be summarised as:

- inspection
- palpation
- percussion
- auscultation.

Initial observations

The physical examination begins as soon as you see the patient. Start with a rapid assessment of how unwell the patient is, since the clinical assessment may have to be adjusted for a deteriorating or dying patient, and any abnormal physiology may need to be addressed urgently before the actual diagnosis is found (pp. 341 and 348). Early warning scoring systems (which include assessment of vital signs: pulse, blood pressure, respiratory rate and oxygen saturations, temperature, conscious level and pain score) are used routinely to assess unwell patients and these clinical measurements aid decisions about illness severity and urgency of assessment (p. 340). If your patient is distressed or in pain, giving effective analgesia may take priority before undertaking a more structured evaluation, although a concurrent evaluation for the cause of the pain is clearly important.

For the stable or generally well patient, a more measured assessment can begin. Observe the patient before the consultation begins. Do they look generally well or unwell? What is their demeanour? Are they sitting up comfortably reading or on the telephone to a relative, or do they seem withdrawn, distressed or confused?

Notice the patient's attire. Are they dressed appropriately? Clothing gives clues about personality, state of mind and social circumstances, as well as a patient's physical state. Patients with recent weight loss may be wearing clothes that look very baggy and loose. Are there signs of self-neglect (which may be underpinned by other factors such as cognitive impairment, immobility or drug or alcohol dependence) or inappropriate attire? For example, a patient with thyrotoxicosis may come to see you dressed for summer in the depths of winter due to heat intolerance.

Often there will be clues to the patient's underlying medical condition either about the person (for example, they may be wearing a subcutaneous insulin pump to treat their type 1 diabetes, or carrying a portable oxygen cylinder if they have significant pulmonary fibrosis) or by the bedside (look on the bedside table for a hearing aid, peak flow meter or inhaler device, and note any walking aid, commode and wheelchair, which provide clues to the patient's functional status). Patients may be wearing a medical identity bracelet or other jewellery alerting you to an underlying medical condition or life-sustaining treatment. Note any tattoos or piercings; as well as there being possible associated infection risks, these can provide important background information (Fig. 3.2). Be sure to look for any venepuncture marks of intravenous drug use or linear (usually transverse) scars from recent or previous deliberate self-harm (Figs 3.3 and 3.4).

Gait and posture

If patients are ambulant, watch how they rise from a chair and walk towards you. Are they using a walking aid? Is the gait

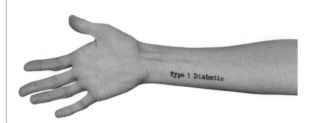

Fig. 3.2 **Tattoos can be revealing.**

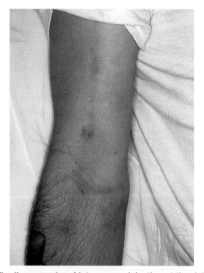

Fig. 3.3 **The linear marks of intravenous injection at the right antecubital fossa.**

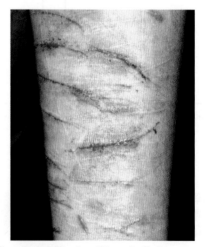

Fig. 3.4 **Scars from deliberate self-harm (cutting).**

normal or is there evidence of pain, immobility or weakness? Abnormalities of gait can be pathognomonic signs of neurological or musculoskeletal disease: for example, the hemiplegic gait after stroke, the ataxic gait of cerebellar disease or the *marche à petits pas* ('walk of little steps') gait in a patient with diffuse

3.3 Facial expression as a guide to diagnosis

Features	Diagnosis
Poverty of expression	Parkinsonism
Startled expression	Hyperthyroidism
Apathy, with poverty of expression and poor eye contact	Depression
Apathy, with pale and puffy skin	Hypothyroidism
Agitated expression	Anxiety, hyperthyroidism, hypomania

cerebrovascular disease or Parkinsonism (see Fig. 7.17D). Notice any abnormal movements such as tremor (in alcohol withdrawal, for example), dystonia (perhaps as a side effect of neuroleptic therapy) or chorea (jerky, involuntary movements, characteristic of Huntington's disease). Abnormalities of posture and movement can also be a clue to the patient's overall wellbeing, and may represent pain, weakness or psychological or emotional disturbance.

Facial expression and speech

As with gait and posture, a patient's facial expression and how they interact with you can provide clues to their physical and psychological wellbeing (Box 3.3). Reluctance to engage in the consultation may indicate underlying depression, anxiety, fear, anger or grief, and it is important to recognise these emotions to ensure that both the physical and the emotional needs of the patient are addressed effectively. Some people conceal anxieties and depression with inappropriate cheerfulness. Illness itself may alter demeanour: frontal lobe disease or bipolar disorders may lead to animated disinhibition, whereas poverty of expression may occur in depression or Parkinson's disease. Physical signs in the face that are associated with specific diagnoses are covered later (see Box 3.9).

Be vigilant for abnormalities in the character of speech, such as slurring (due to alcohol, for example, or dysarthria caused by motor neurone disease; p. 125), hoarseness (which can represent recurrent laryngeal nerve damage; p. 186) or abnormality of speech cadence (which could be caused by pressure of speech in hyperthyroidism or slowing of speech in myxoedema; p. 197).

Hands

Starting your physical contact with a patient with a handshake not only is polite but also may reveal relevant signs (see Box 3.1). The rare disease myotonic dystrophy (which is over-represented in candidate assessments) causes a patient to fail to release the handgrip (due to delayed muscle relaxation). A patient with neurological disease may be unable to shake your hand, or may have signs of muscle wasting or tremor. Detailed examination of the hands is described on page 265 but even a brief inspection and palpation may be very revealing.

Deformity

Deformity may indicate nerve palsies or arthritic changes (such as ulnar deviation at the metacarpophalangeal joints in longstanding rheumatoid arthritis; see Fig. 13.22). Arthritis frequently involves the small joints of the hands. Rheumatoid arthritis typically affects

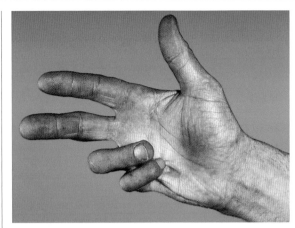

Fig. 3.5 **Dupuytren's contracture.**

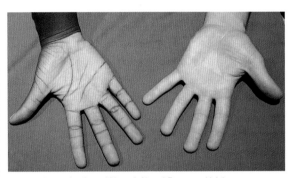

Fig. 3.6 **Normal palms.** African (left) and European (right).

metacarpophalangeal and proximal interphalangeal joints (see Fig. 13.22), and osteoarthritis and psoriatic arthropathy affect the distal interphalangeal joints (see Fig. 13.8). Small-muscle wasting of the hands is common in rheumatoid arthritis, producing 'dorsal guttering' of the hands, and also occurs in cervical spondylosis with nerve root entrapment. In carpal tunnel syndrome, median nerve compression leads to wasting of the thenar muscles, also seen in damage affecting the T1 nerve root (see Fig. 13.23).

Dupuytren's contracture is a thickening of the palmar fascia causing fixed flexion deformity, and usually affects the little and ring fingers (Fig. 3.5). Arachnodactyly (long, thin fingers) is typical of Marfan's syndrome (see Fig. 3.21B). Trauma is the most common cause of hand deformity.

Colour

Colour changes in the hands may also be revealing. Look for peripheral cyanosis in the nail bed and tobacco staining of the fingers (see Fig. 5.8). Examine the skin creases for pigmentation, although pigmentation is normal in many non-Caucasian races (Fig. 3.6).

Temperature

The temperature of the patient's hand is a good guide to peripheral perfusion. In chronic obstructive pulmonary disease the hands may be cyanosed due to reduced arterial oxygen saturation but warm due to vasodilatation from elevated arterial carbon dioxide levels. In heart failure the hands are often cold and cyanosed because of vasoconstriction in response to a low cardiac output. If they are warm, heart failure may be due to a high-output state, such as hyperthyroidism.

3.4 The nails in systemic disease

Nail changes	Description of nail	Differential diagnosis
Beau's lines	Transverse grooves (see Fig. 3.7B)	Sequella of any severe systemic illness that affects growth of the nail matrix
Clubbing	Loss of angle between nail fold and nail plate (see Fig. 3.8)	Serious cardiac, respiratory or gastrointestinal disease (see Box 3.5)
Leuconychia	White spots, ridges or complete discoloration of nail (see Fig. 3.7C)	Trauma, infection, poisoning, chemotherapy, vitamin deficiency
Lindsay's nails	White/brown 'half-and-half' nails (see Fig. 12.7)	Chronic kidney disease
Koilonychia	Spoon-shaped depression of nail plate (see Fig. 3.7D)	Iron deficiency anaemia, lichen planus, repeated exposure to detergents
Muehrcke's lines	Narrow, white transverse lines (see Fig. 12.6)	Decreased protein synthesis or protein loss
Nail-fold telangiectasia	Dilated capillaries and erythema at nail fold (see Fig. 14.13B)	Connective tissue disorders, including systemic sclerosis, systemic lupus erythematosus, dermatomyositis
Onycholysis	Nail separates from nail bed (see Fig. 3.7A)	Psoriasis, fungal infection, trauma, thyrotoxicosis, tetracyclines (photo-onycholysis)
Onychomycosis	Thickening of nail plate with white, yellow or brown discoloration	Fungal infection
Pitting	Fine or coarse pits in nail (see Fig. 3.7A)	Psoriasis (onycholysis, thickening and ridging may also be present), eczema, alopecia areata, lichen planus
Splinter haemorrhages	Small red streaks that lie longitudinally in nail plate (see Fig. 4.5B)	Trauma, infective endocarditis
Yellow nails	Yellow discoloration and thickening (see Fig. 14.13C)	Yellow nail syndrome

Skin

Skin changes in the hands can indicate systemic disease, as in the coarse skin and broad hands of a patient with acromegaly (see Fig. 10.8), or the tight, contracted skin (scleroderma) and calcium deposits associated with systemic sclerosis (see Figs 3.30C and 13.6). Clues about lifestyle can also be seen in the hands: manual workers may have specific callosities due to pressure at characteristic sites, while disuse results in soft, smooth skin.

Nails

Nail changes occur in a wide variety of systemic diseases. Box 3.4 and Fig. 3.7 summarise nail changes seen on general examination that may indicate underlying systemic disease.

Finger clubbing describes painless soft tissue swelling of the terminal phalanges and increased convexity of the nail (Fig. 3.8). Clubbing usually affects the fingers symmetrically. It may also involve the toes and can be unilateral if caused by a proximal vascular condition, such as arteriovenous shunts for dialysis. It is sometimes congenital but in over 90% of patients it heralds a serious underlying disorder (Box 3.5). Clubbing may recede if the underlying condition resolves.

Examination sequence

- Look across the nail bed from the side of each finger. Observe the distal phalanges, nail and nail bed:
  - Estimate the interphalangeal depth at the level of the distal interphalangeal joint (this is the anteroposterior thickness of the digit rather than the width). Repeat at the level of the nail bed.
  - Assess the nail-bed (hyponychial) angle (Fig. 3.9A).
- Ask the patient to place the nails of corresponding (ring) fingers back to back and look for the normal 'diamond-shaped' gap between the nail beds (Schamroth's window sign; Fig. 3.9B).

3.5 Causes of clubbing

Congenital or familial (5–10%)

Acquired
- Thoracic (~70%):
  - Lung cancer
  - Chronic suppurative conditions: pulmonary tuberculosis, bronchiectasis, lung abscess, empyema, cystic fibrosis
  - Mesothelioma
  - Fibroma
  - Pulmonary fibrosis
- Cardiovascular:
  - Cyanotic congenital heart disease
  - Infective endocarditis
  - Arteriovenous shunts and aneurysms
- Gastrointestinal:
  - Cirrhosis
  - Inflammatory bowel disease
  - Coeliac disease
- Others:
  - Thyrotoxicosis (thyroid acropachy)
  - Primary hypertrophic osteoarthropathy

- Place your thumbs under the pulp of the distal phalanx and use your index fingers alternately to see if there is fluctuant movement of the nail on the nail bed (Fig. 3.9C).

Finger clubbing is likely if:
- the interphalangeal depth ratio is >1 (that is, the digit is thicker at the level of the nail bed than the level of the distal interphalangeal joint; Fig. 3.9A)
- the nail fold angle is >190 degrees (Fig. 3.9A)
- Schamroth's window sign is absent (Fig. 3.9B).

Increased nail-bed fluctuation may be present and may support the finding of clubbing, but its presence is subjective and less discriminatory than the above features.

3

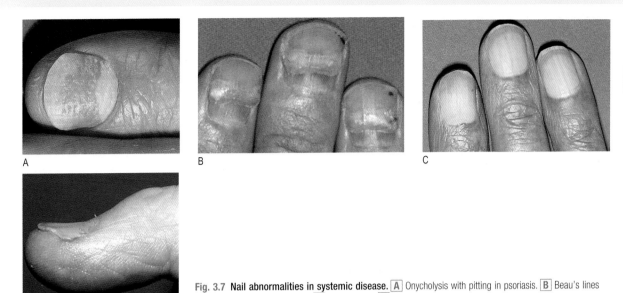

Fig. 3.7 Nail abnormalities in systemic disease. **A** Onycholysis with pitting in psoriasis. **B** Beau's lines seen after acute severe illness. **C** Leuconychia. **D** Koilonychia. *(A) From Innes JA. Davidson's Essentials of Medicine. 2nd edn. Edinburgh: Churchill Livingstone; 2016.*

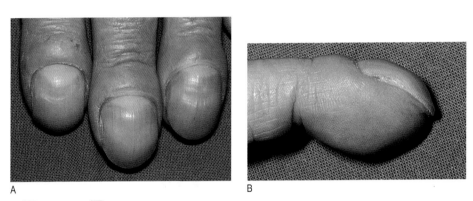

Fig. 3.8 Clubbing. **A** Anterior view. **B** Lateral view.

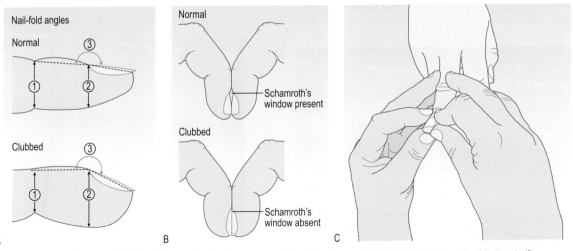

Fig. 3.9 Examining for finger clubbing. **A** Assessing interphalangeal depth at (**1**) interphalangeal joint and (**2**) nail bed, and nail-bed angle (**3**). **B** Schamroth's window sign. **C** Assessing nail-bed fluctuation.

Skin

A detailed approach to examination of the skin is described on page 286. In everyday practice the skin can provide insights into present and past medical·disorders, as well as information about the patient's social or mental status.

The skin should be exposed where appropriate and inspected carefully for any abnormalities of pigmentation. Skin colour is determined by pigments in the skin – melanin, an endogenous brown pigment, and carotene, an exogenous yellow pigment (mainly derived from ingestion of carrots and other vegetables) – as well as by the amount of oxyhaemoglobin (red) and deoxyhaemoglobin (blue) circulating in the dermis.

Depigmentation occurs in the autoimmune condition vitiligo, in which there is often bilateral symmetrical depigmentation, commonly of the face, neck and extensor aspects of the limbs, resulting in irregular pale patches of skin (Fig. 3.10). It is associated with other autoimmune diseases like diabetes mellitus, thyroid and adrenal disorders, and pernicious anaemia. Hypopituitarism also results in pale skin due to reduced production of melanotrophic peptides (see Fig. 10.10). Albinism is an inherited disorder in which patients have little or no melanin in their skin or hair. The amount of pigment in the iris varies; some individuals have reddish eyes but most have blue.

Hyperpigmentation can be due to excess of the pituitary hormone adrenocorticotrophic hormone (ACTH), as in adrenal insufficiency (or the very rare condition Nelson's syndrome, in which there is ACTH overproduction following bilateral adrenalectomy for pituitary Cushing's disease). It produces brown pigmentation, particularly in skin creases, recent scars, sites overlying bony prominences, areas exposed to pressure such as belts and bra straps, and the mucous membranes of the lips and mouth, where it results in muddy brown patches (see Fig. 10.12B). Pregnancy and oral contraceptives may also cause blotchy hyperpigmentation on the face, known as chloasma, and pregnancy may increase pigmentation of the areolae, axillae, genital skin and linea alba (producing a dark line in the midline of the lower abdomen, called a 'linea nigra').

Haemochromatosis

This inherited condition of excessive iron absorption results in skin hyperpigmentation due to iron deposition and increased melanin production (Fig. 3.11). When iron deposition in the pancreas also causes diabetes mellitus, this is called 'bronze diabetes'.

Haemosiderin

This product of haemoglobin breakdown is deposited in the skin of the lower legs following subcutaneous extravasation of blood due to venous insufficiency. Local deposition of haemosiderin (erythema ab igne or 'granny's tartan') occurs with heat damage to the skin from sitting too close to a fire or from applying local heat, such as a hot water bottle, to the site of pain (Fig. 3.12).

Easy bruising

Easy bruising can be a reflection of skin and connective tissue fragility due to advancing age or glucocorticoid usage, or a more serious coagulopathy.

Hypercarotenaemia

Hypercarotenaemia occurs due to excessive ingestion of carotene-containing vegetables or in situations of impaired metabolism such as hypothyroidism or anorexia nervosa. A yellowish discoloration is seen on the face, palms and soles but not the sclera or conjunctiva, and this distinguishes it from jaundice (Fig. 3.13).

Discoloration

Skin discoloration can also occur due to abnormal pigments such as the sallow yellow-brownish tinge in chronic kidney disease. A bluish tinge is produced by abnormal haemoglobins, such as sulphaemoglobin or methaemoglobin (see the section on cyanosis later), or by drugs such as dapsone. Some drug metabolites cause

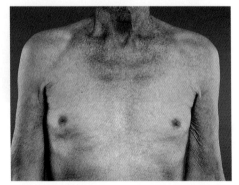

Fig. 3.11 Haemochromatosis with increased skin pigmentation.

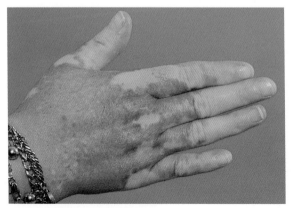

Fig. 3.10 Vitiligo.

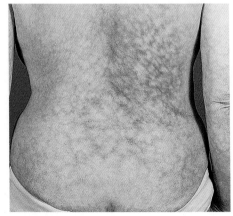

Fig. 3.12 Erythema ab igne.

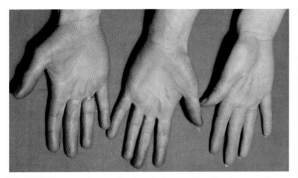

Fig. 3.13 **Hypercarotenaemia.** A control normal hand is shown on the right for comparison.

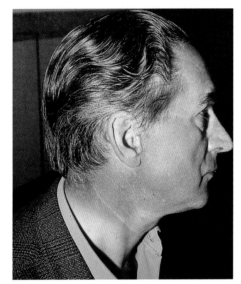

Fig. 3.14 **Phenothiazine-induced pigmentation.**

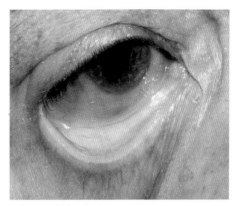

Fig. 3.15 **Conjunctival pallor.**

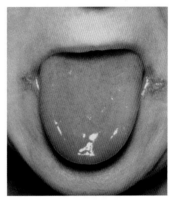

Fig. 3.16 **Smooth red tongue (glossitis) and angular stomatitis of iron deficiency.**

3.6 Conditions associated with facial flushing
Physiological
• Fever
• Exercise
• Heat exposure
• Emotional
Drugs (e.g. glyceryl trinitrate, calcium channel blockers, nicotinic acid)
Anaphylaxis
Endocrine
• Menopause
• Androgen deficiency (in men)
• Carcinoid syndrome
• Medullary thyroid cancer
Others
• Serotonin syndrome
• Food/alcohol ingestion
• Neurological (e.g. Frey's syndrome)
• Rosacea
• Mastocytoses

strikingly abnormal coloration of the skin, particularly in areas exposed to light: for example, mepacrine (yellow), amiodarone (bluish-grey) and phenothiazines (slate-grey; Fig. 3.14).

Jaundice

Jaundice is an abnormal yellow discoloration of the skin, sclera and mucous membranes. It is usually detectable when serum bilirubin concentration rises above 50 μmol/L (3 mg/dL) as a result of parenchymal liver disease, biliary obstruction or haemolysis (see Fig. 6.8).

Pallor

Pallor can result from anaemia, in which there is a reduction in circulating oxyhaemoglobin in the dermal and subconjunctival capillaries, or from vasoconstriction due to cold exposure or sympathetic activation. The best sites to assess for the pallor of anaemia are the conjunctiva (specifically the anterior rim; Fig. 3.15), the palmar skin creases and the face in general, although absence of pallor does not exclude anaemia. Nail-bed pallor lacks diagnostic value for predicting anaemia but is still often assessed by clinicians. In significant iron deficiency anaemia there may be additional findings of angular stomatitis, glossitis (Fig. 3.16), koilonychia (spoon-shaped nails) and blue sclerae.

Conversely, vasodilatation, or flushing, may produce a pink complexion, even in anaemia, and may be due to fever, heat, exercise, food, drugs and other neurological or hormonal disturbances (Fig. 3.17 and Box 3.6). Facial plethora is caused by raised haemoglobin concentration with elevated haematocrit (polycythaemia); it may be primary or may indicate an underlying

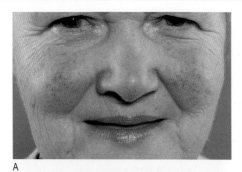

A

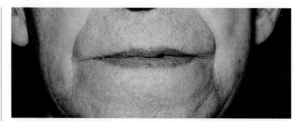

Fig. 3.18 Central cyanosis of the lips.

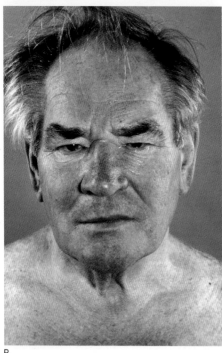

B

Fig. 3.17 Flushing due to carcinoid syndrome. [A] Acute carcinoid flush. [B] Chronic telangiectasia.

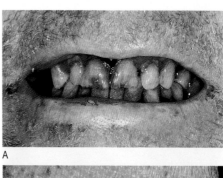

A

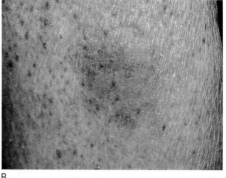

B

Fig. 3.19 Scurvy. [A] Bleeding gums. [B] Bruising and perifollicular haemorrhages.

disease resulting in chronic hypoxia or excess erythropoietin production. Plethora of the head and neck only may indicate superior vena cava obstruction (p. 86).

Cyanosis

Cyanosis is a blue discoloration of the skin and mucous membranes that occurs when the absolute concentration of deoxygenated haemoglobin is increased. It can be difficult to detect, particularly in black and Asian patients, but is most easily seen where the subepidermal vessels are close to the skin surface, as in the lips, mucous membranes, nose, cheeks, ears, hands and feet. Rarely, cyanosis can be due to excessive circulating methaemoglobin (which can be congenital or acquired, most often due to drug therapy) or sulphaemoglobin (usually due to drug therapy), and typically does not resolve with oxygen administration.

Central cyanosis

Central cyanosis can be seen in the lips, tongue and buccal or sublingual mucosa (Fig. 3.18; see Fig. 5.12), and can accompany any disease (usually cardiac or respiratory) that results in hypoxia

sufficient to raise the capillary deoxyhaemoglobin concentration above 50 g/L (5 g/dL). Since the detection of cyanosis relies on the presence of an absolute concentration of deoxyhaemoglobin, it may be absent in anaemic or hypovolaemic patients despite the presence of hypoxia. Conversely, cyanosis may manifest at relatively mild levels of hypoxia in polycythaemic patients.

Peripheral cyanosis

Peripheral cyanosis is seen in the distal extremities and may simply be a result of cold exposure, when prolonged peripheral capillary flow allows greater oxygen extraction and hence increased levels of deoxyhaemoglobin. As the patient is warmed and the circulation improves, so does the cyanosis. Pathological causes of peripheral cyanosis include low cardiac output states, arterial disease and venous stasis or obstruction.

Characteristic skin changes

Characteristic skin changes also occur in other conditions such as scurvy (Fig. 3.19), neurofibromatosis (Fig. 3.20) and acanthosis nigricans (see Fig. 10.15A).

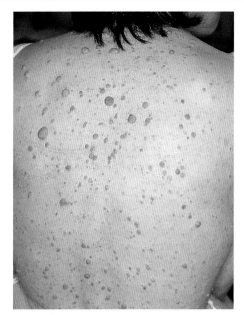

Fig. 3.20 Neurofibromatosis.

3.7 The relationship between body mass index (BMI), nutritional status and ethnic group		
Nutritional status	BMI non-Asian	BMI Asian
Underweight	<18.5	<18.5
Normal	18.5–24.9	18.5–22.9
Overweight	25–29.9	23–24.9
Obese	30–39.9	25–29.9
Morbidly obese	≥40	≥30

Tongue

In addition to revealing central cyanosis, examination may uncover the smooth tongue of iron deficiency (see Fig. 3.16), enlargement in acromegaly, or wasting and fasciculation in motor neurone disease.

Odours

Odours can provide clues to a patient's social or behavioural habits; the smell of alcohol, tobacco or cannabis may be readily apparent. Stale urine and anaerobic skin infections also produce distinctive smells. Halitosis (bad breath) can be due to poor dental hygiene, gingivitis, stomatitis, atrophic rhinitis, tumours of the nasal passages or suppurative lung conditions such as lung abscess or bronchiectasis.

Other characteristic odours include:

- ketones: a sweet smell (like nail varnish remover) due to acetone in diabetic ketoacidosis or starvation
- fetor hepaticus: the stale, 'mousy' smell of the volatile amine dimethylsulphide in patients with liver failure
- uraemic fetor: a fishy or ammoniacal smell on the breath in uraemia
- foul-smelling belching in patients with gastric outlet obstruction
- a faecal smell in patients with gastrocolic fistula.

Body habitus and nutrition

Weight

Weight is an important indicator of general health and nutrition, and serial weight measurements can be useful in monitoring

both acute and chronic disease. The body mass index (BMI; calculated from the formula weight(kg)/height(m)^2) is more useful than weight alone, as it allows for differing height. Normal values for different ethnicities are available (Box 3.7).

Obesity

Obesity is associated with an increased risk of malignancy, particularly oesophageal and renal cancer in both sexes, thyroid and colon cancer in men, and endometrial and gallbladder cancer in women, as well as hypertension, hyperlipidaemia, type 2 diabetes mellitus, gastro-oesophageal reflux, gallbladder disease, osteoarthritis and sleep apnoea. While it is usually the result of excessive calorie intake relative to calories expended, it can rarely be secondary to hypothyroidism, Cushing's syndrome, hypothalamic disease or drugs such as oral hypoglycaemic agents, insulin and antipsychotics.

Note the distribution of fat, since central obesity (as judged by the waist circumference: the maximum abdominal girth at the midpoint between the lower costal margin and the iliac crest) correlates with increased visceral adiposity and has worse health outcomes due to its association with hypertension, insulin resistance, type 2 diabetes mellitus and coronary artery disease. Waist-to-hip ratio can also be a useful assessment of adipose distribution: gluteal–femoral obesity or the 'pear shape' (waist : hip ratio of ≤0.8 in females or <0.9 in males) has a better prognosis, whereas 'apple-shaped' patients with a greater waist : hip ratio have an increased risk of coronary artery disease and the 'metabolic syndrome'.

Weight loss

Weight loss or malnutrition (p. 94) may be due to inadequate energy consumption or utilisation (such as malabsorption, anorexia, glycosuria) or to conditions in which nutritional demand is increased (such as fever, infection, thyrotoxicosis, malignancy, surgery). Psychiatric disease and alcohol or drug dependency may also result in weight loss. Useful markers of malnutrition include arm muscle circumference and grip strength. Malnutrition may also be associated with biochemical and physical evidence of hypoproteinaemia and/or vitamin deficiencies. Malnutrition lengthens recovery time from illness and surgery, and delays wound healing.

Stature

Short stature

Short stature may reflect general nutritional state or significant illness during childhood, although it may be familial (ask about the height of the patient's parents and siblings; p. 310). Loss of height is part of normal ageing but is accentuated by compression fractures of the spine due to osteoporosis, particularly in women. In postmenopausal women, loss of >5 cm height is an indication to investigate for osteoporosis.

Tall stature

Tall stature is less common than short stature and is usually familial. Most individuals with heights above the 95th centile are not abnormal so ask about the height of close relatives. Pathological causes of increased height include Marfan's syndrome, prepubertal hypogonadism and gigantism. In Marfan's syndrome the limbs are long in relation to the length of the trunk, and the arm span exceeds height (Fig. 3.21A). Additional features include long, slender fingers (arachnodactyly; Fig. 3.21B), narrow feet, a high-arched palate (Fig. 3.21C), upward dislocation of the lenses of the eyes (Fig. 3.21D), cardiovascular abnormalities such as mitral valve prolapse, and dilatation of the aortic root with aortic regurgitation.

During puberty, the epiphyses close in response to stimulation from the sex hormones, so in some patients with hypogonadism the limbs continue to grow for longer than usual (as in Klinefelter's syndrome). Gigantism is a very rare cause of tall stature due to excessive growth hormone secretion (from a pituitary adenoma) before epiphyseal fusion has occurred.

Hydration

Assessment of a patient's hydration is particularly important, especially in the acutely unwell patient. Look for evidence of dehydration or generalised oedema (pp. 240 and 244).

Localised oedema

Localised oedema (an excess of interstitial fluid) is most commonly caused by venous disease but may also develop in lymphatic, inflammatory or allergic disorders.

Venous causes

Increased venous pressure raises hydrostatic pressure within capillaries, producing oedema in the area drained by that vein. Venous causes include deep vein thrombosis, external pressure from a tumour or pregnancy, or venous valvular incompetence from previous thrombosis or surgery (Fig. 3.22). Conditions that impair the normal muscle pumping action, such as hemiparesis and forced immobility, increase venous pressure by impairing venous return. As a result, oedema may occur in immobile, bed-ridden patients, in a paralysed limb, or in a healthy person sitting for long periods such as during travel.

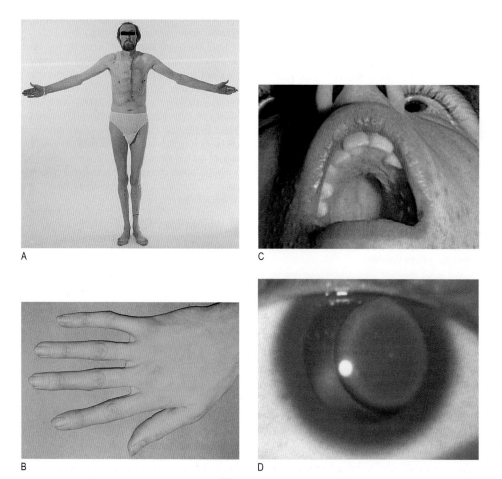

A

B

C

D

Fig. 3.21 Marfan's syndrome, an autosomal dominant condition. A Tall stature, with the torso shorter than the legs (note surgery for aortic dissection). B Long fingers. C High-arched palate. D Dislocation of the lens in the eye. *(A–D) From Forbes CD, Jackson WF. Color Atlas of Clinical Medicine. 3rd edn. Edinburgh: Mosby; 2003.*

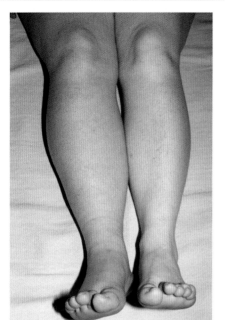

Fig. 3.22 **Swollen right leg, suggesting deep vein thrombosis or inflammation.** Causes include soft tissue infection or a ruptured Baker's cyst.

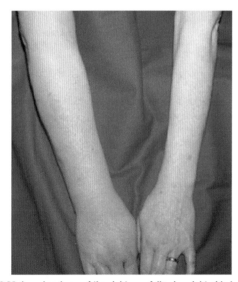

Fig. 3.23 **Lymphoedema of the right arm following right-sided mastectomy and radiotherapy.**

Lymphatic causes

Normally, interstitial fluid returns to the central circulation via the lymphatic system. Any obstruction to lymphatic flow may produce localised oedema (lymphoedema; Fig. 3.23). If the condition persists, fibrous tissue proliferates in the interstitial space and the affected area becomes hard and no longer pits on pressure. In the UK the most common cause of chronic leg lymphoedema is congenital hypoplasia of leg lymphatics (Milroy's disease); in the arm, lymphoedema usually follows radical mastectomy and/ or irradiation for breast cancer. Lymphoedema is common in some tropical countries because of lymphatic obstruction by filarial worms (elephantiasis).

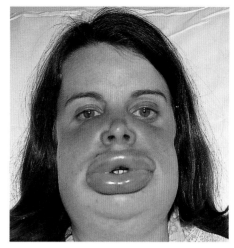

Fig. 3.24 **Angio-oedema following a wasp sting.**

3.8 Features to note in any lump or swelling (SPACESPIT)	
• <u>S</u>ize	• <u>P</u>ulsation, thrills and bruits
• <u>P</u>osition	• <u>I</u>nflammation:
• <u>A</u>ttachments	○ Redness
• <u>C</u>onsistency	○ Tenderness
• <u>E</u>dge	○ Warmth
• <u>S</u>urface and shape	• <u>T</u>ransillumination

Inflammatory causes

Any cause of tissue inflammation, including infection or injury, liberates mediators such as histamine, bradykinin and cytokines, which cause vasodilatation and increase capillary permeability. Inflammatory oedema is accompanied by the other features of inflammation (redness, tenderness and warmth) and is therefore painful.

Allergic causes

Increased capillary permeability occurs in acute allergic conditions: for example, an insect bite in an allergic individual. The affected area is usually red and pruritic (itchy) because of local release of histamine and other inflammatory mediators but, in contrast to inflammation, is not painful.

Angio-oedema is a severe form of allergic oedema affecting the face, lips and mouth, most commonly caused by insect bites, food allergy or drug reactions (Fig. 3.24). Swelling may develop rapidly and become life-threatening if the upper airway is involved.

Lumps and lymph nodes

Patients often present with a lump or enlarged lymph nodes (lymphadenopathy), which, while usually benign, can herald a serious underlying infective or malignant process. Alternatively, when examining a patient you may find a lump of which they were unaware.

Lumps

Ask about the rapidity of onset of the lump and the presence of any associated pain, tenderness or colour change. Document the following features (Box 3.8):

Size

Measure the size of any lump (preferably using callipers).

Position

The source of some lumps may be obvious from position, such as in the breast, thyroid or parotid gland; in other sites, such as the abdomen, this is less clear. Multiple lumps may occur in neurofibromatosis (see Fig. 3.20), skin metastases, lipomatosis and lymphomas.

Attachment

Malignant masses commonly infiltrate adjacent tissues, causing them to feel fixed and immobile.

Lymphatic obstruction may cause skin swelling with fine dimpling where the skin is tethered by hair follicles, giving it an 'orange peel' appearance (*peau d'orange*; see Fig. 11.5). This is common in malignant disease when attachment to deeper structures, such as underlying muscle, may also occur.

Consistency

The consistency of a lump can vary from soft to 'stony' hard. Very hard swellings are usually malignant, calcified or dense fibrous tissue. Fluctuation indicates the presence of fluid, as in an abscess, cyst or blister (Fig. 3.25), or in soft, encapsulated tumours, such as lipoma.

Edge

The margin may be well delineated or ill defined, regular or irregular, and sharp or rounded. The margins of enlarged organs, such as the thyroid gland, liver, spleen or kidney, can usually be defined more clearly than those of inflammatory or malignant masses. An indefinite margin suggests infiltrating malignancy, in contrast to the clearly defined edge of a benign tumour.

Surface and shape

The surface and shape of a swelling can be characteristic. In the abdomen, examples include an enlarged spleen or liver, a distended bladder or the uterine fundus in pregnancy. The surface may be smooth or irregular: for example, the surface of the liver is smooth in acute hepatitis but is often nodular in metastatic disease.

Pulsations, thrills and bruits

Arterial swellings (aneurysms) and highly vascular tumours are pulsatile, expanding in time with the arterial pulse. Other swellings may transmit pulsation if they lie over a major blood vessel. If the blood flow through a lump is increased, a systolic murmur (bruit) may be auscultated; occasionally, with sufficient flow, a thrill may be palpable. Bruits are also heard over arterial aneurysms and arteriovenous malformations due to turbulent flow.

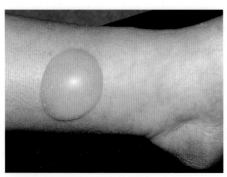

Fig. 3.25 Blister on a leg.

Inflammation

Redness, tenderness and warmth suggest inflammation:

- Redness (erythema): the skin over acute inflammatory lesions is usually red due to vasodilatation. In haematomas the pigment from extravasated blood may produce the range of colours in a bruise (ecchymosis).
- Tenderness: inflammatory lumps such as boils or abscesses are usually tender or painful, while non-inflamed swellings such as lipomas, skin metastases and neurofibromas are characteristically painless.
- Warmth: inflammatory lumps and some tumours, especially if rapidly growing, may feel warm due to increased blood flow.

Transillumination

In a darkened room, press the lighted end of a pen torch on to one side of the swelling. A cystic swelling, such as a testicular hydrocoele, will light up if the fluid is translucent, providing the covering tissues are not too thick (see Fig. 15.9).

Examination sequence

- Inspect the lump, noting any change in the colour or texture of the overlying skin.
- Define the site and shape of the lump.
- Measure its size and record the findings diagrammatically.
- Gently palpate for tenderness or change in skin temperature.
- Feel the lump for a few seconds to determine if it is pulsatile.
- Assess the consistency, surface texture and margins of the lump.
- Try to pick up an overlying fold of skin to assess whether the lump is fixed to the skin.
- Try to move the lump in different planes relative to the surrounding tissues to see if it is fixed to deeper structures.
- Compress the lump on one side; see and feel if a bulge occurs on the opposite side (fluctuation). Confirm the fluctuation in two planes. Fluctuation usually indicates that the lump contains fluid, although some soft lipomas can feel fluctuant.
- Auscultate for vascular bruits.
- Transilluminate.

Lymph nodes

Palpable lymphadenopathy (enlarged peripheral lymph nodes) may be local or generalised, and is of diagnostic and prognostic significance in the staging of lymphoproliferative and other malignancies. Lymph nodes may also be palpable in normal people, especially in the submandibular, axilla and groin regions (Fig. 3.26).

As with any lump, note the size and position of the nodes (normal nodes in adults are <0.5 cm in diameter) and assess fixation to deeper structures (lymph nodes fixed to deep structures or skin suggest malignancy). Assess consistency: normal nodes feel soft. In Hodgkin's lymphoma, they are characteristically 'rubbery', in tuberculosis they may be 'matted', and in metastatic cancer they feel hard. Acute viral or bacterial infection, including infectious mononucleosis, dental sepsis and tonsillitis, causes tender, variably enlarged lymph nodes.

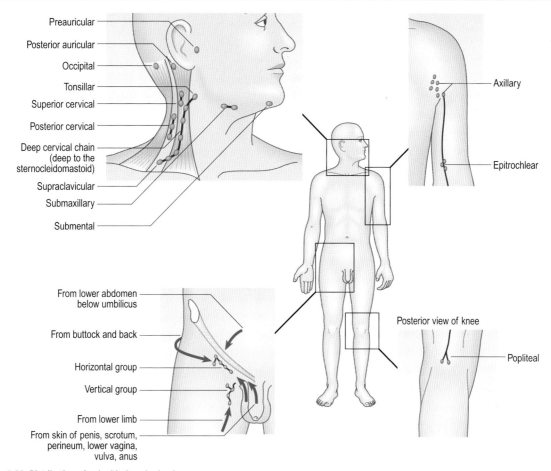

Fig. 3.26 **Distribution of palpable lymph glands.**

Examination sequence

General principles

- Inspect for visible lymphadenopathy.
- Palpate one side at a time, using the fingers of each hand in turn.
- Compare with the nodes on the contralateral side.
- Assess:
  - Site
  - Size.
- Determine whether the node is fixed to:
  - Surrounding and deep structures
  - Skin.
- Check consistency.
- Check for tenderness.

Cervical nodes

- Examine the cervical and axillary nodes with the patient sitting.
- From behind, examine the submental, submandibular, preauricular, tonsillar, supraclavicular and deep cervical nodes in the anterior triangle of the neck (Fig. 3.27A).
- Palpate for the scalene nodes by placing your index finger between the sternocleidomastoid muscle and clavicle. Ask the patient to tilt their head to the same side and press firmly down towards the first rib (Fig. 3.27B).

- From the front of the patient, palpate the posterior triangles, up the back of the neck and the posterior auricular and occipital nodes (Fig. 3.27C).

Axillary nodes

- To palpate the right axilla, support the patient's right arm with your right arm to relax their shoulder muscles and explore the axilla with your left hand (Fig. 3.28A; follow a mirror image for other side).
- Gently place your fingertips into the apex of the axilla and then draw them downwards, feeling the medial, anterior and posterior axillary walls in turn.

Epitrochlear nodes

- Support the patient's right wrist with your left hand, hold their partially flexed elbow with your right hand, and use your thumb to feel for the epitrochlear node. Examine the left epitrochlear node with your left thumb (Fig. 3.28B).

Inguinal nodes

- Examine for the inguinal and popliteal nodes with the patient lying down.
- Palpate over the horizontal chain, which lies just below the inguinal ligament, and then over the vertical chain along the line of the saphenous vein (Fig. 3.28C).

If you find localised lymphadenopathy, examine the areas that drain to that site. Infection commonly causes lymphadenitis (localised tender lymphadenopathy); in acute tonsillitis, for example,

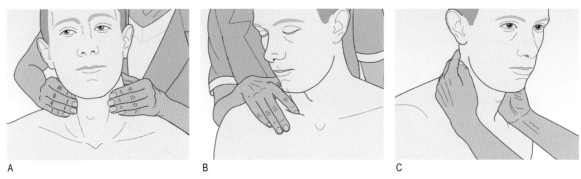

Fig. 3.27 Palpation of the cervical glands. [A] Examine the glands of the anterior triangle from behind, using both hands. [B] Examine for the scalene nodes from behind with your index finger in the angle between the sternocleidomastoid muscle and the clavicle. [C] Examine the glands in the posterior triangle from the front.

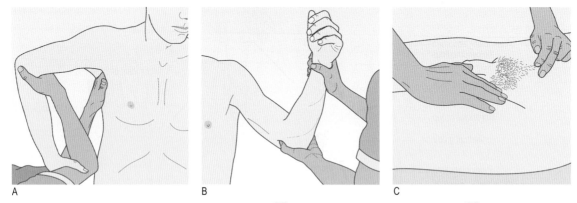

Fig. 3.28 Palpation of the axillary, epitrochlear and inguinal glands. [A] Examination for right axillary lymphadenopathy. [B] Examination of the left epitrochlear glands. [C] Examination of the left inguinal glands.

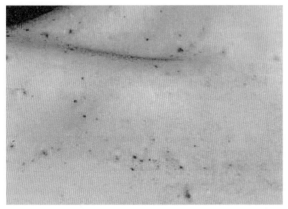

Fig. 3.29 Petechiae.

the submandibular nodes are involved. If the lymphadenopathy is non-tender, look for a malignant cause, tuberculosis or features of human immunodeficiency virus (HIV) infection. Generalised lymphadenopathy occurs in a number of conditions, including lymphoma, tuberculosis, HIV and systemic inflammatory disorders such as sarcoidosis. Examine for enlargement of the liver and spleen, and for other haematological features such as purpura (bruising under the skin), which can be large (ecchymoses) or pinpoint (petechiae; Fig. 3.29).

Spot diagnoses

Several disorders have characteristic physical or facial features (Box 3.9) that allow a diagnosis to be made by observation alone. These conditions, together with those that have a more generalised distinctive physical phenotype, are often over-represented in candidate assessments, where they are referred to as 'spot diagnoses'.

Osteogenesis imperfecta is an autosomal dominant condition causing fragile and brittle bones; the sclerae (Fig. 3.30A) are blue due to abnormal collagen formation. Hereditary haemorrhagic telangiectasia is an autosomal dominant condition associated with small, dilated capillaries or terminal arteries (telangiectasia), most commonly on the lips and tongue (Fig. 3.30B). In systemic sclerosis the skin is thickened and tight, causing loss of the normal wrinkles and skin folds, 'beaking' of the nose, and narrowing and puckering of the mouth (Fig. 3.30C). Myotonic dystrophy, mentioned previously in the context of delayed relaxation of grip after a handshake, is an autosomal dominant condition with characteristic features of frontal balding and bilateral ptosis (Fig. 3.30D).

Major chromosomal abnormalities

There are several genetic or chromosomal syndromes that are easily identified on first contact with the patient.

3.9 Conditions with characteristic facial appearances

Diagnosis	Facial features
Hypothyroidism (see Fig. 10.5)	Sparse, coarse hair and eyebrows, periorbital puffiness, dry, waxy skin, apathetic expression, macroglossia
Graves' disease (autoimmune thyrotoxicosis) (see Fig. 10.2A)	Staring appearance due to lid retraction, proptosis, evidence of weight loss
Hypopituitarism (see Fig. 10.10A)	Pale, often unwrinkled skin with loss of hair
Acromegaly (see Fig. 10.9A)	Thickened, coarse skin with enlarged nose and frontal bones, prognathism (lower jaw protrusion), widely spaced teeth, macroglossia
Cushing's syndrome (see Fig. 10.11A)	Moon-shaped plethoric facies
Osteogenesis imperfecta (see Fig. 3.30A)	Blue sclerae
Hereditary haemorrhagic telangiectasia (see Fig. 3.30B)	Telangiectasia on and around lips
Systemic sclerosis (see Fig. 3.30C)	Tight skin constricting mouth, 'beaking' of nose, loss of nasolabial folds
Myotonic dystrophy (see Fig. 3.30D)	Frontal balding, paucity of expression, bilateral ptosis
Down's syndrome (see Fig. 3.31)	Flat facial profile, up-slanting palpebral fissures, small, low-set ears, macroglossia, Brushfield spots in iris
Systemic lupus erythematosus	'Butterfly' erythematous rash on cheeks

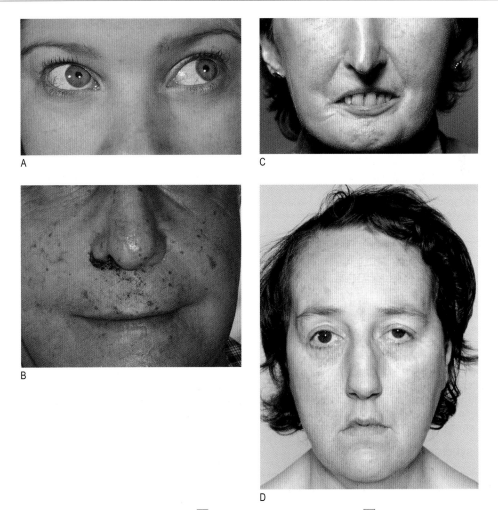

Fig. 3.30 Characteristic facial features of some disorders. A Blue sclerae of osteogenesis imperfecta. B Telangiectasia around the mouth, typical of hereditary haemorrhagic telangiectasia. C Systemic sclerosis with 'beaking' of the nose and taut skin around the mouth. D Myotonic dystrophy with frontal balding and bilateral ptosis.

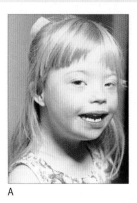

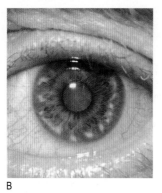

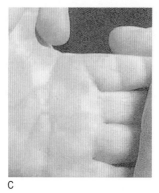

A   B   C

Fig. 3.31 Down's syndrome.
A Typical facial appearance.
B Brushfield spots: grey–white areas of depigmentation in the iris. C Single palmar crease.
A *From Kerryn Phelps, Craig Hassed; Genetic conditions. In General Practice: The Integrative Approach, 1e, Churchill Livingstone; 2011.*

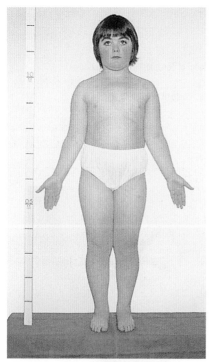

Fig. 3.32 Turner's syndrome. *From Henry M. Seidel, Jane Ball, Joyce Dain, G. William Benedict. Growth and measurement. In: Mosby's Guide to Physical Examination, 6e; 2006.*

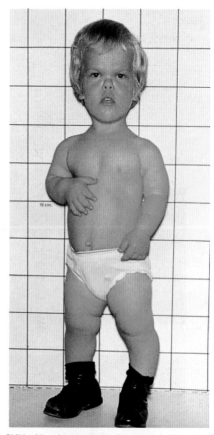

Fig. 3.33 Child with achondroplasia. *From Keith L. Moore, T. V. N. Persaud. Congenital Anatomic Anomalies or Human Birth Defects. in the Developing Human: Clinically Oriented Embryology, 8e; 2008.*

Down's syndrome (trisomy 21 – 47XX/XY + 21)

Down's syndrome is characterised by typical physical features, including short stature, a small head with flat occiput, up-slanting palpebral fissures, epicanthic folds, a small nose with a poorly developed bridge and small, low-set ears (Fig. 3.31A). Grey–white areas of depigmentation are seen in the iris (Brushfield spots; Fig. 3.31B). The hands are broad with a single palmar crease (Fig. 3.31C), the fingers are short and the little finger is curved. Trisomy 21 is also associated with characteristic cognitive, cardiac, gastrointestinal, ophthalmic, ocular, endocrine and haematological disorders, for which patients should be screened.

Turner's syndrome (45X0)

Turner's syndrome (Fig. 3.32) is due to loss of an X chromosome. It occurs in 1: 2500 live female births and is a cause of delayed puberty in girls. Typical features include short stature, webbing of the neck, small chin, low-set ears, low hairline, short fourth finger, increased carrying angle at the elbows and widely spaced nipples ('shield-like chest').

Klinefelter's syndrome (47XXY)

This chromosomal abnormality results in tall stature, gynaecomastia, reduced pubic hair and small testes (see Fig. 10.13). It is the most common cause of primary hypogonadism in men.

Achondroplasia

This is an autosomal dominant disease of cartilage caused by mutation of the fibroblast growth factor gene. Although the trunk is of normal length, the limbs are very short and broad (Fig. 3.33). The vault of the skull is enlarged, the face is small and the bridge of the nose is flat.

Section 2

System-based examination

Nicholas L Mills
Alan G Japp
Jennifer Robson

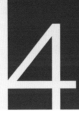

The cardiovascular system

HEART

Anatomy and physiology

The heart comprises two muscular pumps working in series, covered in a serous sac (pericardium) that allows free movement with each heart beat and respiration (Fig. 4.1). The right heart (right atrium and ventricle) pumps deoxygenated blood returning from the systemic veins into the pulmonary circulation at relatively low pressures. The left heart (left atrium and ventricle) receives blood from the lungs and pumps it round the body to the tissues at higher pressures (Fig. 4.2). Atrioventricular valves (tricuspid on the right side, mitral on the left) separate the atria from the ventricles. The pulmonary valve on the right side of the heart and the aortic valve on the left separate the ventricles from the pulmonary and systemic arterial systems, respectively. Cardiac contraction is coordinated by specialised groups of cells. The cells in the sinoatrial node normally act as the cardiac pacemaker. Subsequent spread of impulses through the heart ensures that atrial contraction is complete before ventricular contraction (systole) begins. At the end of systole the ventricles relax and the atrioventricular valves open, allowing them to refill with blood from the atria (diastole).

The history

Common presenting symptoms

Cardiovascular disease may present with a number of diverse symptoms; non-cardiac causes must also be considered (Box 4.1).

Chest pain

Intermittent chest pain

Chest pain due to intermittent myocardial ischaemia (angina pectoris) is typically a dull discomfort, often described as a tight or pressing 'band-like' sensation akin to a heavy weight. It tends to be felt diffusely across the anterior chest and may radiate down one or both arms and into the throat, jaw or teeth. In stable angina (caused by chronic narrowing in one or more coronary arteries), episodes of pain are precipitated by exertion and may occur more readily when walking in cold or windy weather, after

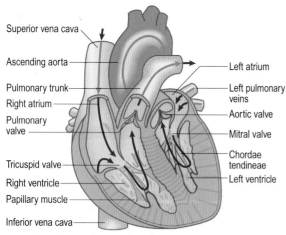

Fig. 4.1 The heart chambers and valves.

- Superior vena cava
- Ascending aorta
- Pulmonary trunk
- Right atrium
- Pulmonary valve
- Tricuspid valve
- Right ventricle
- Papillary muscle
- Inferior vena cava
- Left atrium
- Left pulmonary veins
- Aortic valve
- Mitral valve
- Chordae tendineae
- Left ventricle

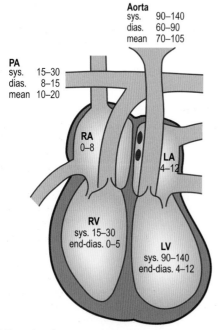

Aorta
sys. 90–140
dias. 60–90
mean 70–105

PA
sys. 15–30
dias. 8–15
mean 10–20

RA
0–8

LA
4–12

RV
sys. 15–30
end-dias. 0–5

LV
sys. 90–140
end-dias. 4–12

Fig. 4.2 Normal resting pressures (mmHg) in the heart and great vessels. *dias.*, diastolic; *LA*, left atrium; *LV*, left ventricle; *PA*, pulmonary artery; *RA*, right atrium; *RV*, right ventricle; *sys.*, systolic.

4.1 Common symptoms of heart disease

Symptom	Cardiovascular causes	Other causes
Chest discomfort	Myocardial infarction Angina Pericarditis Aortic dissection	Oesophageal spasm Pneumothorax Musculoskeletal pain
Breathlessness	Heart failure Valvular disease Angina Pulmonary embolism Pulmonary hypertension	Respiratory disease Anaemia Obesity Anxiety
Palpitation	Tachyarrhythmias Ectopic beats	Anxiety Hyperthyroidism Drugs
Syncope/presyncope	Arrhythmias Postural hypotension Aortic stenosis Hypertrophic cardiomyopathy Atrial myxoma	Simple faints Epilepsy Anxiety
Oedema	Heart failure Constrictive pericarditis Venous stasis Lymphoedema	Nephrotic syndrome Liver disease Drugs Immobility

a large meal or while carrying a heavy load; the pain is promptly relieved by rest and/or sublingual glyceryl nitrate (GTN) spray, and typically lasts for less than 10 minutes. The degree of physical exertion required to precipitate symptoms is a better guide to disease severity than the intensity of discomfort (Box 4.2). In unstable angina (caused by a sudden severe narrowing in a coronary artery), there is usually an abrupt onset or worsening

of chest pain episodes that may occur on minimal exertion or at rest. It may be difficult to distinguish between angina and non-cardiac causes of episodic chest pain, such as oesophageal pain or musculoskeletal problems (Box 4.3). The latter may occur at any site over the chest, often vary with posture or specific movements (such as twisting or turning), and may be associated with tenderness to palpation.

Ask about:
- site, onset, severity and character of the pain, and whether the pain radiates anywhere
- associated symptoms such as breathlessness
- aggravating and relieving factors, especially their relationship to exertion
- frequency and duration of symptoms, and any recent change in pattern
- degree of limitation caused by symptoms.

Acute chest pain

Myocardial infarction causes symptoms that are similar to, but more severe and prolonged than, those of angina pectoris. Associated features include restlessness, breathlessness and a feeling of impending death (*angor animi*). Autonomic stimulation may result in sweating, pallor, nausea and vomiting.

Pericardial pain is typically a constant anterior central chest pain that may radiate to the shoulders. It tends to be sharp or

4.2 Canadian Cardiovascular Society: functional classification of stable angina	
Grade	Description
1	Ordinary physical activity, such as walking and climbing stairs, does not cause angina. Angina with strenuous, rapid or prolonged exertion at work or during recreation
2	Slight limitation of ordinary activity. Walking or climbing stairs rapidly, walking uphill, walking or climbing stairs after meals, in cold, in wind, or when under emotional stress, or only during the few hours after awakening
3	Marked limitation of ordinary physical activity. Walking 1–2 blocks on the level and climbing less than one flight in normal conditions
4	Inability to carry on any physical activity without discomfort; angina may be present at rest

4.3 Cardiovascular causes of chest pain and their characteristics					
	Angina	Myocardial infarction	Aortic dissection	Pericardial pain	Oesophageal pain
Site	Retrosternal	Retrosternal	Interscapular/retrosternal	Retrosternal or left-sided	Retrosternal or epigastric
Onset	Progressive increase in intensity over 1–2 minutes	Rapid over a few minutes	Very sudden	Gradual; postural change may suddenly aggravate	Over 1–2 minutes; can be sudden (spasm)
Character	Constricting, heavy	Constricting, heavy	Tearing or ripping	Sharp, 'stabbing', pleuritic	Gripping, tight or burning
Radiation	Sometimes arm(s), neck, epigastrium	Often to arm(s), neck, jaw, sometimes epigastrium	Back, between shoulders	Left shoulder or back	Often to back, sometimes to arms
Associated features	Breathlessness	Sweating, nausea, vomiting, breathlessness, feeling of impending death (angor animi)	Sweating, syncope, focal neurological signs, signs of limb ischaemia, mesenteric ischaemia	Flu-like prodrome, breathlessness, fever	Heartburn, acid reflux
Timing	Intermittent, with episodes lasting 2–10 minutes	Acute presentation; prolonged duration	Acute presentation; prolonged duration	Acute presentation; variable duration	Intermittent, often at night-time; variable duration
Exacerbating/ relieving factors	Triggered by emotion, exertion, especially if cold, windy Relieved by rest, nitrates	'Stress' and exercise rare triggers, usually spontaneous Not relieved by rest or nitrates	Spontaneous No manoeuvres relieve pain	Sitting up/lying down may affect intensity NSAIDs help	Lying flat/some foods may trigger Not relieved by rest; nitrates sometimes relieve
Severity	Mild to moderate	Usually severe	Very severe	Can be severe	Usually mild but oesophageal spasm can mimic myocardial infarction
Cause	Coronary atherosclerosis, aortic stenosis, hypertrophic cardiomyopathy	Plaque rupture and coronary artery occlusion	Thoracic aortic dissection rupture	Pericarditis (usually viral, also post myocardial infarction)	Oesophageal spasm, reflux, hiatus hernia

NSAIDs, *non-steroidal anti-inflammatory drugs.*

stabbing in character, exacerbated by inspiration or lying down, and relieved by sitting forwards. It is caused by inflammation of the pericardium secondary to viral infection, connective tissue disease or myocardial infarction, or after surgery, catheter ablation or radiotherapy.

Aortic dissection (a tear in the intima of the aorta) is usually associated with abrupt onset of very severe, tearing chest pain that can radiate to the back (typically the interscapular region) and may be associated with profound autonomic stimulation. If the tear involves the cranial or upper limb arteries, there may be associated syncope, stroke or upper limb pulse asymmetry. Predisposing factors include hypertension and connective tissue disorders, such as Marfan's syndrome (see Fig. 3.21A–D).

As with intermittent chest pain, explore the characteristics of the pain, and ask specifically about associated symptoms that may guide you to a likely diagnosis, such as interscapular pain, sweating, nausea, vomiting, syncope or neurological features (Box 4.3).

Dyspnoea (breathlessness)

Heart failure is the most common cardiovascular cause of both acute and chronic dyspnoea (Box 4.4). Other cardiovascular causes of acute breathlessness include pulmonary embolism and arrhythmias. Patients with acute heart failure and pulmonary oedema (accumulation of fluid in the alveoli) usually prefer to be upright, while patients with massive pulmonary embolism are often more comfortable lying flat and may faint (syncope) if made to sit upright.

Exertional dyspnoea is the symptomatic hallmark of chronic heart failure. The New York Heart Association grading system is used to assess the degree of symptomatic limitation caused by the exertional breathlessness of heart failure (Box 4.5). Dyspnoea caused by myocardial ischaemia is known as 'angina equivalent'. It may occur instead of, or with, chest discomfort, especially in patients who are elderly or who have diabetes. It has identical precipitants to angina and may be relieved by GTN.

Orthopnoea, dyspnoea on lying flat, may occur in patients with heart failure, where it signifies advanced disease or incipient decompensation. Lying flat increases venous return and in patients with left ventricular impairment may precipitate pulmonary oedema. The severity can be graded by the number of pillows used at night: 'three-pillow orthopnoea', for example. Paroxysmal nocturnal dyspnoea is caused by the same mechanism, resulting in sudden breathlessness that wakes the patient from sleep (Fig. 4.3). Patients may choke or gasp for air, sit on the edge of the bed and open windows in an attempt to relieve their distress. It may be confused with asthma, which can also cause night-time dyspnoea, chest tightness, cough and wheeze, but patients with heart failure may also produce frothy white or blood-stained sputum.

4.4 Some mechanisms and causes of heart failure

Mechanism	Cause
Reduced ventricular contractility (systolic dysfunction)	Myocardial infarction Dilated cardiomyopathy, e.g. genetic, idiopathic, alcohol excess, cytotoxic drugs, peripartum cardiomyopathy Myocarditis
Impaired ventricular filling (diastolic dysfunction)	Left ventricular hypertrophy Constrictive pericarditis Hypertrophic or restrictive cardiomyopathy
Increased metabolic and cardiac demand (rare)	Thyrotoxicosis Arteriovenous fistulae Paget's disease
Valvular or congenital lesions	Mitral and/or aortic valve disease Tricuspid and/or pulmonary valve disease (rare) Ventricular septal defect Patent ductus arteriosus

4.5 New York Heart Association classification of heart failure symptom severity

Class	Description
I	No limitations. Ordinary physical activity does not cause undue fatigue, dyspnoea or palpitation (asymptomatic left ventricular dysfunction)
II	Slight limitation of physical activity. Such patients are comfortable at rest. Ordinary physical activity results in fatigue, palpitation, dyspnoea or angina pectoris (symptomatically 'mild' heart failure)
III	Marked limitation of physical activity. Less than ordinary physical activity will lead to symptoms (symptomatically 'moderate' heart failure)
IV	Symptoms of congestive heart failure are present, even at rest. With any physical activity, increased discomfort is experienced (symptomatically 'severe' heart failure)

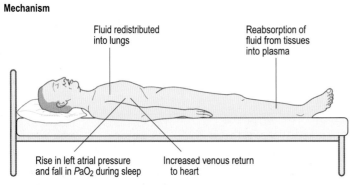
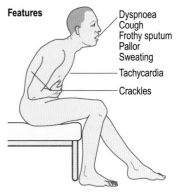

Mechanism — Fluid redistributed into lungs — Reabsorption of fluid from tissues into plasma — Rise in left atrial pressure and fall in PaO_2 during sleep — Increased venous return to heart

Features — Dyspnoea / Cough / Frothy sputum / Pallor / Sweating — Tachycardia — Crackles

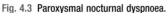

Fig. 4.3 Paroxysmal nocturnal dyspnoea.

In acute dyspnoea, ask about:

- duration of onset
- background symptoms of exertional dyspnoea and usual exercise tolerance
- associated symptoms: chest pain, syncope, palpitation or respiratory symptoms (such as cough, sputum, wheeze or haemoptysis; p. 79).

In patients with chronic symptoms, ask about:

- relationship between symptoms and exertion
- degree of limitation caused by symptoms and their impact on everyday activities
- effect of posture on symptoms and/or episodes of nocturnal breathlessness
- associated symptoms: ankle swelling, cough, wheeze or sputum.

Palpitation

Palpitation is an unexpected or unpleasant awareness of the heart beating in the chest. Detailed history taking can help to distinguish the different types of palpitation (Box 4.6).

Ask about:

- nature of the palpitation: is the heart beat rapid, forceful or irregular? Can the patient tap it out?
- timing of symptoms: speed of onset and offset; frequency and duration of episodes
- precipitants for symptoms or relieving factors
- associated symptoms: presyncope, syncope or chest pain
- history of underlying cardiac disease.

Healthy people are occasionally aware of their heart beating with normal (sinus) rhythm, especially after exercise or in stressful situations such as when waiting for an interview or examination. The sensation is often more common in bed at night and slim people may notice it when lying on their left side.

Ectopic beats (extrasystoles) are a benign cause of palpitation at rest and are abolished by exercise. The premature ectopic beat produces a small stroke volume and an impalpable impulse due to incomplete left ventricular filling. The subsequent compensatory pause leads to ventricular overfilling and a forceful contraction with the next beat. Accordingly, patients often describe 'missed beats', sometimes followed by a particularly strong heart beat ('jolt' or 'thump').

Supraventricular tachycardia produces sudden paroxysms of rapid, regular palpitation that can sometimes be terminated with vagal stimulation using Valsalva breathing manœuvres or carotid sinus pressure. It often affects young patients with no other underlying cardiac disease. Ventricular tachycardia can produce similar symptoms but is more commonly associated with presyncope or syncope, and tends to affect patients with cardiomyopathy or previous myocardial infarction.

High-risk features that increase the likelihood of a life-threatening arrhythmia such as ventricular tachycardia include:

- previous myocardial infarction or cardiac surgery
- associated syncope or severe chest pain
- family history of sudden death
- Wolff–Parkinson–White syndrome
- significant structural heart disease such as hypertrophic cardiomyopathy or aortic stenosis.

Syncope and presyncope

Syncope is a transient loss of consciousness due to transient cerebral hypoperfusion. Causes include postural hypotension, neurocardiogenic syncope, arrhythmias and mechanical obstruction to cardiac output. The same mechanisms may lead to a sensation of lightheadedness and impending loss of consciousness without progressing to actual loss of consciousness (presyncope). The main differential diagnosis of syncope is seizure (p. 122), while lightheadedness and presyncope must be distinguished from dizziness or vertigo due to non-cardiovascular causes (p. 123).

In patients who present with syncope, ask about:

- circumstances of the event and any preceding symptoms: palpitation, chest pain, lightheadedness, nausea, tinnitus, sweating or visual disturbance
- duration of loss of consciousness, appearance of the patient while unconscious and any injuries sustained (a detailed witness history is extremely helpful)
- time to recovery of full consciousness and normal cognition
- current driving status, including occupational driving.

4.6 Descriptions of arrhythmias					
	Extrasystoles	Sinus tachycardia	Supraventricular tachycardia	Atrial fibrillation	Ventricular tachycardia
Site	–	–	–	–	–
Onset	Sudden	Gradual	Sudden, with 'jump'	Sudden	Sudden
Character	'Jump', missed beat or flutter	Regular, fast, 'pounding'	Regular, fast	Irregular, usually fast; slower in elderly	Regular, fast
Radiation	–	–	–	–	–
Associated features	Nil	Anxiety	Polyuria, lightheadedness, chest tightness	Polyuria, breathlessness Syncope uncommon	Presyncope, syncope, chest tightness
Timing	Brief	A few minutes	Minutes to hours	Variable	Variable
Exacerbating/ relieving factors	Fatigue, caffeine, alcohol may trigger Often relieved by walking (increases sinus rate)	Exercise or anxiety may trigger	Usually at rest, trivial movements, e.g. bending, may trigger Vagal manœuvres may relieve	Exercise or alcohol may trigger; often spontaneous	Exercise may trigger; often spontaneous
Severity	Mild (usually)	Mild to moderate	Moderate to severe	Very variable, may be asymptomatic	Often severe

4.7 Symptoms related to medication	
Symptom	**Medication**
Angina	Aggravated by thyroxine or drug-induced anaemia, e.g. aspirin or NSAIDs
Dyspnoea	Beta-blockers in patients with asthma Exacerbation of heart failure by beta-blockers, some calcium channel antagonists (verapamil, diltiazem), NSAIDs
Palpitation	Tachycardia and/or arrhythmia from thyroxine, β_2 stimulants, e.g. salbutamol, digoxin toxicity, hypokalaemia from diuretics, tricyclic antidepressants
Syncope/ presyncope	Vasodilators, e.g. nitrates, alpha-blockers, ACE inhibitors and angiotensin II receptor antagonists Bradycardia from rate-limiting agents, e.g. beta-blockers, some calcium channel antagonists (verapamil, diltiazem), digoxin, amiodarone
Oedema	Glucocorticoids, NSAIDs, some calcium channel antagonists, e.g. nifedipine, amlodipine

ACE, angiotensin-converting enzyme; NSAIDs, non-steroidal anti-inflammatory drugs.

In patients with presyncopal symptoms of lightheadedness or dizziness, ask about:

- exact nature of symptoms and associated features such as palpitation
- precipitants for symptoms, such as postural change, prolonged standing, intense emotion or exertion
- frequency of episodes and impact on lifestyle
- possible contributing medications, such as antihypertensive agents (Box 4.7).

Postural hypotension, a fall of more than 20 mmHg in systolic blood pressure on standing, may lead to syncope or presyncope. It can be caused by hypovolaemia, drugs (Box 4.7) or autonomic neuropathy and is common in the elderly, affecting up to one-third of individuals over 65 years.

In simple faint and other forms of reflex syncope or presyncope, abnormal autonomic reflexes produce a sudden slow heart rate (bradycardia) and/or vasodilatation. These may be triggered in healthy people forced to stand for a long time in a warm environment or subject to painful or emotional stimuli, such as the sight of blood. There is typically a prodrome of lightheadedness, tinnitus, nausea, sweating and facial pallor, and a darkening of vision from the periphery as the retinal blood supply (the most oxygen-sensitive part of the nervous system) is reduced. The person then slides to the floor, losing consciousness. When laid flat to aid cerebral circulation the individual wakes up, often flushing from vasodilatation and nauseated or even vomiting due to vagal overactivity. If the person is held upright by misguided bystanders, continued cerebral hypoperfusion delays recovery and may lead to a seizure and a mistaken diagnosis of epilepsy. In patients with hypersensitive carotid sinus syndrome, pressure over the carotid sinus may lead to reflex bradycardia and syncope.

Arrhythmias can cause syncope or presyncope. The most common cause is bradyarrhythmia caused by sinoatrial disease or atrioventricular block: Stokes–Adams attacks. Rate-limiting drugs are a common cause of bradyarrhythmia. Supraventricular tachyarrhythmias, like atrial fibrillation, rarely cause syncope whereas ventricular tachycardia often causes syncope or presyncope, especially in patients with impaired left ventricular function.

Mechanical obstruction to left ventricular outflow, including severe aortic stenosis and hypertrophic cardiomyopathy, can cause syncope or presyncope, especially on exertion, when cardiac output cannot meet the increased metabolic demand. Massive pulmonary embolism can lead to syncope by obstructing outflow from the right ventricle; associated features are usually apparent and include acute dyspnoea, chest pain and hypoxia. Cardiac tumours, such as atrial myxoma, and thrombosis or failure of prosthetic heart valves are rare causes of syncope.

Oedema

Excess fluid in the interstitial space causes oedema (tissue swelling). It is usually gravity-dependent and so is seen especially around the ankles, or over the sacrum in patients lying in bed. Unilateral lower limb oedema may occur in deep vein thrombosis (p. 70). Heart failure is a common cause of bilateral lower limb oedema but other causes include chronic venous disease, vasodilating calcium channel antagonists (such as amlodipine) and hypoalbuminaemia. An elevated jugular venous pressure strongly suggests a cardiogenic cause of oedema. Enquire about other symptoms of fluid overload, including dyspnoea, orthopnoea and abdominal distension.

Other symptoms of cardiac disease

Infective endocarditis, microbial infection of a heart valve, frequently presents with non-specific symptoms, including weight loss, tiredness, fever and night sweats.

Embolisation of intracardiac thrombus, tumour (such as atrial myxoma) or infective 'vegetations' (Fig. 4.4) may produce symptoms of stroke (p. 123), acute limb ischaemia (p. 65) or acute mesenteric ischaemia (p. 66).

Advanced heart failure may result in either abdominal distension due to ascites, or weight loss and muscle wasting ('cardiac cachexia') due to a prolonged catabolic state.

Past medical history

Obtaining a detailed record of any previous cardiac disease, investigations and interventions is essential (Box 4.8). You may need to consult the patient, family members and electronic case records.

Also ask about:

- conditions associated with increased risk of vascular disease such as hypertension, diabetes mellitus and hyperlipidaemia
- rheumatic fever or heart murmurs during childhood
- potential causes of bacteraemia in patients with suspected infective endocarditis, such as skin infection, recent dental work, intravenous drug use or penetrating trauma
- systemic disorders with cardiovascular manifestations such as connective tissue diseases (pericarditis and Raynaud's phenomenon), Marfan's syndrome (aortic dissection) and myotonic dystrophy (atrioventricular block).

Drug history

Drugs may cause or aggravate symptoms such as breathlessness, chest pain, oedema, palpitation or syncope (see Box 4.7). Ask about 'over-the-counter' purchases, such as non-steroidal anti-inflammatory drugs (NSAIDs) and alternative and herbal medicines, as these may have cardiovascular actions.

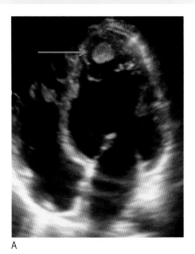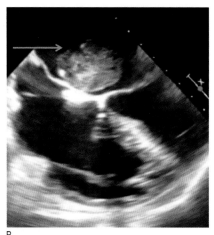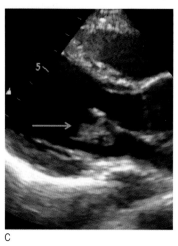

A   B   C

Fig. 4.4 Cardiac sources of systemic embolism: echocardiographic images. [A] A large apical thrombus in the left ventricle *(arrow)*. [B] An atrial myxoma attached to the interatrial septum *(arrow)*. [C] A vegetation on the mitral valve *(arrow)* in infective endocarditis. Because all of these lesions are located within the left side of the heart, emboli would flow to the systemic (or coronary) circulation. Conversely, emboli from the right side of the heart would flow to the pulmonary circulation.

4.8 Key elements of the past cardiac history			
	Ischaemic heart disease	**Heart failure**	**Valvular disease**
Baseline symptoms	Exertional angina? If so, ascertain functional limitation (see Box 4.2)/response to GTN spray	Dyspnoea, fatigue, ankle swelling Record usual functional status (see Box 4.5)	Often asymptomatic Exertional dyspnoea (common), chest pain or syncope
Major events	Previous myocardial infarction/unstable angina	Hospitalisation for decompensated heart failure Ventricular arrhythmias	Infective endocarditis Previous rheumatic fever
Investigations	Coronary angiography (invasive or computed tomography): presence, extent and severity of coronary artery disease Exercise electrocardiogram (or other stress test): evidence of inducible ischaemia? Exercise capacity and symptoms	Echocardiogram (± cardiac magnetic resonance imaging): left ventricular size, wall thickness and systolic function; valvular disease; right ventricular function	Echocardiogram (transthoracic ± transoesophageal): nature and severity of valve lesion; ventricular size and function
Procedures	Percutaneous coronary intervention (angioplasty and stenting) Coronary artery bypass graft surgery	Implantable cardioverter–defibrillator Cardiac resynchronisation therapy	Surgical valve repair or replacement (note whether mechanical or bioprosthetic) Transcatheter valve procedures
GTN, *glyceryl trinitrate*.			

Family history

Many cardiac disorders such as cardiomyopathies have a genetic component. Ask about premature coronary artery disease in first-degree relatives (<60 years in a female or <55 years in a male); sudden unexplained death at a young age may raise the possibility of a cardiomyopathy or inherited arrhythmia. Patients with venous thrombosis may have inherited thrombophilia, such as a factor V Leiden mutation. Familial hypercholesterolaemia is associated with premature arterial disease.

Social history

Smoking is the strongest risk factor for coronary and peripheral arterial disease. Take a detailed smoking history (p. 14). Alcohol can induce atrial fibrillation and, in excess, is associated with obesity, hypertension and dilated cardiomyopathy. Recreational drugs such as cocaine and amphetamines can cause arrhythmias,

chest pain, occlusive and aneurysmal peripheral arterial disease and even myocardial infarction. Heart disease may have important consequences for employment. Patients with limiting exertional symptoms may struggle to perform jobs that entail a high degree of physical activity. In addition, some diagnoses such as ischaemic heart disease or cardiac arrhythmia may impact on eligibility for certain occupations that have implications for public safety, such as commercial drivers and pilots.

The physical examination

Tailor the sequence and extent of examination to the patient's condition. If you suspect that the person may be unstable, deteriorating or critically unwell (breathless, distressed, cyanosed or obtunded, for example), adopt an ABCDE approach initially (p. 341) and defer detailed examination until stabilised. In stable patients, perform a detailed and comprehensive physical examination.

General examination

Look at the patient's general appearance. Do they look unwell, frightened or distressed? Are there any signs of breathlessness or cyanosis? Is the patient overweight or cachectic? Are there any features of conditions associated with cardiovascular disease such as Marfan's (p. 30), Down's (p. 36) or Turner's syndrome (p. 36), or ankylosing spondylitis (p. 262)?

Conclude by examining the entire skin surface for petechiae, checking the temperature (p. 345) and performing urinalysis (p. 246). Fever is a feature of infective endocarditis and pericarditis, and may occur after myocardial infarction. Urinalysis is necessary to check for haematuria (endocarditis, vasculitis), glucosuria (diabetes) and proteinuria (hypertension and renal disease).

Hands

Examination sequence

- Feel the temperature of the hands and measure capillary refill time (p. 343).
- Examine the hands for tobacco staining (see Fig. 5.8), skin crease pallor (anaemia) or peripheral cyanosis.
- Look at the nails for finger clubbing (p. 24) and for splinter haemorrhages: linear, reddish-brown marks along the axis of the fingernails and toenails (Fig. 4.5B).

- Examine the extensor surface of the hands for tendon xanthomata: hard, slightly yellowish masses over the extensor tendons of the hand from lipid deposits (Fig. 4.6B).
- Examine the palmar aspect of the hands for:
  - Janeway lesions: painless, blanching red macules on the thenar/hypothenar eminences (Fig. 4.5A)
  - Osler's nodes: painful raised erythematous lesions, typically on the pads of the fingers (Fig. 4.5C).

The hands usually feel dry and warm at ambient temperature. Normal capillary refill time is 2 seconds or less. Cool extremities and prolonged capillary refill time signify impaired peripheral

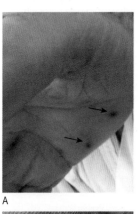

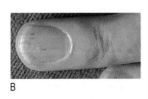
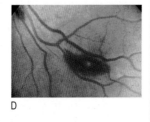
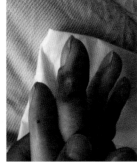
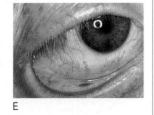

Fig. 4.5 Peripheral signs that may be present in infective endocarditis. [A] Janeway lesions on the hypothenar eminence *(arrows).* [B] Splinter haemorrhages. [C] Osler's nodes. [D] Roth's spot on fundoscopy. [E] Petechial haemorrhages on the conjunctiva. *(B and E) From Walker BR, Colledge NR, Ralston SR, Penman ID, eds. Davidson's Principles and Practice of Medicine. 22nd edn. Edinburgh: Churchill Livingstone; 2014. (D) From Forbes CD, Jackson WF. Color Atlas of Clinical Medicine. 3rd edn. Edinburgh: Mosby; 2003.*

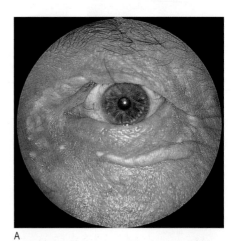

A

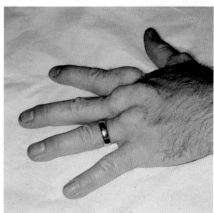

B

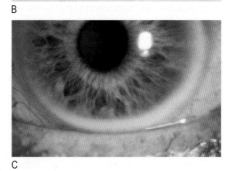

C

Fig. 4.6 Features of hyperlipidaemia. [A] Xanthelasmata. [B] Tendon xanthomata. [C] Corneal arcus. *(B) From Swartz M. Textbook of Physical Diagnosis. 6th edn. Philadelphia: Saunders; 2009. (C) From Kanski J. Clinical Diagnosis in Ophthalmology. London: Mosby; 2006.*

perfusion, which may occur in shock (p. 343) or chronic conditions associated with a low cardiac output state (as in severe aortic stenosis, mitral stenosis or pulmonary hypertension).

One or two isolated splinter haemorrhages from trauma are common in healthy individuals, especially in manual workers. Splinter haemorrhages (Fig. 4.5B) are found in infective endocarditis and some vasculitic disorders. A petechial rash (caused by vasculitis), most often present on the legs and conjunctivae (Fig. 4.5E), is a transient finding in endocarditis and can be confused with the rash of meningococcal disease. Janeway lesions and Osler's nodes (Fig. 4.5A and C) are features of endocarditis but are rare in the modern era.

Tendon xanthomata (Fig. 4.6) are a sign of familial hypercholesterolaemia, a genetic disorder associated with severe elevations in serum cholesterol and premature coronary artery disease.

Face

Examination sequence

- Look in the mouth for central cyanosis: a purplish blue discoloration of the lips and underside of the tongue (see Fig. 5.11).
- Examine the eyelids for xanthelasmata: soft, yellowish plaques found periorbitally and on the medial aspect of the eyelids (Fig. 4.6A).
- Look at the iris for corneal arcus: a creamy yellow discoloration at the boundary of the iris and cornea (Fig. 4.6C).
- Examine the fundi (p. 164) for features of hypertension (p. 165), diabetes (p. 165) or Roth's spots (flame-shaped retinal haemorrhages with a 'cotton-wool' centre; Fig. 4.5D).

Cardiac causes of central cyanosis include heart failure sufficient to cause pulmonary congestion and oedema impairing gas exchange, or, rarely, congenital heart disease, in which case it is associated with right-to-left shunting and finger clubbing (p. 24).

Xanthelasmata and corneal arcus (Fig. 4.6A and C) are associated with hyperlipidaemia but also occur frequently in normolipidaemic patients. The presence of xanthelasma is an independent risk factor for coronary heart disease and myocardial infarction but corneal arcus has no independent prognostic value.

Arterial pulses

The palpable pulse in an artery reflects the pressure wave generated by the ejection of blood into the circulation from the left ventricle.

When taking a pulse, assess:
- rate: the number of pulses occurring per minute
- rhythm: the pattern or regularity of pulses
- volume: the perceived degree of pulsation
- character: an impression of the pulse waveform or shape.

The rate and rhythm of the pulse are usually determined at the radial artery; use the larger pulses (brachial, carotid or femoral) to assess the pulse volume and character.

Examination sequence

Radial pulse
- Place the pads of your index and middle fingers over the right wrist, just lateral to the flexor carpi radialis tendon (Fig. 4.7A).
- Assess the rhythm of the pulse and count the number over 15 seconds; multiply by 4 to obtain the rate in beats per minute (bpm).
- To detect a collapsing pulse: first, check that the patient has no shoulder or arm pain or restriction on movement; next, feel the pulse with the base of your fingers, then raise the patient's arm vertically above their head (Fig. 4.7B).
- Palpate both radial pulses simultaneously, assessing any delay between the two.

Brachial pulse
- Use your index and middle fingers to palpate the pulse in the antecubital fossa, just medial to the biceps tendon (Fig. 4.7C). Assess the character and volume of the pulse.

Carotid pulse
- Explain what you are going to do.
- With the patient semirecumbent, place the tips of your fingers between the larynx and the anterior border of the sternocleidomastoid muscle (Fig. 4.7D).
- Palpate the pulse gently to avoid a vagal reflex, and never assess both carotids simultaneously.
- Listen for bruits over both carotid arteries, using the diaphragm of your stethoscope in held inspiration.

Rate and rhythm

Resting heart rate is normally 50–95 bpm but should be considered in the clinical context. A pulse rate of 40 bpm can be normal in a fit young adult, whereas a pulse rate of 65 bpm may be abnormally low in acute heart failure. Bradycardia is defined as a pulse rate of <60 bpm; tachycardia is a rate of >100 bpm. The most common causes of bradycardia are medication, athletic conditioning and sinoatrial or atrioventricular node dysfunction.

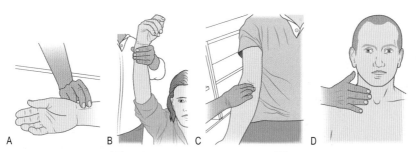

Fig. 4.7 The radial, brachial and carotid pulses. [A] Locating and palpating the radial pulse. [B] Feeling for a collapsing radial pulse. [C] Assessing the brachial pulse. [D] Locating the right carotid pulse with the fingers.

4.9 Causes of abnormal pulse rate or rhythm

Abnormality	Sinus rhythm	Arrhythmia

Fast rate (tachycardia, >100 bpm)	Exercise
	Pain
	Excitement/anxiety
	Fever
	Hyperthyroidism
	Medication:
	  Sympathomimetics,
	  e.g. salbutamol
	  Vasodilators
		Atrial fibrillation
		Atrial flutter
		Supraventricular tachycardia
		Ventricular tachycardia

Slow rate (bradycardia, <60 bpm)	Sleep
	Athletic training
	Hypothyroidism
	Medication:
	  Beta-blockers
	  Digoxin
	  Verapamil, diltiazem
		Carotid sinus hypersensitivity
		Sick sinus syndrome
		Second-degree heart block
		Complete heart block

Irregular pulse	Sinus arrhythmia Atrial extrasystoles Ventricular extrasystoles	Atrial fibrillation Atrial flutter with variable response Second-degree heart block with variable response

4.10 Haemodynamic effects of respiration

	Inspiration	Expiration
Pulse/heart rate	Accelerates	Slows
Systolic blood pressure	Falls (up to 10 mmHg)	Rises
Jugular venous pressure	Falls	Rises
Second heart sound	Splits	Fuses

4.11 Common causes of atrial fibrillation

- Hypertension
- Heart failure
- Myocardial infarction
- Thyrotoxicosis
- Alcohol-related heart disease
- Mitral valve disease
- Infection, e.g. respiratory, urinary
- Following surgery, especially cardiothoracic surgery

Sinus rhythm

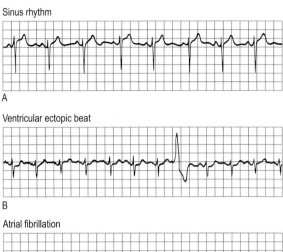

A

Ventricular ectopic beat

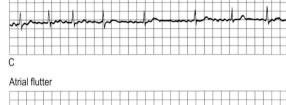

B

Atrial fibrillation

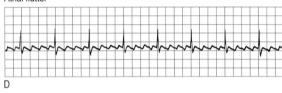

C

Atrial flutter

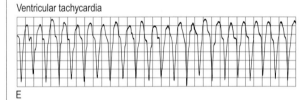

D

Ventricular tachycardia

E

Fig. 4.8 Electrocardiogram rhythm strips. A Sinus rhythm. B Ventricular ectopic beat. C Atrial fibrillation with 'controlled' ventricular response. D Atrial flutter: note the regular 'saw-toothed' atrial flutter waves at about 300/min. E Ventricular tachycardia, with a ventricular rate of about 200/min.

The most common cause of tachycardia is sinus tachycardia (Box 4.9).

The pulse may be regular or irregular (Box 4.9). Sinus rhythm is regular (Fig. 4.8A) but heart rate varies with the respiratory cycle, particularly in children, young adults or athletes (sinus arrhythmia). During inspiration, parasympathetic tone falls and the heart rate increases; on expiration, the heart rate decreases (Box 4.10). With intermittent extrasystoles (Fig. 4.8B) or second-degree atrioventricular block, there may be an underlying regularity to the pulse, interspersed with periods of irregularity (sometimes referred to as 'regularly irregular'). In atrial fibrillation the pulse has no appreciable pattern and is often described as 'irregularly irregular' (Fig. 4.8C and Box 4.11). The rate in atrial fibrillation depends on the number of beats conducted by the atrioventricular node. Untreated, the ventricular rate may be very fast (up to 200 bpm). The variability of the pulse rate (and therefore ventricular filling) explains why the pulse volume varies and there may be a pulse deficit, with some cycles not felt at the radial artery. The pulse deficit can be calculated by counting the radial pulse rate and subtracting this from the apical heart rate, assessed by auscultation.

Volume and character

The ventricles fill during diastole. Longer diastolic intervals are associated with increased stroke volume, which is reflected by increased pulse volume on examination. Abnormalities of pulse volume and character are highly subjective, however, and tend to have poor interobserver agreement.

A large pulse volume is a reflection of a large pulse pressure, which can be physiological or pathological (Box 4.12).

Low pulse volume may result from severe heart failure and conditions associated with inadequate ventricular filling such as hypovolaemia, cardiac tamponade and mitral stenosis. Asymmetric pulses may represent occlusive peripheral arterial disease or

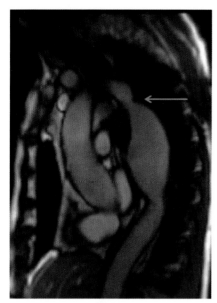

Fig. 4.9 Coarctation of the aorta. Magnetic resonance image showing the typical site of aortic coarctation, just distal to the origin of the left subclavian artery *(arrow)*. This explains why there is synchrony of the radial pulses but radiofemoral delay.

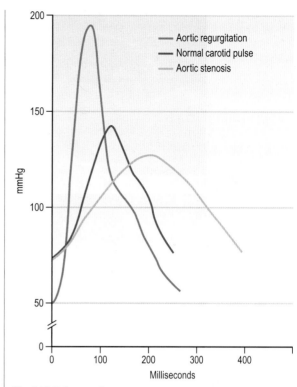

Fig. 4.10 Pulse waveforms.

4.12 Causes of increased pulse volume	
Physiological	
• Exercise	• Increased environmental
• Pregnancy	temperature
• Advanced age	
Pathological	
• Hypertension	• Aortic regurgitation
• Fever	• Paget's disease of bone
• Thyrotoxicosis	• Peripheral atrioventricular
• Anaemia	shunt

stenosis and, rarely, aortic dissection. Coarctation is a congenital narrowing of the aorta, usually distal to the left subclavian artery (Fig. 4.9); it may produce reduced-volume lower limb pulses, which are also delayed relative to the upper limb pulses (radiofemoral delay). In adults, coarctation usually presents with hypertension and heart failure.

A slow-rising pulse has a gradual upstroke with a reduced peak occurring late in systole, and is a feature of severe aortic stenosis (Fig. 4.10).

A collapsing pulse may occur with severe aortic regurgitation. The peak of the pulse wave arrives early and is followed by a rapid fall in pressure (Fig. 4.10) as blood flows back into the left ventricle, resulting in a wide pulse pressure (systolic – diastolic blood pressure >80 mmHg). This rapid fall imparts the 'collapsing' sensation, and is exaggerated by raising the patient's arm above the level of the heart (see Fig. 4.7B).

Pulsus bisferiens, an increased pulse with a double systolic peak separated by a distinct mid-systolic dip, is classically produced by concomitant aortic stenosis and regurgitation. Pulsus alternans, beat-to-beat variation in pulse volume with a normal rhythm, may occur in advanced heart failure. Both

of these signs are rare, however, and of limited relevance in contemporary practice.

Pulsus paradoxus is an exaggeration of the normal variability of pulse volume with breathing. Pulse volume normally increases in expiration and decreases during inspiration due to intrathoracic pressure changes affecting venous return to the heart. This variability is exaggerated when ventricular diastolic filling is impeded by elevated intrapericardial pressure. This is usually due to accumulation of pericardial fluid (cardiac tamponade; Fig. 4.11) but can occur to a lesser extent with pericardial constriction and in acute severe asthma. If suspected, pulsus paradoxus can be confirmed using a blood pressure cuff (see later and Fig. 4.12); a fall of >10 mmHg between the cuff pressure at which Korotkoff sounds appear in expiration only and the cuff pressure at which Korotkoff sounds persist throughout the respiratory cycle is diagnostic.

Blood pressure

Blood pressure (BP) is a measure of the pressure that the circulating blood exerts against the arterial walls. Systolic pressure is the maximal pressure that occurs during ventricular contraction (systole). During ventricular filling (diastole), arterial pressure is maintained at a lower level by the elasticity and compliance of the vessel wall. The lowest value (diastolic pressure) occurs immediately before the next cycle.

BP is usually measured using a sphygmomanometer (Fig. 4.12). In certain situations, such as the intensive care unit, it is measured invasively using an indwelling intra-arterial catheter connected to a pressure sensor.

BP is measured in mmHg and recorded as systolic pressure/ diastolic pressure, together with a note of where and how the

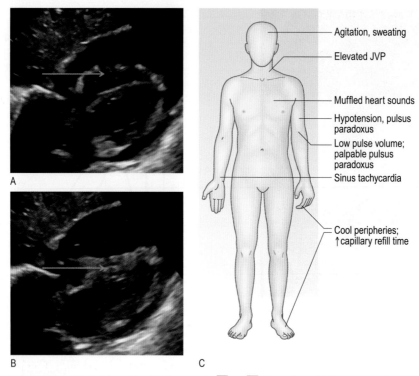

Fig. 4.11 Clinical and echocardiographic features of cardiac tamponade. [A] and [B] Echocardiographic images taken from the subcostal position at the onset of systole (A) and in early diastole (B). The right ventricle *(arrows)* is collapsed in the early phase of diastole due to the elevated intrapericardial pressure; this is an important echo finding in tamponade. In both images there is a large pericardial effusion adjacent to the right ventricle. [C] Clinical features. *JVP,* jugular venous pressure.

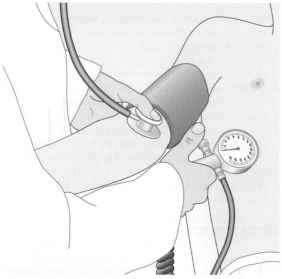

Fig. 4.12 Measuring the blood pressure.

4.13 British Hypertension Society classification of blood pressure (BP) levels		
BP	**Systolic BP (mmHg)**	**Diastolic BP (mmHg)**
Optimal	<120	<80
Normal	<130	<85
High normal	130–139	85–89
Hypertension Grade 1 (mild) Grade 2 (moderate) Grade 3 (severe)	 140–159 160–179 >180	 90–99 100–109 >110
Isolated systolic hypertension Grade 1 Grade 2	 140–159 >160	 <90 <90

Reproduced by kind permission of the British and Irish Hypertension Society.

reading was taken: for example, BP 146/92 mmHg, right arm, supine.

BP provides vital information on the haemodynamic condition of acutely ill or injured patients. Over the longer term it is also an important guide to cardiovascular risk. BP constantly varies and rises with stress, excitement and environment. 'White coat hypertension' refers to a transient increase in BP caused by the stress of being in a healthcare setting. Ambulatory BP measurement, using a portable device at intervals during normal daytime activity and at night, is better at determining cardiovascular risk.

Hypertension

Although any threshold for distinguishing abnormal elevation of BP from normal BP is somewhat arbitrary, hypertension is widely defined as a systolic pressure of ≥140 mmHg and/or a diastolic pressure ≥90 mmHg (Box 4.13). Hypertension is associated with significant morbidity and mortality from vascular disease (heart failure, coronary artery disease, cerebrovascular disease and chronic kidney disease). It is almost invariably asymptomatic, although, rarely and in severe hypertension, headaches and visual disturbances can occur. In most hypertensive patients there is no identifiable cause – so-called 'essential hypertension'. Secondary hypertension is rare, occurring in <1% of the hypertensive population (Box 4.14).

Assess the hypertensive patient for:

- potential underlying causes (Box 4.14)
- end-organ damage:
  - cardiac: heart failure
  - renal: chronic kidney disease, proteinuria
  - eye: hypertensive retinopathy (see Fig. 8.18).

Korotkoff sounds

These sounds are produced when the cuff pressure is between systolic and diastolic because the artery collapses completely and reopens with each heart beat, producing a snapping or knocking sound (Fig. 4.13). The first appearance of sounds (phase 1) during cuff deflation indicates systole. As pressure is gradually reduced, the sounds muffle (phase 4) and then disappear (phase 5).

4.14 Clinical clues to secondary hypertension

Clinical feature	Cause
Widespread vascular disease Renal bruit	Renovascular disease, including renal artery stenosis
Episodes of sweating, headache and palpitation	Phaeochromocytoma
Hypokalaemia	Primary aldosteronism
Cushingoid facies, central obesity, abdominal striae, proximal muscle weakness Chronic glucocorticoid use	Cushing's syndrome
Low-volume femoral pulses with radiofemoral delay	Coarctation of the aorta
Bilateral palpable kidneys	Adult polycystic kidney disease (p. 243)

Phase	Korotkoff sounds	
		——— 120 mmHg systolic
1	A thud	
		——— 110 mmHg
2	A blowing noise	
		——— 100 mmHg
3	A softer thud	
		——— 90 mmHg diastolic (1st)
4	A disappearing blowing noise	
		——— 80 mmHg diastolic (2nd)
5	Nothing	

Fig. 4.13 Korotkoff sounds.

Examination sequence

- Rest the patient for 5 minutes.
- Ideally, measure BP in both arms (brachial arteries); the higher of the two is closest to central aortic pressure and should be used to determine treatment.
- With the patient seated or lying down, support their arm comfortably at about heart level, with no tight clothing constricting the upper arm.
- Apply an appropriately sized cuff to the upper arm, with the centre of the bladder over the brachial artery.
- Palpate the brachial pulse.
- Inflate the cuff until the pulse is impalpable. Note the pressure on the manometer; this is a rough estimate of systolic pressure.
- Inflate the cuff another 30 mmHg and listen through the diaphragm of the stethoscope placed over the brachial artery.
- Deflate the cuff slowly (2–3 mmHg/s) until you hear a regular tapping sound (phase 1 Korotkoff sounds). Record the reading to the nearest 2 mmHg. This is the systolic pressure.
- Continue to deflate the cuff slowly until the sounds disappear.
- Record the pressure at which the sounds completely disappear as the diastolic pressure (phase 5). If muffled sounds persist (phase 4) and do not disappear, use the point of muffling as the diastolic pressure.

Common problems in BP measurement

- Different BP in each arm: a difference of >10 mmHg on repeated measurements suggests the presence of aortic or subclavian artery disease. Record the highest pressure and use this to guide management.
- Wrong cuff size: the bladder should be approximately 80% of the length and 40% of the width of the upper arm circumference. A standard adult cuff has a bladder that measures approximately 13×30 cm and suits an arm circumference of 22–26 cm. In obese patients a standard adult cuff will overestimate BP, so use a large adult (bladder 16×38 cm) or thigh cuff (20×42 cm).
- Auscultatory gap: up to 20% of elderly hypertensive patients have Korotkoff sounds that appear at systolic pressure and disappear for an interval between systolic and diastolic pressure. If the first appearance of the sound is missed, the systolic pressure will be recorded at a falsely low level. Avoid this by palpating the systolic pressure first.
- Patient's arm at the wrong level: the patient's elbow should be level with the heart. Hydrostatic pressure causes a change of approximately 5 mmHg in recorded systolic and diastolic BP for a 7 cm change in arm elevation.
- Postural change: the pulse increases by about 11 bpm, systolic BP falls by 3–4 mmHg and diastolic BP rises by 5–6 mmHg when a healthy person stands. The BP stabilises after 1–2 minutes. Check the BP after a patient has been standing for 2 minutes; a drop of >20 mmHg on standing is postural hypotension.
- Atrial fibrillation: in this condition, stroke volume and BP vary from beat to beat, making accurate measurement challenging, so extra care is needed. Reducing cuff

pressure slowly and repeating the measurement more than once will allow an acceptable average value of BP to be obtained.

Jugular venous pressure and waveform

Estimate the jugular venous pressure (JVP) by observing the level of pulsation in the internal jugular vein. The vein runs deep to the sternomastoid muscle and enters the thorax between the sternal and clavicular heads. The normal waveform has two main peaks per cycle, which helps to distinguish it from the carotid arterial pulse (Box 4.15). The external jugular vein is more superficial, prominent and easier to see. It can be kinked or obstructed as it traverses the deep fascia of the neck but, when visible and pulsatile, can be used to estimate the JVP in difficult cases.

The JVP level reflects right atrial pressure (normally <7 mmHg/9 cmH$_2$O). The sternal angle is approximately 5 cm above the right atrium, so the JVP in health should be ≤4 cm above this angle when the patient lies at 45 degrees (see Fig. 4.15B later). If right atrial pressure is low, the patient may have to lie flat for the JVP to be seen; if high, the patient may need to sit upright (Fig. 4.14).

4.15 Differences between carotid artery and jugular venous pulsation	
Carotid	**Jugular**
Rapid outward movement	Rapid inward movement
One peak per heart beat	Two peaks per heart beat (in sinus rhythm)
Palpable	Impalpable
Pulsation unaffected by pressure at the root of the neck	Pulsation diminished by pressure at the root of the neck
Independent of respiration	Height of pulsation varies with respiration
Independent of the position of the patient	Varies with the position of the patient
Independent of abdominal pressure	Rises with abdominal pressure

Examination sequence

The JVP is usually best seen on the patient's right side.

- Position the patient supine, reclined at 45 degrees, with the head resting on a pillow and turned slightly to the left. The JVP is seen best if the sternocleidomastoid muscles and overlying skin are relaxed, so ensure the head is supported and avoid excessive head turning or elevation of the chin.
- Look across the patient's neck from the right side (Fig. 4.15A). Use oblique lighting if the JVP is difficult to see.
- Identify the jugular vein pulsation behind the sternocleidomastoid muscle (usually just above the clavicle, unless it is elevated).
- If a pulsation is visualised, use the abdominojugular test and/or occlusion to help confirm that it is the JVP.
- The JVP is the vertical height in centimetres between the upper limit of the venous pulsation and the sternal angle (junction of the manubrium and sternum at the level of the second costal cartilages; Fig. 4.15B).
- Identify the timing and waveform of the pulsation and note any abnormality.

It can be difficult to differentiate the jugular venous waveform from arterial pulsation (Box 4.15). If that is the case, the following may help:

- Abdominojugular test: press firmly over the abdomen. This increases venous return to the right side of the heart temporarily and the JVP normally rises.
- Changes with respiration: the JVP normally falls with inspiration due to decreased intrathoracic pressure.
- Waveform: the normal JVP waveform has two distinct peaks per cardiac cycle (Fig. 4.15C):
  - The 'a' wave corresponds to right atrial contraction and occurs just before the first heart sound. In atrial fibrillation the 'a' wave is absent.
  - The 'v' wave is caused by atrial filling during ventricular systole when the tricuspid valve is closed.
  - Rarely, a third peak ('c' wave) may be seen due to closure of the tricuspid valve.
- Occlusion: the JVP waveform is obliterated by gently occluding the vein at the base of the neck with your finger.
- Changes with position: the JVP will vary with the position of the patient (see Fig. 4.14).

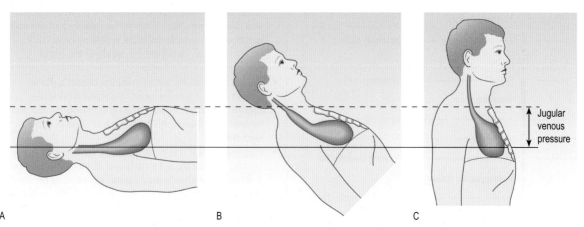

A   B   C

Fig. 4.14 Jugular venous pressure in a healthy subject. [A] Supine: jugular vein distended, pulsation not visible. [B] Reclining at 45 degrees: the point of transition between the distended and the collapsed vein can usually be seen to pulsate just above the clavicle. [C] Upright: the upper part of vein is collapsed and the transition point obscured.

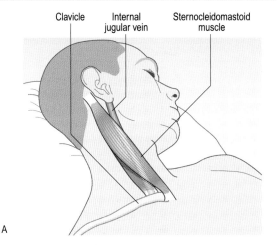

A

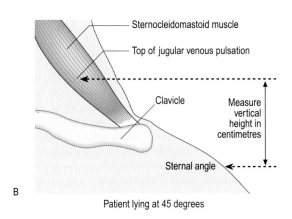

B

Patient lying at 45 degrees

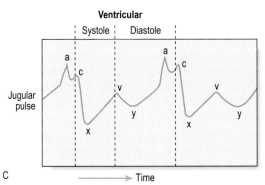

C

Fig. 4.15 Jugular venous pressure. A Inspecting the jugular venous pressure from the side (the internal jugular vein lies deep to the sternocleidomastoid muscle). B Measuring the height of the jugular venous pressure. C Form of the venous pulse wave tracing from the internal jugular vein: *a,* atrial systole; *c,* closure of the tricuspid valve; *v,* peak pressure in the right atrium immediately prior to opening of the tricuspid valve; *a–x,* descent, due to downward displacement of the tricuspid ring during systole; *v–y,* descent at the commencement of ventricular filling.

The JVP provides a guide to central venous pressure. It is elevated in states of fluid overload, particularly heart failure. Examine the patient for pulmonary oedema or pleural effusions (p. 88), ascites (p. 109) and/or peripheral oedema (p. 245). It is also elevated in any condition that leads to high right ventricular filling pressures, such as pulmonary embolism, chronic pulmonary

4.16 Abnormalities of the jugular venous pulse

Condition	Abnormalities
Heart failure	Elevation, sustained abdominojugular reflux >10 seconds
Pulmonary embolism	Elevation
Pericardial effusion	Elevation, prominent 'y' descent
Pericardial constriction	Elevation, Kussmaul's sign
Superior vena cava obstruction	Elevation, loss of pulsation
Atrial fibrillation	Absent 'a' waves
Tricuspid stenosis	Giant 'a' waves
Tricuspid regurgitation	Giant 'v' or 'cv' waves
Complete heart block	'Cannon' waves

hypertension, cardiac tamponade (see Fig. 4.11) or pericardial constriction (Box 4.16). Mechanical obstruction of the superior vena cava (most often caused by lung cancer) may cause extreme, non-pulsatile elevation of the JVP. In this case the JVP no longer reflects right atrial pressure and the abdominojugular test will be negative.

Kussmaul's sign is a paradoxical rise of JVP on inspiration that is seen in pericardial constriction, severe right ventricular failure and restrictive cardiomyopathy.

Prominent 'a' waves are caused by delayed or restricted right ventricular filling, as in pulmonary hypertension or tricuspid stenosis.

Cannon waves (giant 'a' waves) occur when the right atrium contracts against a closed tricuspid valve. Irregular cannon waves are seen in complete heart block and are due to atrioventricular dissociation. Regular cannon waves occur during junctional rhythm and with some ventricular and supraventricular tachycardias.

Tricuspid regurgitation results in prominent systolic 'v' waves, which can fuse with the 'c' wave to produce 'cv' waves; there may be an associated pulsatile liver.

Precordium

The precordium is the anterior chest surface overlying the heart and great vessels (Fig. 4.16).

Learn the surface anatomy and basic physiology of the heart to understand the basis and timing of the heart sounds and murmurs, and why they are heard best in different locations and radiate in a particular direction (Figs 4.16 and 4.17). The optimal sites for auscultation (aortic, pulmonary, apex and left sternal border) do not correspond with the location of cardiac structures but are where the transmitted sounds and murmurs are best heard (Box 4.17). It is important to note that the heart sounds and some murmurs can be heard widely across the precordium, but these sites represent the surface location where the murmur is loudest or easiest to hear.

Inspection

Pectus excavatum (funnel chest; see Fig. 5.6D), a posterior displacement of the lower sternum, and pectus carinatum (pigeon chest; see Fig. 5.6C) may displace the heart and affect palpation and auscultation.

A midline sternotomy scar usually indicates previous valve replacement or coronary artery bypass surgery, in which case

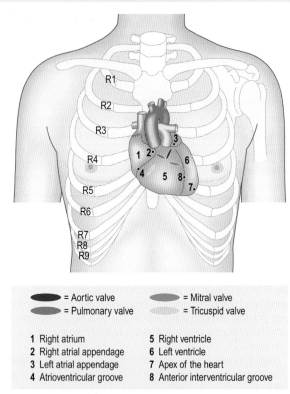

= Aortic valve
= Pulmonary valve
= Mitral valve
= Tricuspid valve

1 Right atrium
2 Right atrial appendage
3 Left atrial appendage
4 Atrioventricular groove
5 Right ventricle
6 Left ventricle
7 Apex of the heart
8 Anterior interventricular groove

Fig. 4.16 Surface anatomy of the chambers and valves of the heart.

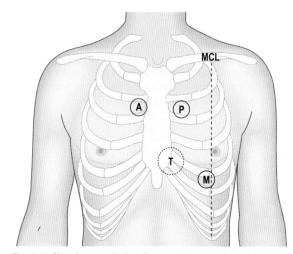

Fig. 4.17 Sites for auscultation. Sites at which murmurs from the relevant valves are usually, but not preferentially, heard. *A*, aortic; *M*, mitral; *MCL*, mid-clavicular line; *P*, pulmonary; *T*, tricuspid.

it may be accompanied by saphenous vein or radial artery graft harvest scars. A left submammary scar is usually the result of mitral valvotomy or transapical transcatheter aortic valve implantation. Infraclavicular scars are seen after pacemaker or defibrillator implantation, and the bulge of the device may be obvious.

Palpation

The apex beat may be visible on inspection but is defined as the most lateral and inferior position at which the cardiac impulse can

4.17 Cardiac auscultation: the best sites for hearing an abnormality	
Site	Sound
Cardiac apex	First heart sound Third and fourth heart sounds Mid-diastolic murmur of mitral stenosis
Lower left sternal border	Early diastolic murmurs of aortic and tricuspid regurgitation Opening snap of mitral stenosis Pansystolic murmur of ventricular septal defect
Upper left sternal border	Second heart sound Pulmonary valve murmurs
Upper right sternal border	Systolic ejection (outflow) murmurs, e.g. aortic stenosis, hypertrophic cardiomyopathy
Left axilla	Radiation of the pansystolic murmur of mitral regurgitation
Below left clavicle	Continuous 'machinery' murmur of a persistent patent ductus arteriosus

be felt. The cardiac impulse results from the left ventricle moving forwards and striking the chest wall during systole. The apex beat is normally in the fifth left intercostal space at, or medial to, the mid-clavicular line (halfway between the suprasternal notch and the acromioclavicular joint), but may be displaced laterally to the anterior or mid-axillary line, or inferiorly to the sixth or seventh intercostal space when the left ventricle is dilated. A heave is a palpable impulse that noticeably lifts your hand. A thrill is the tactile equivalent of a murmur and is a palpable vibration.

Examination sequence

- Explain that you wish to examine the chest and ask the patient to remove all clothing above the waist. Keep a female patient's chest covered with a sheet as far as possible.
- Inspect the precordium with the patient sitting at a 45-degree angle with shoulders horizontal. Look for surgical scars, visible pulsations and chest deformity.
- Place your right hand flat over the precordium to obtain a general impression of the cardiac impulse (Fig. 4.18A).
- Locate the apex beat by laying your fingers on the chest parallel to the rib spaces; if you cannot feel it, ask the patient to roll on to their left side (Fig. 4.18B).
- Assess the character of the apex beat and note its position.
- Apply the heel of your right hand firmly to the left parasternal area and feel for a right ventricle heave. Ask the patient to hold their breath in expiration (Fig. 4.18C).
- Palpate for thrills at the apex and on both sides of the sternum using the flat of your fingers.

A normal apical impulse briefly lifts your fingers and is localised. There should be no parasternal heave or thrill. The apex beat may be impalpable in overweight or muscular people, or in patients with asthma or emphysema because the lungs are hyperinflated. It may be diffusely displaced inferiorly and laterally in left ventricular dilatation, such as after myocardial infarction or in dilated cardiomyopathy, severe aortic regurgitation or decompensated aortic stenosis. In dextrocardia the cardiac apex is palpable on the right side but this condition is uncommon, with a prevalence of 1 : 10,000.

Left ventricular hypertrophy, as in hypertension or severe aortic stenosis, produces a forceful but undisplaced apical impulse. This thrusting apical 'heave' is quite different from the diffuse impulse of left ventricular dilatation. Pulsation over the left parasternal area (right ventricular heave) indicates right ventricular hypertrophy or dilatation, most often accompanying pulmonary hypertension. The 'tapping' apex beat in mitral stenosis represents a palpable first heart sound and is not usually displaced. A double apical impulse is characteristic of hypertrophic cardiomyopathy.

The most common thrill is that of aortic stenosis, which is usually palpable over the upper right sternal border. The thrill caused by a ventricular septal defect is best felt at the left and right sternal edges. Diastolic thrills are very rare.

Auscultation

Correct identification and characterisation of the heart sounds and of any added sounds and/or murmurs require a careful, systematic approach to auscultation.

The diaphragm attenuates all frequencies equally, thus making some low-frequency sounds less audible. Use the diaphragm to identify the first and second heart sounds, and high-pitched sounds such as the early diastolic murmur of aortic regurgitation. Listen with the diaphragm over the whole precordium for a pericardial friction rub.

The bell of the stethoscope transmits all sounds well, but in patients with high-frequency murmurs additional low-frequency sounds may be masked by the high-frequency murmur. The bell is particularly useful at the apex and left sternal edge to listen for the diastolic murmur of mitral stenosis and third and fourth heart sounds.

Examination sequence

Make sure the room is quiet when you auscultate. Your stethoscope should fit comfortably with the earpieces angled slightly forwards. The tubing should be approximately 25 cm long and thick enough to reduce external sound.

- Listen with your stethoscope diaphragm at the:
  - apex
  - lower left sternal border
  - upper right and left sternal borders.
- Listen with your stethoscope bell at the:
  - apex
  - lower left sternal border.

- Listen over the carotid arteries (ejection systolic murmur of aortic stenosis and carotid bruits) and in the left axilla (pansystolic murmur of mitral regurgitation).
- At each site, identify the S_1 and S_2 sounds. Assess their character and intensity; note any splitting of the S_2. Palpate the carotid pulse to time any murmur. The S_1 barely precedes the upstroke of the carotid pulsation, while the S_2 is clearly out of phase with it.
- Concentrate in turn on systole (the interval between S_1 and S_2) and diastole (the interval between S_2 and S_1). Listen for added sounds and then for murmurs. Soft diastolic murmurs are sometimes described as the 'absence of silence'.
- Roll the patient on to their left side. Listen at the apex using light pressure with the bell, to detect the mid-diastolic murmur of mitral stenosis (Fig. 4.19A).
- Ask the patient to sit up and lean forwards, then to breathe out fully and hold their breath (Fig. 4.19B). Listen over the right second intercostal space and over the left sternal edge with the diaphragm for the murmur of aortic regurgitation.
- Note the character and intensity of any murmur heard.
- Develop a routine for auscultation so that you do not overlook subtle abnormalities. Identify and describe the following:
  - the first and second heart sounds (S_1 and S_2)
  - extra heart sounds (S_3 and S_4)
  - additional sounds such as clicks and snaps
  - murmurs in systole and/or diastole (timing, duration, character, pitch, intensity, location and radiation)
  - pericardial rubs.

Heart sounds

Normal heart valves make a sound only when they close. The 'lub-dub' sounds are caused by closure of the atrioventricular (mitral and tricuspid) valves followed by the outlet (aortic and pulmonary) valves.

First heart sound

The first heart sound (S_1), 'lub', is caused by closure of the mitral and tricuspid valves at the onset of ventricular systole. It is best heard at the apex. In mitral stenosis the intensity of S_1 is increased due to elevated left atrial pressure (Box 4.18).

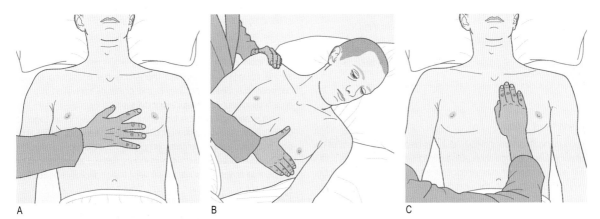

A   B   C

Fig. 4.18 Palpating the heart. $\boxed{A}$ Use your hand to palpate the cardiac impulse. $\boxed{B}$ Localise the apex beat with your finger (if necessary, roll the patient into the left lateral position). $\boxed{C}$ Palpate from apex to sternum for parasternal pulsations.

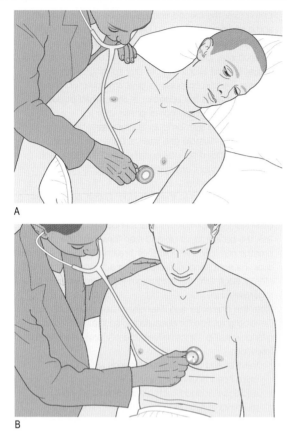

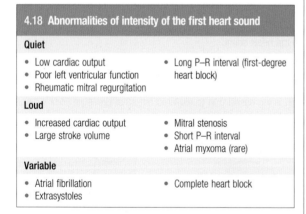

Fig. 4.19 Auscultating the heart. [A] Listen for the murmur of mitral stenosis using the bell lightly applied with the patient in the left lateral position. [B] Listen for the murmur of aortic regurgitation using the diaphragm with the patient leaning forwards.

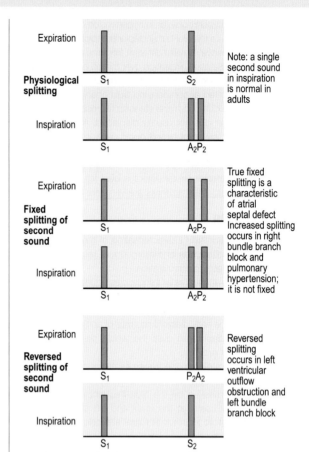

Fig. 4.20 Physiological and pathological splitting of the second heart sound.

4.18 Abnormalities of intensity of the first heart sound	
Quiet	
• Low cardiac output	• Long P–R interval (first-degree
• Poor left ventricular function	heart block)
• Rheumatic mitral regurgitation	
Loud	
• Increased cardiac output	• Mitral stenosis
• Large stroke volume	• Short P–R interval
	• Atrial myxoma (rare)
Variable	
• Atrial fibrillation	• Complete heart block
• Extrasystoles	

Second heart sound

The second heart sound (S_2), 'dub', is caused by closure of the pulmonary and aortic valves at the end of ventricular systole and is best heard at the left sternal edge. It is louder and higher-pitched than the S_1 'lub', and the aortic component is normally louder than the pulmonary component. Physiological splitting of S_2 occurs because left ventricular contraction slightly precedes that of the right ventricle so that the aortic valve closes before the pulmonary valve. This splitting increases at end-inspiration

because increased venous filling of the right ventricle further delays pulmonary valve closure. The separation disappears on expiration (Fig. 4.20). On auscultation, 'lub d-dub' (inspiration) 'lub-dub' (expiration) is heard.

The aortic component of S2 is sometimes quiet or absent in calcific aortic stenosis and reduced in aortic regurgitation (Box 4.19). The aortic component of S_2 is loud in systemic hypertension, and the pulmonary component is increased in pulmonary hypertension.

Wide splitting of S_2, but with normal respiratory variation, occurs in conditions that delay right ventricular emptying, such as right bundle branch block or pulmonary hypertension. Fixed splitting of S_2, with no variation with respiration, is a feature of atrial septal defect (Fig. 4.21). In this condition the right ventricular stroke volume is larger than the left, and the splitting is fixed because the defect equalises the pressure between the two atria throughout the respiratory cycle.

In reversed splitting the two components of S_2 occur together on inspiration and separate on expiration (see Fig. 4.20). This occurs when left ventricular emptying is delayed so that the aortic valve closes after the pulmonary valve. Examples include left bundle branch block and left ventricular outflow obstruction.

Third heart sound

The third heart sound (S_3) is a low-pitched early diastolic sound best heard with the bell at the apex. It coincides with rapid ventricular filling immediately after opening of the atrioventricular

4

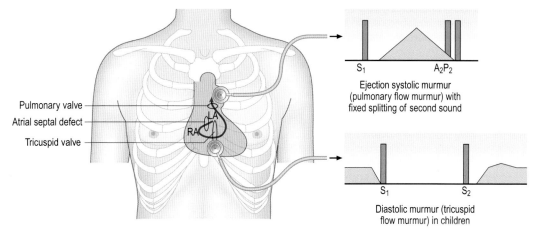

Fig. 4.21 **Atrial septal defect.** *LA,* left atrium; *RA,* right atrium.

4.19 Abnormalities of the second heart sound

Quiet

- Low cardiac output
- Calcific aortic stenosis
- Aortic regurgitation

Loud

- Systemic hypertension (aortic component)
- Pulmonary hypertension (pulmonary component)

Split

Widens in inspiration (enhanced physiological splitting)
- Right bundle branch block
- Pulmonary stenosis
- Pulmonary hypertension
- Ventricular septal defect

Fixed splitting (unaffected by respiration)
- Atrial septal defect

Widens in expiration (reversed splitting)
- Aortic stenosis
- Hypertrophic cardiomyopathy
- Left bundle branch block
- Ventricular pacing

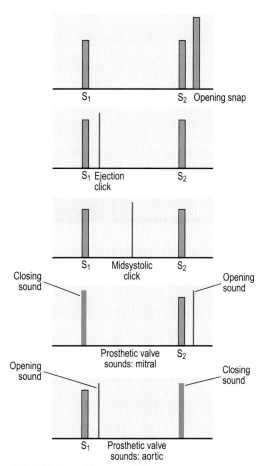

Fig. 4.22 'Added sounds' on auscultation.

valves and is therefore heard after the second heart sound as 'lub-dub-dum'. It is a normal physiological finding in children, young adults and febrile patients, and during pregnancy, but is usually pathological after the age of 40 years. The most common causes are left ventricular failure, when it is an early sign, and mitral regurgitation, due to volume loading of the ventricle. In heart failure, S_3 occurs with a tachycardia, referred to as a 'gallop' rhythm, and S_1 and S_2 are quiet (lub-da-dub).

Fourth heart sound

The fourth heart sound (S_4) is less common. It is soft and low-pitched, best heard with the bell at the apex. It occurs just before S_1 (da-lub-dub). It is always pathological and is caused by forceful atrial contraction against a non-compliant or stiff ventricle. An S_4 is most often heard with left ventricular hypertrophy (due to hypertension, aortic stenosis or hypertrophic cardiomyopathy). It cannot occur when there is atrial fibrillation.

Added sounds

An opening snap is commonly heard in mitral (rarely, tricuspid) stenosis. It results from sudden opening of a stenosed valve and occurs early in diastole, just after the S_2 (Fig. 4.22A). It is best heard with the diaphragm at the apex.

Ejection clicks are high-pitched sounds best heard with the diaphragm. They occur early in systole just after the S_1, in patients with congenital pulmonary or aortic stenosis (Fig. 4.22B). The mechanism is similar to that of an opening snap. Ejection clicks do not occur in calcific aortic stenosis because the cusps are rigid.

Mid-systolic clicks are high-pitched and best heard at the apex with the diaphragm. They occur in mitral valve prolapse (Fig. 4.22C) and may be associated with a late systolic murmur.

Mechanical heart valves can make a sound when they close or open. The closure sound is normally louder, especially with modern valves. The sounds are high-pitched, 'metallic' and often palpable, and may even be heard without a stethoscope. A mechanical mitral valve replacement makes a metallic S_1 and a sound like a loud opening snap early in diastole (Fig. 4.22D). Mechanical aortic valves have a loud, metallic S_2 and an opening sound like an ejection click at the start of systole (Fig. 4.22E). They are normally associated with a flow murmur.

Pericardial rub (friction rub) is a coarse scratching sound, often with systolic and diastolic components. It is best heard using the diaphragm with the patient holding their breath in expiration. It may be audible over any part of the precordium but is often localised, varying in intensity over time and with the position of the patient. It is most often heard in acute pericarditis or a few days after an extensive myocardial infarction. A pleuropericardial rub is a similar sound that occurs in time with the cardiac cycle, but is also influenced by respiration and is pleural in origin. Occasionally, a 'crunching' noise can be heard, caused by gas in the pericardium (pneumopericardium).

Murmurs

Heart murmurs are produced by turbulent flow across an abnormal valve, septal defect or outflow obstruction. 'Innocent' murmurs are caused by increased velocity of flow through a normal valve and occur when stroke volume is increased, as in pregnant women, athletes with resting bradycardia or patients with fever.

Examination sequence

Timing

- Identify the first and second heart sounds, S_1 and S_2, respectively. It may help to palpate the patient's carotid pulse while listening to the precordium to determine the onset of ventricular systole. Determine whether the murmur is systolic or diastolic:
  - Systole begins with S_1 (mitral and tricuspid valve closure). This occurs when left and right ventricular pressures exceed the corresponding atrial pressures. For a short period, all four heart valves are closed (pre-ejection period). Ventricular pressures continue to rise until they exceed those of the aorta and pulmonary artery, causing the aortic and pulmonary valves to open. Systole ends with the closure of these valves, producing S_2.
  - Diastole is the interval between S_2 and S_1. Physiologically, it is divided into three phases: early diastole (isovolumic relaxation), the time from the closure of the aortic and pulmonary valves until the opening of the mitral and tricuspid valves; mid-diastole, the early period of ventricular filling when atrial pressures exceed ventricular pressures; and presystole, coinciding with atrial systole.
- Murmurs of aortic and pulmonary regurgitation start in early diastole and extend into mid-diastole. The murmurs of mitral or tricuspid stenosis cannot start before mid-diastole. S_3 occurs in mid-diastole and S_4 in presystole.

Duration

- The murmurs of mitral and tricuspid regurgitation start with S_1, sometimes muffling or obscuring it, and continue throughout systole (pansystolic; Fig. 4.23). The murmur produced by mitral valve prolapse does not begin until the mitral valve leaflet has prolapsed during systole, producing a late systolic murmur (Fig. 4.23). The ejection systolic murmur of aortic or pulmonary stenosis begins after S_1 reaches maximal intensity in mid-systole, then fades, stopping before S_2 (Fig. 4.24).

Character and pitch

- The quality of a murmur is subjective but terms such as harsh, blowing, musical, rumbling and high- or low-pitched can be useful. High-pitched murmurs often correspond to

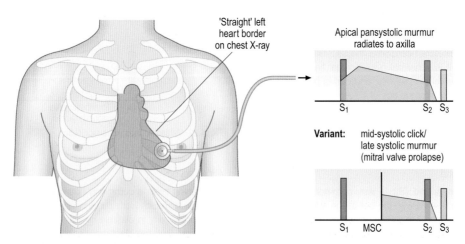

Fig. 4.23 Mitral regurgitation. Mitral regurgitation is caused by dilatation of the left ventricle and failure of leaflets to co-apt. The murmur begins at the moment of valve closure and may obscure the first heart sound. It varies little in intensity throughout systole. In mitral valve prolapse the murmur begins in mid- or late systole and there is often a mid-systolic click (MSC).

4

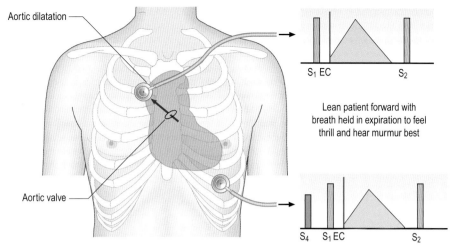

Fig. 4.24 Aortic stenosis. There is a systolic pressure gradient across the stenosed aortic valve. The resultant high-velocity jet impinges on the wall of the aorta *(arrow)*, and is best heard with the diaphragm in the aortic area. Alternatively, the bell may be placed in the suprasternal notch. The ejection systolic murmur follows an ejection click (EC).

4.20 Grades of intensity of murmur	
Grade	**Description**
1	Heard by an expert in optimum conditions
2	Heard by a non-expert in optimum conditions
3	Easily heard; no thrill
4	A loud murmur, with a thrill
5	Very loud, often heard over a wide area, with thrill
6	Extremely loud, heard without a stethoscope

4.21 Causes of systolic murmurs

Ejection systolic murmurs

- Increased flow through normal valves:
  - Severe anaemia, fever, athletes (bradycardia → large stroke volume), pregnancy
  - Atrial septal defect (pulmonary flow murmur)
  - Other causes of flow murmurs (increased stroke volume in aortic regurgitation)
- Normal or reduced flow though a stenotic valve:
  - Aortic stenosis
  - Pulmonary stenosis
- Subvalvular obstruction:
  - Hypertrophic obstructive cardiomyopathy

Pansystolic murmurs

- Mitral regurgitation
- Tricuspid regurgitation
- Ventricular septal defect
- Leaking mitral or tricuspid prosthesis

Late systolic murmurs

- Mitral valve prolapse

high-pressure gradients, so the diastolic murmur of aortic regurgitation is higher-pitched than that of mitral stenosis.

Intensity

- Describe any murmur according to its grade of intensity (Box 4.20). Diastolic murmurs are rarely louder than grade 3. The intensity of a murmur does not correlate with severity of valve dysfunction; for instance, the murmur of critical aortic stenosis can be quiet and occasionally inaudible. Changes in intensity with time are important, as they can denote progression of a valve lesion. Rapidly changing murmurs can occur with infective endocarditis because of valve destruction.

Location

- Record the site(s) where you hear the murmur best. This helps to differentiate diastolic murmurs (mitral stenosis at the apex, aortic regurgitation at the left sternal edge) but is less helpful with systolic murmurs, which are often audible across the precordium (see Fig. 4.17).

Radiation

- Murmurs radiate in the direction of the blood flow to specific sites outside the precordium. Differentiate radiation from location. The pansystolic murmur of mitral regurgitation radiates towards the left axilla, the murmur of ventricular septal defect towards the right sternal edge, and that of aortic stenosis to the suprasternal notch and the carotid arteries.

Systolic murmurs

Ejection systolic murmurs are caused by increased flow through a normal valve (flow or innocent murmur), or by turbulent flow through an abnormal valve, as in aortic or pulmonary stenosis (Box 4.21). An ejection systolic murmur is also a feature of hypertrophic obstructive cardiomyopathy, where it is accentuated by exercise or during the strain phase of the Valsalva manœuvre. An atrial septal defect is characterised by a pulmonary flow murmur during systole.

The murmur of aortic stenosis is often audible all over the precordium (see Fig. 4.24). It is harsh, high-pitched and musical, and radiates to the upper right sternal edge, suprasternal notch and carotid arteries. It is usually loud and there may be a thrill.

Pansystolic murmurs are most commonly caused by mitral regurgitation. The murmur is often loud and blowing in character, and is best heard at the apex and radiating to the axilla. With mitral valve prolapse, regurgitation begins in mid-systole, producing a late systolic murmur (see Fig. 4.23). The murmur of tricuspid regurgitation is heard at the lower left sternal edge; if significant, it is associated with a prominent 'v' wave in the JVP and a pulsatile liver.

Ventricular septal defects also cause a pansystolic murmur. Small congenital defects produce a loud murmur audible at the left sternal border, radiating to the right sternal border and often associated with a thrill. Rupture of the interventricular septum can complicate myocardial infarction, producing a harsh pansystolic murmur. The differential diagnosis of a murmur heard after myocardial infarction includes acute mitral regurgitation due to papillary muscle rupture, functional mitral regurgitation caused by left ventricular dilatation, and a pericardial rub.

Diastolic murmurs

Early diastolic murmurs usually last throughout diastole but are loudest in early diastole, so the term 'early diastolic murmur' is misleading. The murmur is typically caused by aortic regurgitation (Fig. 4.25), and is best heard at the left sternal edge with the patient leaning forwards in held expiration. The duration of the aortic regurgitation murmur is inversely proportional to severity. Since the regurgitant blood must be ejected during the subsequent systolic period, significant aortic regurgitation increases stroke volume is usually associated with a systolic flow murmur.

Pulmonary regurgitation is very uncommon. It may be caused by pulmonary artery dilatation in pulmonary hypertension (Graham Steell murmur) or a congenital defect of the pulmonary valve.

Mid-diastolic murmurs are usually caused by mitral stenosis. This is a low-pitched, rumbling sound that may follow an opening snap (Fig. 4.26). It is best heard with the bell at the apex and the patient positioned on their left side. The murmur is accentuated by exercise. The cadence sounds like 'lup-ta-ta-rru'; 'lup' is the loud S_1, 'ta-ta' the S_2 and opening snap, and 'rru' the mid-diastolic murmur. If the patient is in sinus rhythm, left atrial contraction increases the blood flow across the stenosed valve, leading to presystolic accentuation of the murmur. The murmur of tricuspid stenosis is similar but rare.

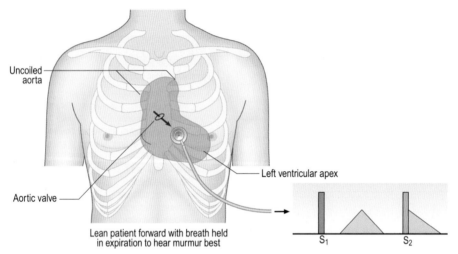

Fig. 4.25 Aortic regurgitation. The pulse pressure is usually increased. The jet from the aortic valve is directed inferiorly towards the left ventricular outflow tract *(arrow)* during diastole, producing an early diastolic murmur, best heard with the diaphragm during held expiration with the patient leaning forward. An associated systolic murmur is common because of the increased flow through the aortic valve in systole.

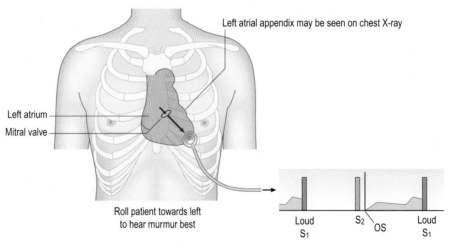

Fig. 4.26 Mitral stenosis. There is a pressure gradient across the mitral valve, giving rise to a low-pitched mid-diastolic murmur that is heard best with the bell at the apex and the patient rolled on to their left-hand side. The jet through the stenosed valve *(arrow)* strikes the endocardium at the cardiac apex. Occasionally, an opening snap (OS) can arise due to the sharp movement of the tethered anterior cusp of the mitral valve at the time when the flow commences.

4

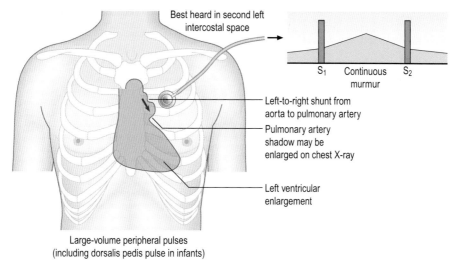

Best heard in second left
intercostal space

S_1 Continuous S_2
murmur

Left-to-right shunt from
aorta to pulmonary artery

Pulmonary artery
shadow may be
enlarged on chest X-ray

Left ventricular
enlargement

Large-volume peripheral pulses
(including dorsalis pedis pulse in infants)

Fig. 4.27 Persistent patent ductus arteriosus. A continuous 'machinery' murmur is heard because aortic pressure always exceeds pulmonary arterial pressure, resulting in continuous ductal flow. The pressure difference is greatest in systole, producing a louder systolic component to the murmur.

An Austin Flint murmur is a mid-diastolic murmur that accompanies aortic regurgitation. It is caused by the regurgitant jet striking the anterior leaflet of the mitral valve, restricting inflow to the left ventricle.

Continuous murmurs

Continuous murmurs are rare in adults. The most common cause is a patent ductus arteriosus. In the fetus this connects the upper descending aorta and pulmonary artery, and normally closes just after birth. The murmur is best heard at the upper left sternal border and radiates over the left scapula. Its continuous character is 'machinery-like'; as aortic pressure always exceeds pulmonary pressure, there is continuous ductal flow, with the greatest pressure difference in systole, resulting in a louder systolic component (Fig. 4.27).

Interpretation of the findings

Auscultation remains an important clinical skill, despite the availability of echocardiography. You must be able to detect abnormal signs to prompt appropriate investigation. Auscultatory signs, such as S_3 or S_4 and pericardial friction rubs, have no direct equivalent on echocardiography but do have diagnostic utility. In addition, some patients, especially those with rheumatic heart disease, have multiple heart valve defects, and the interpretation of more subtle physical signs may be important. For example, a patient with mixed mitral stenosis and regurgitation will probably have dominant stenosis if the S_1 is loud but dominant regurgitation if there is an S_3.

Investigations

Haematology and clinical chemistry

As anaemia can unmask angina or exacerbate heart failure, a full blood count is useful and helps guide the safe use of antiplatelet therapies and anticoagulants. Measurement of the erythrocyte sedimentation rate and serology are indicated if connective tissue disease is suspected. Urea and electrolytes are measured and liver function tests performed prior to starting therapies that may impact on renal function or cause hepatotoxicity. Blood glucose and a lipid profile help identify patients with diabetes mellitus and assess cardiovascular risk. In patients with acute chest pain, cardiac troponin is measured to determine whether there is myocardial injury or infarction.

Electrocardiography

In performing standard 12-lead electrocardiography (ECG; Fig. 4.28), the patient must be resting supine and relaxed to avoid muscle tremor. Good contact between the electrode and skin is important and it may be necessary to shave the chest. The electrodes must be positioned correctly to obtain recordings made from the six precordial electrodes (V_1–V_6) and six recordings from the limb electrodes (left arm, right arm and left leg). The right leg electrode is used as a reference. Confirm that the electrocardiograph is calibrated using a 1 mV signal prior to recording.

Ambulatory ECG monitoring

Continuous ECG recording over 24–48 hours can be used to identify symptomatic or asymptomatic rhythm disturbances in patients with palpitation or syncope. If symptoms are less frequent, it may be necessary to use patient-activated recorders that record the heart rhythm only when the patient is symptomatic; the device is activated by the patient (Fig. 4.29).

Exercise ECG

An exercise ECG is useful in the diagnosis and functional assessment of patients with suspected coronary artery disease. Down-sloping ST segment depression, particularly when it occurs during minor exertion, or ST segment elevation is of prognostic significance and helps inform the need for invasive investigation with coronary angiography.

Ambulatory blood pressure monitoring

A portable device can be worn by the patient at home that takes at least two BP measurements per hour. It is used to confirm the diagnosis of hypertension and provide a more reliable assessment of response to treatment.

A

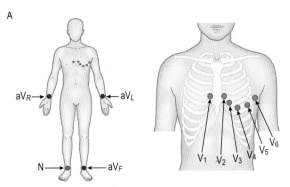

Fig. 4.28 Electrocardiography (ECG). [A] 12-lead ECG lead placement. [B] Normal PQRST complex. [C] Acute anterior myocardial infarction. Note the ST elevation in leads V_1–V_6 and aV_L, and 'reciprocal' ST depression in leads II, III and aV_F.

B

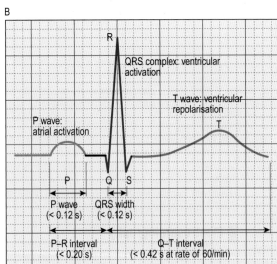

C

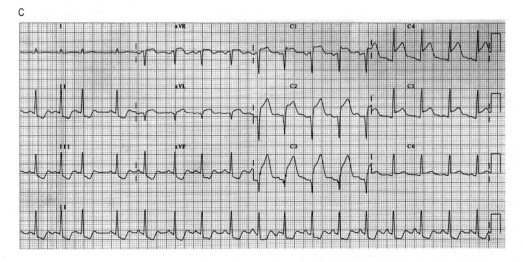

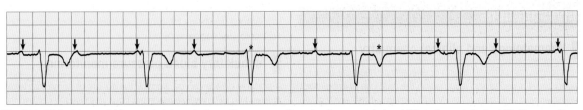

Fig. 4.29 Printout from a 24-hour ambulatory electrocardiogram recording, showing complete heart block. Arrows indicate visible P waves. At times, these are masked by the QRS complex or T wave (*).

Chest X-ray

The maximum width of the heart divided by the maximum width of the thorax on a posteroanterior chest X-ray (the cardiothoracic ratio) should normally be <0.5. An increased cardiothoracic ratio is common in valvular heart disease and heart failure. In heart failure this is often accompanied by distension of the upper lobe pulmonary veins, diffuse shadowing within the lungs due to pulmonary oedema, and Kerley B lines (horizontal, engorged lymphatics at the periphery of the lower lobes; Fig. 4.30A). A widened mediastinum may indicate a thoracic aneurysm.

Echocardiography

Echocardiography uses high-frequency sound waves to evaluate valve abnormalities, ventricular function and blood flow (Doppler echocardiography). Most scans are performed through the anterior chest wall (transthoracic; Fig. 4.30B). Transoesophageal echocardiography requires sedation but gives high resolution

of posterior structures such as the left atrium, mitral valve and descending aorta, and is useful in detecting valvular vegetations in infective endocarditis.

Radionuclide studies

Technetium-99 is injected intravenously and detected using a gamma camera to assess left ventricular function. Thallium and sestamibi are taken up by myocardial cells and indicate myocardial perfusion at rest and exercise.

Cardiac catheterisation

A fine catheter is introduced under local anaesthetic via a peripheral artery (usually the radial or femoral) and advanced to the heart under X-ray guidance. Although measurements of intracardiac pressures, and therefore estimates of valvular and cardiac function, are possible, the primary application of this technique is imaging of the coronary circulation using contrast

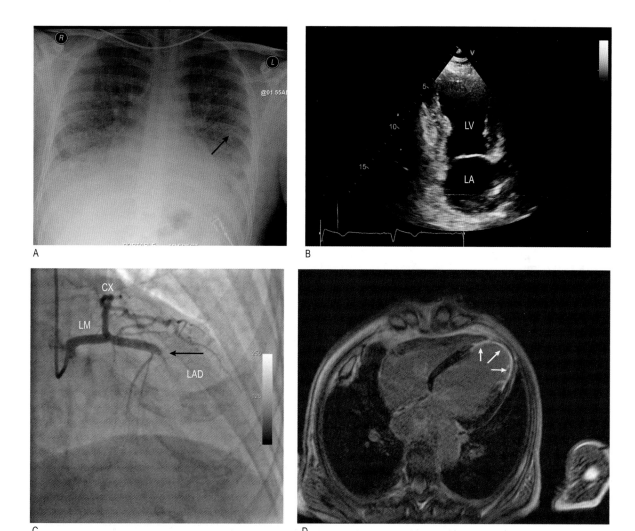

Fig. 4.30 Cardiovascular imaging. A Chest X-ray in heart failure. This shows cardiomegaly with patchy alveolar shadowing of pulmonary oedema and Kerley B lines (engorged lymphatics, *arrow*) at the periphery of both lungs. B Transthoracic echocardiogram in an apical two-chamber view, showing thinning of the left ventricular apex. This is the site of a recent anterior myocardial infarct. *LA*, left atrium; *LV*, left ventricle. C Coronary angiography. The *arrow* indicates an abrupt occlusion of the proximal left anterior descending artery. *CX*, circumflex; *LAD*, left anterior descending; *LM*, left main. D Cardiac magnetic resonance imaging. Gadolinium enhancement image demonstrates regional uptake of gadolinium *(white arrows)* consistent with myocardial fibrosis in the territory of the LAD.

medium. This is performed to inform and guide revascularisation, either by coronary angioplasty or bypass grafting (Fig. 4.30C).

Computed tomography and magnetic resonance imaging

Computed tomography (CT), with its superior temporal resolution of the coronary arteries, is particularly useful for investigating symptomatic patients at low to intermediate risk of coronary artery disease. It can reduce the need for invasive investigation in patients with a low probability of occlusive coronary disease who require valve surgery. Magnetic resonance imaging (MRI) provides superior spatial resolution (Fig. 4.30D) and is the imaging modality of choice for investigating the aetiology of heart muscle diseases (cardiomyopathy).

PERIPHERAL ARTERIAL SYSTEM

Anatomy and physiology

See Fig. 4.31.

The history

Common presenting symptoms

Leg pain

Asymptomatic ischaemia

Approximately 20% of people over 60 years of age in developed countries have peripheral arterial disease (PAD) but only one-quarter of these are symptomatic. The underlying pathology is usually atherosclerosis affecting large and medium-sized vessels.

Haemodynamically significant lower limb ischaemia is defined as an ankle-to-brachial pressure index of <0.9 at rest (p. 69).

Most of these patients are asymptomatic, either because they choose not to walk very far or because their exercise tolerance is limited by other comorbidities. Although asymptomatic, these patients have extensive atherosclerosis, putting them at high risk of major cardiovascular events, and should be treated with best medical therapy to reduce their mortality rate. Furthermore, PAD may affect the medical and surgical treatment for other conditions. For example, wound healing may be impaired in the lower limb.

PAD affects the legs eight times more commonly than the arms. This is partly because the lower limb arteries are more frequently affected by atherosclerosis, but also because the arterial supply to the legs is less well developed in relation to the muscle mass.

The Fontaine classification describes the progression of symptoms that occurs as the atherosclerotic burden increases and the blood supply to the limb diminishes (Box 4.22).

Intermittent claudication

Intermittent claudication is pain felt in the legs on walking due to arterial insufficiency and is the most common symptom of PAD. Patients describe tightness or 'cramp-like' pain that develops after a relatively constant distance; the distance is often shorter if walking uphill, in the cold and after meals. The pain disappears completely within a few minutes of rest but recurs on walking. The 'claudication distance' is how far patients say they can walk before the pain comes on. The 'total walking distance' is how far they can walk before the pain is so bad that they have to stop.

The pain is felt in major muscle groups and its location depends on the level at which the arteries are diseased. The calf muscle is most commonly affected and this is due to femoropopliteal disease, while pain in the thigh suggests common femoral or aortoiliac obstruction. Male patients who have bilateral common iliac or internal iliac artery occlusion may develop Leriche's syndrome, involving buttock claudication and erectile dysfunction.

Claudication is not in itself limb-threatening, although it is a marker for widespread atherosclerotic disease. With best medical therapy and supervised exercise programmes, 50% will improve, 30% will remain stable and only 20% will deteriorate further.

It is important to distinguish claudication due to arterial insufficiency from other causes of lower limb pain, which include

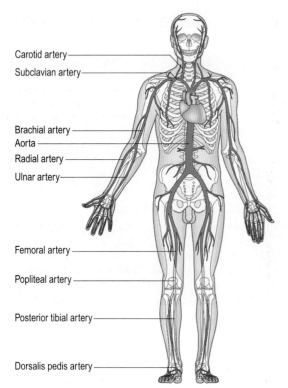

Carotid artery
Subclavian artery

Brachial artery
Aorta
Radial artery
Ulnar artery

Femoral artery

Popliteal artery

Posterior tibial artery

Dorsalis pedis artery

Fig. 4.31 The arterial system.

4.22 Fontaine classification of lower limb ischaemia	
Stage	**Description**
I	Asymptomatic
II	Intermittent claudication
III	Night/rest pain
IV	Tissue loss (ulceration/gangrene)

4.23 The clinical features of arterial, neurogenic and venous claudication

	Arterial	Neurogenic	Venous
Pathology	Stenosis or occlusion of major lower limb arteries	Lumbar nerve root or cauda equina compression (spinal stenosis)	Obstruction to the venous outflow of the leg due to iliofemoral venous occlusion
Site of pain	Muscles, usually the calf but may involve thigh and buttocks	Ill-defined Whole leg May be associated with numbness and tingling	Whole leg 'Bursting' in nature
Laterality	Unilateral or bilateral	Often bilateral	Nearly always unilateral
Onset	Gradual after walking the 'claudication distance'	Often immediate on walking or standing up	Gradual, from the moment walking starts
Relieving features	On stopping walking, the pain disappears completely in 1–2 minutes	Bending forwards and stopping walking Patient may sit down for full relief	Leg elevation
Colour	Normal or pale	Normal	Cyanosed Often visible varicose veins
Temperature	Normal or cool	Normal	Normal or increased
Oedema	Absent	Absent	Always present
Pulses	Reduced or absent	Normal	Present but may be difficult to feel owing to oedema
Straight-leg raising	Normal	May be limited	Normal

osteoarthritis, neurogenic claudication and venous claudication (Box 4.23).

Any intervention for claudication is purely on the basis of symptomatic relief, since only a small minority of patients progress to critical limb ischaemia. The patient's age, occupation and comorbidities are important in determining the extent to which claudication limits their lifestyle. A postal worker who can walk only 200 metres has a serious problem but an elderly person who simply wants to cross the road to the shops may cope well. While absolute distances are important, it may be more helpful to ask specific questions about how symptoms affect the patient's lifestyle:

- Can you walk to the clinic from the bus stop or car park without stopping?
- Can you do your own shopping?
- What are you unable to do because of the pain?

Night pain

The patient goes to bed and falls asleep, but is then woken 1–2 hours later with severe pain in the foot, usually in the instep. The pain is due to poor perfusion, resulting from loss of the beneficial effects of gravity on lying down, and from the reductions in heart rate, BP and cardiac output that occur when sleeping. Patients may find relief by hanging the leg out of bed or by getting up and walking around. On return to bed, however, the pain recurs and patients often choose to sleep in a chair. This leads to dependent oedema, increased interstitial tissue pressure, a further reduction in tissue perfusion and ultimately a worsening of the pain.

Rest pain

Rest pain occurs when blood flow is insufficient to meet the metabolic demands of the tissues, even at rest. Critical ischaemia is defined as rest pain (persisting for more than 2 weeks and requiring opiate analgesia) or tissue loss associated with an ankle pressure of <50 mmHg or a toe pressure of <30 mmHg.

4.24 Signs of acute limb ischaemia

- Pallor
- Pulselessness
- Perishing cold
- Paraesthesia
- Pain (worse when muscle squeezed)
- Paralysis

Rest or night pain indicates severe, multilevel, lower limb PAD and is a 'red flag' symptom that mandates urgent referral to a vascular surgeon, as failure to revascularise the leg usually leads to the development of tissue loss (gangrene, ulceration) and amputation.

In patients with diabetes it may be difficult to differentiate between rest pain and diabetic neuropathy, as both may be worse at night. Neuropathic pain may not be confined to the foot, is associated with burning and tingling, is not relieved by dependency and is accompanied by dysaesthesia (pain or uncomfortable sensations, sometimes described as burning, tingling or numbness). Many patients with neuropathy cannot even bear the pressure of bedclothes on their feet.

Tissue loss (ulceration and/or gangrene)

In patients with severe lower limb PAD, perfusion is inadequate to support the tissues, and areas of tissue loss (gangrene) develop at the tips of the digits, gradually spreading proximally. Furthermore, even trivial injuries do not heal and cause ulceration. Tissue loss often progresses rapidly and, without revascularisation, leads to amputation and/or death.

Acute limb ischaemia

The classical features of acute limb ischaemia are the 'six Ps' (Box 4.24). Paralysis (inability to move the toes/fingers) and paraesthesia (numbness or tingling over the forefoot or dorsum of the hand) are the most important and indicate severe ischaemia affecting nerve and muscle function. Muscle tenderness is a grave sign

4.25 Acute limb ischaemia: embolus versus thrombosis in situ		
	Embolus	Thrombosis
Onset and severity	Acute (seconds or minutes), ischaemia profound (no pre-existing collaterals)	Insidious (hours or days), ischaemia less severe (pre-existing collaterals)
Embolic source	Present	Absent
Previous claudication	Absent	Present
Pulses in contralateral leg	Present	Often absent, reflecting widespread peripheral arterial disease
Diagnosis	Clinical	Angiography
Treatment	Embolectomy and anticoagulation	Medical, bypass surgery, catheter-directed thrombolysis

indicating impending muscle infarction. A limb with these features will usually become irreversibly damaged unless the circulation is restored within a few hours.

It is important to consider the most likely underlying cause:

- Thromboembolism: usually from the left atrium in association with atrial fibrillation or myocardial infarction. There is usually no history of claudication.
- Thrombosis in situ: thrombotic occlusion of an already narrowed atherosclerotic arterial segment (Box 4.25). In this situation the patient is likely to have a past history of claudication.

Compartment syndrome

The perfusion pressure of a muscle is the difference between the mean arterial pressure and the pressure within the fascial compartment within which it lies. Compartment syndrome occurs where there is increased pressure within the fascial compartments of the limb that compromises the perfusion and viability of muscle and nerves. The calf is most commonly affected and the two leading causes are lower limb trauma (such as fractured tibia) and reperfusion injury following treatment of acute lower limb ischaemia. Failure to recognise and treat compartment syndrome may result in limb amputation. The key symptom is severe pain that is often unrelieved by opioids and exacerbated by active or passive movement. It is worth remembering that peripheral pulses are usually present, since the major arteries lie outside the fascial compartments and are not affected by increased compartment pressure. Compartment monitors can be used as an adjunct to measure compartment pressure.

Abdominal pain

Mesenteric ischaemia

Because of the rich collateral circulation of the gut, usually two of the three major visceral arteries (coeliac trunk, superior and inferior mesenteric arteries) must be critically stenosed or occluded before symptoms and signs of chronic mesenteric arterial insufficiency occur. Severe central abdominal pain typically develops 10–15 minutes after eating. The patient becomes scared of eating and significant weight loss is a universal finding. Diarrhoea may also

be present and the non-specific nature of symptoms may result in misdiagnosis; the patient may have had numerous investigations, including laparotomy, before the diagnosis is made.

Acute mesenteric ischaemia is a surgical emergency. It is most commonly caused by an embolus from the heart or by thrombosis in situ of a pre-existing atherosclerotic plaque in one of the mesenteric vessels. It is often hard to diagnose in the early stages, as patients typically present initially with severe abdominal pain that is out of proportion to often unimpressive abdominal signs. Presentation with severe abdominal pain, shock, bloody diarrhoea and profound metabolic acidosis indicates infarction of the bowel, which carries a high mortality rate. Rarely, renal angle pain occurs from renal infarction or ischaemia, and is associated with visible or non-visible haematuria.

Any patient suspected of having visceral ischaemia should undergo urgent CT angiography.

Abdominal aortic aneurysm

Abdominal aortic aneurysm (AAA) is an abnormal focal dilatation of the aorta to at least 150% of its normal diameter (Fig. 4.32). It is often diagnosed incidentally during a CT scan or alternative imaging for other reasons.

Patients may present with abdominal and/or back pain, or occasionally with more subtle signs such as an awareness of abdominal pulsation or observation of ripples in the water when they are in the bath (wave sign). However, most patients are asymptomatic until the aneurysm ruptures.

The classical features of AAA rupture include abdominal/back pain, pulsatile abdominal mass, syncope and shock (hypotension), but these are not always present and it is important to have a low threshold of suspicion and consider early referral and/or CT imaging.

Digital ischaemia

Blue toes

Blue toe syndrome occurs when there is atheroembolism from an AAA or alternative proximal embolic source (such as popliteal aneurysm or atherosclerotic plaque). Patchy bluish discoloration appears over the toes and forefoot of one or both feet. There is usually a full set of pedal pulses. Although seemingly innocuous, this symptom should be taken seriously, as small emboli may herald the risk of a major embolus leading to acute limb ischaemia and even limb loss.

Vasospastic symptoms

Raynaud's phenomenon is digital ischaemia induced by cold and emotion. It has three phases (Fig. 4.33):

- pallor: due to digital artery spasm and/or obstruction
- cyanosis: due to deoxygenation of static venous blood (this phase may be absent)
- redness: due to reactive hyperaemia.

Raynaud's phenomenon may be primary (Raynaud's disease) and caused by idiopathic digital artery vasospasm, or secondary to other conditions (Raynaud's syndrome) such as drugs, connective tissue disease, hyperviscosity syndromes or use of power tools. While for most patients this is a self-limiting condition, a small minority develop tissue loss.

Patients over 40 years old presenting with unilateral Raynaud's phenomenon should be investigated for underlying PAD, especially if they have cardiovascular risk factors, diabetes or a smoking habit.

4

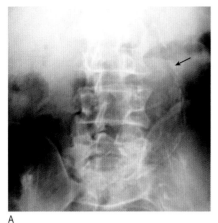

A

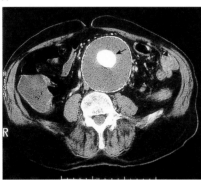

B

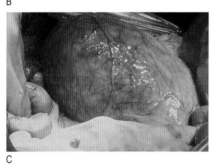

C

Fig. 4.32 Abdominal aortic aneurysm. [A] Abdominal X-ray showing calcification *(arrow).* [B] Computed tomogram of the abdomen showing an abdominal aortic aneurysm *(arrow).* [C] At laparotomy the aorta is seen to be grossly and irregularly dilated.

Stroke

Stroke is a focal neurological deficit that has a vascular cause and is discussed on page 123.

Past medical history

Is the patient known to have established peripheral vascular disease? Ask about previous investigations, operations or procedures. Is there a history of other atherosclerotic conditions such as coronary artery disease or cerebrovascular disease? Ask about risk factors for atherosclerotic disease, including hypertension, hypercholesterolaemia and diabetes mellitus. Are there any other comorbidities (such as severe cardiac or lung disease) that would make any potential operative intervention high-risk or futile?

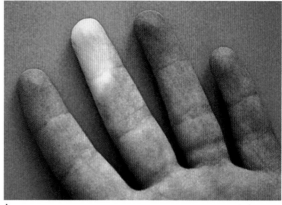

A

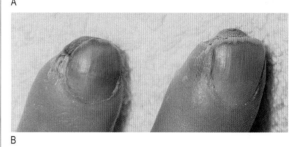

B

Fig. 4.33 Raynaud's syndrome. [A] The acute phase, showing severe blanching of the tip of one finger. [B] Raynaud's syndrome occasionally progresses to fingertip ulceration or even gangrene. *(A and B) From Forbes CD, Jackson WF. Color Atlas of Clinical Medicine. 3rd edn. Edinburgh: Mosby; 2003.*

Drug history

Enquire about medication used for secondary prevention and adherence to these: antiplatelet, lipid-lowering, antihypertensive and diabetes therapies. Patients may be taking vasoactive drugs for claudication (naftidrofuryl or cilostazol, for example), although their efficacy in this setting is not clear. Enquire about other cardiac medications, as these may make symptoms of rest pain worse through their BP-lowering or negatively inotropic effects.

Family history

Ask about a family history of premature coronary or other vascular disease (p. 45). There is a strong familial association for AAAs so, where relevant, a family history should be sought.

Social history

Take a smoking history (p. 14). Enquire about occupation and activities of daily living. How are the patient's symptoms impacting on quality of life or employment?

The physical examination

Follow the routine described for the heart, looking for evidence of anaemia or cyanosis, signs of heart failure, and direct or

4.26 Signs suggesting vascular disease

Sign	Implication
Hands and arms	
Tobacco stains	Smoking
Purple discoloration of the fingertips	Atheroembolism from a proximal subclavian aneurysm
Pits and healed scars in the finger pulps	Secondary Raynaud's syndrome
Calcinosis and visible nail-fold capillary loops	Systemic sclerosis and CREST (calcinosis, Raynaud's phenomenon, oesophageal dysfunction, sclerodactyly, telangiectasia)
Wasting of the small muscles of the hand	Thoracic outlet syndrome
Face and neck	
Corneal arcus and xanthelasma	Hypercholesterolaemia
Horner's syndrome	Carotid artery dissection or aneurysm
Hoarseness of the voice and 'bovine' cough	Recurrent laryngeal nerve palsy from a thoracic aortic aneurysm
Prominent veins in the neck, shoulder and anterior chest	Axillary/subclavian vein occlusion
Abdomen	
Epigastric/umbilical pulsation	Aortoiliac aneurysm
Mottling of the abdomen	Ruptured abdominal aortic aneurysm or saddle embolism occluding aortic bifurcation
Evidence of weight loss	Visceral ischaemia

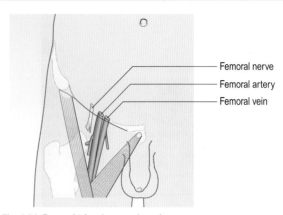

Fig. 4.34 Femoral triangle: vessels and nerves.

- Femoral nerve
- Femoral artery
- Femoral vein

indirect evidence of PAD. Box 4.26 lists some of the direct and indirect signs of peripheral arterial disease.

Perform a detailed examination of the arterial pulses.

Examination sequence

Work down the body, starting with the hands, and using the sequence and principles of inspection, palpation and auscultation for each area.

Arms
- Examine the radial and brachial pulses (p. 47 and see Fig. 4.7).
- Measure the BP in both arms (p. 49 and see Fig. 4.12).

Neck
- Examine the carotid pulses (p. 47 and see Fig. 4.7).

Abdomen
- Inspect from the side for obvious pulsation.
- Palpate over the abdominal aorta. The aortic bifurcation is at the level of the umbilicus, so feel in the epigastrium for a palpable AAA. If you do feel an aneurysm, try to gauge its approximate size by placing the fingers of each hand on either side of it.
- In thin patients a tortuous but normal-diameter aorta can be palpable, but an aneurysm tends to be expansile rather than just pulsatile. A pulsatile mass below the umbilicus suggests an iliac aneurysm.

Clinical examination is unreliable in the detection of AAA since the aorta lies right at the back of the abdominal cavity. If you harbour any suspicion that the patient has an

aneurysm, organise an ultrasound scan to confirm or exclude its presence.

Legs
- Inspect and feel the legs and feet for changes of ischaemia, including temperature and colour changes (see Box 4.23), thin skin, brittle nails and absence of hair.
- Note scars from previous vascular or non-vascular surgery.
- Note the position, margin, depth and colour of any ulceration.
- Look specifically between the toes for ulcers and at the heels for ischaemic changes (the most common site of 'pressure sores').

Femoral pulse
- Ask the patient to lie down and explain what you are going to do.
- Place the pads of your index and middle fingers over the femoral artery. If you are having trouble feeling it (in an obese patient, for example), remember that the femoral artery lies at the mid-inguinal point, halfway between the anterior superior iliac spine and the pubic symphysis (Fig. 4.34).
- Remember that, while it is possible to listen for femoral bruits using the stethoscope diaphragm, the presence or absence of a bruit bears no relation to the likelihood or severity of aortoiliac disease.
- Palpate the femoral and radial pulses simultaneously to assess for radiofemoral delay (Fig. 4.35A).

Popliteal pulse
- With the patient lying down, flex their knee to 30 degrees.
- With your thumbs on the tibial tuberosity and your fingers in the midline posteriorly (2–3 cm below the skin crease), try to compress the artery against the back of the tibia (Fig. 4.35B).

The popliteal artery is usually hard to feel, so if it is readily palpable consider that there may be a popliteal artery aneurysm.

Posterior tibial pulse
- Feel 2 cm below and 2 cm behind the medial malleolus, using the pads of your middle three fingers (Fig. 4.35C).

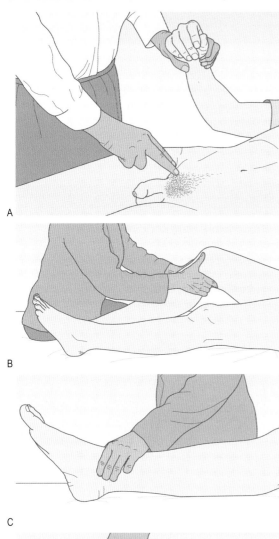

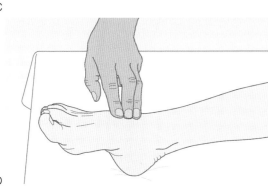

Fig. 4.35 Examination of the femoral, popliteal, posterior tibial and dorsalis pedis arteries. A Examine the femoral artery, while simultaneously checking for radiofemoral delay. B Feel the popliteal artery with your fingertips, having curled the fingers into the popliteal fossa. C Examine the posterior tibial artery. D Examine the dorsalis pedis artery.

Dorsalis pedis pulse

• Using the pads of your middle three fingers, feel at the origin of the first web space just lateral to the tendon of extensor hallucis longus (Fig. 4.35D).

The presence of foot pulses does not completely exclude significant lower limb PAD but they are almost always

diminished or absent. If the history is convincing but pulses are felt, ask the patient to walk on a treadmill until pain develops; if they have flow-limiting PAD, their pulses will disappear and their APBI will fall (see below).

Buerger's test

Examination sequence

• With the patient lying supine, stand at the foot of the bed. Raise the patient's feet and support the legs at 45 degrees to the horizontal for 2–3 minutes.
• Watch for pallor with emptying and 'guttering' of the superficial veins.
• Ask the patient to sit up and hang their legs over the edge of the bed.
• Watch for reactive hyperaemia on dependency due to accumulation of vasoactive metabolites; the loss of pallor and spreading redness make a positive test.

Ankle:brachial pressure index

Assessing pulse status can be unreliable in patients with obesity or oedema. Routinely measure the ankle:brachial pressure index (ABPI) whenever there is difficulty palpating lower limb pulses or when PAD is suspected on the basis of the history.

Examination sequence

• Use a hand-held Doppler probe and a sphygmomanometer.
• Hold the probe over the posterior tibial artery at an angle of 45 degrees.
• Inflate a BP cuff round the ankle.
• Note the pressure at which the Doppler signal disappears. This is the systolic pressure in that artery as it passes under the cuff.
• Repeat, holding the probe over the dorsalis pedis artery.
• Measure the brachial BP in both arms, holding the Doppler probe over the brachial artery at the elbow or the radial artery at the wrist.

The ratio of the highest pedal artery pressure to the highest brachial artery pressure is the ABPI. In health, the ABPI is >1.0 when the patient is supine. An ABPI of <0.9 would be consistent with intermittent claudication and a value <0.4 may indicate critical limb ischaemia. Patients with critical limb ischaemia (rest pain, tissue loss) typically have an ankle BP of <50 mmHg and a positive Buerger's test.

Patients with lower limb PAD, particularly those with diabetes mellitus, often have incompressible, calcified crural arteries that give falsely reassuring pedal pressures and ABPI. Toe pressures may be more accurate in these patients and can be measured using a cuff round the base of the hallux with a laser Doppler probe at the tip of the toe.

Investigations

Further investigations must be carefully selected to provide the most information with the least risk to the patient and at least expense. Duplex ultrasound is often the first-line investigation of choice for unilateral disease, while bilateral symptoms can be investigated using a CT or MR angiogram (Box 4.27).

4.27 Investigations in peripheral arterial disease	
Investigation	Indication/comment
Duplex ultrasound	Carotid artery stenosis, abdominal aortic aneurysm surveillance, peripheral arterial disease
Computed tomography	Abdominal aortic aneurysm, peripheral arterial disease, carotid artery stenosis
Magnetic resonance imaging	Peripheral arterial disease, carotid artery stenosis, arteriovenous malformations
Angiography	Acute and chronic limb ischaemia, carotid artery stenosis Invasive angiography has largely been replaced by computed tomography/magnetic resonance angiography as a diagnostic test

PERIPHERAL VENOUS SYSTEM

Anatomy and physiology

Blood is returned to the heart from the peripheries by a network of deep (90%) and superficial (10%) veins. Venous return from the head and neck is passive, while blood from the legs must be pumped actively back up to the heart against gravity. Pressure on the sole of the foot on walking, together with contraction of muscles in the calf (the 'calf muscle pump') and, to a lesser extent, in the thighs and buttocks, drives blood back up through the veins. Backward flow (reflux) is prevented by valves that divide the long column of blood from the foot to the right atrium into a series of short, low-pressure segments. As a result, the 'ambulatory venous pressure' in the feet in health is usually <20 mmHg.

Deep veins follow the course of the main arteries. Valvular insufficiency causing venous reflux may be primary or post-thrombotic (following deep vein thrombosis, DVT). Following DVT, the vein may remain occluded or recanalise; valve function is usually compromised, however. The combination of deep venous obstruction and reflux leads to the signs and symptoms of post-thrombotic syndrome, including pain, venous claudication, blue discoloration, swelling, dilated superficial veins, skin changes and ulceration.

The long and short saphenous veins are the superficial veins of the lower limb and may also be affected by primary valvular failure and by valvular failure secondary to superficial thrombophlebitis. The long (great) saphenous vein passes anterior to the medial malleolus at the ankle, then up the medial aspect of the calf and thigh to join the common femoral vein in the groin at the saphenofemoral junction (Fig. 4.36).

The short (lesser) saphenous vein passes behind the lateral malleolus at the ankle and up the posterior aspect of the calf. It commonly joins the popliteal vein at the saphenopopliteal junction, which usually lies 2 cm above the posterior knee crease.

There are numerous intercommunications between the long and short saphenous veins, and between the deep and superficial venous systems, via perforator or communicating veins. The venous anatomy of the lower limb is highly variable.

The history

Common presenting symptoms

Lower limb venous disease presents in four ways:
- varicose veins
- deep venous thrombosis

- chronic venous insufficiency and ulceration
- superficial thrombophlebitis.

The severity of symptoms and signs may bear little relationship to the severity of the underlying pathology and the physical signs. Life-threatening DVT may be asymptomatic, while apparently trivial varicose veins may be associated with significant symptoms.

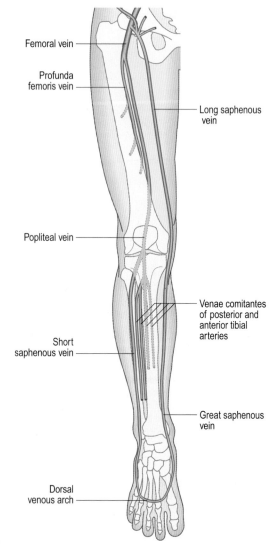

Femoral vein

Profunda femoris vein

Long saphenous vein

Popliteal vein

Venae comitantes of posterior and anterior tibial arteries

Short saphenous vein

Great saphenous vein

Dorsal venous arch

Fig. 4.36 Veins of the lower limb.

Pain

Patients with uncomplicated varicose (dilated, tortuous, superficial) veins often complain of aching leg discomfort, itching and a feeling of swelling (Fig. 4.37A). Symptoms are aggravated by prolonged standing and are often worse towards the end of the day. Once established, DVT causes pain and tenderness in the affected part (usually the calf). Superficial thrombophlebitis produces a red, painful area on the skin overlying the vein involved, and the vein may be palpable as a tender cord. Varicose ulceration may be surprisingly painless; if there is pain, this may be relieved by limb elevation but it is extremely important to exclude coexisting arterial disease (Box 4.28). Graduated compression bandaging is the mainstay of treatment for a venous leg ulcer,

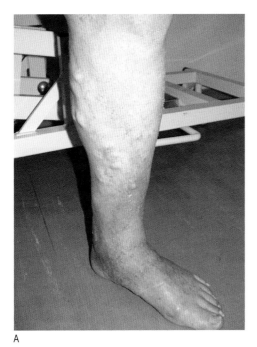
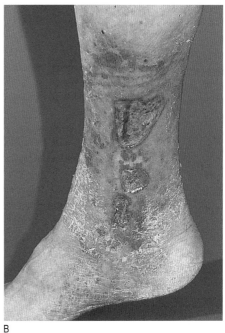

A   B

Fig. 4.37 Lower limb venous disease. A Varicose veins and associated haemosiderin deposition. B Venous ulcer. *(A) From Metcalfe M, Baker D. Varicose veins. Surgery (Oxford) 2008; 26(1):4–7.*

4.28 Clinical features of venous and arterial ulceration

Clinical feature	Venous ulceration	Arterial ulceration	Neuropathic ulceration
Sex	More common in women	More common in men	Equal in men and women
Risk factors	Thrombophilia, family history, previous deep vein thrombosis, varicose veins	Known peripheral vascular disease or risk factors for atherosclerotic disease, e.g. smoking, diabetes, dyslipidaemia, hypertension	Diabetes or other peripheral neuropathy (loss of sensation, loss of intrinsic foot muscle function, autonomic dysregulation)
Pain	Often painless but some patients have some pain that improves with elevating the leg	Severe pain, except in diabetics with neuropathy; improves on dependency	Painless or neuropathic pain
Site	Gaiter areas; 80% medial (long saphenous vein), 20% lateral (short saphenous vein)	Pressure areas (malleoli, heel, fifth metatarsal base, metatarsal heads and toes)	Pressure areas, sole of foot, tips of toes
Appearance	Shallow, irregular margin Slough on granulating base	Regular, 'punched out' Sloughy or necrotic base	Macerated, moist white skin surrounded by callus, often on load-bearing aspects (motor neuropathy)
Surrounding skin	Lipodermatosclerosis always present Oedema	Shiny, hairless, trophic changes	Dry due to reduced sweating (autonomic neuropathy)
Veins	Full and usually varicose	Empty with 'guttering' on elevation	Normal
Temperature	Warm Palpable pulses	Cold Absent pulses	Warm or cold due to autonomic neuropathy Palpable pulses

4.29 Risk factors for deep vein thrombosis

- Obesity
- Smoking
- Recent bed rest or operations (especially to the leg, pelvis or abdomen)
- Recent travel, especially long flights
- Previous trauma to the leg, especially long-bone fractures, plaster of Paris splintage and immobilisation
- Pregnancy or features suggesting pelvic disease
- Malignant disease
- Previous deep vein thrombosis
- Family history of thrombosis
- Inherited thrombophilia, e.g. factor V Leiden
- Recent central venous catheterisation, injection of drug
- Use of oral contraceptive or hormone replacement therapy

but is contraindicated unless there is documented evidence of adequate arterial circulation, which is assessed by feeling the pulses or by measuring the ABPI (see earlier).

Limb swelling

Swelling, or a feeling of swelling, even in the absence of visible signs, may be associated with lower limb venous disease. Enquire about risk factors for DVT (Box 4.29).

In upper limb DVT the arm is swollen and the skin is cyanosed and mottled, especially when dependent. Look for superficial distended veins (acting as collaterals) in the upper arm, over the shoulder region and on the anterior chest wall (Fig. 4.38). Symptoms are often exacerbated by activity, especially when holding the arm overhead.

There may be a history of repetitive trauma at the thoracic outlet due to vigorous, repetitive exercise (swimming, weight lifting, racquet sports). Upper limb DVT may also complicate indwelling subclavian/jugular venous catheters.

Skin changes

Chronic venous insufficiency is often associated with bluish discoloration of the distal extremity. A range of skin changes may be observed (see Fig. 4.37A). Varicose eczema leads to red, itchy, dry areas of skin over the lower leg. Venous hypertension causes extravasation of blood components into surrounding tissues, leading to haemosiderin deposition, which is seen as a brown discoloration of the skin, primarily around the medial aspect of the lower third of the leg. Lipodermatosclerosis occurs when there is an inflammatory response to the haemosiderin and causes red/purple discoloration and induration of the skin. The thickened, fibrotic skin forms a tight band around the lower leg, giving the appearance of an inverted champagne bottle. In *atrophie blanche*, there are multiple, small, white, scarred areas within the affected skin.

Chronic venous ulceration

In developed countries, about 70–80% of lower limb ulceration is primarily due to venous disease. Other causes include pyoderma gangrenosum, syphilis, tuberculosis, leprosy (Hansen's disease), sickle cell disease and tropical conditions. Chronic venous ulceration (see Fig. 4.37B) usually affects the medial aspect of the calf. Ulcers are shallow and pink (granulation tissue) or yellow/green (slough) in colour, with an irregular margin, and are

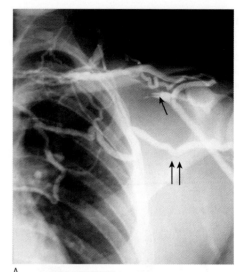

A

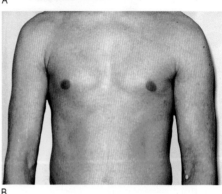

B

Fig. 4.38 Axillary vein thrombosis. [A] Angiogram. *Single arrow* shows site of thrombosis. *Double arrows* show dilated collateral vessels. [B] Clinical appearance with swollen left arm and dilated superficial veins.

usually associated with other skin changes of chronic venous insufficiency (varicose eczema, lipodermatosclerosis).

Superficial venous thrombophlebitis

This condition affects up to 10% of patients with severe varicose veins and is more common during pregnancy. Recurrent superficial venous thrombophlebitis, especially that affecting different areas sequentially and non-varicose veins, may be associated with underlying malignancy. It may propagate into the deep system, leading to DVT and pulmonary embolism.

Past history

Enquire about previous varicose vein surgery and risk factors for DVT (Box 4.29).

The physical examination

Examination sequence

Expose the patient's legs and examine them with the patient standing and then lying supine.

- Inspect the skin for colour changes, swelling and superficial venous dilatation and tortuosity (varicose veins).
- Feel for any temperature difference.
- Press gently with your fingertip over the tibia above the ankle for a few seconds and then see if your finger has left a pit (pitting oedema). Remember to avoid areas that might be tender such as around ulcers.
- If the leg is grossly swollen, press at a higher level to establish how far the oedema extends.
- If you find oedema, check the JVP (p. 52). If the JVP is raised, this suggests cardiac disease or pulmonary hypertension as a cause, especially if both legs are oedematous.

Investigations

Tests such as the tourniquet and the Trendelenburg tests, to assess for saphenofemoral valve incompetence, are now obsolete and have been replaced by hand-held Doppler. With the patient standing, ask them to put their weight on the contralateral foot and position the hand-held Doppler probe over the long saphenous vein or saphenofemoral junction (2 cm below and medial to the mid-inguinal point). Squeeze the calf muscle and listen for blood flowing up through the long saphenous vein. If the valves are competent, you will hear a brief backflow of blood (<0.5 s) only when you release the calf muscle, which is physiological as the valves close. If the valves are incompetent, you will hear the prolonged sound of blood refluxing back down the vein.

OSCE example 1: Chest pain history

Ms McLeod, 62 years old, presents to you with intermittent chest pain.

Please take a history

- Introduce yourself and clean your hands.
- Invite the patient to describe the presenting symptoms, using open questioning.
- Take a detailed history of the presenting symptoms, including the onset, duration, site, quality and severity of the pain and any aggravating or relieving factors, in particular the relationship to exertion. Determine the functional consequences and any change in the pattern of symptoms.
- Ask about relevant past history and vascular risk factors, including hypertension, diabetes and hyperlipidaemia.
- Enquire about drug history or intolerances, including preventative therapies.
- Ask about premature coronary artery disease in first-degree relatives.
- Take a social history, including occupation, smoking and alcohol.
- Conduct a systematic inquiry. In particular, is there associated palpitation, breathlessness, orthopnoea and ankle swelling, or has there been any bleeding?
- Ask about any other patient concerns.
- Thank the patient and clean your hands.

Summarise your findings

Ms McLeod gives a 6-week history of intermittent chest discomfort. She reports a dull central ache that does not radiate to the arms or jaw. It occurs predominantly with effort, is worse on inclines or walking on cold mornings, and resolves at rest after a few minutes. These symptoms make her work as a carer challenging. She has no previous cardiac problems but is known to have hypertension and type 2 diabetes; she takes metformin for the latter. There is no family history of premature coronary artery disease and she has never been a smoker.

Suggest a likely diagnosis

The likely diagnosis is stable angina pectoris.

Suggest further evaluation

Full cardiovascular examination, blood glucose and lipid profile, and a 12-lead electrocardiogram. Consider referral for an exercise tolerance test or coronary angiogram.

OSCE example 2: Cardiac examination

Mr Munro, 82 years old, presents with progressive breathlessness and lightheadedness on exertion.

Please examine his cardiovascular system

- Introduce yourself and clean your hands.
- Carry out general observations. Is the patient tachypnoeic or distressed at rest? Are his hands cool?
- Measure the pulse, blood pressure and jugular venous pressure. Are the pulse volume and systolic pressure reduced? Is the jugular venous pressure elevated?
- Palpate the precordium. Is the apex more forceful or displaced?
- Auscultate over the apex and lower left, upper right and upper left sternal borders for the character of the first and second heart sounds, and the presence and characteristics of any added sounds or murmurs. If a murmur is heard, is there any radiation?
- Examine the chest, sacrum and lower limbs for signs of heart failure.
- Thank the patient and clean your hands.

Summarise your findings

Mr Munro appears comfortable. His heart rate is 80 bpm with a low-volume, slow-rising pulse. His blood pressure is 110/60 mmHg. The jugular venous pressure is not raised. There is an apical heave but the apex is not displaced. The first heart sound is normal but the second is diminished. There is a grade 3 ejection systolic murmur, loudest over the aortic area but heard widely, radiating to the carotids. There are fine end-inspiratory crackles at the lung bases.

Suggest a likely diagnosis

The likely diagnosis is aortic stenosis with left ventricular decompensation and heart failure.

Suggest initial investigations

Twelve-lead electrocardiogram, chest X-ray and transthoracic echocardiogram.

Integrated examination sequence for the cardiovascular system

- Position the patient: supine and reclined at 45 degrees, with the head resting on a pillow.
- Examine the general appearance:
  - Is the patient breathless, cyanosed, sweating or distressed?
  - Note body habitus (overweight or cachectic), Marfanoid features and the presence of radial or saphenous vein harvest scars.
- Check the hands, pulse and blood pressure, face and neck:
  - Hands: colour and temperature, tobacco staining, clubbing, splinter haemorrhages, Janeway lesions or Osler's nodes, tendon xanthomata.
  - Pulse: rate, rhythm, character and synchronicity of radial pulse, collapsing pulse, volume and character of brachial or carotid pulse.
  - Blood pressure: systolic and diastolic pressure at the brachial artery.
  - Face: central cyanosis, xanthelasmata, corneal arcus, petechiae.
  - Neck: timing, waveform and abnormalities of the jugular venous pressure, carotid bruits.
- Examine the precordium:
  - Inspection: look for midline sternotomy or left submammary scars, pacemaker site, visible pulsation.
  - Palpation: define the character and position of the apex beat, parasternal heave, thrills.
  - Auscultation: listen over the apex, lower left sternal border, upper right and left sternal borders, over the carotid arteries and left axilla. Listen with the patient on their left side and leaning forward during expiration.
    - Heart sounds: identify first and second heart sounds (S_1 and S_2), and any extra heart sounds (S_3 or S_4).
    - Additional sounds: clicks and snaps.
    - Murmurs in systole and/or diastole (timing, duration, character, pitch, intensity, location and radiation).
    - Pericardial rub.
- Other:
  - Listen for fine end-inspiratory crackles or pleural effusion at the lung bases.
  - Examine the abdomen for hepatomegaly or pulsatile liver.
  - Check for ankle and sacral oedema.

Peripheral arterial and venous system

- Inspection of the lower limbs:
  - Check temperature and colour, capillary refill time, skin discoloration, ulceration, varicosities, scars.
- Palpation:
  - Examine the abdomen for expansile aortic aneurysm.
  - Identify the femoral, popliteal, posterior tibial and dorsalis pedis pulses.
  - Identify pitting oedema.
  - Perform Buerger's test.
- Auscultation:
  - Listen for bruits over the abdomen and over the femoral arteries.

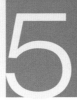

J Alastair Innes
James Tiernan

The respiratory system

Anatomy and physiology

An understanding of the surface anatomy of the lungs (Fig. 5.1) and their relation to closely adjacent structures is essential for the practice of respiratory medicine. At the end of tidal expiration the dome of the diaphragm extends high into the thorax to around the level of the anterior end of the fifth rib, slightly lower on the left. The lower anterior ribs therefore overlie the liver on the right and the stomach and spleen on the left, with the parietal pleura extending lower than the lungs on the lateral chest wall. Posteriorly, the lungs extend much lower, approaching the 12th rib on full inspiration.

The lung apex lies immediately beneath the brachial plexus, so apical lung tumours commonly disrupt T1 root fibres, causing pain and numbness in the inner aspect of the upper arm and wasting of the small hand muscles. The upper thoracic sympathetic outflow to the eye may also be compromised, leading to a constricted pupil and ptosis. In the mid- and lower mediastinum, tumours can invade and compromise the pericardium, atria and oesophagus.

In health, the lungs optimise gas exchange by close matching of regional ventilation and perfusion. Airway and parenchymal lung diseases disrupt this matching, causing hypoxia and cyanosis, and commonly stimulate breathing through lung afferent nerves, leading to a history of breathlessness, and tachypnoea on examination.

The history

Patients use a wide range of terms to describe respiratory symptoms (such as infection, phlegm, catarrh, pleurisy and wheeze). These can be ambiguous and require careful definition to avoid misunderstanding. 'Wheeze' may be used when describing breathlessness, or 'I had a chest infection' may denote a breathless episode actually due to pulmonary embolism.

As with other systems, the respiratory history should start with open questions but should also specifically cover all the areas outlined in Box 5.1.

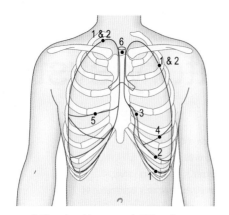

1 Pleural markings	4 Oblique fissure
2 Lung markings	5 Horizontal fissure
3 Cardiac notch	6 Trachea

A

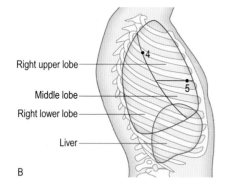

Right upper lobe

Middle lobe

Right lower lobe

Liver

B

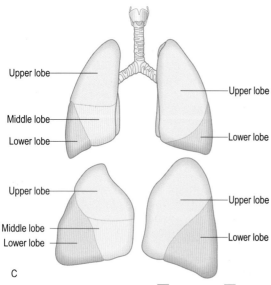

Upper lobe — Upper lobe

Middle lobe — Lower lobe

Lower lobe

Upper lobe — Upper lobe

Middle lobe — Lower lobe

Lower lobe

C

Fig. 5.1 Surface anatomy of the thorax. A Anterior view. B Right lateral view. C Lobar anatomy of the lung surfaces: anterior view (upper), lateral view (lower).

5.1 Respiratory history taking/documentation framework

History of presenting symptoms

Specific respiratory symptoms
- Breathlessness
- Wheeze
- Cough
- Sputum/haemoptysis
- Chest pain
- Fever/rigors/night sweats
- Weight loss
- Sleepiness

Past medical history
- Respiratory disease
- Other illness/hospital encounters

Drug and allergy history
- Drugs causing or relieving respiratory symptoms
- Allergies to pollens/pets/dust; anaphylaxis

Social and family history
- Family history of respiratory disease
- Home circumstances/effect of and on disease
- Smoking
- Occupational history

Systematic review
- Systemic diseases involving the lung
- Risk factors for lung disease

Common presenting symptoms

Breathlessness

Breathlessness (or dyspnoea) denotes the feeling of an 'uncomfortable need to breathe' and is the most commonly reported respiratory symptom. It is also one of the most challenging to quantify, being inherently subjective. Breathlessness may originate from respiratory or cardiac dysfunction, or be a manifestation of psychological distress.

Respiratory disease can cause breathlessness through a range of mechanisms:

- stimulation of intrapulmonary afferent nerves by interstitial inflammation or thromboembolism
- mechanical loading of respiratory muscles by airflow obstruction or reduced lung compliance in fibrosis
- hypoxia due to ventilation/perfusion mismatch, stimulating chemoreceptors.

The Medical Research Council (MRC) breathlessness scale (Box 5.2) is a useful and validated way to document the patient's level of dyspnoea formally.

Specific questions may help to distinguish the causes of breathlessness. Ask in particular:

- How did the breathlessness come on? If the onset was instantaneous, think of pneumothorax, pulmonary embolus or acute allergy. Onset over hours is typical in asthma, acute pulmonary oedema or acute infections, while insidious onset occurs with developing effusions, interstitial diseases and tumours.
- How is your breathing at rest and overnight? Asthma commonly wakes patients, while most patients with chronic obstructive pulmonary disease (COPD) are comfortable at rest and when asleep but struggle with exertion. Breathlessness provoked by lying down (orthopnoea) is a feature of heart failure (p. 42) but also occurs frequently in patients with severe airflow obstruction or diaphragmatic weakness because the weight of the abdominal contents displaces the diaphragm towards the head on lying down, compromising the vital capacity.
- Is your breathing normal some days? Variable breathlessness is the hallmark of asthma, while consistent daily limitation is typical in COPD.
- Tell me something you do that would make you breathless? How far can you walk on a good day? This is useful for quantification and assessment of disease impact

Grade	Degree of breathlessness related to activities
1	Not troubled by breathlessness except on strenuous exercise
2	Short of breath when hurrying on the level or walking up a slight hill
3	Walks slower than most people on the level, stops after a mile or so, or stops after 15 minutes walking at own pace
4	Stops for breath after walking about 100 yds or after a few minutes on level ground
5	Too breathless to leave the house, or breathless when undressing

5.2 Medical Research Council (MRC) breathlessness scale

Used with the permission of the Medical Research Council.

and disability. Record restrictions on normal activity or work and the corresponding MRC breathlessness score (Box 5.2)

- When does the breathlessness come on? Asthma induced by exercise frequently appears only after exercise, during early recovery, because sympathetic drive during exercise defends airway patency.

Certain phrases in the history strongly suggest a psychological aetiology of breathlessness, particularly 'I feel I can't get enough air (or oxygen) into my chest.' In patients with hyperventilation due to anxiety, this symptom is frequently accompanied by a normal measured vital capacity. Associated symptoms induced by hypocapnia in hyperventilation include digital and perioral paraesthesiae, lightheadedness and sometimes chest tightness.

Fig. 5.2 summarises how to use the history and examination findings to distinguish some common causes of breathlessness. Remember that patients rarely report exactly what textbooks describe.

Wheeze

Wheeze describes the high-pitched musical or 'whistling' sounds produced by turbulent air flow through small airways narrowed by bronchospasm and/or airway secretions. It is most commonly heard during expiration, when airway calibre is reduced. Wheeze must be distinguished from the rattling inspiratory and expiratory sounds caused by loose, mobile secretions in the upper airways, and from the louder, dramatic croak of stridor (see later) caused by obstruction in the trachea or large airways.

Identifying wheeze in the patient's history is very important, as true wheeze is typical of small airways diseases. It is most commonly associated with asthma and COPD but can also occur with acute respiratory tract infection or with exacerbations of bronchiectasis (due to a combination of airway narrowing and excessive secretions).

Ask:

- Is the wheeze worse during or after exercise? If it occurs during exercise and limits it, this suggests COPD; in asthma, wheeze and tightness usually appear after exercise.
- Do you wake with wheeze during the night? This suggests asthma.
- Do you have hay fever or other allergies? Atopy is common in allergic asthma. A family history of wheeze or asthma is common in asthma.
- Is it worse on waking in the morning and relieved by clearing sputum? This is common in COPD.
- Do you smoke? Smoking is suggestive of COPD, though patients with asthma occasionally smoke.
- Are there daily volumes of yellow or green sputum, sometimes with blood? This suggests possible bronchiectasis.

Cough

The cough reflex has evolved to dislodge foreign material and secretions from the central airways, and may be triggered by pathology at any level of the bronchial tree. Inspiration is followed by an expiratory effort against a closed glottis. Subsequent sudden opening of the glottis with rapid expiratory flow produces the characteristic sound.

Ask about:

- Duration of the cough.
- Whether it is present every day.

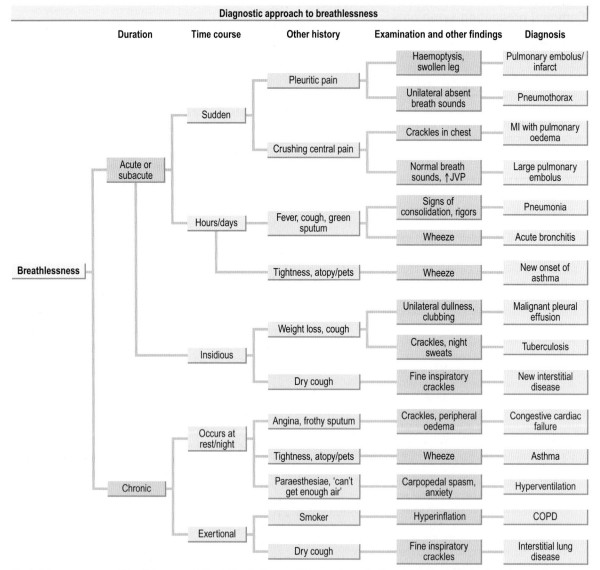

Fig. 5.2 Common causes of breathlessness: distinguishing features on history and examination. *COPD,* chronic obstructive pulmonary disease; *JVP,* jugular venous pressure; *MI,* myocardial infarction.

- If it is intrusive/irresistible or whether the patient coughs deliberately to clear a perceived obstruction (throat clearing).
- Whether it produces sputum. If so, how much and what colour?
- Any triggers (such as during swallowing, in cold air, during exercise).
- Smoking. This increases the likelihood of chronic bronchitis or lung cancer.
- Associated clinical features:
  - Wheeze: may signal cough-variant asthma.
  - Heartburn or reflux: gastro-oesophageal reflux commonly triggers cough.
  - Altered voice or swallowing: consider laryngeal causes.
- Drug history, especially angiotensin-converting enzyme (ACE) inhibitors.

Cough productive of green or yellow sputum suggests bronchial infection. Large volumes of sputum over long periods suggest bronchiectasis. Haemoptysis is covered below.

Cough is most commonly a symptom of acute viral upper respiratory tract infections, which are usually self-limiting over days to weeks.

Cough that fails to settle over weeks may be the presenting feature of bronchial carcinoma. A history of smoking raises further suspicion of malignancy, although chronic cough is a non-specific symptom in smokers. Other investigations, including a chest X-ray, are often required to exclude early cancer. Chronic cough is defined as cough lasting more than 8 weeks and can be debilitating both physically and socially. Causes of chronic cough and features in the history that may indicate the underlying cause are summarised in Box 5.3.

In patients with malignancy at the left hilum, damage to the left recurrent laryngeal nerve may paralyse the left vocal cord, making it impossible for the patient to close the glottis and generate a normal explosive cough. The resulting hoarse forced expiration without the initial explosive glottal opening is termed a 'bovine cough' and is an important symptom warning of possible hilar malignancy.

5.3 Causes of chronic cough and accompanying clues in the history

Pathophysiology	Suggestive features in history/examination
Airways inflammation: Asthma – 'cough-variant asthma'	Affects children and some adults Often present at night Associated wheeze, atopy
Chronic obstructive pulmonary disease	History of smoking and intermittent sputum
Persisting airway reactivity following acute bronchitis	Recent acute-onset cough and sputum
Bronchiectasis	Daily purulent sputum for long periods Pneumonia or whooping cough in childhood Recurrent haemoptysis
Lung cancer	Persistent cough, especially in smokers Any haemoptysis Pneumonia that fails to clear in 4–6 weeks
Rhinitis with postnasal drip	Chronic sneezing, nasal blockage/discharge
Oesophageal reflux	Heartburn or regurgitation of acid after eating, bending or lying Nocturnal as well as daytime cough
Drug effects	Patient on angiotensin-converting enzyme inhibitors
Interstitial lung diseases	Persistent dry cough Fine inspiratory crackles at bases
Idiopathic cough	Long history with no signs and negative investigations – diagnosis of exclusion

Sputum

In health, the airway lining fluid coating the tracheobronchial tree ascends the mucociliary escalator to the larynx, where it mixes with upper respiratory tract secretions and saliva and is swallowed. In acute or chronic airways infection, accumulation of neutrophils, mucus and proteinaceous secretions in the airways results in cough with expectoration of sputum. Ask about the characteristics of sputum to clarify the pathology. A change in colour or consistency, or an increase in volume may indicate a new infection in chronic disease.

Colour

- Clear (mucoid): COPD/bronchiectasis without current infection/rhinitis.
- Yellow (mucopurulent): acute lower respiratory tract infection/asthma.
- Green (purulent): current infection – acute disease or exacerbation of chronic disease, such as COPD.
- Red/brown (rusty): pneumococcal pneumonia (Fig. 5.3B). Try to distinguish between rusty and frank red blood (see below).
- Pink (serous/frothy): acute pulmonary oedema.

In bronchiectasis, the colour of sputum may be used to guide the need for antibiotic treatment (Fig. 5.3A).

Volume

- Establish the volume produced over 24 hours: small amounts into a tissue or enough to fill a spoon(s), eggcup(s) or cup(s).
- Compare the current volume with the patient's baseline or minimal volume.

Consistency

- An increase in stickiness (viscosity) may indicate exacerbation in bronchiectasis.
- Large volumes of frothy secretions over weeks/months are a feature of the uncommon bronchoalveolar cell carcinoma.
- Occasionally, sputum is produced as firm 'plugs' by patients with asthma (Fig. 5.3C), sometimes indicating underlying allergic bronchopulmonary aspergillosis.

Haemoptysis

Haemoptysis means coughing up blood from the respiratory tract. It can complicate any severe forceful cough but is most commonly associated with acute or chronic respiratory tract infections. Haemoptysis may also indicate pulmonary embolism and lung cancer. Never assume haemoptysis has a benign cause until serious pathology has been considered and excluded.

Ask about how it appeared, how much blood there was, whether there are associated features and over what time period it came on:

- Was the blood definitely coughed up from the chest? Blood in the mouth may be vomited, may have come from the nose in epistaxis, or may appear on chewing or tooth brushing in patients with gum disease.
- A short history of streaks of blood with purulent sputum suggests acute bronchitis.
- A sudden episode of a small volume of blood with pleuritic pain and breathlessness suggests pulmonary embolism.
- Recurrent streaks of blood in clear sputum should prompt a search for lung cancer.
- Recurrent blood streaks in purulent sputum over weeks suggest possible tuberculosis or cancer with infection; over years, they suggest bronchiectasis.
- Larger volumes of haemoptysis (>20 mL, for example) suggest specific causes:
  - lung cancer eroding a pulmonary vessel
  - bronchiectasis (such as in cystic fibrosis)
  - cavitatory disease (such as bleeding into an aspergilloma)
  - pulmonary vasculitis
  - pulmonary arteriovenous malformation.

Stridor

This harsh, grating respiratory sound is caused by vibration of the walls of the trachea or major bronchi when the airway lumen is critically narrowed by compression, tumour or inhaled foreign material. Inspiration lowers the pressure inside the extrathoracic trachea, so critical narrowing here leads to inspiratory stridor. In contrast, the intrathoracic large airways are compressed during expiration by positive pressure in the surrounding lung, leading to fixed expiratory wheeze or stridor. Large airway narrowing at the thoracic inlet (for example, tracheal compression by a large goitre) may cause both inspiratory and expiratory stridor. Rapid investigation and treatment are vital when this sign is present.

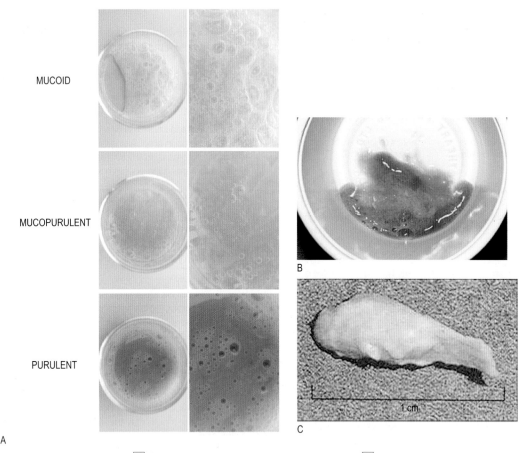

MUCOID

MUCOPURULENT

B

PURULENT

1 cm

C

A

Fig. 5.3 Sputum appearance in disease. [A] Colour chart of sputum purulence used in bronchiectasis. [B] Rusty red sputum of pneumococcal pneumonia. [C] Mucus plug from a patient with asthma. *(A) Courtesy Medical Photography, NHS Lothian.*

Chest pain

Chest pain may originate from musculoskeletal, respiratory, cardiovascular and gastro-oesophageal disease.

Establish:

- Site and severity.
- Character: sharp suggests pleural pain.
- Onset: gradual or rapid?
- Exacerbating or relieving factors: worsening with cough or deep breaths suggests pleural disease.
- Associated symptoms: breathlessness, fever and cough suggest an infective cause.

A large pulmonary embolus can cause angina-like chest pain (p. 40), due to increased right ventricular work together with reduced coronary oxygen delivery caused by hypotension and hypoxaemia, resulting in right ventricular ischaemia.

Besides myocardial ischaemia, chest pain can arise from the chest wall, parietal pleura, mediastinal structures, tracheobronchial tree, pericardium, oesophagus and subdiaphragmatic organs (liver and gallbladder). Pain does not originate in the lung parenchyma or visceral pleura, as they have only an autonomic nerve supply.

Pleuritic pain is worse on inspiration and coughing, and is usually described as sharp, stabbing or knife-like. It is usually sited away from the midline, and may be localised or affect a wide area of chest wall. Disease causes parietal pleural pain in several ways:

- pneumonia and pulmonary infarcts: either direct pleural inflammation or adhesions with pleural traction on respiratory movement
- pneumothorax: mechanical distortion of pleura with lung collapse
- lung cancer: pleural distortion by infiltration, although constant pain is more typical.

Musculoskeletal chest pain is common and may occur with chest trauma, forceful coughing or connective tissue disease. The chest is characteristically tender to local palpation, and the pain can be reproduced by respiratory movements and/or movement of the spine or shoulder muscles. There may be associated soft tissue injury or rib fractures. A detailed history of events preceding the onset is vital, as injury is easily overlooked.

Two other uncommon conditions can cause acute chest pain. Bornholm disease is an infection with an enterovirus (Coxsackie B), which causes acute but self-limiting inflammation of intercostal muscles. Episodes of unilateral severe, stabbing myalgia develop over an intercostal space and settle after a few days. Costochondritis (called Tietze's syndrome when costochondral swelling is present) is idiopathic inflammation of the costochondral cartilages adjoining the sternum and can cause acute localised pain and tenderness. The pain settles with simple analgesia and the passage of time in both of these conditions.

Herpes zoster infection (shingles) may start with superficial itch or burning pain in a thoracic dermatome, followed by the appearance of a vesicular rash. Pain and altered sensation may persist long after the rash has resolved, often with scarring in the dermatomal distribution.

Burning retrosternal pain may indicate oesophagitis but also occurs with myocardial ischaemia. Alteration of discomfort after eating or antacids helps to distinguish oesophageal pain; cardiac pain is described on page 40.

Central, constant, progressive, non-pleuritic chest pain may represent mediastinal disease, particularly malignancy. Similarly, chest wall pain (without trauma) that is constant, progressive and non-pleuritic suggests chest wall invasion by malignancy. Pain-induced sleep disturbance is a feature of such malignant pains.

Fevers/rigors/night sweats

These symptoms are not specific to respiratory medicine but are commonly reported by patients with respiratory diseases. Infection (acute or chronic) is the usual cause but other aetiologies such as lung cancer, lymphoma or vasculitis should also be considered.

Patients use a range of terms to describe fever (such as shivers, chills, being 'hot and bothered', shakes), so ask for a detailed account of their symptoms using common terms.

Rigors are generalised, uncontrollable episodes of vigorous body shaking lasting a few minutes. Despite high fever, the patient may complain of feeling cold and seek extra clothing. Rigors usually indicate bacterial sepsis; lobar pneumonia and acute pyelonephritis are the most common causes. They can be misinterpreted as seizures but the retention of consciousness and associated pyrexia suggest rigors.

Night sweats are more closely associated with chronic infection (such as tuberculosis) and malignancy or lymphoma rather than acute infection. Occasional episodes of a sweaty head or pillow are inconclusive, but if patients report having to change their nightclothes or sheets frequently due to profuse nocturnal sweating over several weeks, this is more likely to indicate underlying disease.

Weight loss

Weight loss is a common feature of several important respiratory diseases:
- lung cancers
- chronic infective diseases (such as tuberculosis and bronchiectasis)
- diseases causing chronic breathlessness (such as COPD and interstitial lung diseases).

The pathophysiology is complex; however, breathlessness is associated with diminished appetite, and the systemic inflammatory response is also thought to contribute to weight loss.

Small amounts of weight loss also occur in acute infection with consequent loss of appetite, particularly during hospitalisation. Ask the patient to estimate the extent and duration of weight loss, and enquire about appetite and dietary intake. Being underweight is a poor prognostic indicator in any chronic respiratory disease.

Sleepiness

Excessive daytime sleepiness may be a symptom of an underlying sleep-related breathing disorder (obstructive sleep apnoea (OSA) or obstructive sleep apnoea/sleep hypopnoea (OSASH)). In these conditions, frequent episodes of upper airway obstruction at night cause repeated microarousals from sleep, leading to complete disruption of normal sleep. Daytime somnolence impairs work and driving performance, causing danger to the patient and others.

Ask about:
- Normal sleeping habit: does the patient keep hours that allow reasonable rest?
- Shift or night work: this can disrupt and prevent healthy sleep patterns.
- Does the person wake refreshed or exhausted? Sleep apnoea patients are exhausted in the morning.
- Have they struggled to stay awake in the day: for example, at work or when driving?

It is vital to advise cessation of driving pending investigation if OSA is suspected.

Ideally, seek a description of any night-time breathing disturbance from a bed partner. In OSA, the partner may observe periodic cessation of breathing, accompanied by increasing respiratory efforts, followed by a sudden and loud resumption of breathing, often with postural repositioning, then repetition of this cycle.

Validated sleepiness scores (such as the Epworth Sleepiness Scale: http://epworthsleepinessscale.com/) can be used to quantify daytime somnolence and are helpful if considering referral to a sleep disorder clinic.

Past medical history

Past illnesses relevant to respiratory disease are summarised in Box 5.4. These include respiratory disease that may recur or cause long-term symptoms, and disease in other systems that may cause, complicate or present with respiratory symptoms, including thromboembolic, cardiovascular, haematological, malignant and connective tissue diseases.

Note prior respiratory treatments (including need for critical care) and the degree of chronic symptoms, such as usual exacerbation frequency, prescription rate and hospitalisation.

Drug and allergy history

Note all drugs that the patient is currently using, including inhalers, nebulised bronchodilators and domiciliary oxygen, non-prescription remedies and recreational drugs. Cross-check the drug names and doses with a separate source such as the general practitioner's records.

Drugs given for other problems commonly cause respiratory side effects; these are summarised in Box 5.5.

Always ask and record whether the patient has any known allergies, as allergic asthma is far more common in those with a history of atopy.

Family history

Ask about a family history of asthma, although this is common in the population and therefore not highly predictive. Respiratory diseases with a known genetic cause are relatively rare. Most patients with cystic fibrosis have unaffected carrier parents but many have affected siblings.

Social history

Always start by identifying the patient's normal level of daily activity and the impact of their recent symptoms on this. Can they still manage their work, their self-care and any caring they deliver?

5.4 Previous illness relevant to respiratory history

History	Current implications
Eczema, hay fever	Allergic tendency relevant to asthma
Childhood asthma	Many wheezy children do not have asthma as adults, yet many adults with asthma had childhood wheeze
Whooping cough, measles, inhaled foreign body	Recognised causes of bronchiectasis, especially if complicated by pneumonia
Pneumonia, pleurisy	Recognised causes of bronchiectasis Recurrent episodes may be a manifestation of bronchiectasis
Tuberculosis	Reactivation if not previously treated effectively Respiratory failure may complicate thoracoplasty Mycetoma in lung cavity may present with haemoptysis
Connective tissue disorders, e.g. rheumatoid arthritis	Lung diseases are recognised complications, e.g. pulmonary fibrosis, effusions, bronchiectasis Immunomodulatory treatments of these diseases may also cause pulmonary toxicity or render patients susceptible to respiratory infection
Previous malignancy	Recurrence, metastatic/pleural disease Chemotherapeutic agents recognised causes of pulmonary fibrosis Radiotherapy-induced pulmonary fibrosis
Cancer, recent travel, surgery or immobility	Pulmonary thromboembolism
Recent surgery, loss of consciousness	Aspiration of foreign body, gastric contents Pneumonia, lung abscess
Neuromuscular disorders	Respiratory failure Aspiration

5.5 Respiratory problems caused by drugs

Respiratory condition	Drug
Bronchoconstriction	Beta-blockers Opioids Non-steroidal anti-inflammatory drugs
Cough	Angiotensin-converting enzyme inhibitors
Bronchiolitis obliterans	Penicillamine
Diffuse parenchymal lung disease	Cytotoxic agents: bleomycin, methotrexate Anti-inflammatory agents: sulfasalazine, penicillamine, gold salts, aspirin Cardiovascular drugs: amiodarone, hydralazine Antibiotics: nitrofurantoin Intravenous drug misuse
Pulmonary thromboembolism	Oestrogens
Pulmonary hypertension	Oestrogens Dexfenfluramine, fenfluramine
Pleural effusion	Amiodarone Nitrofurantoin Phenytoin Methotrexate Pergolide
Respiratory depression	Opioids Benzodiazepines

Systematic enquiry

Ask specifically about any risk factors, such as malignancy for thromboembolism. The remaining history may reveal previously unsuspected pathologies presenting with respiratory symptoms or complicating respiratory illness, such as ovarian malignancy presenting with pleural effusion.

The physical examination

The patient should be reclining on an examination couch or bed at about 45 degrees, with the thorax exposed and the head supported by a pillow.

Inspection

Much can be learned about the respiratory system by careful inspection from the end of the bed. The normal shape and respiratory movements of the chest wall are significantly altered by the hyperinflation that accompanies chronic airflow obstruction (Fig. 5.5). Such obstruction also causes prolonged expiration relative to inspiration, and sometimes 'pursed-lip' breathing on expiration. Forceful inspiration at these very high lung volumes may cause indrawing of the intercostal spaces during mid-inspiration and also the recruitment of muscles not normally involved in breathing ('accessory muscles'). These include the sternocleidomastoid muscles lifting the sternum, and trapezius and the scalenes lifting the shoulder girdle. Patients sometimes sit forwards and brace their arms on a table, allowing them to

Home circumstances

Patients limited by chronic respiratory conditions may become confined to their own homes, particularly if they become too breathless to manage stairs. Ask about their home environment and what support they receive to enable them to function.

Smoking

Obtaining an honest and accurate history of tobacco use is difficult and is covered on page 14. Ask if others smoke in the house; this can be a major obstacle to smoking cessation. Remember also to enquire about the use of cannabis and e-cigarettes.

Occupational history

Many respiratory diseases are caused by occupational or domestic exposure to inhaled substances. Common examples are summarised in Fig. 5.4. Ask the patient what work they have done, starting with their first job. Look out for the occupations listed in Fig. 5.4, and also record the employers' names, the dates and duration of exposure, and whether any protective masks were offered or used.

5

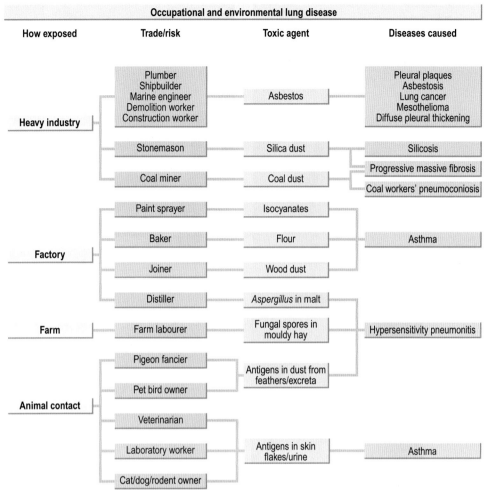

Fig. 5.4 Common occupational and environmental causes of respiratory disease.

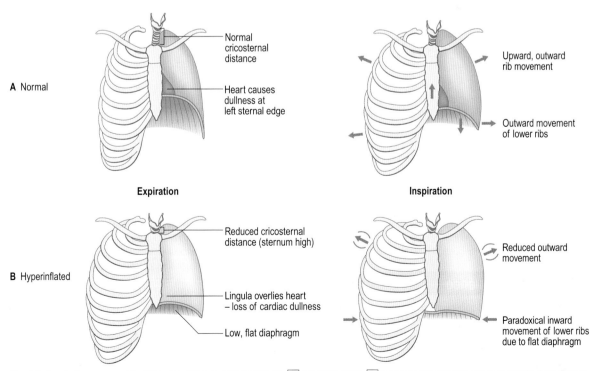

Fig. 5.5 **Respiratory movement of the ribs, sternum and diaphragm.** [A] In normal adults. [B] In chronic hyperinflation due to obstructive lung disease. Hyperinflation causes upward displacement of the sternum and clavicles, increased anteroposterior thoracic diameter, loss of cardiac dullness at the lower left sternal edge, and a low flat diaphragm that pulls the lower ribs in during inspiration.

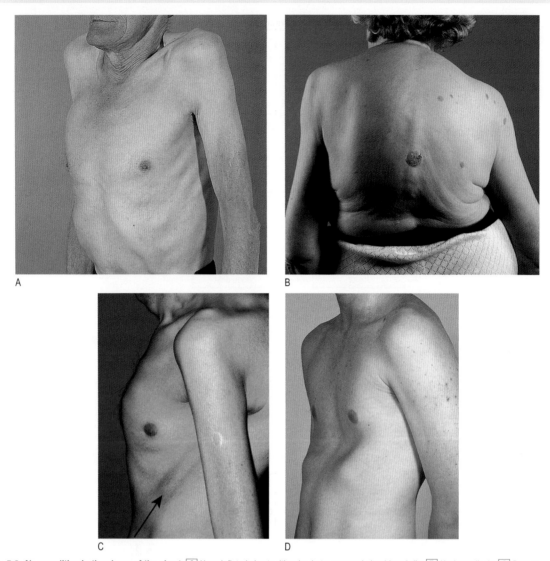

Fig. 5.6 Abnormalities in the shape of the chest. [A] Hyperinflated chest with raised sternum and shoulder girdle. [B] Kyphoscoliosis. [C] Pectus carinatum with Harrison's sulcus *(arrow)*. [D] Pectus excavatum.

use pectoralis major to pull the ribs outwards during inspiration. In contrast to the hyperinflation of obstructive disease, interstitial disease causes small, stiff lungs, diminishes thoracic volume and raises resting respiratory rate.

Chest deformity (Fig. 5.6) may be congenital, as in pectus excavatum, or acquired, as in pectus carinatum. The latter is an inward displacement of the lower ribs with a prominent sternum, caused by severe airflow obstruction in early childhood, when the rib cage is developing. Asymmetry of the chest may be secondary to scoliosis, shrinkage of scarred lung following tuberculous infection, or prior surgical resection of lung and/or ribs.

Examination sequence

- Note the presence of nebulisers or inhalers (indicating obstructive lung disease), oxygen therapy and cyanosis; check sputum pots.
- Look for asymmetry of the chest, deformities, operative scars and chest drains, remembering that thoracotomy scars may be visible only on the lateral and posterior aspects of the chest.
- Quietly observe and time respiratory rate (for example, breaths in 15 seconds × 4) without drawing the patient's attention to it, as this may cause it to change. Feeling the radial pulse, while timing breathing, is a common solution to this problem.
- Inspect the remaining skin for relevant abnormalities.

At rest the rate is normally 12–15 breaths per minute; anxious patients may breathe at 15–20 breaths per minute but a rate of over 20 breaths per minute is abnormal for an adult.

In healthy adults at altitude, elderly people and patients with heart failure, a distinctive pattern of alternating periods of deep and shallow breathing may be seen. This is known as Cheyne–Stokes respiration and is thought to represent abnormal feedback from the carotid chemoreceptors to the respiratory centre.

Subcutaneous metastases from lung tumours (Fig. 5.7A) may be seen and offer the chance for rapid biopsy and diagnosis. In the legs the painful dusky red lesions of erythema nodosum

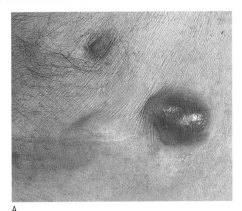

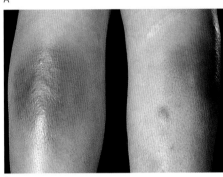

Fig. 5.7 Skin lesions associated with respiratory conditions.
[A] Metastatic nodules of lung cancer. [B] Erythema nodosum on the shins in sarcoidosis.

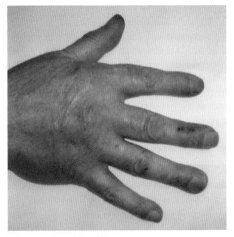

Fig. 5.8 Tobacco 'tar'-stained finger.

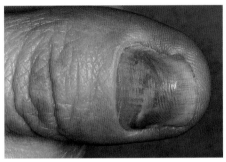

Fig. 5.9 Yellow nail syndrome.

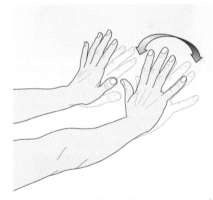

Fig. 5.10 Hand position for testing for the coarse tremor of CO_2 retention.

(Fig. 5.7B) may indicate underlying sarcoidosis, or swelling may signal thromboembolic disease.

Hands and arms

Finger clubbing is due to overgrowth of soft tissue in the terminal phalanx, which increases the lateral and longitudinal curvature of the nail (see Fig. 3.8), raising the nail bed off the underlying bone. It is palpable as a boggy fluctuation of the nail when pressure is applied just proximal to the nail (see Fig. 3.9C). The most common respiratory causes of clubbing are chronic suppurative lung disease (such as bronchiectasis), lung cancer and pulmonary fibrosis (see Box 3.4).

An additional rare complication of lung cancer is hypertrophic pulmonary osteoarthropathy, in which painful, tender swelling of the wrists and ankles accompanies pronounced finger clubbing. X-rays of the distal forearm and lower legs show subperiosteal new bone formation overlying the cortex of the long bones.

Other important signs of respiratory disease in the hands include:

- cyanosis
- tar staining of fingers from tobacco use (Fig. 5.8)
- small-muscle wasting (see Fig. 13.22), which may indicate T1 root damage by an apical lung tumour
- rarely, yellow–brown discoloration of nails in yellow nail syndrome (Fig. 5.9).

Examination sequence

- Examine the hands for finger clubbing (see Fig. 3.9), tar staining, nail discoloration and cyanosis.

- Ask the patient to hold their arms out straight with the wrists extended (Fig. 5.10).
- Check the pulse while examining the hands.
- Check for any tenderness in the distal forearm.

Fine tremor of the outstretched hands is common in respiratory patients and usually due to the direct effect of high-dose beta-agonist bronchodilators on skeletal muscle. A coarse flapping tremor of the outstretched hands is seen in patients with CO_2 retention.

Face

Respiratory disease can cause important signs in the face. Superior vena cava obstruction causes dusky, generalised swelling of the head, neck and face (Fig. 5.11) with subconjunctival oedema (looking like a tear inside the lower lid, but not mobile); this usually indicates tumour invasion of the upper mediastinum. Tumour at the root of the neck may disrupt the sympathetic nerves to the eye, which run from the upper thoracic spinal segments via ganglia in the neck to join the carotid artery sheath. This causes unilateral ptosis and pupillary constriction (Horner's syndrome).

Examination sequence

- Check the conjunctiva of one eye for anaemia, and the colour of the tongue for central cyanosis (Fig. 5.12).
- Check for ptosis and pupil asymmetry.

Remember that cyanosis becomes visible only when a sufficient quantity of deoxyhaemoglobin is circulating, making it hard to detect in anaemia but obvious in polycythaemic patients with only a mild percentage of desaturation.

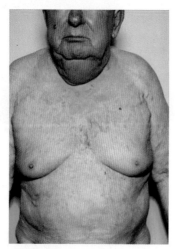

Fig. 5.11 **Superior vena cava obstruction.** Dusky, swollen face and neck, and distended superficial collateral veins on the chest wall. *From Midthun DE, Jett JR. Clinical presentation of lung cancer. In Pass HI, Mitchel JB, Johnson DH, et al. (eds). Lung Cancer: Principles and Practice. Philadelphia: Lippincott–Raven; 1996, p. 421.*

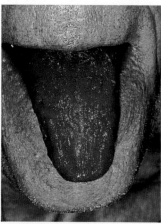

Fig. 5.12 **Central cyanosis of the tongue.**

Neck

Jugular venous pressure (JVP) is raised in many patients with pulmonary hypertension, and may be acutely raised in those with tension pneumothorax or large pulmonary embolism. In superior vena cava obstruction the JVP may be raised above the angle of the jaw, making pulsatility invisible. In those who are using the sternocleidomastoids as accessory muscles (see earlier), it is frequently impossible to see the JVP, as the internal jugular vein lies deep to the active muscle.

Examination sequence

- Support the patient's head with a pillow before examining the neck, to facilitate relaxation of the sternocleidomastoid muscles.
- Examine the JVP (p. 52).
- Check for tracheal deviation by gently advancing a single finger resting in the sternal notch in the midline (Fig. 5.13). If the fingertip meets the centre of the trachea, it is not deviated.
- Check the cricosternal distance (the vertical distance between the sternal notch and the cricoid cartilage, the first prominent ridge felt above the tracheal rings). In health, three average fingers fit between the sternal notch and the cricoid.
- Examine the cervical lymph nodes from behind with the patient sitting forward, as described in full on page 33.

Tracheal deviation away from the affected side is seen acutely in tension pneumothorax. Chronic tracheal deviation towards the affected side occurs with loss of lung volume in upper lobe fibrosis or collapse, and following lobectomy or pneumonectomy.

Reduction in cricosternal distance is a sign of hyperinflation and reflects upward displacement of the sternum (see Fig. 5.5B). Upward movement of the sternum and downward movement of the trachea on inspiration are normal, but may become more obvious with forceful inspiratory efforts in respiratory disease. Rarely, systolic downward movement of the trachea is felt in patients with aortic aneurysm (sometimes called 'tracheal tug'). Cervical lymph nodes are frequently involved in lung neoplasms spreading via the mediastinum.

Thorax

First inspect the chest closely again, in case abnormalities have been missed from the end of the bed. In patients with a thin chest wall and increased respiratory drive (as in exacerbation of

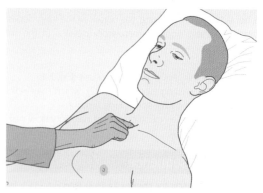

Fig. 5.13 **Examining for tracheal shift.**

asthma or COPD), forced, rapid inspiration often causes visible indrawing of the skin in the intercostal spaces during inspiration, seen more easily with tangential light (see Fig. 5.6A).

Palpation

Examination sequence

- Locate the apex beat, the most inferior and lateral place where the finger is lifted by the twisting systolic movement of the cardiac apex. This is normally in the fifth intercostal space in the mid-clavicular line; count down the intercostal spaces from the second, which is just below the sternal angle.
- Palpate for a right ventricular heave using a straight arm, with the palm over the lower sternum (see Fig. 4.18C).

The apex beat is displaced laterally by dilatation of the ventricles or leftward displacement of the mediastinum. Hyperinflation in obstructive lung disease causes the lingula of the left upper lobe to come between the heart and the chest wall, making the apex beat impalpable and the heart sounds inaudible (see Fig. 5.5B; in this situation the heart sounds are best heard in the epigastrium).

In pulmonary hypertension the lower sternum is lifted by the cardiac cycle (right ventricular heave).

Next assess thoracic expansion in both the upper and lower anterior chest wall.

Examination sequence

- Cup your hands, with fingers spread, round the patient's upper anterior chest wall, pressing the fingertips firmly in the mid-axillary line. Pull your hands medially towards each other to tighten any loose skin, and use your thumbs (off the skin) as pointers to judge how much each hand moves outwards when the patient is instructed to take a full breath in (Fig. 5.14). In a healthy thorax, the ribs move out and up with inspiration.
- Check for any asymmetry. This is more important than the absolute degree of expansion, which will vary between individuals.
- Repeat the process in the lower anterior chest wall.

In COPD with hyperinflation the normal outward movement of the lower ribs on inspiration is replaced by paradoxical inward movement, caused by contraction of the abnormally low flat diaphragm (see Fig. 5.5). This striking sign (paradoxical rib cage movement or 'Hoover's sign') may be missed if expansion is assessed only in the upper chest or from behind.

Palpation of the chest wall may rarely reveal surgical emphysema, indicating air trapped in the subcutaneous tissues (Fig. 5.15). This most commonly complicates pneumothorax with chest drainage or rib fracture, and feels like a palpable crackling under the skin of the upper thorax and neck.

Percussion

Correctly performed, percussion can distinguish areas of the chest wall over air-filled lung from those overlying consolidated lung or fluid. It generates a hollow, ringing sound accompanied by a palpable resonance over air-filled lung, but a dull thud lacking resonance over consolidation or fluid. The absolute quality and volume of the percussed sound vary widely between individuals with differing chest wall thickness, muscularity and subcutaneous fat, and is of little value. The value of percussion lies in detecting asymmetry of resonance between mirror image positions on the right and left sides.

Examination sequence

- To percuss the chest, apply the middle finger of your non-dominant hand firmly to an intercostal space, parallel to the ribs, and drum the middle phalanx with the flexed tip of your dominant index or middle finger (Fig. 5.16A).
- Percuss in sequence, comparing areas on the right with corresponding areas on the left before moving to the next level (Fig. 5.16B).
- Posteriorly, the scapular and spinal muscles obstruct percussion, so position the patient sitting forwards with their arms folded in front to move the scapulae laterally. Percuss a few centimetres lateral to the spinal muscles, taking care to compare positions the same distance from the midline on right and left (Fig. 5.16C).

In healthy people, anterior chest percussion is symmetrical except for the area immediately lateral to the lower left sternal edge, where the right ventricle causes dullness; this 'cardiac dullness' is lost in hyperinflated patients in whom the lingula overlies the heart (see Fig. 5.5). Clear resonance is the usual finding over a pneumothorax, although the difference between normal lung and pneumothorax may be quite subtle because

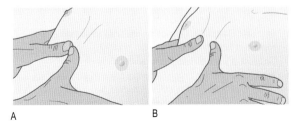

A B

Fig. 5.14 Assessing chest expansion from the front. A Expiration. B Inspiration.

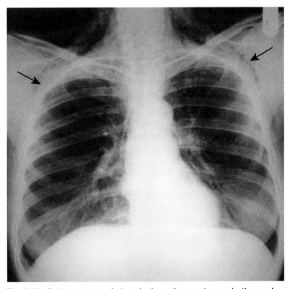

Fig. 5.15 Subcutaneous air (surgical emphysema) seen in the neck and chest wall on chest X-ray *(arrows)*.

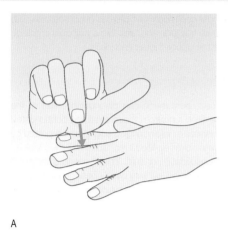
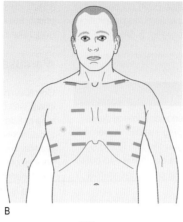
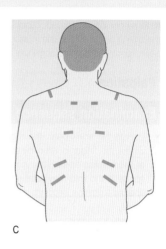

A   B   C

Fig. 5.16 Percussion of the chest. [A] Technique. [B] Anterior and lateral sites. [C] Posterior sites.

normal lung is almost all air. Resonance on percussion together with unilateral absent breath sounds indicates pneumothorax.

Auscultation

To understand chest auscultation it is necessary to understand the origin of breath sounds. The tracheobronchial tree branches 23 times between the trachea and the alveoli. This results in an exponential rise in the number of airways and their combined cross-sectional area moving towards the alveoli. During a maximal breath in and out, the same vital capacity (about 5 L of air in healthy adults) passes through each generation of airway. In the larynx and trachea, this volume must all pass through a cross-sectional area of only a few square centimetres and therefore flow rate is fast, causing turbulence with vibration of the airway wall and generating sound. In the distal airway, the very large total cross-sectional area of the multitude of bronchioles means that 5 L can easily pass at slow flow rates, so flow is normally virtually silent. The harsh 'bronchial' sound generated by the major airways can be appreciated by listening with the diaphragm of the stethoscope applied to the larynx (try this on yourself).

Most of the sound heard when auscultating the chest wall originates in the large central airways but is muffled and deadened by passage through overlying air-filled alveolar tissue; this, together with a small contribution from medium-sized airways, results in 'normal' breath sounds at the chest wall, sometimes termed 'vesicular'. When healthy, air-filled lung becomes consolidated by pneumonia or thickened and stiffened by fibrosis, sound conduction is improved, and the centrally generated 'bronchial' breath sounds appear clearly and loudly on the overlying chest wall. In the same way, with soft speech ('say one, one, one'), the laryngeal sounds are muffled by healthy lung but heard clearly and loudly at the chest wall overlying consolidation and fibrosis, due to improved conduction of major airway sounds through diseased lung.

When there is lobar collapse caused by a proximal bronchial obstruction, the signs are different from those in simple consolidation. The usual findings are diminished expansion, sometimes with chest asymmetry due to loss of volume, dullness to percussion over the collapsed lobe, and reduced breath sounds and vocal resonance.

When the lung tissue is physically separated from the chest wall by intervening air (pneumothorax) or fluid (pleural effusion), sound conduction is greatly impaired and the breath sounds are usually absent. These two causes of absent sounds are readily distinguished by percussion, which will be resonant with pneumothorax and completely dull over pleural fluid.

Use of the stethoscope

Remember to wear the stethoscope with the ear pieces facing forwards to align them with your auditory canal. Normal breath sounds are relatively quiet, so the greater area of contact offered by the diaphragm is usually well adapted to chest auscultation. The two common exceptions are in patients with:

- A cachectic chest wall with sunken intercostal spaces, where it may be impossible to achieve flat skin contact with the diaphragm.
- A hairy chest wall, where movement of chest hairs against the diaphragm are easily mistaken for lung crackles. In these situations, use the stethoscope bell instead to listen to the breath sounds.

Breath sounds

As with percussion, the absolute volume and character of breath sounds in individuals are greatly affected by the thickness, muscularity and fat content of the chest wall. The symmetry of sounds is therefore the key feature.

Examination sequence

- Auscultate the apices, comparing right with left, and changing to the bell if you cannot achieve flat skin contact with the diaphragm.
- Ask the patient to take repeated slow, deep breaths in and out through their open mouth. Auscultate the anterior chest wall from top to bottom, always comparing mirror image positions on right and left before moving down.
- Use the same sequence of sites as for percussion (see Fig. 5.16B and C). Do not waste time by listening to repeated breath cycles at each position, unless you suspect an abnormality and wish to check.
- Note whether the breath sounds are soft and muffled, absent, or loud and harsh (bronchial, like those heard over the larynx). Seek and note any asymmetry and added sounds (see later), deciding which side is abnormal.
- Auscultate the lateral chest wall in the mid-axillary line, again comparing right with left before changing level.

Added sounds

There are three common added sounds: wheezes, crackles and rubs. Wheeze is a musical whistling sound accompanying airflow and usually originates in narrowed small airways. It is most commonly expiratory, due to dynamic airway narrowing on expiration, but can also occur on inspiration. Usually, multiple wheezing sounds are heard together (polyphonic wheeze); this sign is common in asthma, bronchitis and exacerbation of COPD. A solitary wheeze that is present consistently with each breath and does not clear with coughing suggests a possible fixed bronchial obstruction and can be an important sign of underlying cancer.

Crackles accompanying deep breathing are thought to represent the sudden opening of small airways but sometimes may indicate secretions in the airways or underlying lung fibrosis. In healthy people, gravitational compression of the dependent lung bases often causes a few crackles on the first few deep breaths; these are of no pathological significance. Crackles that persist after several breaths and do not clear with a deliberate cough are pathological. They are graded as 'fine', meaning soft, multiple crackles, to 'coarse', indicating loud, scanty crackles that tend to change with each breath. Showers of fine crackles during inspiration, resembling the sound made by peeling a Velcro fastener, are characteristic of interstitial pulmonary fibrosis, and are most commonly heard at the lung bases posteriorly and laterally. Fine crackles also occur in pulmonary oedema and some viral pneumonias. Coarse crackles are generally heard in patients with significant purulent airway secretions such as those with bronchopneumonia or bronchiectasis. Inspiratory crackles are also often heard over the areas of incompletely inflated lung immediately above a pleural effusion.

Pleural rub is a rasping, grating sound occurring with each breath and sounding superficial, just under the stethoscope, like two sheets of sandpaper rubbing together. It indicates pleural inflammation, usually due to infection, and is often accompanied by pleuritic chest pain.

Vocal resonance

Breath sounds normally reveal the presence of consolidation or fibrosis (bronchial breath sounds) or pleural air or fluid (absent breath sounds). These signs can be confirmed by asking the patient to generate laryngeal sounds deliberately ('Please say "one, one, one" each time I move my stethoscope on the skin') and listening on the chest wall in the same sequence of sites used for breath sounds. The spoken sound is muffled and deadened over healthy lung, but the spoken sound is heard loudly and clearly through the stethoscope over consolidation or fibrotic lung scarring. Consistent with absent breath sounds, vocal resonance is absent or greatly diminished over pneumothorax and pleural effusion.

'Whispering pectoriloquy' may be used to confirm the same changes in sound conduction. Whispered speech is muffled to silence by normal lung but may be heard over consolidated or scarred lung.

Interpretation of the findings

Review your findings and assemble the positive features you have uncovered. On completion of the history and examination you should have a broad idea of the category of respiratory illness with which you are dealing. As with any system, consider as you go the likely categories of disease and how these affect presentation. This approach is summarised in Box 5.6.

Investigations

Selecting the relevant investigation depends on the clinical problem revealed on history and examination. Investigations are costly and many carry risks, so choose tests capable of distinguishing the likely diagnoses and prioritise the most decisive ones. In respiratory disease, imaging of the lungs is fundamental, but respiratory function testing is equally important to distinguish obstructive disease of the airways from the restrictive pattern seen in many parenchymal diseases, and to quantify the degree of abnormality. A summary of the appropriate initial investigations according to the type of respiratory presentation is included in Box 5.7.

5.6 Categories of respiratory disease and associated features on history and examination

Category of problem	Suggestive features on history	Suggestive features on examination
Infection: Acute bronchitis Exacerbation of chronic obstructive pulmonary disease Pneumonia	Fever Wheeze, cough, sputum Acute-on-chronic dyspnoea Pleuritic pain, rusty sputum, rigors	 Wheeze Hyperinflation If lobar, dull to percussion and bronchial breathing
Malignancy	Insidious onset, weight loss, persisting pain or cough	Cervical lymphadenopathy, clubbing, signs of lobar/lung collapse ± effusion
Pulmonary fibrosis	Progressive dyspnoea	Tachypnoea, inspiratory fine crackles at bases, cyanosis
Pleural effusion	Progressive dyspnoea	Unilateral basal dullness and reduced breath sounds
Pulmonary embolism: Large Medium Multiple small	 Sudden, severe dyspnoea Episodes of pleural pain, haemoptysis Progressive dyspnoea	 Normal breath sounds Pleural rub, swollen leg if deep vein thrombosis, crackles if infarct Raised jugular venous pressure, right ventricular heave, loud pulmonary second sound
Asthma	Atopy, hay fever, pet ownership, variable wheeze, disturbance of sleep	Polyphonic expiratory wheeze, eczema

5.7 Selecting investigations for different respiratory presentations

Likely problem from history and examination	Appropriate initial investigations	Diagnostic value
Infection (e.g. acute bronchitis, exacerbation of COPD and pneumonia)	Chest X-ray O_2 saturation or ABG Sputum and blood culture Respiratory function WCC, CRP	Consolidation in pneumonia Assessment of respiratory failure Causal infection Quantification of any COPD Degree of inflammation
Malignancy	Chest X-ray CT scan thorax + abdomen Bronchoscopy if central CT-guided biopsy if peripheral Respiratory function	Identification of masses Staging of extent Diagnostic pathology Diagnostic pathology Fitness for radical therapies
Pulmonary fibrosis/interstitial lung disease	Chest X-ray High-resolution CT thorax Respiratory function Autoantibodies	Bi-basal reticular shadows Extent and type of disease Quantification; identification of restrictive pattern Identification of any associated connective tissue disease
Pleural effusion	Chest X-ray Ultrasound-guided aspiration CT thorax + abdomen	Dense basal fluid pool Culture for infection pH low in empyema Glucose low in infection Cytology to identify malignancy Protein to identify transudate or exudate Identification of underlying tumour
Pulmonary embolism	d-Dimer CT pulmonary angiogram Echocardiogram O_2 saturation or ABG	Normal if not pulmonary embolism Detection of emboli Detection of right ventricular strain Assessment of respiratory failure

Asthma	Respiratory function:
	  Peak flow diary
	  FEV_1/reversibility
	O_2 saturation or ABG
	IgE, allergen skin tests
		
		Variable obstruction
		Reversible obstruction
		Assessment of respiratory failure
		Detection of allergic stimuli

ABG, *arterial blood gas;* COPD, *chronic obstructive pulmonary disease;* CRP, *C-reactive protein;* CT, *computed tomography;* FEV_1, *forced expiratory volume in 1 second;* IgE, *immunoglobulin E;* WCC, *white cell count.*

OSCE example 1: Respiratory history

Mrs Walker, 55 years old, presents to the respiratory clinic with cough and wheeze.

Please take a history

- Introduce yourself and clean your hands.
- Ask an open question about why this person has come to the clinic.
- Explore each presenting symptom:
  - Cough:
    - Onset, duration?
    - Productive? If so, characterise sputum volume and colour, and any blood.
    - Triggers? Did it start with an upper respiratory tract infection? Is it provoked by exercise or environment?
    - Time pattern – nocturnal (suggests asthma or reflux)?
    - On angiotensin-converting enzyme inhibitors?
  - Wheeze:
    - What exactly does the patient mean by 'wheeze'?
    - When does it occur – at night or during exercise?
    - Provoking factors – infection, environment, contact with animals, dust, beta-blockers?
    - Any relieving factors – inhalers?
    - Associated respiratory symptoms – breathlessness, chest pain, fevers/rigors, weight loss.
- Ask about past respiratory diagnoses, particularly childhood wheeze or asthma, rhinitis/hay fever and prior respiratory treatments/admissions.
- Explore past non-respiratory illness: for example, eczema (suggests atopy), hypertension or angina (on beta-blockers?), other prior illnesses.
- Take a drug history – prescribed medications, including inhalers/nebulisers and recreational drugs.
- Ask about any known allergies.
- Take a social history: smoking, occupation, contact with animals.

OSCE example 1: Respiratory history – *cont'd*

- Establish whether there is a family history of respiratory disease (including asthma).
- Ask about any other patient concerns.
- Thank the patient and clean your hands.

Summarise your findings

Mrs Walker is a 55-year-old cook who gives a 6-month history of wheeze disturbing her sleep, associated with an unproductive cough. Her symptoms vary from day to day and sometimes make climbing stairs difficult. She smokes 10 cigarettes a day and has a 20-pack-year smoking history.

Suggest a differential diagnosis

The most likely diagnosis is asthma (variable, nocturnal symptoms) and the differential is chronic obstructive pulmonary disease.

Suggest initial investigations

Spirometry and reversibility, peak-flow diary, chest X-ray, blood count for eosinophils, serum immunoglobulin E, and skin tests to common allergens.

5

OSCE example 2: Respiratory examination

Mr Tate, 82 years old, reports increasing breathlessness over several weeks.

Please examine his respiratory system

- Introduce yourself and clean your hands.
- Note clues around the patient, such as oxygen, nebulisers, inhalers or sputum pots.
- Observe from the end of the bed:
  - Scars, chest shape, asymmetry, pattern of breathing, accessory muscle use.
  - Chest wall movement, paradoxical rib movement, intercostal indrawing.
- Examine the hands: clubbing, tar staining, muscle wasting.
- Check for tremor and flap.
- Measure respiratory rate unobtrusively.
- Examine the face: anaemia, cyanosis, Horner's syndrome and superior vena cava obstruction.
- Examine the neck: jugular venous pressure, tracheal deviation, cricosternal distance.
- Examine the anterior chest wall:
  - Palpate: apex beat, right ventricular heave, expansion of the upper and lower chest.
  - Percuss: compare right with left, from top with bottom, then axillae.
  - Auscultate: deep breaths; compare right with left, from top with bottom, then axillae. Repeat, checking vocal resonance.
- Examine the posterior chest wall (commonly in OSCEs, you may be directed to examine either anterior or posterior):
  - Ask the patient to sit forwards.
  - Inspect the back for scars, asymmetry and so on.
  - Palpate:
    - Cervical lymph nodes.
    - Chest expansion of the upper and lower chest.
  - Percuss: ask the patient to fold his arms at the front to part the scapulae; compare right with left, from top to bottom.
  - Auscultate: deep breaths; compare right with left, from top to bottom, then axillae. Repeat, checking vocal resonance.
- Check for pitting oedema over the sacrum and lumbar spine.
- Thank the patient and clean your hands.

Summarise your findings

The patient has finger clubbing, a raised respiratory rate, and diminished expansion with dullness to percussion and loss of breath sounds at the right base. A small scar suggests prior pleural aspiration.

Suggest a differential diagnosis

Signs suggest a large right pleural effusion.
(Away from patient's bedside) A large unilateral effusion with finger clubbing suggests an underlying neoplasm. Alternatives include chronic empyema and tuberculous effusion.

Suggest initial investigations

Chest X-ray to confirm effusion and possibly show an underlying tumour. Ultrasound to reveal pleural disease and loculation, and guide aspiration. Pleural aspiration for cytology, culture and biochemical analysis.

Integrated examination sequence for the respiratory system

- Introduce yourself and seek the patient's consent to chest examination.
- Position the patient: resting comfortably, with the chest supported at about 45 degrees and the head resting on a pillow.
- Carry out general observations: note any clues around the patient, such as oxygen, nebulisers, inhalers, sputum pots, etc.
- Observe from the end of the bed:
  - Scars.
  - Chest shape, asymmetry.
  - Pattern of breathing:
    - Respiratory rate.
    - Time spent in inspiration and expiration.
    - Pursed-lip breathing.
  - Chest wall movement, paradoxical rib movement, intercostal indrawing.
  - Accessory muscle use.
- Examine the hands:
  - Clubbing, tar staining, muscle wasting.
  - Check for tremor and flap.
  - Measure respiratory rate unobtrusively.
- Examine the face:
  - Check for anaemia, cyanosis, Horner's syndrome and signs of superior vena cava obstruction.
- Examine the neck:
  - Jugular venous pressure, tracheal deviation and cricosternal distance.
- Examine the anterior chest wall:
  - Palpate: apex beat, right ventricular heave, expansion of upper and lower chest.
  - Percuss: compare right with left, from top to bottom, then axillae.
  - Auscultate: deep breaths; compare right with left, from top to bottom, then axillae. Repeat positions, asking the patient to say 'one, one, one' for vocal resonance.
- Examine the posterior chest wall: ask the patient to sit forwards so that you can:
  - Inspect the back for scars, asymmetry and so on.
  - Palpate:
    - Cervical lymph nodes.
    - Expansion of the upper and lower chest.
  - Percuss: ask the patient to fold their arms at the front to part the scapulae. Compare right with left, from top to bottom (see Fig. 5.16A–C for positions).
  - Auscultate: deep breaths; compare right with left, from top to bottom, then axillae. Repeat positions, asking the patient to say 'one, one, one' for vocal resonance.
- Check for pitting oedema over the sacrum and lumbar spine.

John Plevris
Rowan Parks

The gastrointestinal system

Anatomy and physiology

The gastrointestinal system comprises the alimentary tract, the liver, the biliary system, the pancreas and the spleen. The alimentary tract extends from the mouth to the anus and includes the oesophagus, stomach, small intestine or small bowel (comprising the duodenum, jejunum and ileum), colon (large intestine or large bowel) and rectum (Figs 6.1–6.2 and Box 6.1).

The abdominal surface can be divided into nine regions by the intersection of two horizontal and two vertical planes (Fig. 6.1C).

The history

Gastrointestinal symptoms are common and are often caused by functional dyspepsia and irritable bowel syndrome. Symptoms suggesting a serious alternative or coexistent diagnosis include persistent vomiting, dysphagia, gastrointestinal bleeding, weight loss, painless, watery, high-volume diarrhoea, nocturnal symptoms, fever and anaemia. The risk of serious disease increases with age. Always explore the patient's ideas, concerns and expectations about the symptoms (p. 5) to understand the clinical context.

Common presenting symptoms

Mouth symptoms

Bad breath (halitosis) due to gingival, dental or pharyngeal infection and dry mouth (xerostomia) are common mouth symptoms. Rarely, patients complain of altered taste sensation (dysgeusia) or of a foul taste in the mouth (cacogeusia).

Anorexia and weight loss

Anorexia is loss of appetite and/or a lack of interest in food. In addition to enquiring about appetite, ask 'Do you still enjoy your food?'

Weight loss, in isolation, is rarely associated with serious organic disease. Ask how much weight has been lost, over what time. Loss of <3 kg in the previous 6 months is rarely significant. Weight loss is usually the result of reduced energy intake, not increased energy expenditure. It does not specifically indicate gastrointestinal disease, although it is common in many gastrointestinal disorders, including malignancy and liver disease. Energy requirements average 2500 kcal/day for males

and 2000 kcal/day for females. Reduced energy intake arises from dieting, loss of appetite, malabsorption or malnutrition. Increased energy expenditure occurs in hyperthyroidism, fever or the adoption of a more energetic lifestyle. A net calorie deficit of 1000 kcal/day results in weight loss of approximately

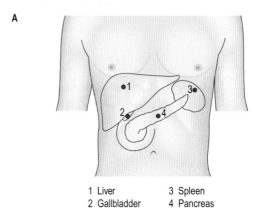

A

1 Liver   3 Spleen
2 Gallbladder   4 Pancreas

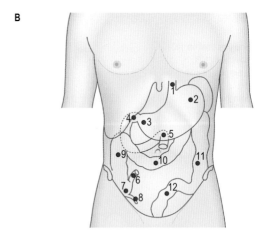

B

1 Oesophagus	7 Caecum
2 Stomach	8 Appendix (in pelvic position)
3 Pyloric antrum	9 Ascending colon
4 Duodenum	10 Transverse colon
5 Duodenojejunal flexure	11 Descending colon
6 Terminal ileum	12 Sigmoid colon

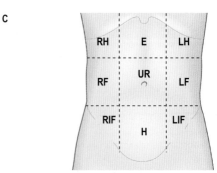

C

Fig. 6.1 Surface anatomy. A Abdominal surface markings of non-alimentary tract viscera. B Surface markings of the alimentary tract. C Regions of the abdomen. *E,* epigastrium; *H,* hypogastrium or suprapubic region; *LF,* left flank or lumbar region; *LH,* left hypochondrium; *LIF,* left iliac fossa; *RF,* right flank or lumbar region; *RH,* right hypochondrium; *RIF,* right iliac fossa; *UR,* umbilical region.

6.1 Surface markings of the main non-alimentary tract abdominal organs	
Structure	**Position**
Liver	Upper border: fifth right intercostal space on full expiration Lower border: at the costal margin in the mid-clavicular line on full inspiration
Spleen	Underlies left ribs 9–11, posterior to the mid-axillary line
Gallbladder	At the intersection of the right lateral vertical plane and the costal margin, i.e. tip of the ninth costal cartilage
Pancreas	Neck of the pancreas lies at the level of L1; head lies below and right; tail lies above and left
Kidneys	Upper pole lies deep to the 12th rib posteriorly, 7 cm from the midline; the right is 2–3 cm lower than the left

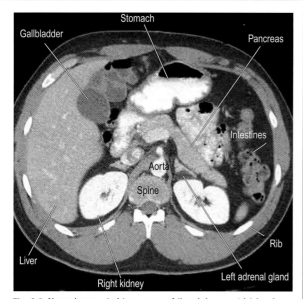

Fig. 6.2 **Normal computed tomogram of the abdomen at L1 level.**

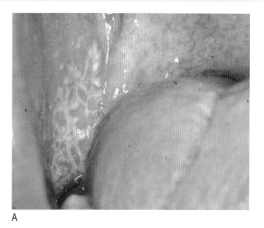

A

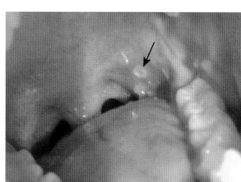

B

Fig. 6.3 **Some causes of a painful mouth.** A Lichen planus. B Small, 'punched-out' aphthous ulcer *(arrow)*.

1 kg/week (7000 kcal ≅ 1 kg of fat). Greater weight loss during the initial stages of energy restriction arises from salt and water loss and depletion of hepatic glycogen stores, not from fat loss. Rapid weight loss over days suggests loss of body fluid as a result of vomiting, diarrhoea or diuretics (1 L of water = 1 kg). Check current and previous weight records to confirm apparent weight loss on examination (loose-fitting clothes, for example).

Pain

Painful mouth

Causes of sore lips, tongue or buccal mucosa include:
- deficiencies, including iron, folate, vitamin B_{12} or C
- dermatological disorders, including lichen planus (Fig. 6.3A)
- chemotherapy
- aphthous ulcers (Fig. 6.3B)
- infective stomatitis
- inflammatory bowel disease and coeliac disease, associated with mouth ulcers.

Heartburn and reflux

Heartburn is a hot, burning retrosternal discomfort.

To differentiate heartburn from cardiac chest pain, ask about associated features:
- character of pain: burning
- radiation: upward
- precipitating factors: lying flat or bending forward
- associated symptoms:
  - waterbrash (sudden appearance of fluid in the mouth due to reflex salivation as a result of gastro-oesophageal reflux disease (GORD) or, rarely, peptic ulcer disease)
  - the taste of acid appearing in the mouth due to reflux/regurgitation.

When heartburn is the principal symptom, GORD is the most likely diagnosis.

Dyspepsia

Dyspepsia is pain or discomfort centred in the upper abdomen. In contrast, 'indigestion' is a term commonly used by patients for ill-defined symptoms from the upper gastrointestinal tract.

Ask about:
- site of pain
- character of pain
- exacerbating and relieving factors, such as food and antacid
- associated symptoms, such as nausea, belching, bloating and premature satiety.

Clusters of symptoms are used to classify dyspepsia:
- reflux-like dyspepsia (heartburn-predominant dyspepsia)
- ulcer-like dyspepsia (epigastric pain relieved by food or antacids)
- dysmotility-like dyspepsia (nausea, belching, bloating and premature satiety).

Often there is no structural cause and the dyspepsia is functional. There is considerable overlap, however, and it is impossible to diagnose functional dyspepsia on history alone without investigation. Dyspepsia that is worse with an empty stomach and eased by eating is typical of peptic ulceration. The patient may indicate a single localised point in the epigastrium (pointing sign), and complain of nausea and abdominal fullness

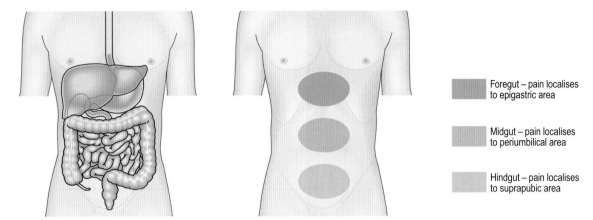

Fig. 6.4 Abdominal pain. Perception of visceral pain is localised to the epigastric, umbilical or suprapubic region, according to the embryological origin of the affected organ.

that is worse after fatty or spicy meals. 'Fat intolerance' is common with all causes of dyspepsia, including gallbladder disease.

Odynophagia

Odynophagia is pain on swallowing, often precipitated by drinking hot liquids. It can be present with or without dysphagia (see below) and may indicate oesophageal ulceration or oesophagitis from gastro-oesophageal reflux or oesophageal candidiasis. It implies intact mucosal sensation, making oesophageal cancer unlikely.

Abdominal pain

Characterise the pain using SOCRATES (see Box 2.2). Ask about the characteristics described here.

Site

Visceral abdominal pain from distension of hollow organs, mesenteric traction or excessive smooth-muscle contraction is deep and poorly localised in the midline. The pain is conducted via sympathetic splanchnic nerves. Somatic pain from the parietal peritoneum and abdominal wall is lateralised and localised to the inflamed area. It is conducted via intercostal nerves.

Pain arising from foregut structures (stomach, pancreas, liver and biliary system) is localised above the umbilicus (Fig. 6.4). Central abdominal pain arises from midgut structures, such as the small bowel and appendix. Lower abdominal pain arises from hindgut structures, such as the colon. Inflammation may cause localised pain: for example, left iliac fossa pain due to diverticular disease of the sigmoid colon.

Pain from an unpaired structure, such as the pancreas, is midline and radiates through to the back. Pain from paired structures, such as renal colic, is felt on and radiates to the affected side (Fig. 6.5). Torsion of the testis may present with abdominal pain (p. 232). In females, consider gynaecological causes like ruptured ovarian cyst, pelvic inflammatory disease, endometriosis or ectopic pregnancy (p. 218).

Onset

Sudden onset of severe abdominal pain, rapidly progressing to become generalised and constant, suggests a hollow viscus perforation (usually due to colorectal cancer, diverticular disease or peptic ulceration), a ruptured abdominal aortic aneurysm or mesenteric infarction.

Torsion of the caecum or sigmoid colon (volvulus) presents with sudden abdominal pain associated with acute intestinal obstruction.

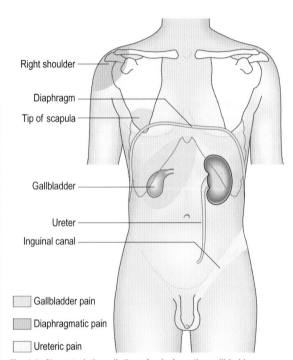

Fig. 6.5 Characteristic radiation of pain from the gallbladder, diaphragm and ureters.

Character

Colicky pain lasts for a short time (seconds or minutes), eases off and then returns. It arises from hollow structures, as in small or large bowel obstruction, or the uterus during labour.

Biliary and renal 'colic' are misnamed, as the pain is rarely colicky; pain rapidly increases to a peak and persists over several hours before gradually resolving. Dull, constant, vague and poorly localised pain is more typical of an inflammatory process or infection, such as salpingitis, appendicitis or diverticulitis (Box 6.2).

Radiation

Pain radiating from the right hypochondrium to the shoulder or interscapular region may reflect diaphragmatic irritation, as in acute cholecystitis (see Fig. 6.5). Pain radiating from the loin to the groin and genitalia is typical of renal colic. Central upper abdominal pain radiating through to the back, partially relieved by

6.2 Diagnosing abdominal pain

	Disorder			
	Peptic ulcer	Biliary colic	Acute pancreatitis	Renal colic
Site	Epigastrium	Epigastrium/right hypochondrium	Epigastrium/left hypochondrium	Loin
Onset	Gradual	Rapidly increasing	Sudden	Rapidly increasing
Character	Gnawing	Constant	Constant	Constant
Radiation	Into back	Below right scapula	Into back	Into genitalia and inner thigh
Associated symptoms	Non-specific	Non-specific	Non-specific	Non-specific
Timing Frequency/periodicity Special times Duration	Remission for weeks/months Nocturnal and especially when hungry ½–2 hours	Attacks can be enumerated Unpredictable 4–24 hours	Attacks can be enumerated After heavy drinking >24 hours	Usually a discrete episode Following periods of dehydration 4–24 hours
Exacerbating factors	Stress, spicy foods, alcohol, non-steroidal anti-inflammatory drugs	Eating – unable to eat during bouts	Alcohol Eating – unable to eat during bouts	–
Relieving factors	Food, antacids, vomiting	–	Sitting upright	–
Severity	Mild to moderate	Severe	Severe	Severe

sitting forward, suggests pancreatitis. Central abdominal pain that later shifts into the right iliac fossa occurs in acute appendicitis. The combination of severe back and abdominal pain may indicate a ruptured or dissecting abdominal aortic aneurysm.

Associated symptoms

Anorexia, nausea and vomiting are common but non-specific symptoms. They may accompany any very severe pain but conversely may be absent, even in advanced intra-abdominal disease. Abdominal pain due to irritable bowel syndrome, diverticular disease or colorectal cancer is usually accompanied by altered bowel habit. Other features such as breathlessness or palpitation suggest non-alimentary causes (Box 6.3).

Hypotension and tachycardia following the onset of pain suggest intra-abdominal sepsis or bleeding: for example, from a peptic ulcer, a ruptured aortic aneurysm or an ectopic pregnancy.

Timing

During the first 1–2 hours after perforation, a 'silent interval' may occur when abdominal pain resolves transiently. The initial chemical peritonitis may subside before bacterial peritonitis becomes established. For example, in acute appendicitis, pain is initially periumbilical (visceral pain) and moves to the right iliac fossa (somatic pain) when localised inflammation of the parietal peritoneum becomes established. If the appendix ruptures, generalised peritonitis may develop. Occasionally, a localised appendix abscess develops, with a palpable mass and localised pain in the right iliac fossa.

Change in the pattern of symptoms suggests either that the initial diagnosis was wrong or that complications have developed. In acute small bowel obstruction, a change from typical intestinal colic to persistent pain with abdominal tenderness suggests intestinal ischaemia, as in strangulated hernia, and is an indication for urgent surgical intervention.

Abdominal pain persisting for hours or days suggests an inflammatory disorder, such as acute appendicitis, cholecystitis or diverticulitis.

6.3 Non-alimentary causes of abdominal pain

Disorder	Clinical features
Myocardial infarction	Epigastric pain without tenderness *Angor animi* (feeling of impending death) Hypotension Cardiac arrhythmias
Dissecting aortic aneurysm	Tearing interscapular pain *Angor animi* Hypotension Asymmetry of femoral pulses
Acute vertebral collapse	Lateralised pain restricting movement Tenderness overlying involved vertebra
Cord compression	Pain on percussion of thoracic spine Hyperaesthesia at affected dermatome with sensory loss below Spinal cord signs
Pleurisy	Lateralised pain on coughing Chest signs, e.g. pleural rub
Herpes zoster	Hyperaesthesia in dermatomal distribution Vesicular eruption
Diabetic ketoacidosis	Cramp-like pain Vomiting Air hunger Tachycardia Ketotic breath
Salpingitis or tubal pregnancy	Suprapubic and iliac fossa pain, localised tenderness Nausea, vomiting Fever
Torsion of testis/ovary	Lower abdominal pain Nausea, vomiting Localised tenderness

Exacerbating and relieving factors

Pain exacerbated by movement or coughing suggests inflammation. Patients tend to lie still to avoid exacerbating the pain. People with colic typically move around or draw their knees up towards the chest during spasms.

Severity

Excruciating pain, poorly relieved by opioid analgesia, suggests an ischaemic vascular event, such as bowel infarction or ruptured abdominal aortic aneurysm. Severe pain rapidly eased by potent analgesia is more typical of acute pancreatitis or peritonitis secondary to a ruptured viscus.

Features of the pain can help distinguish between possible causes (Box 6.3).

The acute abdomen

The majority of general surgical emergencies are patients with sudden severe abdominal pain (an 'acute abdomen'). Patients may be so occupied by recent and severe symptoms that they forget important details of the history unless asked directly. Seek additional information from family or friends if severe pain, shock or altered consciousness makes it difficult to obtain a history from the patient. Note any relevant past history, such as acute perforation in a patient with known diverticular disease. Causes range from self-limiting to severe life-threatening diseases (Box 6.4). Evaluate patients rapidly, and then resuscitate critically ill patients immediately before undertaking further assessment and surgical intervention. Parenteral opioid analgesia to alleviate severe abdominal pain will help, not hinder, clinical assessment. In patients with undiagnosed acute abdominal pain, reassess their clinical state regularly, undertake urgent investigations and consider surgical intervention before administering repeat analgesia.

▌Dysphagia

Patients with dysphagia complain that food or drink sticks when they swallow.

Ask about:

- onset: recent or longstanding
- nature: intermittent or progressive
- difficulty swallowing solids, liquids or both
- the level the patient feels food sticks at
- any regurgitation or reflux of food or fluid
- any associated pain (odynophagia), heartburn or weight loss.

Do not confuse dysphagia with early satiety, the inability to complete a full meal because of premature fullness, or with globus, which is a feeling of a lump in the throat. Globus does not interfere with swallowing and is not related to eating.

Neurological dysphagia resulting from bulbar or pseudobulbar palsy (p. 129) is worse for liquids than solids, and may be accompanied by choking, spluttering and fluid regurgitating from the nose.

Neuromuscular dysphagia, or oesophageal dysmotility, presents in middle age, is worse for solids and may be helped by liquids and sitting upright. Achalasia, when the lower oesophageal sphincter fails to relax normally, leads to progressive oesophageal dilatation above the sphincter. Overflow of secretions and food into the respiratory tract may then occur, especially at night when the patient lies down, causing aspiration pneumonia. Oesophageal dysmotility can cause oesophageal spasm and central chest pain, which may be confused with cardiac pain.

A pharyngeal pouch may cause food to stick or be regurgitated, and may lead to recurrent chest infections due to chronic silent aspiration.

6.4 Typical clinical features in patients with an 'acute abdomen'

Condition	History	Examination
Acute appendicitis	Nausea, vomiting, central abdominal pain that later shifts to right iliac fossa	Fever, tenderness, guarding or palpable mass in right iliac fossa, pelvic peritonitis on rectal examination
Perforated peptic ulcer with acute peritonitis	Vomiting at onset associated with severe acute-onset abdominal pain, previous history of dyspepsia, ulcer disease, non-steroidal anti-inflammatory drugs or glucocorticoid therapy	Shallow breathing with minimal abdominal wall movement, abdominal tenderness and guarding, board-like rigidity, abdominal distension and absent bowel sounds
Acute pancreatitis	Anorexia, nausea, vomiting, constant severe epigastric pain, previous alcohol abuse/cholelithiasis	Fever, periumbilical or loin bruising, epigastric tenderness, variable guarding, reduced or absent bowel sounds
Ruptured aortic aneurysm	Sudden onset of severe, tearing back/loin/abdominal pain, hypotension and past history of vascular disease and/or high blood pressure	Shock and hypotension, pulsatile, tender, abdominal mass, asymmetrical femoral pulses
Acute mesenteric ischaemia	Anorexia, nausea, vomiting, bloody diarrhoea, constant abdominal pain, previous history of vascular disease and/or high blood pressure	Atrial fibrillation, heart failure, asymmetrical peripheral pulses, absent bowel sounds, variable tenderness and guarding
Intestinal obstruction	Colicky central abdominal pain, nausea, vomiting and constipation	Surgical scars, hernias, mass, distension, visible peristalsis, increased bowel sounds
Ruptured ectopic pregnancy	Premenopausal female, delayed or missed menstrual period, hypotension, unilateral iliac fossa pain, pleuritic shoulder-tip pain, 'prune juice'-like vaginal discharge	Suprapubic tenderness, periumbilical bruising, pain and tenderness on vaginal examination (cervical excitation), swelling/fullness in fornix on vaginal examination
Pelvic inflammatory disease	Sexually active young female, previous history of sexually transmitted infection, recent gynaecological procedure, pregnancy or use of intrauterine contraceptive device, irregular menstruation, dyspareunia, lower or central abdominal pain, backache, pleuritic right upper quadrant pain (Fitz-Hugh–Curtis syndrome)	Fever, vaginal discharge, pelvic peritonitis causing tenderness on rectal examination, right upper quadrant tenderness (perihepatitis), pain/tenderness on vaginal examination (cervical excitation), swelling/fullness in fornix on vaginal examination

'Mechanical' dysphagia is often due to oesophageal stricture but can be caused by external compression. With weight loss, a short history and no reflux symptoms, suspect oesophageal cancer. Longstanding dysphagia without weight loss but accompanied by heartburn is more likely to be due to benign peptic stricture. Record the site at which the patient feels the food sticking; this is not a reliable guide to the site of oesophageal obstruction, however.

Nausea and vomiting

Nausea is the sensation of feeling sick. Vomiting is the expulsion of gastric contents via the mouth. Both are associated with pallor, sweating and hyperventilation.

Ask about:

- relation to meals and timing, such as early morning or late evening
- associated symptoms, such as dyspepsia and abdominal pain, and whether they are relieved by vomiting
- whether the vomit is bile-stained (green), blood-stained or faeculent
- associated weight loss
- the patient's medications.

Nausea and vomiting, particularly with abdominal pain or discomfort, suggest upper gastrointestinal disorders. Dyspepsia causes nausea without vomiting. Peptic ulcers seldom cause painless vomiting unless they are complicated by pyloric stenosis, which causes projectile vomiting of large volumes of gastric content that is not bile-stained. Obstruction distal to the pylorus produces bile-stained vomit. Severe vomiting without significant pain suggests gastric outlet or proximal small bowel obstruction. Faeculent vomiting of small bowel contents (not faeces) is a late feature of distal small bowel or colonic obstruction. In peritonitis, the vomitus is usually small in volume but persistent. The more distal the level of intestinal obstruction, the more marked the accompanying abdominal distension and colic.

Vomiting is common in gastroenteritis, cholecystitis, pancreatitis and hepatitis. It is typically preceded by nausea but in raised intracranial pressure may occur without warning. Severe pain may precipitate vomiting, as in renal or biliary colic or myocardial infarction.

Anorexia nervosa and bulimia are eating disorders characterised by undisclosed, self-induced vomiting. In bulimia, weight is maintained or increased, unlike in anorexia nervosa, where profound weight loss is common.

Other non-gastrointestinal causes of nausea and vomiting include:

- drugs, such as alcohol, opioids, theophyllines, digoxin, cytotoxic agents or antidepressants
- pregnancy
- diabetic ketoacidosis
- renal or liver failure
- hypercalcaemia
- Addison's disease
- raised intracranial pressure (meningitis, brain tumour)
- vestibular disorders (labyrinthitis and Ménière's disease).

Wind and flatulence

Belching, excessive or offensive flatus, abdominal distension and borborygmi (audible bowel sounds) are often called 'wind' or flatulence. Clarify exactly what the patient means. Belching is due to air swallowing (aerophagy) and has no medical significance.

It may indicate anxiety but sometimes occurs in an attempt to relieve abdominal pain or discomfort, and accompanies GORD.

Normally, 200–2000 mL of flatus is passed each day. Flatus is a mixture of gases derived from swallowed air and from colonic bacterial fermentation of poorly absorbed carbohydrates. Excessive flatus occurs particularly in lactase deficiency and intestinal malabsorption.

Borborygmi result from movement of fluid and gas along the bowel. Loud borborygmi, particularly if associated with colicky discomfort, suggest small bowel obstruction or dysmotility.

Abdominal distension

Abdominal girth slowly increasing over months or years is usually due to obesity but in a patient with weight loss it suggests intra-abdominal disease. The most common causes of abdominal distension are:

- fat in obesity
- flatus in pseudo-obstruction or bowel obstruction
- faeces in subacute obstruction or constipation
- fluid in ascites (accumulation of fluid in the peritoneal cavity; Fig. 6.6), tumours (especially ovarian) or distended bladder
- fetus
- functional bloating (fluctuating abdominal distension that develops during the day and resolves overnight, usually occurring in irritable bowel syndrome).

Altered bowel habit

Diarrhoea

Clarify what patients mean by diarrhoea. They may complain of frequent stools or of a change in consistency of the stools. Normal frequency ranges from three bowel movements daily to once every 3 days. Diarrhoea is the frequent passage of loose stools. Steatorrhoea is diarrhoea associated with fat malabsorption. The stools are greasy, pale and bulky, and they float, making them difficult to flush away.

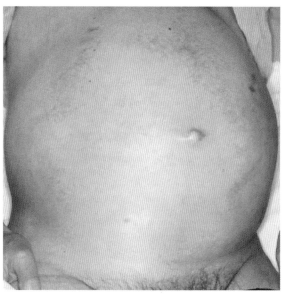

Fig. 6.6 Abdominal distension due to ascites.

Ask about:

- onset of diarrhoea: acute, chronic or intermittent
- stool:
  - frequency
  - volume
  - colour
  - consistency: watery, unformed or semisolid
  - contents: red blood, mucus or pus
- associated features: urgency, faecal incontinence or tenesmus (the sensation of needing to defecate, although the rectum is empty), abdominal pain, vomiting, sleep disturbance
- recent travel and where to
- recent medication, in particular any antibiotics.

High-volume diarrhoea (>1 L per day) occurs when stool water content is increased (the principal site of physiological water absorption being the colon) and may be:

- secretory, due to intestinal inflammation, as in infection or inflammatory bowel disease
- osmotic, due to malabsorption, drugs (as in laxative abuse) or motility disorders (autonomic neuropathy, particularly in diabetes).

If the patient fasts, osmotic diarrhoea stops but secretory diarrhoea persists. The most common cause of acute diarrhoea is infective gastroenteritis due to norovirus, *Salmonella* species or *Clostridium difficile*. Infective diarrhoea can become chronic (>4 weeks) in cases of parasitic infestations (such as giardiasis (*Giardia lamblia*), amoebiasis or cryptosporidiosis). Steatorrhoea is common in coeliac disease, chronic pancreatitis and pancreatic insufficiency due to cystic fibrosis. Bloody diarrhoea may be caused by inflammatory bowel disease, colonic ischaemia or infective gastroenteritis. Change in the bowel habit towards diarrhoea can be a manifestation of colon cancer, in particular cancer of the right side of the colon and in patients over 50 years. Thyrotoxicosis is often accompanied by secretory diarrhoea or steatorrhoea and weight loss.

Low-volume diarrhoea is associated with irritable bowel syndrome. Abdominal pain, bloating, dyspepsia and non-alimentary symptoms commonly accompany irritable bowel symptoms. Criteria have been developed to define irritable bowel syndrome more precisely, taking account of the duration of symptoms, the presence of abdominal pain and its relationship to defecation, and the frequency and consistency of stools (see Rome IV criteria for irritable bowel syndrome).

Constipation

Clarify what the patient means by constipation. Use the Bristol stool form scale (Fig. 6.7) to describe the stools. Constipation is the infrequent passage of hard stools.

Ask about:

- onset: lifelong or of recent onset
- stool frequency: how often the patient moves their bowels each week and how much time is spent straining at stool
- shape of the stool: for example, pellet-like
- associated symptoms, such as abdominal pain, anal pain on defecation or rectal bleeding
- drugs that may cause constipation.

Constipation may be due to lack of dietary fibre, impaired colonic motility, mechanical intestinal obstruction, impaired rectal sensation or anorectal dysfunction impairing the process of defecation. Constipation is common in irritable bowel syndrome. Other important causes include colorectal cancer, hypothyroidism,

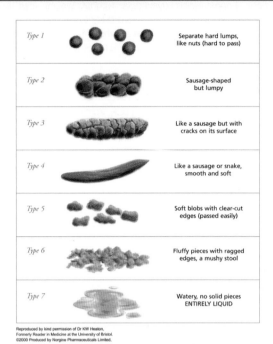

Fig. 6.7 **Bristol stool form scale.** *Reproduced with kind permission of Dr KW Heaton, formerly Reader in Medicine at the University of Bristol. ©2000, Norgine group of companies.*

hypercalcaemia, drugs (opiates, iron) and immobility (Parkinson's disease, stroke). Absolute constipation (no flatus or bowel movements) suggests intestinal obstruction and is usually associated with pain, vomiting and distension. Tenesmus suggests rectal inflammation or tumour. Faecal impaction can occasionally present as overflow diarrhoea.

Bleeding

Haematemesis

Haematemesis is the vomiting of blood.

Ask about:

- Colour: is the vomitus fresh red blood or dark brown, resembling coffee grounds?
- Onset: was haematemesis preceded by intense retching or was blood staining apparent in the first vomit?
- History of dyspepsia, peptic ulceration, gastrointestinal bleeding or liver disease.
- Alcohol, non-steroidal anti-inflammatory drugs (NSAIDs) and glucocorticoid ingestion.

If the source of bleeding is above the gastro-oesophageal sphincter, as with oesophageal varices, fresh blood may well up in the mouth, as well as being actively vomited. With a lower oesophageal mucosal tear due to the trauma of forceful retching (Mallory–Weiss syndrome), fresh blood appears only after the patient has vomited forcefully several times.

6.5 Prediction of the risk of mortality in patients with upper gastrointestinal bleeding: Rockall score

Criterion	Score
Age	
<60 years	0
60–79 years	1
>80 years	2
Shock	
None	0
Pulse >100 beats per minute and systolic blood pressure >100 mmHg	1
Systolic blood pressure <100 mmHg	2
Comorbidity	
None	0
Heart failure, ischaemic heart disease or other major illness	2
Renal failure or disseminated malignancy	3
Endoscopic findings	
Mallory–Weiss tear and no visible bleeding	0
All other diagnoses	1
Upper gastrointestinal malignancy	2
Major stigmata of recent haemorrhage	
None	0
Visible bleeding vessel/adherent clot	2
Total score	
Pre-endoscopy (maximum score = 7)	Score 4 = 14% mortality pre-endoscopy
Post-endoscopy (maximum score = 11)	Score 8+ = 25% mortality post-endoscopy

Reproduced from Rockall TA, Logan RF, Devlin HB, et al. Risk assessment after acute upper gastrointestinal haemorrhage. Journal of the British Society of Gastroenterology 1996; 38(3):316, with permission from BMJ Publishing Group Ltd.

Melaena

Melaena is the passage of tarry, shiny black stools with a characteristic odour and results from upper gastrointestinal bleeding. Distinguish this from the matt black stools associated with oral iron or bismuth therapy.

Peptic ulceration (gastric or duodenal) is the most common cause of upper gastrointestinal bleeding and can manifest with melaena, haematemesis or both. Excessive alcohol ingestion may cause haematemesis from erosive gastritis, Mallory–Weiss tear or bleeding oesophagogastric varices in cirrhotic patients. Oesophageal or gastric cancer and gastric angioectasias (Dieulafoy lesion) are rare causes of upper gastrointestinal bleeding.

The Rockall and Blatchford scores are used to assess the risk in gastrointestinal bleeding (Box 6.5). A profound upper gastrointestinal bleed may lead to the passage of purple stool or, rarely, fresh blood.

Rectal bleeding

Establish whether the blood is mixed with stool, coats the surface of otherwise normal stool or is seen on the toilet paper or in the pan. Fresh rectal bleeding (haematochezia) usually indicates a disorder in the anal canal, rectum or colon. During severe upper gastrointestinal bleeding, however, blood may pass through the intestine unaltered, causing fresh rectal bleeding. Common causes of rectal bleeding include haemorrhoids, anal fissures (blood on the toilet paper or in the pan), complicated diverticular disease,

6.6 Common causes of jaundice

Increased bilirubin production
- Haemolysis (unconjugated hyperbilirubinaemia)

Impaired bilirubin excretion
- Congenital:
  - Gilbert's syndrome (unconjugated)
- Hepatocellular:
  - Viral hepatitis
  - Cirrhosis
  - Drugs
  - Autoimmune hepatitis
- Intrahepatic cholestasis:
  - Drugs
  - Primary biliary cirrhosis
- Extrahepatic cholestasis:
  - Gallstones
  - Cancer: pancreas, cholangiocarcinoma

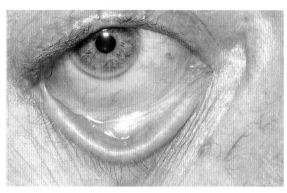

Fig. 6.8 Yellow sclera of jaundice.

colorectal cancer or colonic polyps, inflammatory bowel disease, ischaemic colitis and colonic angioectasias.

Jaundice

Jaundice is a yellowish discoloration of the skin, sclerae (Fig. 6.8) and mucous membranes caused by hyperbilirubinaemia (Box 6.6). There is no absolute level at which jaundice is clinically detected but, in good light, most clinicians will recognise jaundice when bilirubin levels exceed 50 μmol/L (2.92 mg/dL).

Ask about:
- associated symptoms: abdominal pain, fever, weight loss, itching
- colour of stools (normal or pale) and urine (normal or dark)
- alcohol intake
- travel history and immunisations
- use of illicit or intravenous drugs
- sexual history
- previous blood transfusions
- recently prescribed drugs.

Unconjugated bilirubin is insoluble and binds to plasma albumin; it is therefore not filtered by the renal glomeruli. In jaundice from unconjugated hyperbilirubinaemia, the urine is a normal colour (acholuric jaundice; Box 6.7).

Bilirubin is conjugated to form bilirubin diglucuronide in the liver and excreted in bile, producing its characteristic green colour. In conjugated hyperbilirubinaemia, the urine is dark brown due to the presence of bilirubin diglucuronide. In the colon, conjugated bilirubin is metabolised by bacteria to stercobilinogen and stercobilin, which contribute to the brown colour of stool. Stercobilinogen is absorbed from the bowel and excreted in the urine as urobilinogen, a colourless, water-soluble compound.

6.7 Urine and stool analysis in jaundice

	Urine			Stools
	Colour	Bilirubin	Urobilinogen	Colour
Unconjugated	Normal	–	++++	Normal
Hepatocellular	Dark	++	++	Normal
Obstructive	Dark	++++	–	Pale

6.8 Examples of drug-induced gastrointestinal conditions

Symptom	Drug
Weight gain	Oral glucocorticoids
Dyspepsia and gastrointestinal bleeding	Aspirin Non-steroidal anti-inflammatory drugs
Nausea	Many drugs, including selective serotonin reuptake inhibitor antidepressants
Diarrhoea (pseudomembranous colitis)	Antibiotics Proton pump inhibitors
Constipation	Opioids
Jaundice: hepatitis	Paracetamol (overdose) Pyrazinamide Rifampicin Isoniazid
Jaundice: cholestatic	Flucloxacillin Chlorpromazine Co-amoxiclav
Liver fibrosis	Methotrexate

Prehepatic jaundice

In haemolytic disorders, anaemic pallor combined with jaundice may produce a pale lemon complexion. The stools and urine are normal in colour. Gilbert's syndrome is common and causes unconjugated hyperbilirubinaemia. Serum liver enzyme concentrations are normal and jaundice is mild (plasma bilirubin <100 µmol/L (5.85 mg/dL)) but increases during prolonged fasting or intercurrent febrile illness.

Hepatic jaundice

Hepatocellular disease causes hyperbilirubinaemia that is both unconjugated and conjugated. Conjugated bilirubin leads to dark brown urine. The stools are normal in colour.

Posthepatic/cholestatic jaundice

In biliary obstruction, conjugated bilirubin in the bile does not reach the intestine, so the stools are pale. Obstructive jaundice may be accompanied by pruritus (generalised itch) due to skin deposition of bile salts. Obstructive jaundice with abdominal pain is usually due to gallstones; if fever or rigors also occur (Charcot's triad), ascending cholangitis is likely. Painless obstructive jaundice suggests malignant biliary obstruction, as in cholangiocarcinoma or cancer of the head of the pancreas. Obstructive jaundice can be due to intrahepatic as well as extrahepatic cholestasis, as in primary biliary cirrhosis, certain hepatotoxic drug reactions (Box 6.8) and profound hepatocellular injury.

Groin swellings and lumps

Ask about:

- associated pain
- precipitating/exacerbating factors, such as straining due to chronic constipation, chronic cough, heavy manual labour and relationship with micturition
- timing: when the symptoms are worse.

Hernias are common causes of groin lumps and frequently present with dull, dragging discomfort (rather than acute pain), which is often exacerbated by straining and after long periods of standing or activity. Patients can often manually reduce the hernia by applying gentle pressure over the swelling or by lying flat. Other causes of groin swellings include lymph nodes, skin and subcutaneous lumps and, less commonly, saphena varix (a varicosity of the long saphenous vein), hydrocoele of the spermatic cord, undescended testis, femoral aneurysm and psoas abscess.

Past medical history

History of a similar problem may suggest the diagnosis: for example, pancreatitis, bleeding peptic ulcer or inflammatory bowel disease. Coexisting peripheral vascular disease, hypertension, heart failure or atrial fibrillation may suggest aortic aneurysm or mesenteric ischaemia as the cause of acute abdominal pain. Primary biliary cirrhosis and autoimmune hepatitis are associated with thyroid disease, and non-alcoholic fatty liver disease (NAFLD) is associated with diabetes and obesity. Ask about previous abdominal surgery.

Drug history

Ask about all prescribed medications, over-the-counter medicines and herbal preparations. Many drugs affect the gastrointestinal tract (Box 6.8) and are hepatotoxic.

Family history

Inflammatory bowel disease is more common in patients with a family history of either Crohn's disease or ulcerative colitis. Colorectal cancer in a first-degree relative increases the risk of colorectal cancer and polyps. Peptic ulcer disease is familial but this may be due to environmental factors, such as transmission of *Helicobacter pylori* infection. Gilbert's syndrome is an autosomal dominant condition; haemochromatosis and Wilson's disease are autosomal recessive disorders. Autoimmune diseases, particularly thyroid disease, are common in relatives of those with primary biliary cirrhosis and autoimmune hepatitis. A family history of diabetes is frequently seen in the context of NAFLD.

Social history

Ask about:

- Dietary history: assess the intake of calories and sources of essential nutrients. For guidance, there are 9 kcal per g of fat and 4 kcal per g of carbohydrates and protein.
- Food intolerances: patients with irritable bowel syndrome often report specific food intolerances, including wheat, dairy products and others. Painless diarrhoea may indicate high alcohol intake, lactose intolerance or coeliac disease.

- Alcohol consumption: calculate the patient's intake in units (p. 15).
- Smoking: this increases the risk of oesophageal cancer, colorectal cancer, Crohn's disease and peptic ulcer, while patients with ulcerative colitis are less likely to smoke.
- Stress: many disorders, particularly irritable bowel syndrome and dyspepsia, are exacerbated by stress and mental disorders.
- Foreign travel: this is particularly relevant in liver disease and diarrhoea.
- Risk factors for liver disease: these include intravenous drug use, tattoos, foreign travel, blood transfusions, and sex between men or with prostitutes and multiple sexual partners. Hepatitis B and C may present with chronic liver disease or cancer decades after the primary infection, so enquire about risk factors in the distant as well as the recent past.

The physical examination

General examination

Examination sequence

- Note the patient's demeanour and general appearance. Are they in pain, cachectic, thin, well nourished or obese? Record height, weight, waist circumference and body mass index (p. 29). Note whether obesity is truncal or generalised. Look for abdominal striae or loose skin folds.
- Inspect the patient's hands for clubbing, koilonychia (spoon-shaped nails) and signs of chronic liver disease (Fig. 6.9), including leuconychia (white nails) and palmar erythema.

6

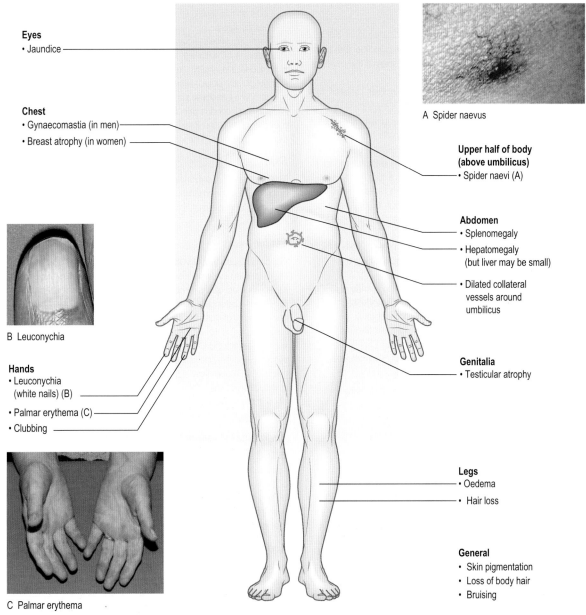

Eyes
- Jaundice

A Spider naevus

Chest
- Gynaecomastia (in men)
- Breast atrophy (in women)

Upper half of body (above umbilicus)
- Spider naevi (A)

Abdomen
- Splenomegaly
- Hepatomegaly (but liver may be small)
- Dilated collateral vessels around umbilicus

B Leuconychia

Hands
- Leuconychia (white nails) (B)
- Palmar erythema (C)
- Clubbing

Genitalia
- Testicular atrophy

Legs
- Oedema
- Hair loss

General
- Skin pigmentation
- Loss of body hair
- Bruising

C Palmar erythema

Fig. 6.9 Features of chronic liver disease.

- Inspect the mouth, throat and tongue.
- Ask the patient to look down and retract the upper eyelid to expose the sclera; look to see if it is yellow in natural light (see Fig. 6.8).
- Examine the cervical, axillary and inguinal lymph nodes (p. 33).

Striae indicate rapid weight gain, previous pregnancy or, rarely, Cushing's syndrome. Loose skin folds signify recent weight loss.

Stigmata of iron deficiency include angular cheilitis (painful cracks at the corners of the mouth) and atrophic glossitis (pale, smooth tongue). The tongue has a beefy, raw appearance in folate and vitamin B_{12} deficiency. Mouth and throat aphthous ulcers are common in coeliac and inflammatory bowel disease (see Fig. 6.3B).

Gastric and pancreatic cancer may spread to cause enlargement of the left supraclavicular lymph nodes (Troisier's sign). More widespread lymphadenopathy with hepatosplenomegaly suggests lymphoma.

Liver disease

Do not confuse the diffuse yellow sclerae of jaundice with small, yellowish fat pads (pingueculae) sometimes seen at the periphery of the sclerae.

Certain signs (stigmata) suggest chronic liver disease (see Fig. 6.9):

- Palmar erythema and spider naevi are caused by excess oestrogen associated with reduced hepatic breakdown of sex steroids. Spider naevi are isolated telangiectasias that characteristically fill from a central vessel and are found in the distribution of the superior vena cava (upper trunk, arms and face). Women may have up to five spider naevi in health; palmar erythema and numerous spider naevi are normal during pregnancy. In men, these signs suggest chronic liver disease.
- Gynaecomastia (breast enlargement in males), with loss of body hair and testicular atrophy, may occur due to reduced breakdown of oestrogens.
- Leuconychia, caused by hypoalbuminaemia, may also occur in protein calorie malnutrition (kwashiorkor), malabsorption due to protein-losing enteropathy, as in coeliac disease, or heavy and prolonged proteinuria (nephrotic syndrome).
- Finger clubbing is found in liver cirrhosis, inflammatory bowel disease and malabsorption syndromes.

Other signs that may be associated with liver disease include:

- Dupuytren's contracture of the palmar fascia (see Fig. 3.5): linked with alcohol-related chronic liver disease
- bilateral parotid swelling due to sialoadenosis: may be a feature of chronic alcohol abuse.

Signs that suggest liver failure include:

- asterixis, a coarse flapping tremor when the arms are outstretched and hands dorsiflexed, which occurs with hepatic encephalopathy
- fetor hepaticus, a distinctive 'mousy' odour of dimethyl sulphide on the breath, which is evidence of portosystemic shunting (with or without encephalopathy)
- altered mental state, varying from drowsiness with the day/night pattern reversed, through confusion and disorientation, to unresponsive coma
- jaundice
- ascites

- late neurological features, which include spasticity, extension of the arms and legs, and extensor plantar responses.

In a jaundiced patient, spider naevi, palmar erythema and ascites all strongly suggest chronic liver disease rather than obstructive jaundice.

Abdominal examination

Examine the patient in good light and warm surroundings, positioned comfortably supine with the head resting on only one or two pillows to relax the abdominal wall muscles. Use extra pillows to support a patient with kyphosis or breathlessness.

Inspection

Examination sequence

- Look at the teeth, tongue and buccal mucosa; check for mouth ulcers.
- Note any smell, including alcohol, fetor hepaticus, uraemia, melaena or ketones.
- Expose the abdomen from the xiphisternum to the symphysis pubis, leaving the chest and legs covered.

The normal abdomen is flat or slightly scaphoid and symmetrical. At rest, respiration is principally diaphragmatic; the abdominal wall moves out and the liver, spleen and kidneys move downwards during inspiration. The umbilicus is usually inverted.

Skin

In older patients, seborrhoeic warts, ranging from pink to brown or black, and haemangiomas (Campbell de Morgan spots) are common and normal, but note any striae, bruising or scratch marks.

Visible veins

Abnormally prominent veins on the abdominal wall suggest portal hypertension or vena cava obstruction. In portal hypertension, recanalisation of the umbilical vein along the falciform ligament produces distended veins that drain away from the umbilicus: the 'caput medusae'. The umbilicus may appear bluish and distended due to an umbilical varix. In contrast, an umbilical hernia is a distended and everted umbilicus that does not appear vascular and may have a palpable cough impulse. Dilated tortuous veins with blood flow superiorly are collateral veins caused by obstruction of the inferior vena cava. Rarely, superior vena cava obstruction gives rise to similarly distended abdominal veins, but these all flow inferiorly.

Abdominal swelling

Diffuse abdominal swelling could be due to ascites or intestinal obstruction. If localised, it could be caused by urinary retention, a mass or an enlarged organ such as the liver. In obesity, the umbilicus is usually sunken; in ascites, it is flat or, more commonly, everted. Look tangentially across the abdomen and from the foot of the bed for any asymmetry suggesting a localised mass.

Abdominal scars and stomas

Note any surgical scars or stomas and clarify what operations have been undertaken (Figs 6.10 and 6.11). A small infraumbilical incision usually indicates a previous laparoscopy. Puncture scars from laparoscopic surgical ports may be visible. An incisional hernia at the site of a scar is palpable as a defect in the abdominal

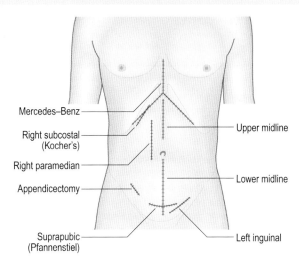

Fig. 6.10 Some abdominal incisions. The midline and oblique incisions avoid damage to innervation of the abdominal musculature and later development of incisional hernias. These incisions have been widely superseded by laparoscopic surgery, however.

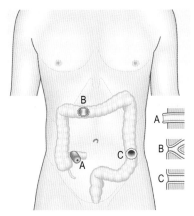

Fig. 6.11 Surgical stomas. [A] An ileostomy is usually in the right iliac fossa and is formed as a spout. [B] A loop colostomy is created to defunction the distal bowel temporarily. It is usually in the transverse colon and has afferent and efferent limbs. [C] A colostomy may be terminal: that is, resected distal bowel. It is usually flush and in the left iliac fossa.

wall musculature and becomes more obvious as the patient raises their head off the bed or coughs.

Palpation

Examination sequence

- Ensure your hands are warm and clean.
- If the bed is low, kneel beside it but avoid touching the floor to prevent infection.
- Ask the patient to show you where any pain is and to report any tenderness during palpation.
- Ask the patient to place their arms by their sides to help relax the abdominal wall.
- Use your right hand, keeping it flat and in contact with the abdominal wall.
- Observe the patient's face throughout for any sign of discomfort.

- Begin with light superficial palpation away from any site of pain.
- Palpate each region in turn, and then repeat with deeper palpation.
- Test abdominal muscle tone using light, dipping finger movements.
- Describe any mass using the basic principles outlined in Box 3.8. Describe its site, size, surface, shape and consistency, and note whether it moves on respiration. Is the mass fixed or mobile?
- To determine if a mass is superficial and in the abdominal wall rather than within the abdominal cavity, ask the patient to tense their abdominal muscles by lifting their head. An abdominal wall mass will still be palpable, whereas an intra-abdominal mass will not.
- Decide whether the mass is an enlarged abdominal organ or separate from the solid organs.

Tenderness

Discomfort during palpation may vary and may be accompanied by resistance to palpation. Consider the patient's level of anxiety when assessing the severity of pain and degree of tenderness elicited. Tenderness in several areas on minimal pressure may be due to generalised peritonitis but is more often caused by anxiety. Severe superficial pain with no tenderness on deep palpation or pain that disappears if the patient is distracted also suggests anxiety. With these exceptions, tenderness usefully indicates underlying pathology.

Voluntary guarding is the voluntary contraction of the abdominal muscles when palpation provokes pain. Involuntary guarding is the reflex contraction of the abdominal muscles when there is inflammation of the parietal peritoneum. If the whole peritoneum is inflamed (generalised peritonitis) due to a perforated viscus, the abdominal wall no longer moves with respiration; breathing becomes increasingly thoracic and the anterior abdominal wall muscles are held rigid (board-like rigidity).

The site of tenderness is important. Tenderness in the epigastrium suggests peptic ulcer; in the right hypochondrium, cholecystitis; in the left iliac fossa, diverticulitis; and in the right iliac fossa, appendicitis or Crohn's ileitis (Fig. 6.12). Ask the patient to cough or gently percuss the abdomen to elicit any pain or tenderness 'Rebound tenderness', when rapidly removing your hand after deep palpation increases the pain, is a sign of intra-abdominal disease but not necessarily of parietal peritoneal inflammation (peritonism). Specific abdominal signs are shown in Box 6.9. Typical findings may be masked in patients taking glucocorticoids, immunosuppressants or anti-inflammatory drugs, in alcohol intoxication or in altered states of consciousness.

Palpable mass

A pulsatile mass palpable in the upper abdomen may be normal aortic pulsation in a thin person, a gastric or pancreatic tumour transmitting underlying aortic pulsation, or an aortic aneurysm.

A pathological mass can usually be distinguished from normal palpable structures by site (Fig. 6.13), and from palpable faeces as these can be indented and may disappear following defecation. A hard subcutaneous nodule at the umbilicus may indicate metastatic cancer ('Sister Mary Joseph's nodule').

Enlarged organs

Examine the liver, gallbladder, spleen and kidneys in turn during deep inspiration. Keep your examining hand still and wait for the organ to move with breathing. Do not start palpation too

6.9 Specific signs in the 'acute abdomen'

Sign	Disease associations	Examination
Murphy's	Acute cholecystitis: Sensitivity 50–97% Specificity 50–80%	As the patient takes a deep breath in, gently palpate in the right upper quadrant of the abdomen; the acutely inflamed gallbladder contacts the examining fingers, evoking pain with the arrest of inspiration
Rovsing's	Acute appendicitis: Sensitivity 20–70% Specificity 40–96%	Palpation in the left iliac fossa produces pain in the right iliac fossa
Iliopsoas	Retroileal appendicitis, iliopsoas abscess, perinephric abscess	Ask the patient to flex their thigh against the resistance of your hand; a painful response indicates an inflammatory process involving the right psoas muscle
Grey Turner's and Cullen's	Haemorrhagic pancreatitis, aortic rupture and ruptured ectopic pregnancy (see Fig. 6.25)	Bleeding into the falciform ligament; bruising develops around the umbilicus (Cullen) or in the loins (Grey Turner)

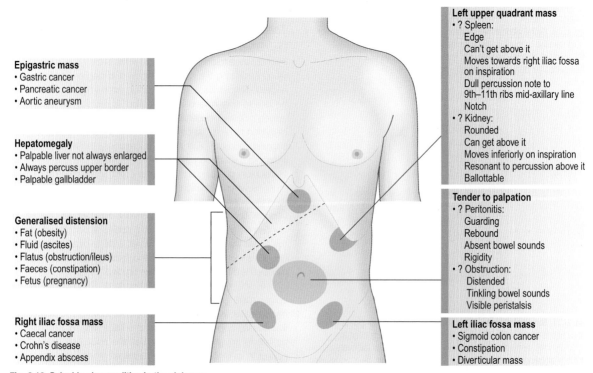

Epigastric mass
- Gastric cancer
- Pancreatic cancer
- Aortic aneurysm

Hepatomegaly
- Palpable liver not always enlarged
- Always percuss upper border
- Palpable gallbladder

Generalised distension
- Fat (obesity)
- Fluid (ascites)
- Flatus (obstruction/ileus)
- Faeces (constipation)
- Fetus (pregnancy)

Right iliac fossa mass
- Caecal cancer
- Crohn's disease
- Appendix abscess

Left upper quadrant mass
- ? Spleen:
  Edge
  Can't get above it
  Moves towards right iliac fossa on inspiration
  Dull percussion note to 9th–11th ribs mid-axillary line
  Notch
- ? Kidney:
  Rounded
  Can get above it
  Moves inferiorly on inspiration
  Resonant to percussion above it
  Ballottable

Tender to palpation
- ? Peritonitis:
  Guarding
  Rebound
  Absent bowel sounds
  Rigidity
- ? Obstruction:
  Distended
  Tinkling bowel sounds
  Visible peristalsis

Left iliac fossa mass
- Sigmoid colon cancer
- Constipation
- Diverticular mass

Fig. 6.12 Palpable abnormalities in the abdomen.

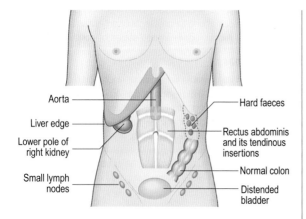

Aorta
Liver edge
Lower pole of right kidney
Small lymph nodes

Hard faeces
Rectus abdominis and its tendinous insertions
Normal colon
Distended bladder

Fig. 6.13 Palpable masses that may be physiological rather than pathological.

close to the costal margin, missing the edge of the liver or spleen.

Hepatomegaly

Examination sequence

- Place your hand flat on the skin of the right iliac fossa.
- Point your fingers upwards and your index and middle fingers lateral to the rectus muscle, so that your fingertips lie parallel to the rectus sheath (Fig. 6.14). Keep your hand stationary.
- Ask the patient to breathe in deeply through the mouth.
- Feel for the liver edge as it descends on inspiration.
- Move your hand progressively up the abdomen, 1 cm at a time, between each breath the patient takes, until you reach the costal margin or detect the liver edge.

- If you feel a liver edge, describe:
  - size
  - surface: smooth or irregular
  - edge: smooth or irregular; define the medial border
  - consistency: soft or hard
  - tenderness
  - pulsatility.
- To examine for gallbladder tenderness, ask the patient to breathe in deeply, then gently palpate the right upper quadrant in the mid-clavicular line.

Percussion

Examination sequence

- Ask the patient to hold their breath in full expiration.
- Percuss downwards from the right fifth intercostal space in the mid-clavicular line, listening for dullness indicating the upper border of the liver.
- Measure the distance in centimetres below the costal margin in the mid-clavicular line or from the upper border of dullness to the palpable liver edge.

In the normal abdomen, you may feel:
- the liver edge below the right costal margin
- the aorta as a pulsatile swelling above the umbilicus

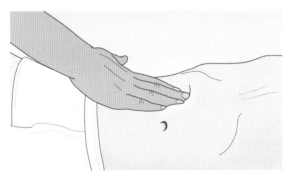

Fig. 6.14 Palpation of the liver.

- the lower pole of the right kidney in the right flank
- faecal scybala (hardened masses of faeces) in the sigmoid colon in the left iliac fossa
- a full bladder arising out of the pelvis in the suprapubic region.

The normal liver is identified as an area of dullness to percussion over the right anterior chest between the fifth rib and the costal margin.

The liver may be enlarged (Fig. 6.15A) or displaced downwards by hyperinflated lungs.

Hepatic enlargement can result from chronic parenchymal liver disease from any cause (Box 6.10). The liver is enlarged in early cirrhosis but often shrunken in advanced cirrhosis. Fatty liver (hepatic steatosis) can cause marked hepatomegaly. Hepatic enlargement due to metastatic tumour is hard and irregular. An enlarged left lobe may be felt in the epigastrium or even the left hypochondrium. In right heart failure the congested liver is usually soft and tender; a pulsatile liver indicates tricuspid regurgitation. A bruit over the liver may be heard in acute alcoholic hepatitis, hepatocellular cancer and arteriovenous malformation. The most

6.10 Causes of hepatomegaly	
Chronic parenchymal liver disease	
• Alcoholic liver disease	• Viral hepatitis
• Hepatic steatosis	• Primary biliary cirrhosis
• Autoimmune hepatitis	
Malignancy	
• Primary hepatocellular cancer	• Secondary metastatic cancer
Right heart failure	
Haematological disorders	
• Lymphoma	• Myelofibrosis
• Leukaemia	• Polycythaemia
Rarities	
• Amyloidosis	• Sarcoidosis
• Budd–Chiari syndrome	• Glycogen storage disorders

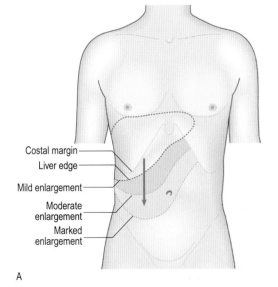

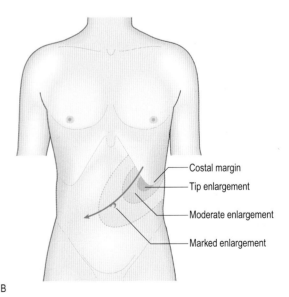

A

B

Fig. 6.15 **Patterns of progressive enlargement of liver and of spleen.** A Direction of enlargement of the liver. B Direction of enlargement of the spleen. The spleen moves downwards and medially during inspiration.

common reason for an audible bruit over the liver, however, is a transmitted heart murmur. Liver failure produces additional symptoms of encephalopathy, which can be graded (Box 6.11).

Resonance below the fifth intercostal space suggests hyperinflated lungs or occasionally the interposition of the transverse colon between the liver and the diaphragm (Chilaiditi's sign).

In a patient with right upper quadrant pain, test for Murphy's sign (see Box 6.9); a positive modestly increases the probability of acute cholecystitis. Palpable distension of the gallbladder is rare and has a characteristic globular shape. It results from either obstruction of the cystic duct, as in mucocoele or empyema of the gallbladder, or obstruction of the common bile duct with a patent cystic duct, as in pancreatic cancer. In a jaundiced patient a palpable gallbladder is likely to be due to extrahepatic obstruction, such as from pancreatic cancer or, very rarely, gallstones (Courvoisier's sign). In gallstone disease the gallbladder may be tender but impalpable because of fibrosis of the gallbladder wall.

Splenomegaly

The spleen has to enlarge threefold before it becomes palpable, so a palpable spleen always indicates splenomegaly. It enlarges from under the left costal margin down and medially towards the umbilicus (Fig. 6.15B). A characteristic notch may be palpable midway along its leading edge, helping differentiate it from an enlarged left kidney (Box 6.12).

Examination sequence

- Place your hand over the patient's umbilicus. With your hand stationary, ask the patient to inhale deeply through the mouth.
- Feel for the splenic edge as it descends on inspiration.
- Move your hand diagonally upwards towards the left hypochondrium (Fig. 6.16A), 1 cm at a time between each breath the patient takes.
- Feel the costal margin along its length, as the position of the spleen tip is variable.
- If you cannot feel the splenic edge, palpate with your right hand, placing your left hand behind the patient's left lower

6.11 Grading of hepatic encephalopathy (West Haven)	
Stage	**State of consciousness**
0	No change in personality or behaviour No asterixis (flapping tremor)
1	Impaired concentration and attention span Sleep disturbance, slurred speech Euphoria or depression Asterixis present
2	Lethargy, drowsiness, apathy or aggression Disorientation, inappropriate behaviour, slurred speech
3	Confusion and disorientation, bizarre behaviour Drowsiness or stupor Asterixis usually absent
4	Comatose with no response to voice commands Minimal or absent response to painful stimuli

Reproduced from Conn HO, Leevy CM, Vlahcevic ZR, et al. Comparison of lactulose and neomycin in the treatment of chronic portal-systemic encephalopathy. A double blind controlled trial. Gastroenterology 1977; 72(4):573, with permission from Elsevier Inc.

6.12 Differentiating a palpable spleen from the left kidney		
Distinguishing feature	**Spleen**	**Kidney**
Mass is smooth and regular in shape	More likely	Polycystic kidneys are bilateral irregular masses
Mass descends in inspiration	Yes, travels superficially and diagonally	Yes, moves deeply and vertically
Ability to feel deep to the mass	Yes	No
Palpable notch on the medial surface	Yes	No
Bilateral masses palpable	No	Sometimes, e.g. polycystic kidneys
Percussion resonant over the mass	No	Sometimes
Mass extends beyond the midline	Sometimes	No (except with horseshoe kidney)

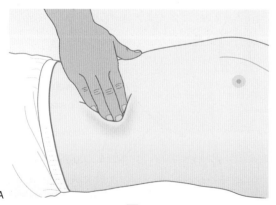
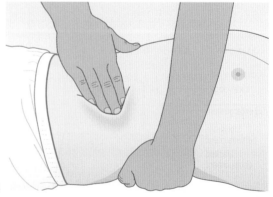

A   B

Fig. 6.16 Palpation of the spleen. **A** Initial palpation for the splenic edge moving diagonally from the umbilicus to the left hypochondrium. **B** If the spleen is impalpable by the method shown in A, use your left hand to pull the ribcage forward and elevate the spleen, making it more likely to be palpable by your right hand.

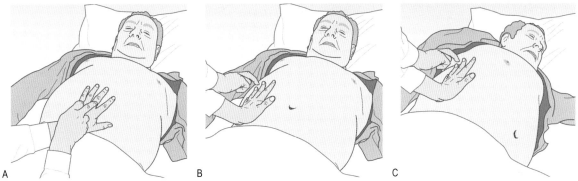

6

Fig. 6.17 **Percussing for ascites.** [A] and [B] Percuss towards the flank from resonant to dull. [C] Then ask the patient to roll on to their other side. In ascites the note then becomes resonant.

6.13 Causes of splenomegaly

Haematological disorders
- Lymphoma and lymphatic leukaemias
- Myeloproliferative diseases, polycythaemia rubra vera and myelofibrosis
- Haemolytic anaemia, congenital spherocytosis

Portal hypertension

Infections
- Glandular fever
- Malaria, kala-azar (leishmaniasis)
- Bacterial endocarditis
- Brucellosis, tuberculosis, salmonellosis

Rheumatological conditions
- Rheumatoid arthritis (Felty's syndrome)
- Systemic lupus erythematosus

Rarities
- Sarcoidosis
- Amyloidosis
- Glycogen storage disorders

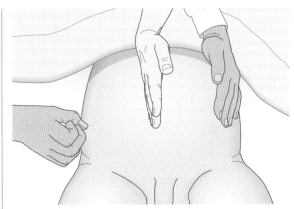

Fig. 6.18 **Eliciting a fluid thrill.**

- Keep your finger on the site of dullness in the flank and ask the patient to turn on to their opposite side.
- Pause for 10 seconds to allow any ascites to gravitate, then percuss again. If the area of dullness is now resonant, shifting dullness is present, indicating ascites.

Fluid thrill
- If the abdomen is tensely distended and you are uncertain whether ascites is present, feel for a fluid thrill.
- Place the palm of your left hand flat against the left side of the patient's abdomen and flick a finger of your right hand against the right side of the abdomen.
- If you feel a ripple against your left hand, ask an assistant or the patient to place the edge of their hand on the midline of the abdomen (Fig. 6.18). This prevents transmission of the impulse via the skin rather than through the ascites. If you still feel a ripple against your left hand, a fluid thrill is present (detected only in gross ascites).

Causes of ascites are shown in Box 6.14.

ribs and pulling the ribcage forward (Fig. 6.16B), or ask the patient to roll towards you and on to their right side and repeat the above.
- Feel along the left costal margin and percuss over the lateral chest wall. The normal spleen causes dullness to percussion posterior to the left mid-axillary line beneath the 9th–11th ribs.

There are many causes of splenomegaly (Box 6.13). Massive enlargement in the developed world is usually due to myeloproliferative disease or haematological malignancy; worldwide, malaria is a common cause.

Important causes of hepatosplenomegaly include lymphoma or myeloproliferative disorders, cirrhosis with portal hypertension, amyloidosis, sarcoidosis and glycogen storage disease.

Ascites

Ascites is the accumulation of intraperitoneal fluid (see Fig. 6.6).

Examination sequence

Shifting dullness
- With the patient supine, percuss from the midline out to the flanks (Fig. 6.17). Note any change from resonant to dull, along with areas of dullness and resonance.

Auscultation

Examination sequence

- With the patient supine, place your stethoscope diaphragm to the right of the umbilicus and do not move it.
- Listen for up to 2 minutes before concluding that bowel sounds are absent.
- Listen above the umbilicus over the aorta for arterial bruits.

6.14 Causes of ascites

Diagnosis	Comment
Common	
Hepatic cirrhosis with portal hypertension	Transudate
Intra-abdominal malignancy with peritoneal spread	Exudate, cytology may be positive
Uncommon	
Hepatic vein occlusion (Budd–Chiari syndrome)	Transudate in acute phase
Constrictive pericarditis and right heart failure	Check jugular venous pressure and listen for pericardial rub
Hypoproteinaemia (nephrotic syndrome, protein-losing enteropathy)	Transudate
Tuberculous peritonitis	Low glucose content
Pancreatitis, pancreatic duct disruption	Very high amylase content

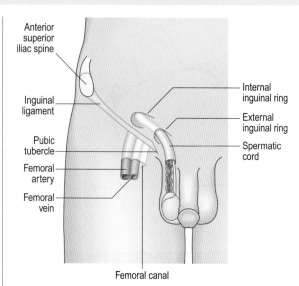

Fig. 6.19 **Anatomy of the inguinal canal and femoral sheath.**

- Now listen 2–3 cm above and lateral to the umbilicus for bruits from renal artery stenosis.
- Listen over the liver for bruits.
- Test for a succussion splash; this sounds like a half-filled water bottle being shaken. Explain the procedure to the patient, then shake their abdomen by rocking their pelvis using both hands.

Normal bowel sounds are gurgling noises from the normal peristaltic activity of the gut. They normally occur every 5–10 seconds but the frequency varies.

Absence of bowel sounds implies paralytic ileus or peritonitis. In intestinal obstruction, bowel sounds occur with increased frequency and volume, and have a high-pitched, tinkling quality. Bruits suggest an atheromatous or aneurysmal aorta or superior mesenteric artery stenosis. A friction rub, which sounds like rubbing your dry fingers together, may be heard over the liver (perihepatitis) or spleen (perisplenitis). An audible splash more than 4 hours after the patient has eaten or drunk anything indicates delayed gastric emptying, as in pyloric stenosis.

Hernias

The inguinal canal extends from the pubic tubercle to the anterior superior iliac spine (Fig. 6.19). It has an internal ring at the mid-inguinal point (midway between the pubic symphysis and the anterior superior iliac spine) and an external ring at the pubic tubercle. The femoral canal lies below the inguinal ligament and lateral to the pubic tubercle.

Hernias are common and typically occur at openings of the abdominal wall, such as the inguinal, femoral and obturator canals, the umbilicus and the oesophageal hiatus. They may also occur at sites of weakness of the abdominal wall, as in previous surgical incisions.

An external abdominal hernia is an abnormal protrusion of bowel and/or omentum from the abdominal cavity. External hernias are more obvious when the pressure within the abdomen rises, such as when the patient is standing, coughing or straining at stool. Internal hernias occur through defects of the mesentery or into the retroperitoneal space and are not visible.

An impulse can often be felt in a hernia during coughing (cough impulse). Identify a hernia from its anatomical site and characteristics, and attempt to differentiate between direct and indirect inguinal hernias.

Examination sequence

- Examine the groin with the patient standing upright.
- Inspect the inguinal and femoral canals and the scrotum for any lumps or bulges.
- Ask the patient to cough; look for an impulse over the femoral or inguinal canal and scrotum.
- Identify the anatomical relationships between the bulge, the pubic tubercle and the inguinal ligament to distinguish a femoral from an inguinal hernia.
- Palpate the external inguinal ring and along the inguinal canal for possible muscle defects. Ask the patient to cough and feel for a cough impulse.
- Now ask the patient to lie down and establish whether the hernia reduces spontaneously.
- If so, press two fingers over the internal inguinal ring at the mid-inguinal point and ask the patient to cough or stand up while you maintain pressure over the internal inguinal ring. If the hernia reappears, it is a direct hernia. If it can be prevented from reappearing, it is an indirect inguinal hernia.
- Examine the opposite side to exclude the possibility of asymptomatic hernias.

An indirect inguinal hernia bulges through the internal ring and follows the course of the inguinal canal. It may extend beyond the external ring and enter the scrotum. Indirect hernias comprise 85% of all hernias and are more common in younger men.

A direct inguinal hernia forms at a site of muscle weakness in the posterior wall of the inguinal canal and rarely extends into the scrotum. It is more common in older men and women (Fig. 6.20).

A femoral hernia projects through the femoral ring and into the femoral canal. Inguinal hernias are palpable above and medial to the pubic tubercle. Femoral hernias are palpable below the inguinal ligament and lateral to the pubic tubercle.

In a reducible hernia the contents can be returned to the abdominal cavity, spontaneously or by manipulation; if they cannot, the hernia is irreducible. An abdominal hernia has a covering sac of peritoneum and the neck of the hernia is a common site of compression of the contents (Fig. 6.21). If the

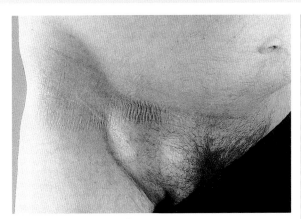

Fig. 6.20 **Right inguinal hernia.**

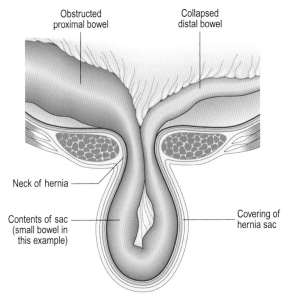

Fig. 6.21 **Hernia: anatomical structure.**

Obstructed proximal bowel

Collapsed distal bowel

Neck of hernia

Contents of sac (small bowel in this example)

Covering of hernia sac

hernia contains bowel, obstruction may occur. If the blood supply to the contents of the hernia (bowel or omentum) is restricted, the hernia is strangulated. It is tense, tender and has no cough impulse, there may be bowel obstruction and, later, signs of sepsis and shock. A strangulated hernia is a surgical emergency and, if left untreated, will lead to bowel infarction and peritonitis.

Rectal examination

Digital examination of the rectum is important (Box 6.15). Do not avoid it because you or the patient finds it disagreeable. The patient's verbal consent is needed, however, and the examination should be carried out in the presence of a chaperone.

The normal rectum is usually empty and smooth-walled, with the coccyx and sacrum lying posteriorly. In the male, anterior to the rectum from below upwards, lie the membranous urethra, the prostate and the base of the bladder. The normal prostate is smooth and firm, with lateral lobes and a median groove between them. In the female, the vagina and cervix lie anteriorly. The upper end of the anal canal is marked by the puborectalis muscle, which is readily palpable and contracts as a reflex action

6.15 Indications for rectal examination

Alimentary
- Suspected appendicitis, pelvic abscess, peritonitis, lower abdominal pain
- Diarrhoea, constipation, tenesmus or anorectal pain
- Rectal bleeding or iron deficiency anaemia
- Unexplained weight loss
- Bimanual examination of lower abdominal mass for diagnosis or staging
- Malignancies of unknown origin

Genitourinary
- Assessment of prostate in prostatism or suspected prostatic cancer
- Dysuria, frequency, haematuria, epididymo-orchitis
- Replacement for vaginal examination when this would be inappropriate

Miscellaneous
- Unexplained bone pain, backache or lumbosacral nerve root pain
- Pyrexia of unknown origin
- Abdominal, pelvic or spinal trauma

on coughing or on conscious contraction by the patient. Beyond the anal canal, the rectum passes upwards and backwards along the curve of the sacrum.

Spasm of the external anal sphincter is common in anxious patients. When associated with local pain, it is probably due to an anal fissure (a mucosal tear). If you suspect an anal fissure, give the patient a local anaesthetic suppository 10 minutes before the examination to reduce the pain and spasm, and to aid examination.

Examination sequence

- Explain what you are going to do and why it is necessary, and ask for permission to proceed. Tell the patient that the examination may be uncomfortable but should not be painful.
- Offer a chaperone; record a refusal. Make a note of the name of the chaperone.
- Position the patient in the left lateral position with their buttocks at the edge of the couch, their knees drawn up to their chest and their heels clear of the perineum (Fig. 6.22).
- Put on gloves and examine the perianal skin, using an effective light source.
- Look for skin lesions, external haemorrhoids, fissures and fistulae.
- Lubricate your index finger with water-based gel.
- Place the pulp of your forefinger on the anal margin and apply steady pressure on the sphincter to push your finger gently through the anal canal into the rectum (Fig. 6.23).
- If anal spasm occurs, ask the patient to breathe in deeply and relax. If necessary, use a local anaesthetic suppository or gel before trying again. If pain persists, examination under general anaesthesia may be necessary.
- Ask the patient to squeeze your finger with their anal muscles and note any weakness of sphincter contraction.

- Palpate systematically around the entire rectum; note any abnormality and examine any mass (Fig. 6.24). Record the percentage of the rectal circumference involved by disease and its distance from the anus.
- Identify the uterine cervix in women and the prostate in men; assess the size, shape and consistency of the prostate and note any tenderness.
- If the rectum contains faeces and you are in doubt about palpable masses, repeat the examination after the patient has defecated.
- Slowly withdraw your finger. Examine it for stool colour and the presence of blood or mucus (Box 6.16).

Haemorrhoids ('piles', congested venous plexuses around the anal canal) are usually palpable if thrombosed. In patients with chronic constipation the rectum is often loaded with faeces. Faecal masses are frequently palpable, should be movable and can be indented. In women a retroverted uterus and the normal cervix are often palpable through the anterior rectal wall and a vaginal tampon may be confusing. Cancer of the lower rectum is palpable as a mucosal irregularity. Obstructing cancer of the upper rectum may produce ballooning of the empty rectal cavity below. Metastases or colonic tumours within the pelvis may be mistaken for faeces and vice versa. Lateralised tenderness suggests pelvic peritonitis. Gynaecological malignancy may cause a 'frozen pelvis' with a hard, rigid feel to the pelvic organs due to extensive peritoneal disease, such as post-radiotherapy or in metastatic cervical or ovarian cancer.

Benign prostatic hyperplasia often produces palpable symmetrical enlargement, but not if the hyperplasia is confined

6.16 Causes of abnormal stool appearance

Stool appearance	Cause
Abnormally pale	Biliary obstruction
Pale and greasy	Steatorrhoea
Black and tarry (melaena)	Bleeding from the upper gastrointestinal tract
Grey/black	Oral iron or bismuth therapy
Silvery	Steatorrhoea plus upper gastrointestinal bleeding, e.g. pancreatic cancer
Fresh blood in or on stool	Large bowel, rectal or anal bleeding
Stool mixed with pus	Infective colitis or inflammatory bowel disease
Rice-water stool (watery with mucus and cell debris)	Cholera

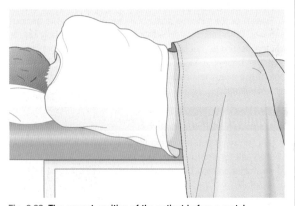

Fig. 6.22 **The correct position of the patient before a rectal examination.**

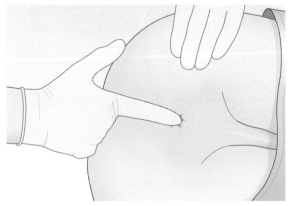

Fig. 6.23 **Rectal examination.** The correct method for inserting your index finger in rectal examination.

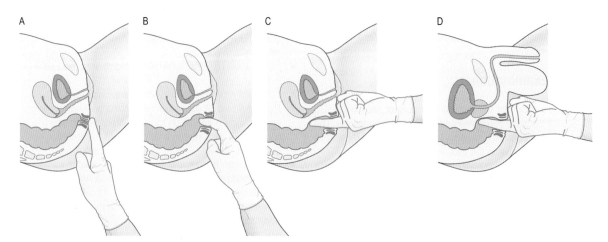

Fig. 6.24 **Examination of the rectum.** [A] and [B] Insert your finger, then rotate your hand. [C] The most prominent feature in the female is the cervix. [D] The most prominent feature in the male is the prostate.

to the median lobe. A hard, irregular or asymmetrical gland with no palpable median groove suggests prostate cancer. Tenderness accompanied by a change in the consistency of the gland may be caused by prostatitis or prostatic abscess. The prostate is abnormally small in hypogonadism.

Proctoscopy

Proctoscopy is visual examination of the anal canal; it is an invasive procedure and should only be practised after appropriate training. Always undertake digital rectal examination first. If examination of the rectal mucosa is required, perform flexible sigmoidoscopy rather than proctoscopy.

Examination sequence

- Place the patient in the left lateral position, as for digital rectal examination.
- With gloved hands, separate the buttocks with the forefinger and thumb of one hand. With your other hand, gently insert a lubricated proctoscope with its obturator in place into the anal canal and rectum in the direction of the umbilicus.

- Remove the obturator and carefully examine the anal canal under good illumination, noting any abnormality. Check for fissures, particularly if the patient reports pain during the procedure.
- Ask the patient to strain down as you slowly withdraw the instrument to detect any degree of rectal prolapse and the presence and severity of any haemorrhoids.

Proctoscopic examination of the anus and lower rectum can confirm or exclude the presence of haemorrhoids, anal fissures and rectal prolapse. Rectal mucosa looks like buccal mucosa, apart from the presence of prominent submucosal veins. During straining, haemorrhoids distend with blood and may prolapse. If the degree of protrusion is more than 3–4 cm, a rectal prolapse may be present.

Investigations

Selecting the relevant investigation depends on the clinical problem revealed on history and examination. Investigations are costly and many carry risks, so choose tests capable of distinguishing the likely diagnoses and prioritise the most decisive ones (Box 6.17 and Figs 6.26–30).

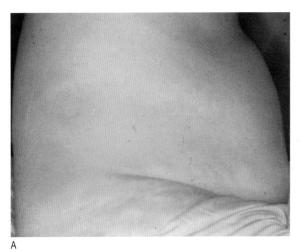
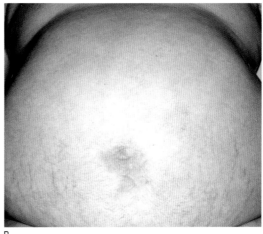

A   B

Fig. 6.25 Acute pancreatitis. A Bruising over the flanks (Grey Turner's sign). B Bruising round the umbilicus (Cullen's sign).

6.17 Investigations in gastrointestinal and hepatobiliary disease	
Investigation	**Indication/comment**
Clinical samples	
Stool:	
Faecal occult blood	Gastrointestinal haemorrhage; sensitive but not specific; used as population screening tool for colorectal cancer
Faecal calprotectin	Inflammatory bowel disease – raised
Urine: dipstick or biochemistry	Jaundice (see Box 6.7)
	Acute abdominal pain
Ascitic fluid: diagnostic tap	Clear/straw-coloured – normal
	Uniformly blood-stained – malignancy
	Turbid – infection
	Chylous – lymphatic obstruction
	High protein (exudate) – inflammation or malignancy
	Low protein (transudate) – cirrhosis and portal hypertension

Continued

6.17 Investigations in gastrointestinal and hepatobiliary disease—cont'd

Investigation	Indication/comment
Radiology	
Chest X-ray	Suspected acute abdomen, suspected perforated viscus or subphrenic abscess
	Pneumonia, free air beneath diaphragm, pleural effusion, elevated diaphragm
Abdominal X-ray	Intestinal obstruction, perforation, renal colic
	Fluid levels, air above liver, urinary tract stones
Barium meal	Rarely indicated unless gastroscopy not possible and there is suspicion of pharyngeal or gastric outlet obstruction on clinical symptoms (dysphagia or vomiting)
	Oesophageal obstruction (endoscopy preferable, especially if previous gastric surgery)
Small bowel follow-through	Subacute small bowel obstruction, duodenal diverticulosis
Small bowel magnetic resonance imaging or magnetic resonance enteroclysis (real-time imaging of liquid moving through the small bowel)	Crohn's disease, lymphoma, obscure gastrointestinal bleeding
CT colonography	Altered bowel habit, iron deficiency anaemia, rectal bleeding: alternative to colonoscopy in the frail, sick patient, if colonoscopy is unsuccessful or if not acceptable to patient to diagnose colon cancer, inflammatory bowel disease or diverticular disease; useful in colon cancer screening
Abdominal ultrasound scan	Biliary colic, jaundice, pancreatitis, malignancy
	Gallstones, liver metastases, cholestasis, pancreatic calcification, subphrenic abscess
Abdominal CT	Acute abdomen, suspected pancreatic or renal mass, tumour staging, abdominal aortic aneurysm
	Confirms or excludes metastatic disease and leaking from aortic aneurysm
MR cholangiopancreatography (MRCP)	Obstructive jaundice, acute and chronic pancreatitis
Pelvic ultrasound scan	Pelvic masses, inflammatory diseases, ectopic pregnancy, polycystic ovary syndrome
	Pelvic structures and abnormalities
	Ascitic fluid
Invasive procedures	
Upper gastrointestinal endoscopy	Dysphagia, dyspepsia, gastrointestinal bleeding, gastric ulcer, malabsorption
	Gastric and/or duodenal biopsies are useful
Lower gastrointestinal endoscopy (colonoscopy)	Rectal bleeding, obscure gastrointestinal bleeding, altered bowel habit, iron deficiency anaemia
	Able to biopsy lesions and remove polyps
Video capsule endoscopy	Obscure gastrointestinal bleeding with bidirectional negative endoscopies, suspected small bowel disease (vascular malformations, inflammatory bowel disease)
Endoscopic retrograde cholangiopancreatography (ERCP)	Obstructive jaundice, acute and chronic pancreatitis
	Mainly therapeutic role
	Stenting strictures and removing stones
Endoscopic ultrasound ± fine-needle aspiration (FNA) or Tru-Cut needle biopsy	Staging of upper gastrointestinal or pancreatobiliary cancer
	Drainage of pancreatic pseudocysts
Laparoscopy	Suspected appendicitis or perforated viscus, suspected ectopic pregnancy, chronic pelvic pain (e.g. due to endometriosis or pelvic inflammatory disease), suspected ovarian disease (e.g. ruptured ovarian cyst), peritoneal and liver disease
Ultrasound- or CT-guided aspiration cytology and biopsy	Liver metastases, intra-abdominal or retroperitoneal tumours
Liver biopsy	Parenchymal disease of liver
	Tissue biopsy by percutaneous, transjugular or laparoscopic route
Others	
Pancreatic function tests	Stool elastase, pancreolauryl test

CT, *computed tomography.*

6

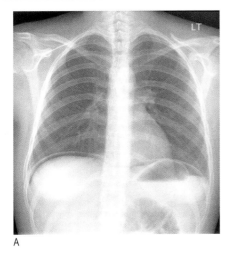

A

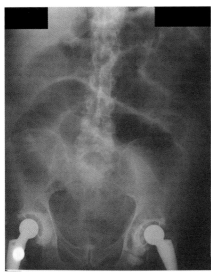

B

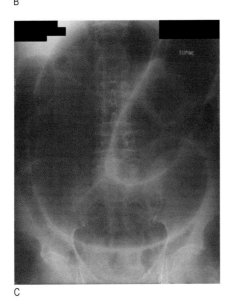

C

Fig. 6.26 Radiography in gastrointestinal disease. **A** Air under the diaphragm on chest X-ray due to a perforated duodenal ulcer. **B** Dilated small bowel due to acute intestinal obstruction. **C** Dilated loop of large bowel due to sigmoid volvulus.

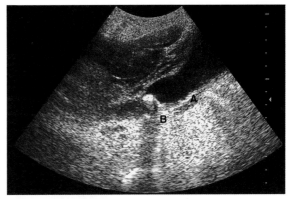

Fig. 6.27 Ultrasound scan of the gallbladder. *A*, Thick-walled gallbladder containing gallstones. *B*, Posterior acoustic shadowing.

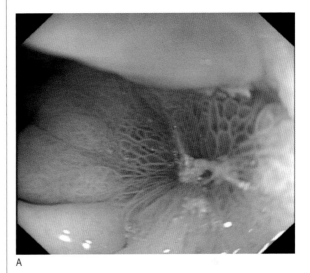

A

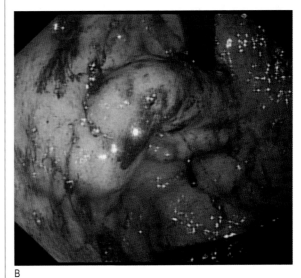

B

Fig. 6.28 Gastrointestinal endoscopy. **A** Gastric ulcer. **B** Gastric varices.

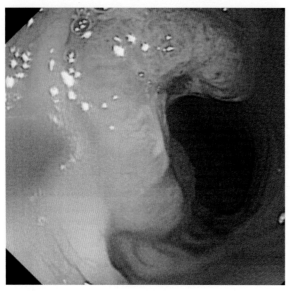

Fig. 6.29 **Colonoscopy.** Colon cancer.

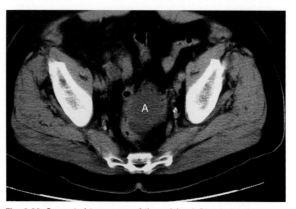

Fig. 6.30 **Computed tomogram of the pelvis.** *A,* Diverticular abscess.

OSCE example 1: Abdominal pain and diarrhoea

Mr Reid, 29 years old, presents with a 6-month history of anorexia, 7 kg weight loss, abdominal pains and diarrhoea (liquid stool). He underwent appendicectomy 4 months ago following severe right iliac fossa pain.

Please examine the gastrointestinal system

- Introduce yourself and clean your hands.
- Start with a general inspection: body habitus, signs of dehydration, fever and pallor.
- Inspect the hands: palmar erythema, finger clubbing, leuconychia, koilonychia, nicotine stains and swollen finger or wrist joints.
- Inspect the face: signs of anaemia (pallor, angular stomatitis), swollen lips and aphthous mouth ulcers.
- Inspect the skin: erythema nodosum or pyoderma gangrenosum.
- Inspect the abdomen: laparotomy scars or skin fistulae.
- Palpate for right iliac fossa tenderness or the presence of a firm, non-tender mass.
- Offer to examine the perianal area for the presence of dusky blue discoloration, oedematous skin tags and the presence of fissures, fistulae or ulcerations.
- Thank the patient and clean your hands.

Summarise your findings

This 29-year-old man with a history of weight loss and diarrhoea appears comfortable at rest but looks thin. He has a recently healed appendicectomy scar, mild periumbilical and left iliac fossa tenderness, and normal bowel sounds.

Suggest a differential diagnosis

The differential diagnosis is Crohn's disease and irritable bowel syndrome.

Suggest initial investigations

Full blood count, C-reactive protein, liver function tests, urea, creatinine and electrolytes, iron studies, vitamin B_{12} and folate levels, ileocolonoscopy and small bowel magnetic resonance imaging, faecal calprotectin.

OSCE example 2: Jaundice

Mr MacDonald, a 61-year-old retired salesman, presents with increasing tiredness and loss of appetite over 4 months. Two weeks ago he noticed dark urine and pale stools, and his friends have remarked that his eyes have become yellow. He has drunk a litre of whisky a day for the last 5 years, although recently he has cut down to a bottle of whisky every 3 days.

Please examine this patient's abdomen

- Introduce yourself and clean your hands.
- Unless prompted otherwise, proceed to peripheral examination prior to concentrating on the abdomen.
- Carry out a general inspection: body habitus, evidence of malnutrition, pallor or jaundice, scratch marks on the forearm and back, bruising.
- Examine the hands: palmar erythema, finger clubbing, leuconychia, Dupuytren's contractures.
- Check for flapping tremor.
- Examine the face: telangiectasias, xanthelasmas, bilateral parotid enlargement and jaundice (yellow sclera of the eyes and skin).
- Smell for alcohol or fetor hepaticus.
- Inspect the neck and chest for spider naevi, gynaecomastia; look for axillary and chest hair loss.
- Inspect the abdomen for distension, everted umbilicus, caput medusae or scars of recent drain insertion.
- Palpate and percuss the abdomen for hepatomegaly and splenomegaly.
- Percuss for shifting dullness.
- Auscultate for hepatic bruits.
- Look for peripheral oedema.
- Thank the patient and your clean hands.

Summarise your findings

This patient is jaundiced with multiple spider naevi on the chest and abdomen. He has generalised abdominal swelling with shifting dullness and a firm liver edge palpable 2 cm below the costal margin.

Suggest a differential diagnosis

The differential diagnosis is alcoholic cirrhosis, chronic hepatitis and hepatoma.

Suggested initial investigations

Liver function tests, ferritin, viral hepatitis screen, full blood count and prothrombin time, urea, creatinine and electrolytes, alpha-fetoprotein, abdominal ultrasound scan and upper digestive endoscopy (to check for oesophagogastric varices).

Integrated examination sequence for the gastrointestinal system

- Position the patient: supine and comfortable on the examination couch. Expose the abdomen from the xiphisternum to the pubic symphysis.
- Inspection: start with general observation, then inspect the skin, face, neck and chest, and finally the abdomen.
- Palpation:
  - Begin with light, superficial palpation away from any site of pain, then repeat with deeper palpation.
  - Describe any mass and decide whether there is an enlarged abdominal organ.
- Palpation for hepatomegaly:
  - Ask the patient to breathe in deeply through the mouth and feel for descent of the liver edge on inspiration.
  - Move your hand progressively up the abdomen, between each breath, until you reach the costal margin or detect the liver edge.
- Percussion to confirm hepatomegaly:
  - Ask the patient to hold their breath in full expiration.
  - Percuss for liver dullness and measure the distance in centimetres below the costal margin.
- Palpation and percussion for splenomegaly:
  - Start with your hand over the umbilicus, moving diagonally up and left to feel for the splenic edge as it descends and moves towards the midline on inspiration.
- Check for ascites (shifting dullness):
  - Percuss from the midline out to the flanks for dullness.
  - Keep your finger on the site of dullness in the flank; ask the patient to turn on to their opposite side and then percuss again. If the area of dullness is now resonant, shifting dullness is present.
- Check for a fluid thrill:
  - Place the palm of your left hand flat against the left side of the patient's abdomen and flick a finger of your right hand against the right side of the abdomen. If you still feel a ripple against your left hand, a fluid thrill is present.
- Auscultation:
  - Listen to the right of the umbilicus for bowel sounds, above the umbilicus over the aorta for arterial bruits, lateral to the umbilicus for bruits from renal artery stenosis, and over the liver for hepatic bruits.
- Check for peripheral oedema.
- Consider a rectal examination (always with a chaperone).

Richard Davenport
Hadi Manji

7

The nervous system

Anatomy and physiology

The nervous system consists of the brain and spinal cord (central nervous system, CNS) and the peripheral nerves (peripheral nervous system, PNS). The PNS includes the autonomic nervous system, responsible for control of involuntary functions.

The neurone is the functional unit of the nervous system. Each neurone has a cell body and axon terminating at a synapse, supported by astrocytes and microglial cells. Astrocytes provide the structural framework for the neurones, control their biochemical environment and form the blood–brain barrier. Microglial cells are blood-derived mononuclear macrophages with immune and scavenging functions. In the CNS, oligodendrocytes produce and maintain a myelin sheath around the axons. In the PNS, myelin is produced by Schwann cells.

The brain consists of two cerebral hemispheres, each with four lobes (frontal, parietal, temporal and occipital), the brainstem and the cerebellum. The brainstem comprises the midbrain, pons and medulla. The cerebellum lies in the posterior fossa, with two hemispheres and a central vermis attached to the brainstem by three pairs of cerebellar peduncles. Between the brain and the skull are three membranous layers called the meninges: dura mater next to the bone, arachnoid and pia mater next to the nervous tissue. The subarachnoid space between the arachnoid and pia is filled with cerebrospinal fluid (CSF) produced by the choroid plexuses. The total volume of CSF is between 140 and 270 mL and there is a turnover of the entire volume 3–4 times a day; thus CSF is produced at a rate of approximately 700 mL per day.

The spinal cord contains afferent and efferent fibres arranged in discrete bundles (pathways running to and from the brain), which are responsible for the transmission of motor and sensory information. Peripheral nerves have myelinated and unmyelinated axons. The sensory cell bodies of peripheral nerves are situated in the dorsal root ganglia. The motor cell bodies are in the anterior horns of the spinal cord (Fig. 7.1).

The history

For many common neurological symptoms such as headache, numbness, disturbance/loss of consciousness and memory loss, the history is the key to diagnosis, as the examination may be either normal or unhelpful. Some symptoms, including loss of consciousness or amnesia, require an additional witness history; make every effort to contact such witnesses.

Remember the two key questions: where (in the nervous system) is the lesion and what is the lesion?

Neurological symptoms may be difficult for patients to describe, so clarify exactly what they tell you. Words such as 'blackout', 'dizziness', 'weakness' and 'numbness' may have different meanings for different patients, so ensure you understand what the person is describing.

Ask patients what they think or fear might be wrong with them, as neurological symptoms cause much anxiety. Patients commonly research their symptoms on the internet; searches on common benign neurological symptoms, like numbness or weakness, usually list the most alarming (and unlikely) diagnoses such multiple sclerosis, motor neurone disease or brain tumours first, and almost never mention more common conditions such as carpal tunnel syndrome or functional disorders.

Time relationships

The onset, duration and pattern of symptoms over time often provide diagnostic clues: for example, in assessing headache (Box 7.1) or vertigo (see Box 9.3).

Ask:

- When did the symptoms start (or when was the patient last well)?
- Are they persistent or intermittent?
- If persistent, are they getting better, getting worse or staying the same?

7.1 Clinical characteristics of headache syndromes

	Onset	Duration/periodicity	Pain location	Associated features
Primary syndromes				
Migraine	Evolves over 30–120 mins	Usually last <24 h, recurrent with weeks/months symptom-free	Classically unilateral but may be anywhere including face/neck	Aura (usually visual), nausea/vomiting, photophobia and phonophobia
Cluster headache	Rapid onset, often waking patient from sleep	30–120 mins, 1–4 attacks within 24 h, clusters usually last weeks to months, with months to years of remission	Orbital/retro-orbital; always same side during cluster, may switch sides between clusters	Autonomic features, including conjunctival injection, tearing, nasal stuffiness, ptosis, miosis, agitation
Stabbing headache	Abrupt, rarely from sleep	Very brief, seconds or less	Anywhere over head	Common in migraineurs
Secondary syndromes				
Meningitis	Usually evolves over a day or two, can be abrupt	Depends on cause and treatment, usually days to weeks	Global, including neck stiffness	Fever, meningism, rash, false localising signs, signs of raised intracranial pressure
Subarachnoid haemorrhage	Abrupt, immediately maximal, rare from sleep	May be fatal at onset, usually days to weeks	Anywhere, poor localising value	20% isolated headache only; nausea/vomiting, reduced consciousness, false localising signs, III nerve palsies
Temporal arteritis	Gradual onset of temple pain and scalp tenderness	Continuous	Temple and scalp	Usually in those >55 years; unwell, jaw pain on chewing, visual symptoms, tender temporal arteries, elevated erythrocyte sedimentation rate and C-reactive protein

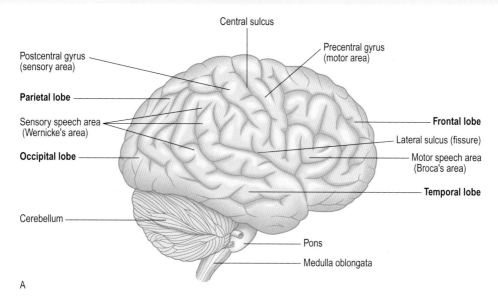

7

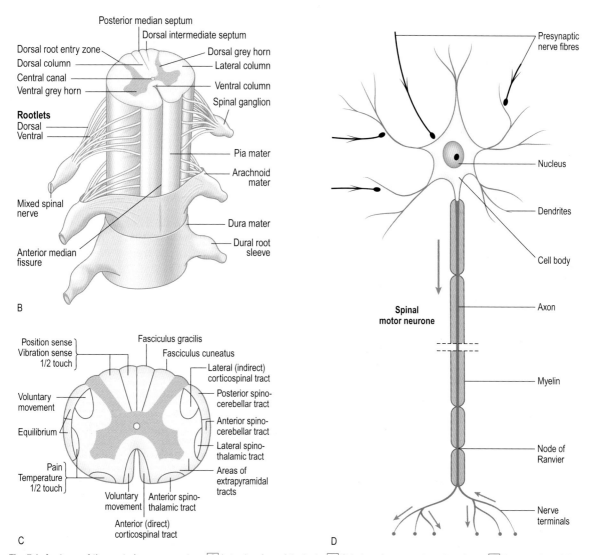

Fig. 7.1 **Anatomy of the central nervous system.** A Lateral surface of the brain. B Spinal cord, nerve roots and meninges. C Cross-section of the spinal cord. D Spinal motor neurone. The terminals of presynaptic neurones form synapses with the cell body and dendrites of the motor neurones.

- If intermittent, how long do they last, and how long does the patient remain symptom-free in between episodes?
- Was the onset sudden or gradual/evolving?

Precipitating, exacerbating or relieving factors

- What was the patient doing when the symptoms occurred?
- Does anything make the symptoms better or worse, such as time of day, menstrual cycle, posture or medication?

Associated symptoms

Associated symptoms can aid diagnosis. For example, headache may be associated with nausea, vomiting, photophobia (aversion to light) and/or phonophobia (aversion to sound) in migraine; headache with neck stiffness, fever and rash may be associated with meningitis (Box 7.1).

Common presenting symptoms

Headache

Headache is the most common neurological symptom and may be either primary or secondary to other pathology. Primary (idiopathic) causes include:

- migraine
- tension-type headache
- trigeminal autonomic cephalalgias (including cluster headache)
- primary stabbing, cough, exertional or sex headache
- primary thunderclap headache
- new daily persistent headache.

Secondary (or symptomatic) headaches are less common, but include potentially life-threatening or disabling causes such as subarachnoid haemorrhage or temporal arteritis. One of the key history aspects is rapidity of onset; isolated headache with a truly abrupt onset may represent a potentially serious cause such as subarachnoid haemorrhage or cerebral vein thrombosis, whereas recurrent headache is much more likely to be migraine, particularly if associated with other migrainous features like aura, nausea and/or vomiting, photophobia and phonophobia (Box 7.1). Asking patents what they do when they have a headache can be instructive. For example, abandoning normal tasks and seeking a bed in a dark, quiet room suggest migraine, whereas pacing around the room in an agitated state, or even head banging, suggests cluster headache.

Transient loss of consciousness

Syncope is loss of consciousness due to inadequate cerebral perfusion and is the most common cause of transient loss of consciousness (TLOC). Vasovagal (or reflex) syncope (fainting) is the most common type and precipitated by stimulation of the parasympathetic nervous system, as with pain or intercurrent illness. Exercise-related syncope, or syncope with no warning or trigger, suggests a possible cardiac cause. TLOC on standing is suggestive of orthostatic (postural) hypotension and may be caused by drugs (antihypertensives or levodopa) or associated with autonomic neuropathies, which may complicate conditions such as diabetes.

Seizure

An epileptic seizure is caused by paroxysmal electrical discharges from either the whole brain (generalised seizure) or part of the brain (focal seizure). A tonic–clonic seizure (convulsion) is the most common form of generalised seizure, and typically follows a stereotyped pattern with early loss of consciousness associated with body stiffening (tonic phase) succeeded by rhythmical jerking crescendoing and subsiding over 30–120 seconds (clonic phase); this is followed by a period of unresponsiveness (often with heavy breathing, the patient appearing to be deeply asleep) and finally confusion as the patient reorientates (postictal phase). The history from the patient and witnesses can help distinguish syncope from epilepsy (Box 7.2). Focal seizures may or may not involve loss of awareness (complete loss of consciousness is less typical) and are characterised by whichever part of the brain is involved: for example, a focal motor seizure arising from the motor cortex, or temporal lobe seizures characterised by autonomic and/or psychic symptoms, often associated with automatisms such as lip smacking or swallowing. Functional dissociative attacks (also known as non-epileptic or psychogenic attacks, or pseudoseizures) are common, and may be difficult to distinguish from epileptic seizures. These attacks are often more frequent than epilepsy, sometimes occurring multiple times in a day, and may last considerably longer, with symptoms waxing and waning. Other features may include asynchronous movements, pelvic thrusts, side-to-side rather than flexion/extension movements and absence of postictal confusion. The widespread availability of videophones allows witnesses to capture such events and may prove invaluable.

7.2 Features that help discriminate vasovagal syncope from epileptic seizure		
Feature	**Vasovagal syncope**	**Seizure**
Triggers	Typically pain, illness, emotion	Often none (sleep deprivation, alcohol, drugs)
Prodrome	Feeling faint/lightheaded, nausea, tinnitus, vision dimming	Focal onset (not always present)
Duration of unconsciousness	<60 s	1–2 mins
Convulsion	May occur but usually brief myoclonic jerks	Usual, tonic–clonic 1–2 mins
Colour	Pale/grey	Flushed/cyanosed, may be pale
Injuries	Uncommon, sometimes biting of tip of tongue	Lateral tongue biting, headache, generalised myalgia, back pain (sometimes vertebral compression fractures), shoulder fracture/dislocation (rare)
Recovery	Rapid, no confusion	Gradual, over 30 mins; patient is often confused, sometimes agitated/aggressive, amnesic

Stroke and transient ischaemic attack

A stroke is a focal neurological deficit of rapid onset that is due to a vascular cause. A transient ischaemic attack (TIA) is the same but symptoms resolve within 24 hours. TIAs are an important risk factor for impending stroke and demand urgent assessment and treatment. Hemiplegia following middle cerebral artery occlusion is a typical example but symptoms are dictated by the vascular territory involved. Much of the cerebral hemispheres are supplied by the anterior circulation (the anterior and middle cerebral arteries are derived from the internal carotid artery), while the occipital lobes and brainstem are supplied by the posterior (vertebrobasilar) circulation (Fig. 7.2).

A useful and simple clinical system for classifying stroke is shown in Box 7.3.

Isolated vertigo, amnesia or TLOC are rarely, if ever, due to stroke. In industrialised countries about 80% of strokes are ischaemic, the remainder haemorrhagic. Factors in the history or examination that increase the likelihood of haemorrhage rather than ischaemia include use of anticoagulation, headache, vomiting, seizures and early reduced consciousness. Haemorrhagic stroke is much more frequent in Asian populations. Spinal strokes are very rare; patients typically present with abrupt bilateral paralysis, depending on the level of spinal cord affected. The anterior spinal artery syndrome is most common and causes loss of motor function and pain/temperature sensation, with relative sparing of joint position and vibration sensation below the level of the lesion.

Dizziness and vertigo

Patients use 'dizziness' to describe many sensations. Recurrent 'dizzy spells' affect approximately 30% of those over 65 years and can be due to postural hypotension, cerebrovascular disease, cardiac arrhythmia or hyperventilation induced by anxiety and panic. Vertigo (the illusion of movement) specifically indicates a problem in the vestibular apparatus (peripheral) or, much less commonly, the brain (central) (see Box 9.3 and p. 174). TIAs do not cause isolated vertigo. Identifying a specific cause of dizziness is often challenging but may be rewarding in some cases, including benign paroxysmal positional vertigo (BPPV), which is eminently treatable. As a guide, recurrent episodes of vertigo lasting a few seconds are most likely to be due to BPPV; vertigo lasting minutes or hours may be caused by Ménière's disease (with associated symptoms including hearing loss, tinnitus, nausea and vomiting) or migrainous vertigo (with or without headache).

Functional neurological symptoms

Many neurological symptoms are not due to disease. These symptoms are often called 'functional' but other (less useful and more pejorative) terms include psychogenic, hysterical, somatisation or conversion disorders. Presentations include blindness, tremor, weakness and collapsing attacks, and patients will often describe numerous other symptoms, with fatigue, lethargy, pain, anxiety and other mood disorders commonly associated. Diagnosing functional symptoms requires experience and patience (p. 363). Clues include symptoms not compatible with disease (such as retained awareness of convulsing during non-epileptic attacks, or being able to walk normally backwards but not forwards), considerable variability in symptoms (such as intermittent recovery of a hemiparesis), multiple symptoms (often with numerous previous assessments by other specialties, particularly gynaecology, gastroenterology, ear, nose and throat and cardiorespiratory) and multiple unremarkable investigations, leading to numerous different diagnoses. The size of a patient's case notes can sometimes be a clue in itself! Beware of labelling symptoms as functional simply because they appear odd or inexplicable. Like disease, most functional neurological disorders follow recognisable patterns, so be cautious when the pattern is atypical.

Past medical history

Symptoms that the patient has forgotten about or overlooked may be important; for example, a history of previous visual loss (optic neuritis) in someone presenting with numbness suggests multiple sclerosis. Birth history and development may be significant, as in epilepsy. Contact parents or family doctors to obtain such information. If considering a vascular cause of neurological symptoms, ask about important risk factors, such as other vascular disease, hypertension, family history and smoking.

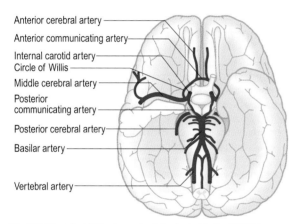

Anterior cerebral artery
Anterior communicating artery
Internal carotid artery
Circle of Willis
Middle cerebral artery
Posterior communicating artery
Posterior cerebral artery
Basilar artery
Vertebral artery

Fig. 7.2 The arterial blood supply of the brain (circle of Willis).

7.3 Clinical classification of stroke

Total anterior circulation syndrome (TACS)

- Hemiparesis, hemianopia and higher cortical deficit (e.g. dysphasia or visuospatial loss)

Partial anterior circulation syndrome (PACS)

- Two of the three components of a TACS
- OR isolated higher cortical deficit
- OR motor/sensory deficit more restricted than LACS (see below)

Posterior circulation syndrome (POCS)

- Ipsilateral cranial nerve palsy with contralateral motor and/or sensory deficit
- OR bilateral motor and/or sensory deficit
- OR disorder of conjugate eye movement
- OR cerebellar dysfunction without ipsilateral long-tract deficits
- OR isolated homonymous visual field defect

Lacunar syndrome (LACS)

- Pure motor > 2 out of 3 of face, arm, leg
- OR pure sensory > 2 out of 3 of face, arm, leg
- OR pure sensorimotor > 2 out of 3 of face, arm, leg
- OR ataxic hemiparesis

Drug history

Always enquire about drugs, including prescribed, over-the-counter, complementary and recreational/illegal ones, as they can give rise to many neurological symptoms (for example, phenytoin toxicity causing ataxia; excessive intake of simple analgesia causing medication overuse headache; use of cocaine provoking convulsions).

Family history

Obtain a family history for at least first-degree relatives: parents, siblings and children. In some communities, parental consanguinity is common, increasing the risk of autosomal recessive conditions, so you may need to enquire sensitively about this. Many neurological disorders are caused by single-gene defects, such as myotonic dystrophy or Huntington's disease. Others have important polygenic influences, as in multiple sclerosis or migraine. Some conditions have a variety of inheritance patterns; for example, Charcot–Marie–Tooth disease may be autosomal dominant, autosomal recessive or X-linked. Mitochondria uniquely have their own DNA, and abnormalities in this DNA can cause a range of disorders that manifest in many different systems (such as diabetes, short stature and deafness), and may cause common neurological syndromes such as migraine or epilepsy. Some diseases, such as Parkinson's or motor neurone disease, may be either due to single-gene disorders or sporadic.

Social history

Social circumstances are relevant. How are patients coping with their symptoms? Are they able to work and drive? What are their support circumstances, and are these adequate?

Alcohol is the most common neurological toxin and damages both the CNS (ataxia, seizures, dementia) and the PNS (neuropathy). Poor diet with vitamin deficiency may compound these problems and is relevant in areas affected by famine and alcoholism or dietary exclusion. Vegetarians may be susceptible to vitamin B_{12} deficiency. Recreational drugs may affect the nervous system; for example, nitrous oxide inhalation causes subacute combined degeneration of the cord due to dysfunction of the vitamin B_{12} pathway, and smoking contributes to vascular and malignant disease. Always consider sexually transmitted or blood-borne infection, such as human immunodeficiency virus (HIV) or syphilis, as both can cause a wide range of neurological symptoms and are treatable. A travel history may give clues to the underlying diagnosis, such as Lyme disease (facial palsy), neurocysticercosis (brain lesions and epilepsy) or malaria (coma).

Occupational history

Occupational factors are relevant to several neurological disorders. For example, toxic peripheral neuropathy, due to exposure to heavy or organic metals like lead, causes a motor neuropathy; manganese causes Parkinsonism. Some neurological diagnoses may adversely affect occupation, such as epilepsy in anyone who needs to drive or operate dangerous machinery. For patients with cognitive disorders, particularly dementias, it may be necessary to advise on whether to stop working.

The physical examination

Neurological assessment begins with your first contact with the patient and continues during the history. Note facial expression, demeanour, dress, posture, gait and speech. Mental state examination (p. 320) and general examination (p. 20) are integral parts of the neurological examination.

Assessment of conscious level

Consciousness has two main components:

- The state of consciousness depends largely on integrity of the ascending reticular activating system, which extends from the brainstem to the thalamus.
- The content of consciousness refers to how aware the person is and depends on the cerebral cortex, the thalamus and their connections.

Do not use ill-defined terms such as stuporose or obtunded. Use the Glasgow Coma Scale (see Box 18.5), a reliable and reproducible tool, to record conscious level.

Meningeal irritation

Meningism (inflammation or irritation of the meninges) can lead to increased resistance to passive flexion of the neck (neck stiffness) or the extended leg (Kernig's sign). Patients may lie with flexed hips to ease their symptoms. Meningism suggests infection (meningitis) or blood within the subarachnoid space (subarachnoid haemorrhage) but can occur with non-neurological infections, such as urinary tract infection or pneumonia. Conversely, absence of meningism does not exclude pathology within the subarachnoid space. In meningitis, neck stiffness has relatively low sensitivity but higher specificity. The absence of all three signs of fever, neck stiffness and altered mental state virtually eliminates the diagnosis of meningitis in immunocompetent individuals.

Examination sequence

- Position the patient supine with no pillow.
- Expose and fully extend both of the patient's legs.

Neck stiffness

- Place your hands on either side of the patient's head, supporting the occiput.
- Flex the patient's head gently until their chin touches their chest.
- Ask the patient to hold that position for 10 seconds. If neck stiffness is present, the neck cannot be passively flexed and you may feel spasm in the neck muscles.
- Flexion of the hips and knees in response to neck flexion is Brudzinski's sign.

Kernig's sign

- Flex one of the patient's legs to 90 degrees at both the hip and the knee, with your left hand placed over the medial hamstrings (Fig. 7.3).
- Extend the knee while the hip is maintained in flexion. Look at the other leg for any reflex flexion. Kernig's sign is positive when extension is resisted by spasm in the hamstrings. Kernig's sign is absent with local causes of neck stiffness, such as cervical spine disease or raised intracranial pressure.

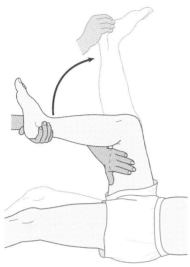

Fig. 7.3 Testing for meningeal irritation: Kernig's sign.

Speech

Dysarthria refers to slurred or 'strangulated' speech caused by articulation problems due to a motor deficit.

Dysphonia describes loss of volume caused by laryngeal disorders.

Examination sequence

- Listen to the patient's spontaneous speech, noting volume, rhythm and clarity.
- Ask the patient to repeat phrases such as 'yellow lorry' to test lingual (tongue) sounds and 'baby hippopotamus' for labial (lip) sounds, then a tongue twister such as 'The Leith police dismisseth us.'
- Ask the patient to count to 30 to assess fatigue.
- Ask the patient to cough and to say 'Ah'; observe the soft palate rising bilaterally.

Disturbed articulation (dysarthria) may result from localised lesions of the tongue, lips or mouth, ill-fitting dentures or neurological dysfunction. This may be due to pathology anywhere in the upper and lower motor neurones, cerebellum, extrapyramidal system, or nerve, muscle or neuromuscular junction.

Bilateral upper motor neurone lesions of the corticobulbar tracts cause a pseudobulbar dysarthria, characterised by a slow, harsh, strangulated speech with difficulty pronouncing consonants, and may be accompanied by a brisk jaw jerk and emotional lability. The tongue is contracted and stiff.

Bulbar palsy (see Box 7.5 later) results from bilateral lower motor neurone lesions affecting the same group of cranial nerves (IX, X, XI, XII). The nature of the speech disturbance is determined by the specific nerves and muscles involved. Weakness of the tongue results in difficulty with lingual sounds, while palatal weakness gives a nasal quality to the speech.

Cerebellar dysarthria may be slow and slurred, similar to alcohol intoxication. Myasthenia gravis causes fatiguing speech, becoming increasing nasal, and may disappear altogether. Parkinsonism may cause dysarthria and dysphonia, with a low-volume, monotonous voice, words running into each other (festination of speech), and marked stuttering/hesitation.

Dysphonia usually results from either vocal cord pathology, as in laryngitis, or damage to the vagal (X) nerve supply to the vocal cords (recurrent laryngeal nerve). Inability to abduct one of the vocal cords leads to a 'bovine' (and ineffective) cough.

Dysphasias

Dysphasia is a disturbance of language resulting in abnormalities of speech production and/or understanding. It may involve other language symptoms, such as writing and/or reading problems, unlike dysarthria and dysphonia.

Anatomy

The language areas are located in the dominant cerebral hemisphere, which is the left in almost all right-handed people and most left-handed people.

Broca's area (inferior frontal region) is concerned with word production and language expression.

Wernicke's area (superior posterior temporal lobe) is the principal area for comprehension of spoken language. Adjacent regions of the parietal lobe are involved in understanding written language and numbers.

The arcuate fasciculus connects Broca's and Wernicke's areas.

Examination sequence

- During spontaneous speech, listen to the fluency and appropriateness of the content, particularly paraphasias (incorrect words) and neologisms (nonsense or meaningless new words).
- Show the patient a common object, such as a coin or pen, and ask them to name it.
- Give a simple three-stage command, such as 'Pick up this piece of paper, fold it in half and place it under the book.'
- Ask the patient to repeat a simple sentence, such as 'Today is Tuesday.'
- Ask the patient to read a passage from a newspaper.
- Ask the patient to write a sentence; examine the handwriting.

Expressive (motor) dysphasia results from damage to Broca's area. It is characterised by reduced verbal output with non-fluent speech and errors of grammar and syntax. Comprehension is intact.

Receptive (sensory) dysphasia occurs due to dysfunction in Wernicke's area. There is poor comprehension, and although speech is fluent, it may be meaningless and contain paraphasias and neologisms.

Global dysphasia is a combination of expressive and receptive difficulties caused by involvement of both areas.

Dysphasia (a focal sign) is frequently misdiagnosed as confusion (non-focal). Always consider dysphasia before assuming confusion, as this fundamentally alters the differential diagnosis and management.

Dominant parietal lobe lesions affecting the supramarginal gyrus may cause dyslexia (difficulty comprehending written language), dyscalculia (problems with simple addition and subtraction) and dysgraphia (impairment of writing). Gerstmann's syndrome is the combination of dysgraphia, dyscalculia, finger agnosia (inability to recognise the fingers) and inability to distinguish left from right. It localises to the left parietal lobe in the region of the angular gyrus.

Cortical function

Thinking, emotions, language, behaviour, planning and initiation of movements, and perception of sensory information are functions of the cerebral cortex and are central to awareness of, and interaction with, the environment. Certain cortical areas are associated with specific functions, so particular patterns of dysfunction can help localise the site of pathology (Fig. 7.4A). Assessment of higher cortical function can be difficult and time-consuming but is essential in patients with cognitive symptoms. There are various tools, all primarily developed as screening and assessment tools for dementia. For the bedside the Mini-Mental State Examination (MMSE) and Montreal Cognitive Assessment (MoCA) are quick to administer, while the Addenbrooke's Cognitive Examination is more detailed but takes longer. None of these bedside tests is a substitute for detailed neuropsychological assessment. The assessment of cognitive function is covered in more detail on page 323.

2 Parietal lobe

Dominant side		Non-dominant side	
FUNCTION Calculation Language Planned movement Appreciation of size, shape, weight and texture	LESIONS Dyscalculia Dysphasia Dyslexia Apraxia Agnosia Homonymous hemianopia	FUNCTION Spatial orientation Constructional skills	LESIONS Neglect of non-dominant side Spatial disorientation Constructional apraxia Dressing apraxia Homonymous hemianopia

1 Frontal lobe

FUNCTION
Personality
Emotional response
Social behaviour

LESIONS
Disinhibition
Lack of initiative
Antisocial behaviour
Impaired memory
Incontinence
Grasp reflexes
Anosmia

3 Occipital lobe

FUNCTION
Analysis of vision

LESIONS
Homonymous hemianopia
Hemianopic scotomas
Visual agnosia
Impaired face recognition
(prosopagnosia)
Visual hallucinations
(lights, lines and zigzags)

4 Temporal lobe

Dominant side		Non-dominant side	
FUNCTION Auditory perception Speech, language Verbal memory Smell	LESIONS Dysphasia Dyslexia Poor memory Complex hallucinations (smell, sound, vision) Homonymous hemianopia	FUNCTION Auditory perception Music, tone sequences Non-verbal memory (faces, shapes, music) Smell	LESIONS Poor non-verbal memory Loss of musical skills Complex hallucinations Homonymous hemianopia

A

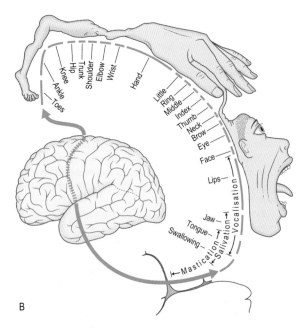

B

Fig. 7.4 Cortical function. A Features of localised cerebral lesions. B Somatotopic homunculus.

Frontal lobe

The posterior part of the frontal lobe is the motor strip (precentral gyrus), which controls voluntary movement. The motor strip is organised somatotopically (Fig. 7.4B). The area anterior to the precentral gyrus is concerned with personality, social behaviour, emotions, cognition and expressive language, and contains the frontal eye fields and cortical centre for micturition (Fig. 7.4A).

Frontal lobe damage may cause:

- personality and behaviour changes, such as apathy or disinhibition
- loss of emotional responsiveness, or emotional lability
- cognitive impairments, such as memory, attention and concentration
- dysphasia (dominant hemisphere)
- conjugate gaze deviation to the side of the lesion
- urinary incontinence
- primitive reflexes, such as grasp
- focal motor seizures (motor strip).

Temporal lobe

The temporal lobe contains the primary auditory cortex, Wernicke's area and parts of the limbic system. The latter is crucially important in memory, emotion and smell appreciation. The temporal lobe also contains the lower fibres of the optic radiation and the area of auditory perception.

Temporal lobe dysfunction may cause:

- memory impairment
- focal seizures with psychic symptoms
- contralateral upper quadrantanopia (see Fig. 8.5(4))
- receptive dysphasia (dominant hemisphere).

Parietal lobe

The postcentral gyrus (sensory strip) is the most anterior part of the parietal lobe and is the principal destination of conscious sensations. The upper fibres of the optic radiation pass through it. The dominant hemisphere contains aspects of language function and the non-dominant lobe is concerned with spatial awareness.

Features of parietal lobe dysfunction include:

- cortical sensory impairments
- contralateral lower quadrantanopia (see Fig. 8.5(5))
- dyslexia, dyscalculia, dysgraphia
- apraxia (an inability to carry out complex tasks despite having an intact sensory and motor system)
- focal sensory seizures (postcentral gyrus)
- visuospatial disturbance (non-dominant parietal lobe).

Occipital lobe

The occipital lobe blends with the temporal and parietal lobes and forms the posterior part of the cerebral cortex. Its main function is analysis of visual information.

Occipital lobe damage may cause:

- visual field defects: hemianopia (loss of part of a visual field) or scotoma (blind spot) (see Fig. 8.5(6)).
- visual agnosia: the inability to recognise visual stimuli
- disturbances of visual perception, such as macropsia (seeing things larger) or micropsia (seeing things smaller)
- visual hallucinations.

Cranial nerves

The 12 pairs of cranial nerves (with the exception of the olfactory (I) pair) arise from the brainstem (Fig. 7.5 and Box 7.4). Cranial nerves II, III, IV and VI relate to the eye (Ch. 8) and the VIII nerve to hearing and balance (Ch. 9).

Olfactory (I) nerve

The olfactory nerve conveys the sense of smell.

Anatomy

Bipolar cells in the olfactory bulb form olfactory filaments with small receptors projecting through the cribriform plate high in the nasal cavity. These cells synapse with second-order neurones, which project centrally via the olfactory tract to the medial temporal lobe and amygdala.

Examination sequence

Bedside testing of smell is of limited clinical value, and rarely performed, although objective 'scratch and sniff' test cards, such as the University of Pennsylvania Smell Identification Test (UPSIT), are available. You can ask patients if they think their sense of smell is normal, although self-reporting can be surprisingly inaccurate.

7.4 Summary of the 12 cranial nerves		
Nerve	Examination	Abnormalities/symptoms
I	Sense of smell, each nostril	Anosmia/parosmia
II	Visual acuity	Partial sight/blindness
	Visual fields	Scotoma; hemianopia
	Pupil size and shape	Anisocoria
	Pupil light reflex	Impairment or loss
	Fundoscopy	Optic disc and retinal changes
III	Light and accommodation reflex	Impairment or loss
III, IV and VI	Eye position and movements	Strabismus, diplopia, nystagmus
V	Facial sensation	Impairment, distortion or loss
	Corneal reflex	Impairment or loss
	Muscles of mastication	Weakness of chewing movements
	Jaw jerk	Increase in upper motor neurone lesions
VII	Muscles of facial expression	Facial weakness
	Taste over anterior two-thirds of tongue	Ageusia (loss of taste)
VIII	Whisper and tuning fork tests	Impaired hearing/deafness
	Vestibular tests	Nystagmus and vertigo
IX	Pharyngeal sensation	Not routinely tested
X	Palate movements	Unilateral or bilateral impairment
XI	Trapezius and sternomastoid	Weakness of scapular and neck movement
XII	Tongue appearance and movement	Dysarthria and chewing/swallowing difficulties

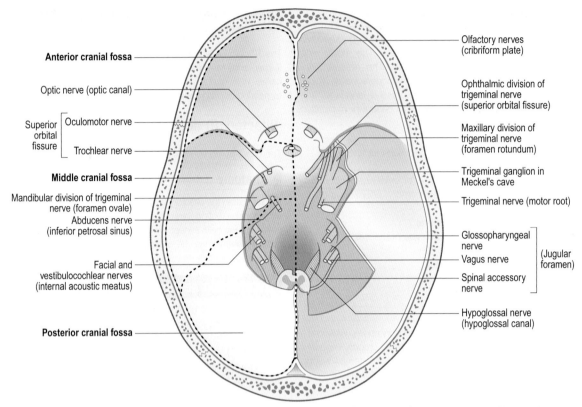

Fig. 7.5 Base of the cranial cavity. The dura mater, with the cranial nerves and their exits from the skull. On the right side, part of the tentorium cerebelli and the roof of the trigeminal cave have been removed.

Hyposmia or anosmia (reduction or loss of the sense of smell) may result from upper respiratory infection, sinus disease, damage to the olfactory filaments after head injury or infection, local compression (by olfactory groove meningioma, for example; see Fig. 7.29C) or invasion by basal skull tumours. Disturbance of smell may also occur very early in Parkinson's and Alzheimer's diseases. Patients often note hypogeusia/ageusia (altered taste) with anosmia too, as taste is crucially influenced by the sense of smell.

Parosmia is the perception of pleasant odours as unpleasant; it may occur with head trauma or sinus infection, or be an adverse effect of drugs. Olfactory hallucinations may occur in Alzheimer's disease and focal epilepsies.

Optic (II), oculomotor (III), trochlear (IV) and abducens (VI) nerves

See Chapter 8.

Trigeminal (V) nerve

The V nerve conveys sensation from the face, mouth and part of the dura, and provides motor supply to the muscles of mastication.

Anatomy

The cell bodies of the sensory fibres are located in the trigeminal (Gasserian) ganglion, which lies in a cavity (Meckel's cave) in the petrous temporal dura (see Fig. 7.5). From the trigeminal

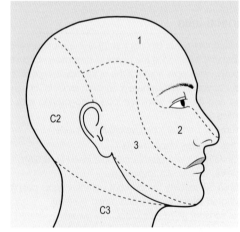

Fig. 7.6 The sensory distribution of the three divisions of the trigeminal nerve. 1, Ophthalmic division. **2,** Maxillary division. **3,** Mandibular division.

ganglion, the V nerve passes to the pons. From here, pain and temperature pathways descend to the C2 segment of the spinal cord, so ipsilateral facial numbness may occur with cervical cord lesions.

There are three major branches of V (Fig. 7.6):

- ophthalmic (V_1): sensory
- maxillary (V_2): sensory
- mandibular (V_3): sensory and motor.

The ophthalmic branch leaves the ganglion and passes forward to the superior orbital fissure via the wall of the cavernous sinus (see Fig. 8.3). In addition to the skin of the upper nose, upper eyelid, forehead and scalp, V_1 supplies sensation to the eye (cornea and conjunctiva) and the mucous membranes of the sphenoidal and ethmoid sinuses and upper nasal cavity.

The maxillary branch (V_2) passes from the ganglion via the cavernous sinus to leave the skull by the foramen rotundum. It contains sensory fibres from the mucous membranes of the upper mouth, roof of pharynx, gums, teeth and palate of the upper jaw and the maxillary, sphenoidal and ethmoid sinuses.

The mandibular branch (V_3) exits the skull via the foramen ovale and supplies the floor of the mouth, sensation (but not taste) to the anterior two-thirds of the tongue, the gums and teeth of the lower jaw, mucosa of the cheek and the temporomandibular joint, in addition to the skin of the lower lips and jaw area, but not the angle of the jaw (see Fig. 7.6).

The motor fibres of V run in the mandibular branch (V_3) and innervate the muscles of mastication: temporalis, masseter and medial and lateral pterygoids.

Examination sequence

Four aspects need to be assessed: sensory, motor and two reflexes.

Sensory

- Ask the patient to close their eyes and say 'yes' each time they feel a light touch (you use a cotton-wool tip for this test). Do this in the areas of V_1, V_2 and V_3.
- Repeat using a fresh neurological pin, such as a Neurotip, to test superficial pain.
- Compare both sides. If you identify an area of reduced sensation, map it out. Does it conform to the distribution of the trigeminal nerve or branches? Remember the angle of the jaw is served by C2 and not the trigeminal nerve, but V_1 extends towards the vertex (see Fig. 7.6).
- 'Nasal tickle' test: use a wisp of cotton wool to 'tickle' the inside of each nostril and ask the patient to compare. The normal result is an unpleasant sensation easily appreciated by the patient.

Motor (signs rare)

- Inspect for wasting of the muscles of mastication (most apparent in temporalis).
- Ask the patient to clench their teeth; feel the masseters, estimating their bulk.
- Ask the patient to open their jaw and note any deviation; the jaw may deviate to the paralysed side due to contraction of the intact contralateral pterygoid muscle.

Corneal reflex

Routine testing of the corneal reflex is unnecessary, but may be relevant when the history suggests a lesion localising to the brainstem or cranial nerves V, VII or VIII. The afferent limb is via the trigeminal nerve, the efferent limb via the facial nerve.

- Explain to the patient what you are going to do and ask them to remove their contact lenses, if relevant.
- Gently depress the lower eyelid while the patient looks up.
- Lightly touch the lateral edge of the cornea with a wisp of damp cotton wool (Fig. 7.7).
- Look for both direct and consensual blinking.

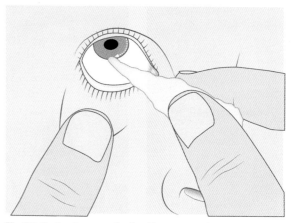

Fig. 7.7 Testing the corneal reflex. The cotton-wool wisp should touch the cornea overlying the iris, not the conjunctiva, and avoid visual stimulus.

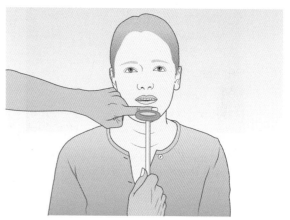

Fig. 7.8 Eliciting the jaw jerk.

7.5 Comparison of bulbar and pseudobulbar palsy		
	Bulbar palsy	**Pseudobulbar palsy**
Level of motor lesion	Lower motor neurone	Upper motor neurone
Speech	Dysarthria	Dysarthria and dysphonia
Swallowing	Dysphagia	Dysphagia
Tongue	Weak, wasted and fasciculating	Spastic, slow-moving
Jaw jerk	Absent	Present/brisk
Emotional lability	Absent	May be present
Causes	Motor neurone disease	Cerebrovascular disease, motor neurone disease, multiple sclerosis

Jaw jerk

- Ask the patient to let their mouth hang loosely open.
- Place your forefinger in the midline between lower lip and chin.
- Percuss your finger gently with the tendon hammer in a downward direction (Fig. 7.8), noting any reflex closing of the jaw.
- An absent, or just present, reflex is normal. A brisk jaw jerk occurs in pseudobulbar palsy (Box 7.5).

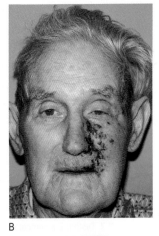

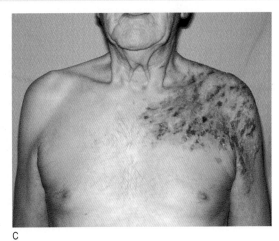

A   B   C

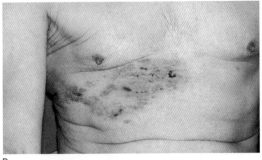

D

Fig. 7.9 Herpes zoster. [A] The ophthalmic division of the left trigeminal (V) nerve is involved. [B] The maxillary division of the left V nerve. [C] Cervical spinal root left C5. [D] Thoracic spinal root right T8.

Sensory symptoms include facial numbness and pain. Unilateral loss of sensation in one or more branches of the V nerve may result from direct injury in association with facial fractures (particularly V_2), local invasion by cancer or Sjögren's syndrome. Lesions in the cavernous sinus often cause loss of the corneal reflex and V_1 or V_2 cutaneous sensory loss. Cranial nerves III, IV and VI may also be involved (see Fig. 8.3). Trigeminal neuralgia causes severe, lancinating pain, typically in the distribution of V_2 or V_3. Reactivation of herpes varicella zoster virus (chickenpox) can affect any sensory nerve, but typically either V_1 or a thoracic dermatome (Fig. 7.9). In herpes zoster ophthalmicus (affecting V_1) there is a risk of sight-threatening complications. Hutchinson's sign, vesicles on the side or tip of the nose, may be present.

Clinically significant weakness of the muscles of mastication is unusual but may occur in myasthenia gravis, with fatigable chewing.

Facial (VII) nerve

The facial nerve supplies the muscles of facial expression (frontalis, orbicularis oculi, buccinators, orbicularis oris and platysma) and carries parasympathetic fibres to the lacrimal, submandibular and sublingual salivary glands (via nervus intermedius). It receives taste sensation from the anterior two-thirds of the tongue (via the chorda tympani; Fig. 7.10).

Anatomy

From its motor nucleus in the lower pons, fibres of the VII nerve pass back to loop around the VI nerve nucleus before emerging from the lateral pontomedullary junction in close association with the VIII nerve (Fig. 7.11); together they enter the internal acoustic meatus (see Fig. 7.5). At the lateral end of the meatus the VII nerve continues in the facial canal within the temporal bone, exiting the skull via the stylomastoid foramen. Passing through the parotid gland, it gives off its terminal branches. In its course in the facial canal it gives off branches to the stapedius muscle and its parasympathetic fibres, as well as being joined by the taste fibres of the chorda tympani (see Fig. 7.10).

Examination sequence

Examination is usually confined to motor function; taste is rarely tested.

Motor function
- Inspect the face for asymmetry or differences in blinking or eye closure on one side. Note that minor facial asymmetry is common and rarely pathological.
- Watch for spontaneous or involuntary movement.
- For the following actions it is often easiest to demonstrate the actions yourself and ask the patient to copy you, observing for any asymmetry.
- Ask the patient to raise their eyebrows and observe for symmetrical wrinkling of the forehead (frontalis muscle).
- Ask the patient to screw their eyes tightly shut and resist you opening them (orbicularis oculi).
- Ask the patient to bare their teeth (orbicularis oris).
- Ask the patient to blow out their cheeks with their mouth closed (buccinators and orbicularis oris).

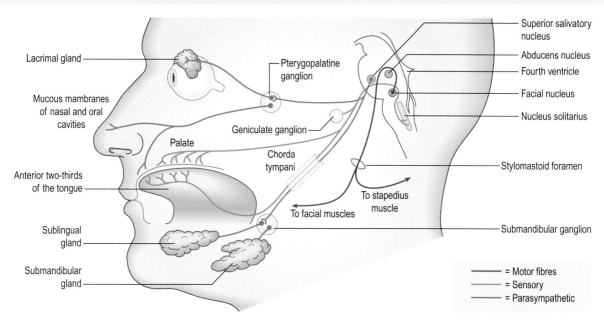

Fig. 7.10 Component fibres of the facial nerve and their peripheral distribution.

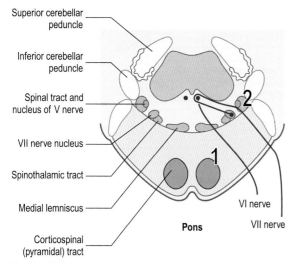

Fig. 7.11 **Lesions of the pons.** Lesions at (1) may result in ipsilateral VI and VII nerve palsies and contralateral hemiplegia. At (2) ipsilateral cerebellar signs and impaired sensation on the ipsilateral side of the face and on the contralateral side of the body may occur.

In a unilateral lower motor neurone VII nerve lesion, there is weakness of both upper and lower facial muscles. Bell's palsy is the term used to describe an idiopathic acute lower motor neurone VII nerve paralysis, often preceded by mastoid pain. It may be associated with impairment of taste and hyperacusis (high-pitched sounds appearing unpleasantly louder than normal). Bell's phenomenon occurs when a patient closes their eyes: as eye closure is incomplete the globe can be seen to roll upwards, to avoid corneal exposure (Fig. 7.12A). Ramsay Hunt syndrome occurs in herpes zoster infection of the geniculate (facial) ganglion. This produces a severe lower motor neurone facial palsy, ipsilateral loss of taste and buccal ulceration, and a painful vesicular eruption in the external auditory meatus. Other causes of a lower motor neurone VII lesion include cerebellopontine

angle tumours (including acoustic neuroma), trauma and parotid tumours. Synkinesis (involuntary muscle contraction accompanying a voluntary movement: most commonly, twitching of the corner of the mouth with ipsilateral blinking) is a sign of aberrant reinnervation and may be seen in recovering lower motor neurone VII lesions.

In unilateral VII nerve upper motor neurone lesions, weakness is marked in the lower facial muscles with relative sparing of the upper face. This is because there is bilateral cortical innervation of the upper facial muscles. The nasolabial fold may be flattened and the corner of the mouth drooped, but eye closure is usually preserved (Fig. 7.12B). Hemifacial spasm presents with synchronised twitching of the ipsilateral eye and mouth.

Bilateral facial palsies are less common, but occasionally occur, as in Guillain–Barré syndrome, sarcoidosis, or infection such as Lyme disease, HIV or leprosy. Facial weakness, especially with respect to eye closure, can also be found in some congenital myopathies (facioscapulohumeral or myotonic dystrophies). Distinct from VII nerve palsies, Parkinson's disease can cause loss of spontaneous facial movements, including a slowed blink rate, and involuntary facial movements (levodopa-induced dyskinesias) may complicate advanced disease.

Involuntary emotional movements, such as spontaneous smiling, have different pathways and may be preserved in the presence of paresis.

Vestibulocochlear (VIII) nerve

See page 173.

Glossopharyngeal (IX) and vagus (X) nerves

The IX and X nerves have an intimate anatomical relationship. Both contain sensory, motor and autonomic components. The glossopharyngeal (IX) nerve mainly carries sensation from the pharynx and tonsils, and sensation and taste from the posterior one-third of the tongue. The IX nerve also supplies the carotid chemoreceptors. The vagus (X) nerve carries important sensory

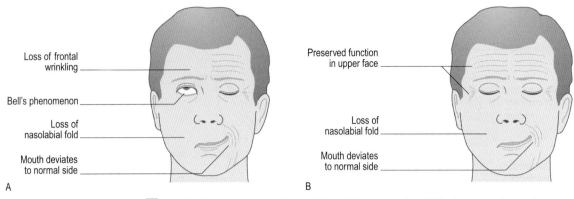

Fig. 7.12 Types of facial weakness. [A] Right-sided lower motor neurone lesion (within facial nerve or nucleus); Bell's phenomenon is also shown. [B] Right-sided upper motor neurone lesion.

information but also innervates upper pharyngeal and laryngeal muscles. The main functions of IX and X that can be tested clinically are swallowing, phonation/articulation and sensation from the pharynx/larynx. In the thorax and abdomen, the vagus (X) nerve receives sensory fibres from the lungs and carries parasympathetic fibres to the lungs, heart and abdominal viscera.

Anatomy

Both nerves arise as several roots from the lateral medulla and leave the skull together via the jugular foramen (see Fig. 7.5). The IX nerve passes down and forwards to supply the stylopharyngeus muscle, the mucosa of the pharynx, the tonsils and the posterior one-third of the tongue, and sends parasympathetic fibres to the parotid gland. The X nerve courses down in the carotid sheath into the thorax, giving off several branches, including pharyngeal and recurrent laryngeal branches, which provide motor supply to the pharyngeal, soft palate and laryngeal muscles. The main nuclei of these nerves in the medulla are the nucleus ambiguus (motor), the dorsal motor vagal nucleus (parasympathetic) and the solitary nucleus (visceral sensation; Fig. 7.13).

Examination sequence

- Assess the patient's speech for dysarthria or dysphonia (p. 125).
- Ask them to say 'Ah'. Look at the movements of the palate and uvula using a torch. Normally, both sides of the palate elevate symmetrically and the uvula remains in the midline.
- Ask the patient to puff out their cheeks with their lips tightly closed. Listen for air escaping from the nose. For the cheeks to puff out, the palate must elevate and occlude the nasopharynx. If palatal movement is weak, air will escape audibly through the nose.
- Ask the patient to cough; assess the strength of the cough.
- Testing pharyngeal sensation and the gag reflex is unpleasant and has poor predictive value for aspiration. Instead, and in fully conscious patients only, use the swallow test. Administer 3 teaspoons of water and observe for absent swallow, cough or delayed cough, or change in voice quality after each teaspoon. If there are no problems, observe again while the patient swallows a glass of water.

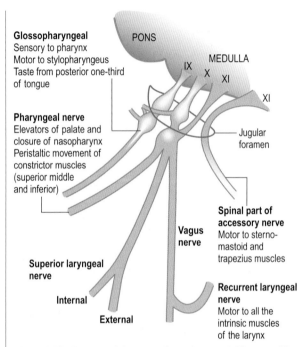

Fig. 7.13 The lower cranial nerves: glossopharyngeal (IX), vagus (X) and accessory (XI).

Isolated unilateral IX nerve lesions are rare. Unilateral X nerve damage leads to ipsilateral reduced elevation of the soft palate, which may cause deviation of the uvula (away from the side of the lesion) when the patient says 'Ah'. Unilateral lesions of IX and X are most commonly caused by strokes, skull-base fractures or tumours. Damage to the recurrent laryngeal branch of the X nerve due to lung cancer, thyroid surgery, mediastinal tumours and aortic arch aneurysms causes dysphonia and a 'bovine' cough. Bilateral X nerve lesions cause dysphagia and dysarthria, and may be due to lesions at the upper motor neurone level (pseudobulbar palsy) or lower motor neurone level (bulbar palsy; see Box 7.5). Less severe cases can result in nasal regurgitation of fluids and nasal air escape when the cheeks are puffed out (dysarthria and nasal escape are often evident during history taking). Always consider myasthenia gravis in patients with symptoms of bulbar dysfunction, even if the examination seems normal.

Accessory (XI) nerve

The accessory nerve has two components:
- a cranial part closely related to the vagus (X) nerve
- a spinal part that provides fibres to the upper trapezius muscles, responsible for elevating (shrugging) the shoulders and elevation of the arm above the horizontal, and the sternomastoid muscles that control head turning and flexing the neck.

The spinal component is discussed here.

Anatomy

The spinal nuclei arise from the anterior horn cells of C1–5. Fibres emerge from the spinal cord, ascend through the foramen magnum and exit via the jugular foramen (see Fig. 7.5), passing posteriorly.

Examination sequence

- Face the patient and inspect the sternomastoid muscles for wasting or hypertrophy; palpate them to assess their bulk.
- Stand behind the patient to inspect the trapezius muscle for wasting or asymmetry.
- Ask the patient to shrug their shoulders, then apply downward pressure with your hands to assess the power.
- Test power in the left sternomastoid by asking the patient to turn their head to the right while you provide resistance with your hand placed on the right side of the patient's chin. Reverse the procedure to check the right sternomastoid.
- Test both sternocleidomastoid muscles simultaneously by asking the patient to flex their neck. Apply your palm to the forehead as resistance.

Isolated XI nerve lesions are uncommon but the nerve may be damaged during surgery in the posterior triangle of the neck, penetrating injuries or tumour invasion. Wasting of the upper fibres of trapezius may be associated with displacement ('winging') of the upper vertebral border of the scapula away from the spine, while the lower border is displaced towards it. Wasting and weakness of the sternomastoids are characteristic of myotonic dystrophy. Weakness of neck flexion or extension, the latter causing head drop, may occur in myasthenia gravis, motor neurone disease and some myopathies. Dystonic head postures causing antecollis (neck flexed), retrocollis (neck extended) or torticollis (neck twisted to one side) are not associated with weakness.

Hypoglossal (XII) nerve

The XII nerve innervates the tongue muscles; the nucleus lies in the dorsal medulla beneath the floor of the fourth ventricle.

Anatomy

The nerve emerges anteriorly and exits the skull in the hypoglossal canal, passing to the root of the tongue (see Fig. 7.5).

Examination sequence

- Ask the patient to open their mouth. Look at the tongue at rest for wasting, fasciculation or involuntary movement.

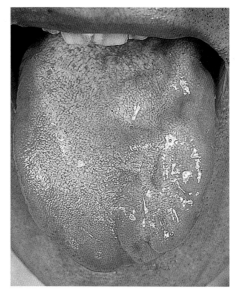

Fig. 7.14 Left hypoglossal nerve lesion. *From Epstein O, Perkin GD, de Bono DP, et al. Clinical Examination. 2nd edn. London: Mosby; 1997.*

- Ask the patient to put out their tongue. Look for deviation or involuntary movement.
- Ask the patient to move their tongue quickly from side to side.
- Test power by asking the patient to press their tongue against the inside of each cheek in turn while you press from the outside with your finger.
- Assess speech by asking the patient to say 'yellow lorry'.
- Assess swallowing with a water swallow test (p. 132).

Unilateral lower motor XII nerve lesions lead to tongue wasting on the affected side and deviation to that side on protrusion (Fig. 7.14). Bilateral lower motor neurone damage results in global wasting, the tongue appears thin and shrunken and fasciculation may be evident. Normal rippling or undulating movements may be mistaken for fasciculation, especially if the tongue is protruded; these usually settle when the tongue is at rest in the mouth. When associated with lesions of the IX, X and XI nerves, typically in motor neurone disease, these features are termed bulbar palsy (see Box 7.5).

Unilateral upper motor XII nerve lesions are uncommon; bilateral lesions lead to a tongue with increased tone (spastic) and the patient has difficulty flicking the tongue from side to side. Bilateral upper motor lesions of the IX–XII nerves are called pseudobulbar palsy (see Box 7.5). Tremor of the resting or protruded tongue may occur in Parkinson's disease, although jaw tremor is more common. Other orolingual dyskinesias (involuntary movements of the mouth and tongue) are often drug-induced and include tardive dyskinesias due to neuroleptics.

Motor system

Anatomy

The principal motor pathway has CNS (corticospinal or pyramidal tract – upper motor neurone) and PNS (anterior horn cell – lower motor neurone) components (Fig. 7.15). Other parts of

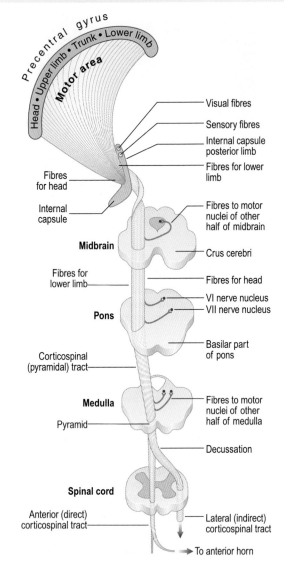

Fig. 7.15 Principal motor pathways.

Labels in figure:
Precentral gyrus — Head • Upper limb • Trunk • Lower limb
Motor area
Visual fibres
Sensory fibres
Internal capsule posterior limb
Fibres for lower limb
Fibres for head
Internal capsule
Midbrain
Fibres to motor nuclei of other half of midbrain
Crus cerebri
Fibres for lower limb
Fibres for head
VI nerve nucleus
VII nerve nucleus
Pons
Basilar part of pons
Corticospinal (pyramidal) tract
Medulla
Pyramid
Fibres to motor nuclei of other half of medulla
Decussation
Spinal cord
Anterior (direct) corticospinal tract
Lateral (indirect) corticospinal tract
To anterior horn

the nervous system, such as the basal ganglia and cerebellum, have important modulating effects on movement. It is important to distinguish upper from lower motor neurone signs to help localise the lesion (Box 7.6).

Upper motor neurone lesions

If the lesion affects the CNS pathways, the lower motor neurones are under the uninhibited influence of the spinal reflex. The motor units then have an exaggerated response to stretch with increased tone (spasticity), clonus and brisk reflexes. There is weakness but not wasting (although atrophy may develop with longstanding lesions). Primitive reflexes, such as the plantar extensor response (Babinski sign), may be present.

Lower motor neurone lesions

Motor fibres, together with input from other systems involved in the control of movement, including extrapyramidal, cerebellar, vestibular and proprioceptive afferents, converge on the cell bodies of lower motor neurones in the anterior horn of the grey matter in the spinal cord (Fig. 7.15).

7.6 Features of motor neurone lesions		
	Upper motor neurone lesion	Lower motor neurone lesion
Inspection	Usually normal (may be disuse wasting in longstanding lesions)	Muscle wasting, fasciculations
Tone	Increased with clonus	Normal or decreased, no clonus
Weakness	Preferentially affects extensors in arms, flexors in leg	Usually more focal, in distribution of nerve root or peripheral nerve
Deep tendon reflexes	Increased	Decreased/absent
Plantar response	Extensor (Babinski sign)	Flexor

The group of muscle fibres innervated by a single anterior horn cell forms a 'motor unit'. A lower motor neurone lesion causes weakness and wasting in these muscle fibres, reduced tone (flaccidity), fasciculation and reduced or absent reflexes.

Basal ganglia lesions

The basal ganglia are connected structures within the cerebral hemispheres and brainstem (Fig. 7.16). They include the caudate nucleus and putamen (collectively known as the striatum), globus pallidus, thalamus, subthalamic nucleus and substantia nigra (the latter in the brainstem). The basal ganglia receive much information from the cortex and are involved in regulating many activities, principally control of movement, but are also involved in eye movement, behaviour and executive function control. Disorders of the basal ganglia may cause reduced movement (typically Parkinsonism; p. 135) or, less commonly, excessive movement such as ballism or tics (p. 137).

Assess the motor system using the following method:

- assessment of stance and gait
- inspection and palpation of muscles
- assessment of tone
- testing movement and power
- examination of reflexes
- testing coordination.

Stance and gait

Stance and gait depend on intact visual, vestibular, sensory, corticospinal, extrapyramidal and cerebellar pathways, together with functioning lower motor neurones and spinal reflexes. Non-neurological gait disorders are discussed in on page 259. Certain abnormal gait patterns are recognisable, suggesting diagnoses (Box 7.7 and Fig. 7.17).

Examination sequence

Stance

- Ask the patient to stand with their (preferably bare) feet close together and eyes open.
- Swaying, lurching or an inability to stand with the feet together and eyes open suggests cerebellar ataxia.
- Ask the patient to close their eyes (Romberg's test) but be prepared to steady/catch them. Repeated falling is a

A

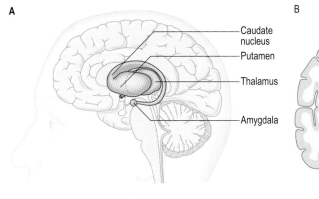

Caudate
nucleus

Putamen

Thalamus

Amygdala

B

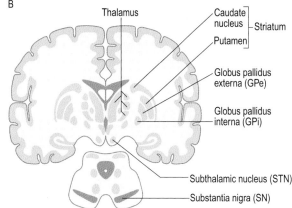

Thalamus

Caudate
nucleus
Striatum

Putamen

Globus pallidus
externa (GPe)

Globus pallidus
interna (GPi)

Subthalamic nucleus (STN)

Substantia nigra (SN)

7

Fig. 7.16 Basal ganglia. [A] Anatomical location. [B] Coronal view.

7.7 Common gait abnormalities		
Gait disturbance	**Description**	**Causes**
Parkinsonian	Stooped posture Shuffling (reduced stride length) Loss of arm swing Postural instability Freezing	Parkinson's disease and other Parkinsonian syndromes
Gait apraxia	Small, shuffling steps (*marche à petits pas*) Difficulty in starting to walk/freezing Better 'cycling' on bed than walking	Cerebrovascular disease Hydrocephalus
Spastic	Stiff 'walking-through-mud' or scissors gait	Spinal cord lesions
Myopathic	Waddling (proximal weakness) Bilateral Trendelenburg signs	Muscular dystrophies and acquired myopathies
Foot drop	Foot slapping	Neuropathies Common peroneal nerve palsy L5 radiculopathy
Central ataxia	Wide-based, 'drunken' Tandem gait poor	Cerebellar disease
Sensory ataxia	Wide-based Positive Romberg sign	Neuropathies Spinal cord disorders
Functional	Variable, often bizarre, inconsistent Knees flexed, buckling Dragging immobile leg behind	Functional neurological disorders

© Crown Copyright.

positive result. Swaying is common and should not be misinterpreted.

- The 'pull test' assesses postural stability. Ask the patient to stand with their feet slightly apart. Inform them that you are going to push them forwards or pull them backwards. They should maintain their position if possible. Standing behind the patient, deliver a brisk push forwards or pull backwards. You must be ready to catch them if they are unable to maintain their balance. If in doubt, have an assistant standing in front of the patient.

Gait

- Look at the patient's shoes for abnormal wear patterns.
- Time the patient walking a measured 10 metres, with a walking aid if needed, turning through 180 degrees and returning.
- Note stride length, arm swing, steadiness (including turning), limping or other difficulties.
- Look for abnormal movements that may be accentuated by walking such as tremor (in Parkinson's disease) or dystonic movements.
- Listen for the slapping sound of a foot-drop gait.
- Ask the patient to walk first on their tiptoes, then heels. Ankle dorsiflexion weakness (foot drop) is much more common than plantar flexion weakness, and makes walking on the heels difficult or impossible.
- Ask the patient to walk heel to toe in a straight line (tandem gait). This emphasises gait ataxia and may be the only abnormal finding in midline cerebellar (vermis) lesions.

Unsteadiness on standing with the eyes open is common in cerebellar disorders. Instability that only occurs, or is markedly worse, on eye closure (Romberg's sign) indicates proprioceptive sensory loss (sensory ataxia) or bilateral vestibular failure. Cerebellar ataxia is not usually associated with a positive Romberg test.

Hemiplegic gait (unilateral upper motor neurone lesion) is characterised by extension at the hip, knee and ankle and circumduction at the hip, such that the foot on the affected side is plantar flexed and describes a semicircle as the patient walks. The upper limb may be flexed (Fig. 7.17A).

Bilateral upper motor neurone damage causes a scissor-like gait due to spasticity. Cerebellar dysfunction leads to a broad-based, unsteady (ataxic) gait, which usually makes walking heel to toe impossible. In Parkinsonism, initiation of walking may be delayed; the steps are short and shuffling with loss/reduction of arm swing (Fig. 7.17D). A tremor may become more apparent. The stooped posture and impairment of postural reflexes can result in a festinant (rapid, short-stepped, hurrying) gait. As a doorway or other obstacle approaches, the patient may freeze. Turning involves many short steps, with the risk of falls. Postural instability on the pull test, especially backwards, occurs in Parkinsonian syndromes. Proximal muscle weakness may lead to a waddling

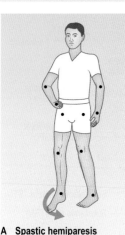

A   Spastic hemiparesis
One arm held immobile and
close to the side with elbow,
wrist and fingers flexed
Leg extended with plantar
flexion of the foot
On walking, the foot is
dragged, scraping the toe
in a circle (circumduction)
Caused by upper motor
neurone lesion, e.g. stroke

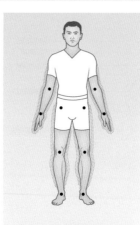

B   Steppage gait
Foot is dragged or lifted high
and slapped on to the floor
Unable to walk on the heels
Caused by foot drop owing to
lower motor neurone lesion

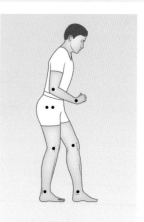

C   Sensory or cerebellar ataxia
Gait is unsteady and wide-
based. Feet are thrown forward
and outward and brought down
on the heels
In sensory ataxia, patients watch
the ground. With their eyes
closed, they cannot stand
steadily (positive Romberg sign)
In cerebellar ataxia, turns are
difficult and patients cannot
stand steadily with feet together
whether eyes are open or
closed
Caused by polyneuropathy or
posterior column damage, e.g.
syphilis

D   Parkinsonian gait
Posture is stooped with head
and neck forwards
Arms are flexed at elbows and
wrists. Little arm swing
Steps are short and shuffling
and patient is slow in getting
started (festinant gait)
Caused by lesions in the basal
ganglia

Fig. 7.17 Abnormalities of gait.

gait with bilateral Trendelenburg signs (see p. 259 and Fig. 13.37). Bizarre gaits, such as when patients drag a leg behind them, are often functional but some diseases, including Huntington's disease, produce unusual and chaotic gaits.

Inspection and palpation of the muscles

Examination sequence

- Completely expose the patient while maintaining their comfort and dignity.
- Look for asymmetry, inspecting both proximally and distally. Note deformities, such as flexion deformities or pes cavus (high foot arches).
- Inspect for wasting or hypertrophy, fasciculation and involuntary movement.

Muscle bulk

Lower motor neurone lesions may cause muscle wasting. This is not seen in acute upper motor neurone lesions, although disuse atrophy may develop with longstanding lesions. A motor neurone lesion in childhood may impair growth (causing a smaller limb or hemiatrophy) or lead to limb deformity, such as pes cavus. Muscle disorders usually result in proximal wasting (the notable exception is myotonic dystrophy, in which it is distal, often with temporalis wasting). People in certain occupations, such as professional sports players, may have physiological muscle hypertrophy. Pseudohypertrophy may occur in muscular dystrophy but the muscles are weak.

Fasciculation

Fasciculations are visible irregular twitches of resting muscles caused by individual motor units firing spontaneously. This occurs in lower motor neurone disease, usually in wasted muscles. Fasciculation is seen, not felt, and you may need to observe carefully for several minutes to be sure that it is not present. Physiological (benign) fasciculation is common, especially in the calves, but is not associated with weakness or wasting. Myokymia – fine, involuntary fascicular contractions – involves rapid bursts of repetitive motor unit activity that often affects orbicularis oculi or the first dorsal interosseus, and is rarely pathological.

Abnormal movements

Myoclonic jerks

These are sudden, shock-like contractions of one or more muscles that may be focal or diffuse and occur singly or repetitively. Healthy people commonly experience these when falling asleep (hypnic jerks). They may also occur pathologically in association with epilepsy, diffuse brain damage and some neurodegenerative disorders such as prion diseases. Negative myoclonus (asterixis) is seen most commonly in liver disease (liver flap).

Tremor

Tremor is an involuntary, oscillatory movement about a joint or a group of joints, resulting from alternating contraction and relaxation of muscles. Tremors are classified according to their frequency, amplitude, position (at rest, on posture or movement) and body part affected.

Physiological tremor is a fine (low-amplitude), fast (high-frequency, 3–30 Hz) postural tremor. A similar tremor occurs in hyperthyroidism and with excess alcohol or caffeine intake, and is a common adverse effect of beta-agonist bronchodilators.

Essential tremor is the most common pathological cause of tremor; it is typically symmetrical in the upper limbs and may involve the head and voice. The tremor is noted on posture and with movement (kinetic). It may be improved by alcohol and often demonstrates an autosomal dominant pattern of inheritance.

Parkinson's disease causes a slow (3–7 Hz), coarse, 'pill-rolling' tremor, worse at rest but reduced with voluntary movement. It is more common in the upper limbs, is usually asymmetrical and does not affect the head, although it may involve the jaw/chin and sometimes the legs.

Isolated head tremor is usually dystonic and may be associated with abnormal neck postures such as torticollis, antecollis or retrocollis.

Intention tremor is absent at rest but maximal on movement and on approaching the target (hunting tremor), and is usually due to cerebellar damage. It is assessed with the finger-to-nose test (p. 141).

Other causes of tremor include hereditary or acquired demyelinating neuropathies (such as Charcot–Marie–Tooth disease) and are termed neuropathic tremors. Drugs commonly causing tremor include sodium valproate, glucocorticoids and lithium.

Movement disorders, including tremor, are common functional symptoms. They are often inconsistent and distractible, with varying frequencies and amplitudes, and may be associated with other functional signs.

Other involuntary movements

These are classified according to their appearance.

Dystonia is caused by sustained muscle contractions, leading to twisting, repetitive movements and sometimes tremor. It may be focal (as in torticollis), segmental (affecting two or more adjacent body parts) or generalised.

Chorea describes brief, jerky, random, purposeless movements that may affect various body parts, commonly the arms.

Athetosis is a slower, writhing movement, more similar to dystonia than chorea.

Ballism refers to violent flinging movements sometimes affecting only one side of the body (hemiballismus).

Tics are repetitive, stereotyped movements that may be briefly suppressed by the patient.

Tone

Tone is the resistance felt by the examiner when moving a joint passively.

Examination sequence

- Ask the patient to lie supine on the examination couch and to relax and 'go floppy'. Enquire about any pain or limitations of movement before proceeding.
- Passively move each joint to be tested through as full a range as possible, both slowly and quickly in all anatomically possible directions. Be unpredictable with these movements, in both direction and speed, to prevent the patient actively moving with you; you want to assess passive tone. It may be helpful to distract the patient by asking them to count backwards from 20 while assessing tone.

Upper limb

- Hold the patient's hand as if shaking hands, using your other hand to support their elbow. Assess tone at the wrist and elbow with supination/pronation and flexion/extension movements.
- Activation (or synkinesis) is a technique used to exaggerate subtle increase in tone, and is particularly useful for assessing extrapyramidal tone increase. Ask the patient to describe circles in the air with the contralateral limb while you assess tone. A transient increase in tone with this manœuvre (Froment's) is normal.

Lower limb

- Roll the leg from side to side and then briskly flip the knee up into a flexed position, observing the movement of the foot. Typically, the heel moves up the bed, but increased tone may cause it to lift off the bed due to failure of relaxation.

Ankle clonus

- Support the patient's leg, with both the knee and the ankle resting in 90-degree flexion.
- Briskly dorsiflex and partially evert the foot, sustaining the pressure. Clonus is felt as repeated beats of dorsiflexion/plantar flexion.

Myotonia

- Ask the patient to make a fist and then to relax and open their hand; watch for the speed of relaxation.
- Using the tendon hammer, percuss the belly of the thenar eminence; this may induce contraction of the muscles, causing the thumb to adduct, and you may witness dimpling of the muscle belly.

Hypotonia

Decreased tone may occur in lower motor neurone lesions and is usually associated with muscle wasting, weakness and hyporeflexia. It may also be a feature of cerebellar disease or signal the early phases of cerebral or spinal shock, when the paralysed limbs are atonic prior to developing spasticity. Reduced tone can be difficult to elicit.

Hypertonia

Increased tone may occur in two main forms: spasticity and rigidity.

Spasticity is velocity-dependent resistance to passive movement: it is detected with quick movements and is a feature of upper motor neurone lesions. It is usually accompanied by weakness, hyper-reflexia, an extensor plantar response and sometimes clonus. In mild forms it is detected as a 'catch' at the beginning or end of passive movement. In severe cases it limits the range of movement and may be associated with contractures. In the upper limbs it may be more obvious on attempted extension; in the legs it is more evident on flexion.

Rigidity is a sustained resistance throughout the range of movement and is most easily detected when the limb is moved slowly. In Parkinsonism this is classically described as 'lead pipe' rigidity. In the presence of a Parkinsonian tremor there may be a regular interruption to the movement, giving it a jerky feel ('cog wheeling').

Clonus

Clonus is a rhythmic series of contractions evoked by a sudden stretch of the muscle and tendon. Unsustained (<6 beats) clonus may be physiological. When sustained, it indicates upper motor neurone damage and is accompanied by spasticity. It is best elicited at the ankle; knee (patella) clonus is rare and not routinely tested.

Myotonia

Myotonia refers to the inability of muscles to relax normally and characterises a group of neuromuscular disorders, the most common of which is myotonic dystrophy. Patients may notice difficulty in letting go of things with their hands, or a stiff gait.

Power

Strength varies with age, occupation and fitness. Grade muscle power using the Medical Research Council (MRC) scale (Box 7.8). Record what patients can do in terms of daily activities; for example, whether they can stand, walk and raise both arms above their head. Lesions at different sites produce different clinical patterns of weakness; examination will help discriminate upper from lower motor neurone lesions.

Examination sequence

- Do not test every muscle in most patients; the commonly tested muscles are listed in Box 7.9.
- Ask about pain that might interfere with testing.
- Observe the patient getting up from a chair and walking.
- Test upper limb power with the patient sitting on the edge of the couch. Test lower limb power with the patient reclining.
- Ask the patient to lift their arms above their head.
- Ask them to 'play the piano'. Check movements of the fingers; asymmetric loss of fine finger movement may be a very early sign of cortical or extrapyramidal disease.
- Observe the patient with their arms outstretched and supinated (palms up) and their eyes closed for 'pronator drift', when one arm starts to pronate.

7.8 Medical Research Council grading of muscle power

Grade	Description
0	No muscle contraction visible
1	Flicker of contraction but no movement
2	Joint movement when effect of gravity eliminated
3	Movement against gravity but not against resistance
4[a]	Movement against resistance but weaker than normal
5	Normal power

[a]May be further classified as 4+ or 4−.

7.9 Nerve and muscle supplies of commonly tested movements

Movement	Muscle	Nerve and root
Shoulder abduction	Deltoid	Axillary C5
Elbow flexion	Biceps[a] Brachioradialis (supinator reflex)[a]	Musculocutaneous C5[a]/6 Radial C6[a]
Elbow extension	Triceps[a]	Radial C7
Wrist extension	Extensor carpi radialis longus	Posterior interosseous C6
Finger extension	Extensor digitorum communis	Posterior interosseous C7
Finger flexion	Flexor pollicis longus (thumb) Flexor digitorum profundus (index and middle fingers) Flexor digitorum profundus (ring and little fingers)	Anterior interosseous C8 Ulnar C8
Finger abduction	First dorsal interosseous	Ulnar T1
Thumb abduction	Abductor pollicis brevis	Median T1
Hip flexion	Iliopsoas	Iliofemoral nerve L1/2
Hip extension	Gluteus maximus	Sciatic L5/S1
Knee flexion	Hamstrings	Sciatic S1
Knee extension	Quadriceps[a]	Femoral L3[a]/4
Ankle dorsiflexion	Tibialis anterior	Deep peroneal L4/5
Ankle plantar flexion	Gastrocnemius and soleus[a]	Tibial S1[a]/2
Great toe extension (dorsiflexion)	Extensor hallucis longus	Deep peroneal L5
Ankle eversion	Peronei	Superficial peroneal L5/S1
Ankle inversion	Tibialis posterior	Tibial nerve L4/5

[a]Indicates nerve root innervation of commonly elicited deep tendon reflexes.

- Assess individual muscles depending on the history. Ask the patient to undertake a movement. First assess whether they can overcome gravity. For example, give the instruction 'Lift your right leg off the bed' to test hip flexion. Then apply resistance to this movement, testing across a single joint; for instance, apply resistance to the thigh in hip flexion, not the lower leg.
- To test truncal strength, ask the patient to sit up from a lying position.

Upper motor neurone lesions produce weakness of a relatively large group of muscles, such as a limb or more than one limb. Lower motor neurone damage can cause paresis of an individual and specific muscle, so more detailed examination of individual muscles is required (Ch. 13). Look for patterns of weakness that may suggest a diagnosis. In pyramidal weakness – after a stroke, for example – the extensors in the upper limbs are weaker than the flexors, and vice versa in the lower limbs. Myopathies tend to cause proximal weakness and neuropathies often give rise to more distal patterns, while mononeuropathies or radiculopathies lead to discrete focal weakness (such as a foot drop caused by a common peroneal nerve palsy or L5 radiculopathy).

Patients may find it difficult to sustain maximum power for reasons other than weakness, most commonly pain. You need only show that the patient can achieve maximum power briefly to be satisfied that the weakness is not neurological. Very few organic diseases cause power to fluctuate; the fatigable weakness of myasthenia is the chief exception. Wildly fluctuating or sudden 'give-way' weakness suggests a functional explanation. Hoover's sign (Fig. 7.18) refers to the improvement of apparently weak hip extension when it is tested at the same time as contralateral hip flexion (as hip flexion is associated with reflex contralateral hip extension), and is often present in functional leg weakness. This is helpful both diagnostically and therapeutically, as you can show patients that their leg is not actually weak using this sign.

Deep tendon reflexes

Anatomy

A tendon reflex is the involuntary contraction of a muscle in response to stretch. It is mediated by a reflex arc consisting of an afferent (sensory) and an efferent (motor) neurone with one synapse between (a monosynaptic reflex). Muscle stretch activates the muscle spindles, which send a burst of afferent signals that lead to direct efferent impulses, causing muscle contraction. These stretch reflex arcs are served by a particular spinal cord segment that is modified by descending upper motor neurones. The most important reflexes are the deep tendon and plantar responses, whereas others, such as abdominal and cremasteric reflexes, are rarely tested and of questionable value. Dermatomal involvement may further help localise a lesion; for example, pain going down one leg, with an absent ankle jerk (S1) and sensory loss on the sole of the foot (S1 dermatome), localises to the S1 root, most commonly due to a prolapsed intervertebral disc (sciatica).

Examination sequence

- Ask the patient to lie supine on the examination couch with the limbs exposed. They should be as relaxed and comfortable as possible, as anxiety and pain can cause an increased response.
- Extend your wrist and allow the weight of the tendon hammer head to determine the strength of the blow. Strike your finger that is palpating the biceps and supinator tendons (otherwise it is painful for the patient), or the tendon itself for the triceps, knee and ankle jerks.
- Record the response as:
  - increased (+++)
  - normal (++)
  - decreased (+)
  - present only with reinforcement (+/-)
  - absent (0).

Principal (deep tendon) reflexes

- Ensure that both limbs are positioned identically with the same amount of stretch. This is especially important for the ankle reflex, where the ankle is passively dorsiflexed before striking the tendon.
- Compare each reflex with the other side; check for symmetry of response (Figs 7.19 and 7.20).
- Use reinforcement whenever a reflex appears to be absent. For knee and ankle reflexes, ask the patient to interlock their fingers and pull one hand against the other on command ('Have a tug of war with yourself'), immediately before you strike the tendon (Jendrassik's manœuvre).
- To reinforce upper limb reflexes, ask the patient to make a fist with the contralateral hand.

Hoffmann's reflex

- Place your right index finger under the distal interphalangeal joint of the patient's middle finger.
- Use your right thumb to flick the patient's finger downwards.
- Look for any reflex flexion of the patient's thumb.

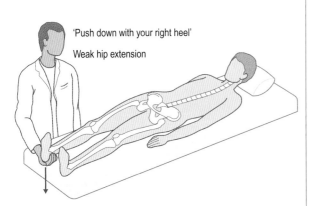

'Push down with your right heel'

Weak hip extension

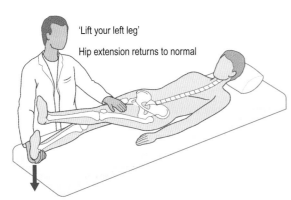

'Lift your left leg'

Hip extension returns to normal

Fig. 7.18 Hoover's sign.

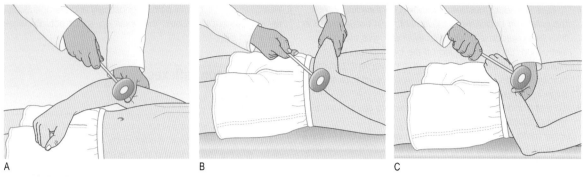

Fig. 7.19 Testing the deep tendon reflexes of the upper limb. [A] Eliciting the biceps jerk, C5. [B] Triceps jerk, C7. [C] Supinator jerk, C6.

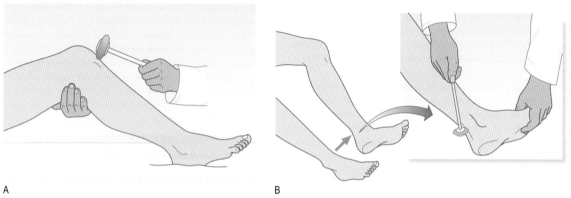

Fig. 7.20 Testing the deep tendon reflexes of the lower limb. [A] Eliciting the knee jerk (note that the patient's legs should not be in contact with each other), L3, L4. [B] Ankle jerk of the recumbent patient, S1.

Finger jerk (C8)

- Place your middle and index fingers across the palmar surface of the patient's proximal phalanges.
- Tap your own fingers with the hammer.
- Watch for flexion of the patient's fingers.

Plantar response (S1–2)

- Run a blunt object (orange stick) along the lateral border of the sole of the foot towards the little toe (Fig. 7.21).
- Watch both the first movement of the great toe and the other leg flexor muscles. The normal response is plantar flexion of the great toe (downward movement).
- A true Babinski sign, signifying an abnormal reflex due to an upper motor neurone lesion:
  - involves activation of the extensor hallucis longus tendon (not movement of the entire foot, a common 'withdrawal' response to an unpleasant stimulus)
  - coincides with contraction of other leg flexor muscles
  - is reproducible.

Abdominal reflexes (T8–12)

- The patient should be supine and relaxed.
- Use an orange stick and briskly but lightly stroke the upper and lower quadrants away from the midline of the relaxed abdomen, watching for a contraction.
- The normal response is contraction of the underlying muscle.

Cremasteric reflex (L1–2): males only

- Explain what you are going to do and why it is necessary.
- Abduct and externally rotate the patient's thigh.

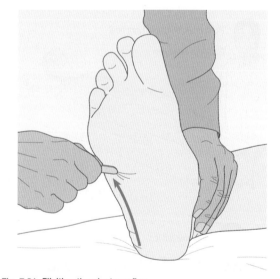

Fig. 7.21 Eliciting the plantar reflex.

- Use an orange stick to stroke the upper medial aspect of the thigh.
- Normally the testis on the side stimulated will rise briskly.

  Hyper-reflexia (abnormally brisk reflexes) is a sign of upper motor neurone damage. Diminished or absent jerks are most commonly due to lower motor neurone lesions. In healthy older people the ankle jerks may be reduced or lost, and in the Holmes–Adie syndrome, myotonic pupils (p. 162) are associated with loss of some reflexes. Isolated loss of a reflex suggests a mononeuropathy or radiculopathy, such as loss of ankle jerk with L5/S1 lumbosacral disc prolapse compressing the S1 nerve root. Reflex patterns are helpful in localising neurological lesions and you should know the nerve roots that serve the commonly tested reflexes (Box 7.9). There are several reflex grading systems but interobserver agreement is poor; record reflexes as present (and, if so, whether normal, increased or decreased) or absent. Never conclude that a reflex is absent until you have used reinforcement.

An 'inverted' biceps reflex is caused by combined spinal cord and root pathology localising to a specific spinal level. It is most common at the C5/6 level. When elicited, the biceps reflex is absent or reduced but finger flexion occurs. This is because the lesion at the C5/6 level affects the efferent arc of the biceps jerk (C5 nerve root), causing it to be reduced or lost, and also the spinal cord, increasing reflexes below this level (including the finger jerks, C8). It is most commonly seen in cervical spondylotic myeloradiculopathy.

A Hoffmann's reflex and increased finger jerks suggest hypertonia; they may occur in healthy individuals but can be informative if asymmetric. In cerebellar disease the reflexes may be pendular and muscle contraction and relaxation tend to be slow, but these are not sensitive or specific cerebellar signs.

An extensor plantar (Babinski) response is a sign of upper motor neurone damage and is usually associated with other upper motor neurone signs, such as spasticity, clonus and hyper-reflexia. Fanning of the toes is normal and not pathological.

Superficial abdominal reflexes (T8–12) are lost in upper motor neurone lesions but are also affected by lower motor neurone damage affecting thoracic roots T8–12. They are usually absent in the obese and the elderly or after abdominal surgery, and are not part of the routine examination.

The cremasteric reflex in males (L1, 2) may be absent on the side of spinal cord or root lesions but this is of little clinical significance.

Primitive reflexes

These are present in normal neonates and young infants but disappear as the nervous system matures (p. 305). People with congenital or hereditary cerebral lesions and a few healthy individuals retain these reflexes, but their return after early childhood is often associated with brain damage or degeneration. Although often referred to as frontal, the primitive reflexes (snout, grasp, palmomental and glabellar tap) have little localising value and in isolation are of little significance, but in combination suggest diffuse or frontal cerebral damage (Box 7.10). Unilateral grasp and palmomental reflexes may occur with contralateral frontal lobe pathology. The glabellar tap is an unreliable sign of Parkinson's disease.

Coordination

Performing complex movements smoothly and efficiently depends on intact sensory and motor function and an intact cerebellum.

Anatomy

The cerebellum lies in the posterior fossa and consists of two hemispheres with a central vermis. Afferent and efferent pathways convey information to and from the cerebral motor cortex, basal ganglia, thalamus, vestibular and other brainstem nuclei and the spinal cord. In general, midline structures, such as the vermis,

7.10 Primitive reflexes

Snout reflex
• Lightly tap the lips. Lip pouting is an abnormal response

Grasp reflex
• Firmly stroke the palm from the radial side. In an abnormal response, your finger is gripped by the patient's hand

Palmomental reflex
• Apply firm pressure to the palm next to the thenar eminence with a tongue depressor. An abnormal response is ipsilateral puckering of the chin

Glabellar tap
• Stand behind the patient and tap repeatedly between their eyebrows with the tip of your index finger. Normally, the blink response stops after three or four taps

influence body equilibrium, while each hemisphere controls ipsilateral coordination.

Examination sequence

Test cerebellar function by assessing stance and gait (p. 134), including tandem gait (walking in a straight line, heel to toe), eye movements (looking for nystagmus; p. 164), speech (dysarthria; p. 125) and limb coordination.

Finger-to-nose test
• Ask the patient to touch their nose with the tip of their index finger and then touch your fingertip. Hold your finger at the extreme of the patient's reach (you should make the patient use the arm outstretched).
• Ask them to repeat the movement between nose and target finger as quickly as possible.
• Make the test more sensitive by changing the position of your target finger. Timing is crucial; move your finger just as the patient's finger is about to leave their nose, otherwise you will induce a false-positive finger-to-nose ataxia.
• Some patients are so ataxic that they may injure their eye/face with this test. If so, use your two hands as the targets or ask the patient to touch their chin rather than nose (Fig. 7.22).

Rapid alternating movements
• Demonstrate repeatedly patting the palm of your hand with the palm and then the back of your opposite hand as quickly and regularly as possible.
• Ask the patient to copy your actions.
• Repeat with the opposite hand.
• Alternatively, ask the patient to tap a steady rhythm rapidly with one hand on the other hand or table, and 'listen to the cerebellum'; ataxia makes this task difficult, producing a slower, more irregular rhythm than normal.

Heel-to-shin test
• With the patient lying supine, ask them to lift the heel into the air and to place it on their opposite knee, then slide their heel up and down their shin between knee and ankle (Fig. 7.23).

The finger-to-nose test may reveal a tendency to fall short of or overshoot the examiner's finger (dysmetria or past-pointing).

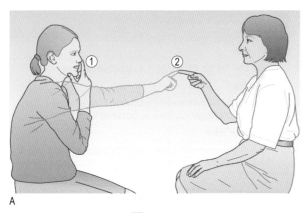 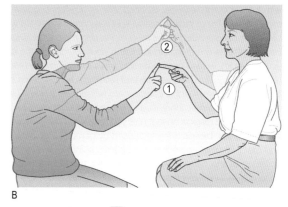

Fig. 7.22 Finger-to-nose test. [A] Ask the patient to touch the tip of their nose (**1**) and then your finger (**2**). [B] Move your finger from one position to another, towards and away from the patient (**1**), as well as from side to side (**2**).

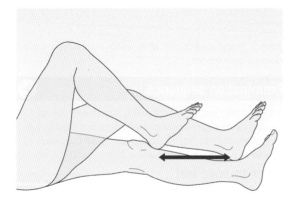

Fig. 7.23 Performing the heel-to-shin test with the right leg.

In more severe cases there may be a tremor (or an increase in amplitude of tremor) of the finger as it approaches the target finger and the patient's own nose (intention or hunting tremor). The movement may be slow, disjointed and clumsy (dyssynergia). The heel-to-shin test is the equivalent test for the legs. It is abnormal if the heel wavers away from the line of the shin. Weakness may produce false-positive finger-to-nose or heel-to-shin tests, so demonstrate that power is normal first.

Dysdiadochokinesis (impairment of rapid alternating movements) is evident as slowness, disorganisation and irregularity of movement. Dysarthria and nystagmus also occur with cerebellar disease. Much less reliable signs of cerebellar disease include the rebound phenomenon (when the displaced outstretched arm may fly up past the original position), pendular reflexes and hypotonia.

In disorders predominantly affecting midline cerebellar structures, such as tumours of the vermis and alcoholic cerebellar damage, the tests described may be normal and truncal ataxia (that is, ataxic gait) may be the only finding. In the most severe cases this may mean that the patient cannot sit unsupported. Cerebellar dysfunction occurs in many conditions, and the differential diagnosis varies with age and speed of presentation.

Apraxia

Apraxia, or dyspraxia, is difficulty or inability to perform a task, despite no sensory or motor abnormalities. It is a sign of higher cortical dysfunction, usually localising to the non-dominant frontal or parietal lobes.

Examination sequence

- Ask the patient to perform an imaginary act, such as drinking a cup of tea, combing their hair, or folding a letter and placing it in an envelope.
- Ask the patient to copy movements you make with your fingers, such as pointing or making a V sign.
- Ask the patient to copy a geometric figure (interlocking pentagons or cube).
- Ask the patient to put on a pyjama top or dressing gown, one sleeve of which has been pulled inside out.
- Ask the patient to lie on the couch and perform cycling movements with their legs.

The patient may be unable to initiate a task or may perform it in an odd or bizarre fashion. Constructional apraxia (difficulty drawing a figure) is a feature of parietal disturbance. Dressing apraxia, often associated with spatial disorientation and neglect, is usually due to parietal lesions of the non-dominant hemisphere. Patients with gait apraxia have difficulty walking but are able to perform cycling movements on the bed surprisingly well.

Sensory system

The sensory system comprises the simple sensations of light touch, pain, temperature and vibration, together with joint position sense (proprioception) and higher cortical sensations, which include two-point discrimination, stereognosis (tactile recognition), graphaesthesia (identification of letters or numbers traced on the skin) and localisation.

Detailed examination of sensation is time-consuming and unnecessary unless the patient volunteers sensory symptoms or you suspect a specific pathology, such as spinal cord compression or mononeuropathy. In patients without sensory symptoms, assessing light touch of all four limbs as a screening process may suffice. It is useful to have a working knowledge of the dermatomal distribution (a dermatome is an area of skin innervated by a single nerve root) and sensory distribution of the more commonly entrapped peripheral nerves (see Figs 7.26 and 7.27 later).

Anatomy

Proprioception and vibration are conveyed in large, myelinated fast-conducting fibres in the peripheral nerves and in the posterior

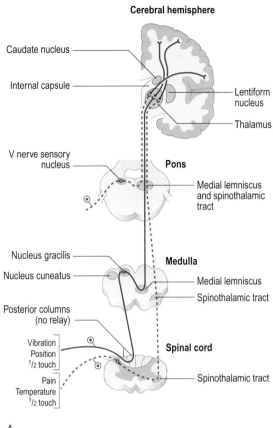

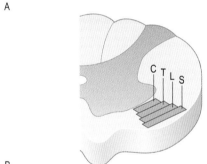

Fig. 7.24 The sensory system. [A] Main sensory pathways.
[B] Spinothalamic tract: layering of the spinothalamic tract in the cervical region. C represents fibres from cervical segments, which lie centrally; fibres from thoracic, lumbar and sacral segments (labelled T, L and S, respectively) lie progressively more laterally.

(dorsal) columns of the spinal cord. Pain and temperature sensation are carried by small, slow-conducting fibres of the peripheral nerves and the spinothalamic tract of the spinal cord. The posterior column remains ipsilateral from the point of entry up to the medulla, but most pain and temperature fibres cross to the contralateral spinothalamic tract within one or two segments of entry to the spinal cord. All sensory fibres relay in the thalamus before sending information to the sensory cortex in the parietal lobe (Fig. 7.24).

Common presenting symptoms

Sensory symptoms are common and it is important to discern what the patient is describing. Clarify that, by 'numbness',

the patient means lack of sensation rather than weakness or clumsiness. Neuropathic pain (pain due to disease or dysfunction of the PNS or CNS) is often severe and refractory to simple analgesia. Reduced ability to feel pain may be accompanied by scars from injuries or burns (trophic injuries). Sensory symptoms are defined as follows:

- paraesthesia: tingling, or pins and needles
- dysaesthesia: unpleasant paraesthesia
- hypoaesthesia: reduced sensation to a normal stimulus
- analgesia: numbness or loss of sensation
- hyperaesthesia: increased sensitivity to a stimulus
- allodynia: painful sensation resulting from a non-painful stimulus
- hyperalgesia: increased sensitivity to a painful stimulus.

Examination sequence

The aim here is to focus the examination. Look for a sensory level if the history and examination suggest spinal cord pathology; a glove and stocking pattern usually starting distally, caused by a peripheral neuropathy; or sensory disturbance in a specific nerve territory or dermatome. Be guided by the history and the examination findings from the motor system and reflexes. It is useful to ask the patient to map out their area(s) of sensory disturbance if they can.

Light touch
- While the patient looks away or closes their eyes, use a wisp of cotton wool (or lightly apply your finger) and ask the patient to say 'yes' to each touch.
- Time the stimuli irregularly and make a dabbing rather than a stroking or tickling stimulus.
- Start distally in the feet and hands; work proximally for a neuropathy or focus on a specific nerve distribution or dermatome.

Superficial pain
- Use a fresh neurological pin, such as a Neurotip, not a hypodermic needle. Dispose of the pin after each patient.
- Explain and demonstrate (on an area of skin not affected by the lesion, such as the sternum) that the ability to feel a sharp pinprick is being tested.
- Map out the boundaries of any area of reduced, absent or increased sensation. Move from reduced to higher sensibility: that is, from hypoaesthesia to normal, or normal to hyperaesthesia.

Temperature
- Touch the patient with a cold metallic object, such as a tuning fork, and ask if it feels cold. More sensitive assessment requires tubes of hot and cold water at controlled temperatures but this is seldom performed.

Vibration
Note that ankle oedema may affect perception. Strike the tuning fork on your own palm; an average healthy person should be able to detect the vibration this causes for over 10 seconds.
- Place a vibrating 128-Hz tuning fork over the patient's sternum.
- Ask the patient, 'Do you feel it buzzing?'
- Place the fork on the patient's big toe. If vibration is not felt, then move it proximally to the medial malleolus; if this is not perceived, move to the patella, then the anterior iliac spine, lower chest wall or clavicle. Repeat on the other

side. Record the level at which vibration is detected by the patient.

- Repeat the process in the upper limb. Start at the distal interphalangeal joint of the forefinger; if sensation is impaired, proceed proximally to the metacarpophalangeal joints, wrist, elbow, shoulder and finally clavicle.
- If in doubt as to the accuracy of the response, ask the patient to close their eyes and to report when you stop the fork vibrating with your fingers.

Joint position sense (proprioception)

- With the patient's eyes open, demonstrate the procedure.
- Lightly hold the distal phalanx of the patient's great toe at the sides. Tell the patient you are going to move their toe up or down, demonstrating as you do so.
- Ask the patient to close their eyes and to identify the direction of small movements in random order.
- If perception is impaired, move to more proximal joints – ankle, knees and hips. Repeat for the other side.
- Repeat for the upper limbs. Start with movements at the distal interphalangeal joint of the index finger; if the movements are not accurately felt, move to the first metacarpophalangeal joint, wrist, elbow and finally shoulder.

Stereognosis and graphaesthesia

- Ask the patient to close their eyes.
- Place a familiar object, such as a coin or key, in their hand and ask them to identify it (stereognosis).
- Use the blunt end of a pencil or orange stick and trace letters or digits on the patient's palm. Ask the patient to identify the figure (graphaesthesia).

Sensory inattention

- Only test if sensory pathways are otherwise intact.
- Ask the patient to close their eyes.
- Touch their arms/legs in turn and ask which side has been touched.
- Now touch both sides simultaneously and ask whether the left side, right side or both sides were touched.

Sensory modalities

In addition to the modalities conveyed in the principal ascending pathways (touch, pain, temperature, vibration and joint position sense), sensory examination includes tests of discriminative aspects of sensation, which may be impaired by lesions of the sensory cortex. Assess these cortical sensory functions only if the main pathway sensations are intact. Consider abnormalities on sensory testing according to whether the lesion (or lesions) is in the peripheral nerve(s), dorsal root(s) or spinal cord, or is intracranial.

Peripheral nerve and dorsal root

Many diseases affect peripheral nerves, generally resulting in peripheral neuropathies or polyneuropathies. Peripheral neuropathies tend to affect the lower limbs, first starting in the toes. In these length-dependent neuropathies the upper limbs may become involved once the symptoms extend above the knees. Symptoms first affecting the upper limbs suggest a demyelinating rather than axonal neuropathy or a disease process in the nerve roots or spinal cord. In many cases, touch and pinprick sensation are lost in a 'stocking-and-glove' distribution (Fig. 7.25A). There

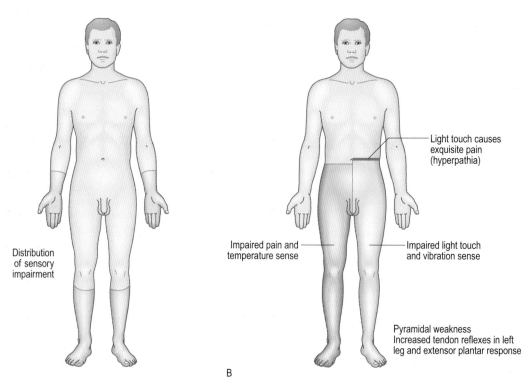

A — Distribution of sensory impairment

B — Light touch causes exquisite pain (hyperpathia)
Impaired pain and temperature sense
Impaired light touch and vibration sense
Pyramidal weakness
Increased tendon reflexes in left leg and extensor plantar response

Fig. 7.25 Patterns of sensory loss. A Length-dependent peripheral neuropathy. B Brown–Séquard syndrome. Note the distribution of corticospinal, posterior column and lateral spinothalamic tract signs. The cord lesion is in the left half of the cord.

may also be autonomic involvement, causing symptoms affecting sweating, sphincter control and the cardiovascular system (such as orthostatic hypotension). In mononeuritis multiplex, different nerves in the upper and lower limbs can be affected in a stepwise fashion.

In 'large-fibre' neuropathies, such as Guillain–Barré syndrome, vibration and joint position sense may be disproportionately affected (reduced vibration sense at the ankle may be normal in people over 60 years). Patients may report staggering when they close their eyes during hair washing or in the dark (Romberg's sign, p. 135). When joint position sense is affected in the arms, pseudoathetosis may be demonstrated by asking the patient to close their eyes and hold their hands outstretched; the fingers/arms will make involuntary, slow, wandering movements, mimicking athetosis. Interpretation of sensory signs requires knowledge of the relevant anatomy of sensory nerves and dermatomes (Figs 7.26 and 7.27). In 'small-fibre' neuropathies, in which pain and temperature sensation are mainly affected, the only finding may be reduced pinprick and temperature sensation; there may also be autonomic involvement. The most common causes worldwide are diabetes mellitus and HIV infection.

Spinal cord

Traumatic and compressive spinal cord lesions cause loss or impairment of sensation in a dermatomal distribution below the level of the lesion. A zone of hyperaesthesia may be found in the dermatomes immediately above the level of sensory loss. Syringomyelia (a fluid-filled cavity within the spinal cord) can result in a dissociated pattern of altered spinothalamic (pain and temperature) sensation and motor function, with sparing of dorsal column (touch and vibration) sensation.

When one-half of the spinal cord is damaged, the Brown–Séquard syndrome may occur. This is characterised by ipsilateral upper motor neurone weakness and loss of touch, vibration and joint position sense, with contralateral loss of pain and temperature (see Fig. 7.25B).

Intracranial lesions

Brainstem lesions are often vascular, and you must understand the relevant anatomy to determine the site of the lesion. Lower brainstem lesions may cause ipsilateral numbness on one side

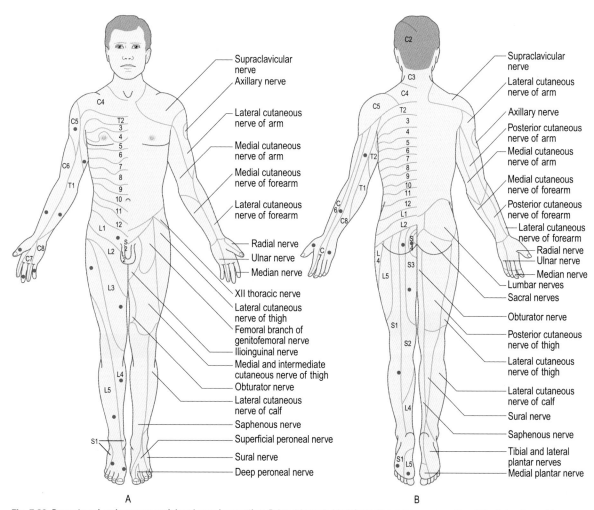

Fig. 7.26 Dermatomal and sensory peripheral map innervation. Points (shown in blue) for testing cutaneous sensation of the limbs. By applying stimuli at the points marked, both the dermatomal and main peripheral nerve distributions are tested simultaneously. [A] Anterior view. [B] Posterior view.

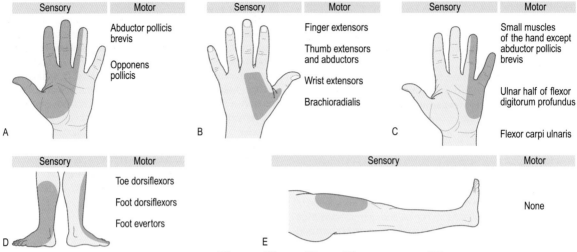

Fig. 7.27 Sensory and motor deficits in nerve lesions. [A] Median. [B] Radial. [C] Ulnar. [D] Common peroneal. [E] Lateral cutaneous of the thigh.

7.11 Common features of carpal tunnel syndrome

- It is more common in women
- There is unpleasant tingling in the hand
- It may not observe anatomical boundaries, radiating up the arm to the shoulder
- Weakness is uncommon; if it does occur, it affects thumb abduction
- Symptoms are frequently present at night, waking the patient from sleep
- The patient may hang the hand and arm out of the bed for relief
- There is thenar muscle wasting (in longstanding cases)
- It is commonly associated with pregnancy, diabetes and hypothyroidism

of the face (V nerve nucleus) and contralateral body numbness (spinothalamic tract).

Thalamic lesions may cause patchy sensory impairment on the opposite side with unpleasant, poorly localised pain, often of a burning quality.

Cortical parietal lobe lesions typically cause sensory inattention but may also affect joint position sense, two-point discrimination, stereognosis (tactile recognition) and localisation of point touch. Two-point discrimination and touch localisation are not helpful signs and tests are not performed routinely.

Peripheral nerves

Peripheral nerves may be damaged individually (mononeuropathy) or multiply (peripheral neuropathy or mononeuritis multiplex). Certain nerves (median nerve at the wrist, common peroneal nerve at the knee) are particularly prone to compression.

Median nerve

The medial nerve may be compressed as it passes between the flexor retinaculum and the carpal bones at the wrist (carpal tunnel syndrome). This is the most common entrapment neuropathy and initially produces sensory symptoms and pain in the hands, occasionally radiating up the arm – typically at night. Carpal tunnel syndrome occurs commonly during pregnancy (Box 7.11).

Examination sequence

- Look for wasting of the thenar eminence.
- Test thumb abduction with the patient's hand held palm up on a flat surface. Ask the patient to move their thumb vertically against your resistance (abductor pollicis brevis).
- Test opposition by asking the patient to touch their thumb and ring finger together while you attempt to pull them apart (opponens pollicis).
- Test for altered sensation over the hand involving the thumb, index and middle fingers and the lateral half of the ring finger – splitting of the ring finger (see Fig. 7.27A).
- Tinel's sign is elicited by tapping the distal wrist crease with the tendon hammer, which may produce tingling in the median nerve territory. Although often used, it has poor sensitivity and specificity.
- Phalen's test is forced flexion of the wrist for up to 60 seconds, to induce symptoms; it also has limited sensitivity and specificity.

Radial nerve

This may be compressed as it runs through the axilla, in the spiral groove of the humerus (Saturday night palsy), or may be injured in fractures of the humerus. It typically causes wrist drop.

Examination sequence

- Test for weakness of brachioradialis (elbow flexor) and the extensors of the arm (triceps), wrist and fingers.
- Look for sensory loss over the dorsum of the hand (see Fig. 7.27B) and loss of triceps tendon jerk.

Ulnar nerve

The ulnar nerve is most often affected at the elbow by external compression as the nerve is exposed, or by injury, as in elbow dislocation/fracture. Compression usually occurs as the nerve passes through the condylar groove behind the medial epicondyle of the humerus or as it passes through the cubital tunnel.

Examination sequence

- Examine the medial elbow, palpating the nerve in the ulnar groove (the most common place of entrapment). Note any scars or other signs of trauma.
- Look for wasting of the interossei (dorsal guttering).
- Test for weakness of finger abduction with the patient's fingers on a flat surface, and ask them to spread the fingers against resistance from your fingers.
- Test adduction by asking them to grip a card placed between their fingers and pulling it out using your own fingers.
- Assess for sensory loss on the ulnar side of the hand, splitting the ring finger (see Fig. 7.27C).

Common peroneal nerve

The nerve may be damaged by fractures as it winds around the fibular head, or it may be compressed, particularly in thin, immobile patients or as a result of repetitive kneeling, squatting or sitting with the legs crossed at the knees. It typically causes a foot drop.

Examination sequence

- Test for weakness of ankle dorsiflexion and eversion; test for extension of the big toe (extensor hallucis longus). Inversion and the ankle reflex will be preserved.
- Test for sensory loss over the dorsum of the foot (see Fig. 7.27D).

Lateral cutaneous nerve of the thigh

This purely sensory nerve may be compressed as it passes under the inguinal ligament, producing paraesthesiae in the lateral thigh (meralgia paraesthetica, which means burning numbness) (see Fig. 7.27E).

Examination sequence

- Ask the patient to map out the area of disturbance.
- Test for disturbed sensation over the lateral aspect of the thigh. Palpate the abdomen and groin for masses or inguinal lymph nodes.

Interpretation of the findings

Having completed the history and examination, first decide whether the symptoms are due to neurological disease, a functional neurological disorder or non-neurological causes. Try to localise the lesion to a single area of the nervous system if possible (Is the lesion in the CNS or PNS?) and then localise in more detail (for example: If the lesion is in the PNS, is it in the root, nerves or neuromuscular junction muscle?). Some conditions, like multiple sclerosis, may give rise to multiple symptoms and signs because they involve several lesions; others, like migraine or functional disorders, do not follow strict neurological and anatomical rules.

Having localised the lesion, consider the likely underlying pathology (What is the lesion?). This will depend on the history (for example, syncope versus seizure; see Box 7.2), and also epidemiology (sudden-onset leg weakness in a 72-year-old man with diabetes and previous angina is unlikely to have the same explanation as a new foot drop in a 20-year-old carpet fitter). Draw up a differential diagnosis and then consider which (if any) investigations are pertinent. Sometimes during the summarising process it may become clear that there are aspects of the history that have not been adequately addressed. Go back and resolve these areas. Time spent reviewing the history is never wasted; undertaking unnecessary tests, on the other hand, is more than just a waste of time.

Do not place undue emphasis on an isolated sign that fails to fit with the history, such as an apparently isolated extensor plantar response in a patient with typical migraine. It is more likely that this is a false-positive sign due to an inept examination/ interpretation of a ticklish patient rather than an indication of underlying pathology.

Investigations

Initial investigations

Not all patients require investigation. Most patients with headache, for example, need no tests, but some do (such as a 75-year-old man with new-onset headache and temporal tenderness on examination, who should have urgent measurement of the erythrocyte sedimentation rate and C-reactive protein and a temporal artery biopsy). Unfortunately, the increasing availability of tests means that many patients are investigated unnecessarily, which creates new problems (such as what to do with the unexpected, and quite incidental, finding of an unruptured intracranial aneurysm identified in a patient with migraine). Avoid doing tests because you can or because you do not know what else to do. Magnetic resonance imaging (MRI) of the brain may unearth incidental findings of no clinical relevance in up to 20%, depending on age, and there is an irony – usually lost on your patient – in attempting reassurance with a scan only to identify an incidental 'abnormality'. Sometimes a single carefully chosen test is all that is necessary to confirm a diagnosis. For example, a patient with chorea, whose father died of Huntington's disease, will almost certainly have the diagnosis confirmed with genetic testing, without the need for imaging or other tests.

Consider your diagnosis and start with any necessary simple blood tests (such as exclusion of metabolic disturbance, including diabetes); then work upwards. If imaging is required, decide what to image using which modality (computed tomography, MRI, ultrasound or functional imaging), and whether any special sequences or techniques are necessary (like intravenous contrast; Figs 7.28–7.30). Discuss the case with the radiologists if you are unsure. For some PNS disorders, nerve conduction studies and electromyography may be helpful. Electroencephalography is perhaps the most misused test in neurology. Think carefully about whether it will add anything to what you already know; it should not be used to *diagnose* epilepsy. The more invasive tests (lumbar puncture, nerve/muscle/brain biopsy) all require careful consideration and should be guided by specialists. Lastly, the worlds of antibody-mediated and genetic diseases are changing rapidly, and you may need to have a discussion with the relevant experts about which specialised test might be most appropriate.

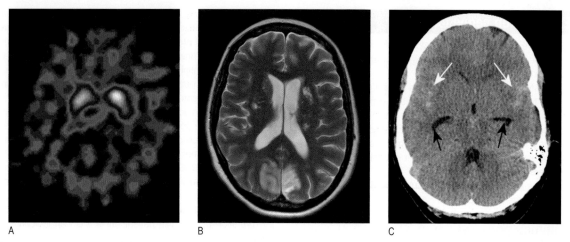

A

B

C

Fig. 7.28 Imaging of the head. [A] DaTscan showing uptake of tracer (dopamine receptors) in the basal ganglia on cross-section of the brain. [B] Magnetic resonance scan showing ischaemic stroke. T2 imaging demonstrates bilateral occipital infarction and bilateral hemisphere lacunar infarction. [C] Unenhanced computed tomogram showing subarachnoid blood in both Sylvian fissures *(white arrows)* and early hydrocephalus. The temporal horns of the lateral ventricles are visible *(black arrows)*.

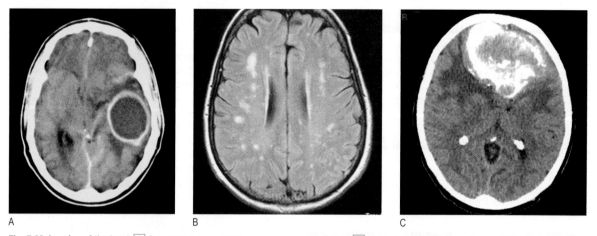

A

B

C

Fig. 7.29 Imaging of the head. [A] Computed tomogram (CT) showing a cerebral abscess. [B] Magnetic resonance scan showing multiple sclerosis with white demyelinating plaques. [C] CT scan showing a large meningioma arising from the olfactory groove.

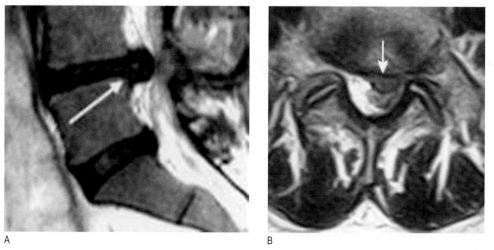

A

B

Fig. 7.30 T2 magnetic resonance images showing a large left paracentral L4–5 disc protrusion *(arrowed)* compressing the L5 nerve root. [A] Sagittal section. [B] Axial section.

Specific investigations

Lumbar puncture

Lumbar puncture is a key investigation in a number of acute and chronic neurological conditions. Always measure the CSF opening pressure (in a lying position, not sitting), using an atraumatic (blunt) needle. CSF is routinely examined for cells, protein content and glucose (compared to simultaneously taken blood glucose); it is also stained and cultured for bacteria. Other specific tests may be carried out, such as analysis for oligoclonal bands, meningococcal and pneumococcal antigens, polymerase chain reaction (PCR) for certain viruses or cytology for malignant cells.

Neurophysiological tests

Electroencephalography (EEG) records spontaneous electrical activity of the brain, using scalp electrodes. It is employed in the investigation of epilepsy, encephalopathies or dementia. Modifications to standard EEG improve sensitivity and include sleep-deprived studies, prolonged videotelemetry and invasive EEG monitoring.

Electromyography (EMG) involves needle electrodes inserted into muscle. Electrical activity is displayed on an oscilloscope and an audio monitor, allowing the neurophysiologist to see and hear the pattern of activity. Neurogenic and myopathic pathology causes characteristic EMG abnormalities.

Nerve conduction studies involve applying electrical stimuli to nerves and measuring the speed of impulse conduction. They are used for both motor and sensory nerves, and are helpful in diagnosing peripheral nerve disorders such as nerve compressions or polyneuropathies. They are also helpful is distinguishing between axonal and demyelinating neuropathies, the underlying causes and management of which are very different.

7

OSCE example 1: Headache history

Miss Bolton, 32 years old, presents acutely with a severe global headache, associated with vomiting and feeling dreadful.

Please take a history from this patient

Confirm:
- Onset – gradual or sudden.
- Site – lateralised or global.
- Severity.
- Aggravating and relieving factors, such as bright light.
- Associated symptoms, such as vomiting, photophobia, neck pain, visual disturbance.
- Relevant family history.

Summarise your findings

This 32-year-old woman's headache began gradually last night and is worse today; she has been in bed in a darkened room, trying to sleep. She has vomited the analgesia she took. She often has headaches at the time of her period but this is the worst headache she has ever experienced. She recalls having one or two migraines as a child, and her mother had migraine. She is otherwise well and takes no medication other than the oral contraceptive. The examination is normal, although she looks tired and distressed.

Suggest a differential diagnosis

The most likely diagnosis is migraine; the headache evolved and worsened over a few hours, with no 'red flags', on a background of a predisposition to migraine. The differential includes more sinister causes such as meningitis, cerebral venous sinus thrombosis or intracranial haemorrhage, but there are no features to support these. The headache is likely to resolve in the next day or two.

Suggest initial investigations

She does not need any tests, as there are no features to suggest she needs brain imaging or lumbar puncture to exclude a subarachnoid haemorrhage or meningitis.

OSCE example 2: Tremor

Mr Anderson, 76 years old, presents with a tremor of his arm.

Please examine his arms

- Introduce yourself and clean your hands.
- Observe the patient sitting at rest; note any tremor, abnormal postures, facial expression, jaw/chin tremor, drooling.
- Listen to his speech.
- Ask him to raise both arms above his head, then to stretch them out in front of him; observe any tremor on posture.
- Ask him to perform piano-playing movements; look carefully for asymmetry and reduced fine finger movements.
- Assess tone, looking specifically for asymmetry, and cog wheeling or lead pipe rigidity in the affected right arm.
- Test power in shoulder abduction, elbow flexion/extension and finger extension.
- Test upper limb deep tendon reflexes (biceps, supinator and triceps).
- Omit sensory testing, as this is unlikely to add anything.
- Test finger-to-nose movements.
- Ask him to walk, observing what happens to the tremor and right arm swing.
- Thank the patient and clean your hands.

Continued

OSCE example 2: Tremor – *cont'd*

Summarise your findings

The patient has an asymmetric pill-rolling rest tremor of the right arm, which briefly disappears on movement but quickly returns (re-emergent tremor). He also has a tremor affecting the jaw/chin. There is a lack of facial expression, drooling, monotonous, hypophonic speech, bradykinesia (reduced fine finger movements, difficulty with repetitive movements), increased tone with cog wheeling, and loss of the right arm swing and increased tremor when walking, with short stride length.

Suggest a diagnosis

These findings are typical of Parkinson's disease.

Suggest initial investigations

A diagnosis of Parkinson's disease is usually based on the clinical features and investigation unnecessary. In selected cases, structural imaging (MR or CT) to rule out the rare mimics of PD, or functional imaging (DaTscan) may be appropriate. Blood tests are rarely helpful, but a strong family history may precipitate consideration of genetic testing.

Integrated examination sequence for the nervous system

A complete neurological examination is demanding for both doctor and patient, and in many cases will not be necessary. The history will dictate a more targeted examination, and time spent on the history is always more productive than an amateur neurological examination.

Cranial nerve examination

- Ask about sense of smell and taste (I).
- Assess visual acuity (using a Snellen chart) and visual fields (by confrontation) (II).
- Observe pupils and test pupillary reactions bilaterally: direct and consensual (II).
- Observe both eyes in the neutral position. Are they orthotropic (both pointing in the same direction)? Test eye movements, observing for completeness of movement in pursuit and looking for nystagmus (III, IV, VI).
- Test facial sensation (V) and corneal reflex (V and VII).
- Observe for facial asymmetry and test facial muscles of the upper and lower parts of the face (VII).
- Perform a bedside test of hearing (VIII).
- Assess speech, swallow and palatal movement (IX, X, XI).
- Inspect the tongue and assess movement (XII).

Neurological examination of the upper limb

- Expose the upper limbs ensuring maintenance of dignity and privacy; request a chaperone if appropriate.
- Inspect for wasting, fasciculations.
- As a screening test ask the patient to hold the arms out (palms up) and close their eyes – watch for pronator drift.
- Assess tone.
- Test muscle power: shoulder abduction (axillary nerve C5), elbow flexion (musculocutaneous nerve, C5, C6) and extension (radial nerve, C7), finger extension (posterior interosseus nerve, C7), index finger abduction (ulnar nerve, T1), little finger abduction (ulnar nerve, T1), thumb abduction (median nerve, T1).
- Assess reflexes at biceps (C5), triceps (C7) and supinator (brachioradialis, C6).
- Test coordination with finger – nose test and look for dysdiodokinesia.
- Test sensory modalities: pinprick, temperature, vibration sense, joint position sense.

Neurological examination of the lower limb

- Undress the patient to expose both lower limbs fully, ensuring maintenance of dignity and privacy; request a chaperone if appropriate.
- Carry out a general inspection, noting walking aids and other associated neurological signs, such as facial droop or ipsilateral arm flexion.
- If the patient is able to do so, ask them to stand and walk so that you can assess stance and gait. Assess tandem gait.
- Inspect both legs, noting any scars, muscle wasting or fasciculations, abnormal postures or movements.
- Assess tone at the hip, knee and ankle. Test for ankle clonus.
- Test muscle power. As a simple screen, assess hip flexion (iliofemoral nerve, L1, 2) and extension (sciatic, L5/S1), knee flexion (sciatic, S1) and extension (femoral, L3, 4), and ankle plantar flexion (tibial, S1, 2) and dorsiflexion (deep peroneal, L4, 5).
- Assess reflexes at the knee (L3) and ankle (S1), comparing sides. Test the plantar response.
- Test coordination via heel-to-shin tests.
- Test sensory modalities: pinprick, temperature, vibration and joint position sense. Map out any symptomatic areas of disturbed sensation.

Shyamanga Borooah
Naing Latt Tint

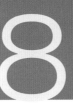

The visual system

Anatomy and physiology

The eye is a complex structure situated in the bony orbit. It is protected by the eyelid, which affords protection against injury as well as helping to maintain the tear film. The upper lid is elevated by the levator palpebrae superioris, innervated by cranial nerve III, and Müller's muscle, innervated by the sympathetic autonomic system. Eyelid closure is mediated by the orbicularis oculi muscle, innervated by cranial nerve VII.

The orbit also contains six extraocular muscles: the superior rectus, medial rectus, lateral rectus, inferior rectus, superior oblique and inferior oblique. In addition, the orbit houses the lacrimal gland, blood vessels, autonomic nerve fibres and cranial nerves II, III, IV and VI. The contents are cushioned by orbital fat, which is enclosed anteriorly by the orbital septum and the eyelids (Fig. 8.1).

The conjunctiva is a thin mucous membrane lining the posterior aspects of the eyelids. It is reflected at the superior and inferior fornices on to the surface of the globe. The conjunctiva is coated in a tear film that protects and nourishes the ocular surface.

Eye

The eyeball is approximately 25 mm in length and comprises three distinct layers. From outside in (Fig. 8.1), these are the:

- Outer fibrous layer: this includes the sclera and the clear cornea. The cornea accounts for two-thirds of the refractive power of the eye, focusing incident light on to the retina.
- Middle vascular layer (uveal tract): anteriorly this consists of the ciliary body and the iris, and posteriorly the choroid.
- Inner neurosensory layer (retina): the retina is the structure responsible for converting light to neurological signals.

Extraocular muscles

The six extraocular muscles are responsible for eye movements (Fig. 8.2). Cranial nerve III innervates the superior rectus, medial rectus, inferior oblique and inferior rectus muscles. Cranial nerve IV innervates the superior oblique muscle and cranial nerve VI innervates the lateral rectus muscle. The cranial nerves originate

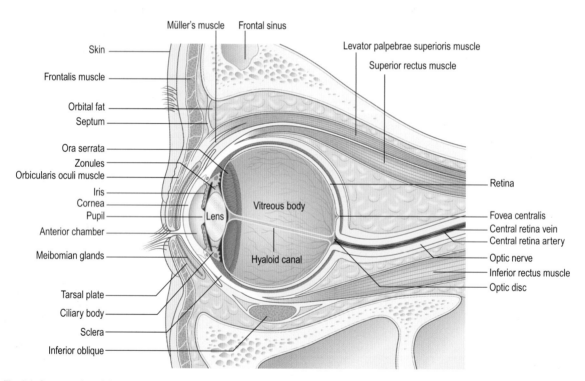

Fig. 8.1 Cross-section of the eye and orbit (sagittal view).

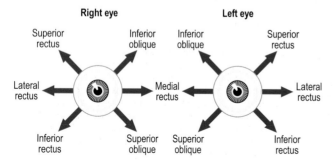

Fig. 8.2 Control of eye movements. The direction of displacement of the pupil by normal contraction of a particular muscle can be used to work out which eye muscle is paretic. For example, a patient whose diplopia is maximal on looking down and to the right has either a weak right inferior rectus or a weak left superior oblique muscle.

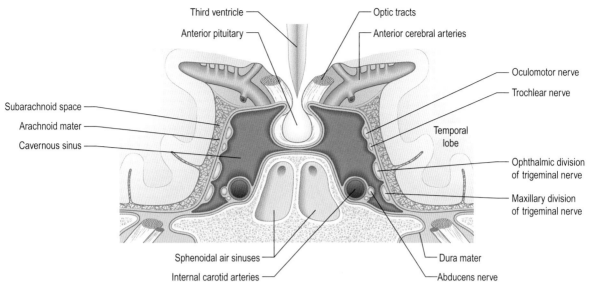

Third ventricle

Anterior pituitary

Optic tracts

Anterior cerebral arteries

Oculomotor nerve

Trochlear nerve

Subarachnoid space

Arachnoid mater

Cavernous sinus

Temporal lobe

Ophthalmic division of trigeminal nerve

Maxillary division of trigeminal nerve

8

Sphenoidal air sinuses

Internal carotid arteries

Dura mater

Abducens nerve

Fig. 8.3 Cavernous sinus (coronal view). Neuroanatomy of cranial nerves III, IV and VI.

in the midbrain and pons and then pass through the cavernous sinus (Fig. 8.3).

Refractive elements of the eye

The major refracting elements of the eye are the tear film, the cornea and the crystalline lens. The cornea possesses the greatest refractive power and is the main refracting element of the eye; the lens provides additional controllable refraction, causing the light to focus on to the retina. When light is precisely focused on to the retina, refraction is called emmetropia (Fig. 8.4A). When the focus point falls behind the retina, the result is hypermetropia (Fig. 8.4B, long-sightedness). When rays focus in front of the retina, the result is myopia (Fig. 8.4C, short-sightedness). These refractive errors can be corrected with lenses or with a pinhole (Fig. 8.4D).

Visual pathway

The visual pathway consists of the retina, optic nerve, optic chiasm, optic tracts, lateral geniculate bodies, optic radiations and visual cortex (Fig. 8.5). Deficits in the visual pathway lead to specific field defects.

Pupillary pathways

The pupil controls the amount of light entering the eye. The intensity of light determines the pupillary aperture via autonomic reflexes. Pupillary constriction is controlled by parasympathetic nerves, and pupillary dilatation is controlled by sympathetic nerves.

For pupillary constriction, the afferent pathway is the optic nerve, synapsing in the pretectal nucleus of the midbrain. Axons synapse in both cranial nerve III (Edinger–Westphal) nuclei, before passing along the inferior division of the oculomotor nerve to synapse in the ciliary ganglion. The efferent postganglionic fibres pass to the pupil via the short ciliary nerves, resulting in constriction (Fig. 8.6A).

For pupillary dilatation, the sympathetic pathway originates in the hypothalamus, passing down to the ciliospinal centre

of Budge at the level of T1. Fibres then pass to, and synapse in, the superior cervical ganglion before joining the surface of the internal carotid artery and passing to the pupil along the nasociliary and the long ciliary nerves (Fig. 8.6B).

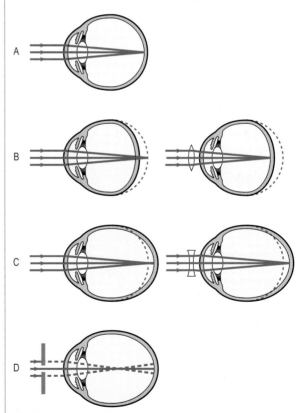

Fig. 8.4 Normal and abnormal refraction by the cornea and lens. **A** Emmetropia (normal refraction). Cornea and lens focus light on retina. **B** Hypermetropia (long-sightedness). The eye is too short and the image on the retina is not in focus. A convex (plus) lens focuses the image on the retina. **C** Myopia (short-sightedness). The eye is too long and the image on the retina is not in focus. A concave (minus) lens focuses the image on the retina. **D** Myopia corrected using a pinhole. This negates the effect of the lens, correcting refractive errors by allowing only rays from directly in front to pass.

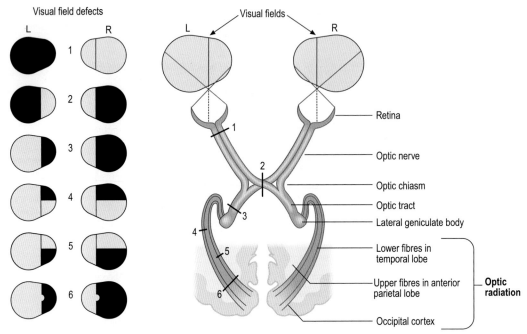

Fig. 8.5 **Visual field defects. 1,** Total loss of vision in one eye because of a lesion of the optic nerve. **2,** Bitemporal hemianopia due to compression of the optic chiasm. **3,** Right homonymous hemianopia from a lesion of the optic tract. **4,** Upper right quadrantanopia from a lesion of the lower fibres of the optic radiation in the temporal lobe. **5,** Lower quadrantanopia from a lesion of the upper fibres of the optic radiation in the anterior part of the parietal lobe. **6,** Right homonymous hemianopia with sparing of the macula due to a lesion of the optic radiation in the occipital lobe.

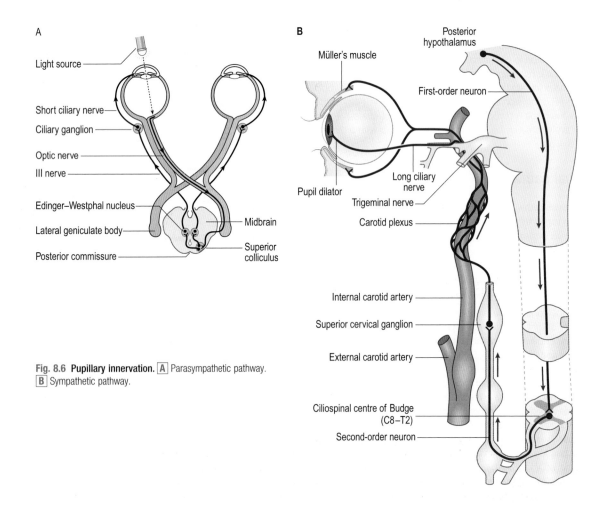

Fig. 8.6 **Pupillary innervation.** [A] Parasympathetic pathway. [B] Sympathetic pathway.

The history

When taking an ophthalmic history, bear in mind the anatomy of the eye and visual pathways. This will enable you to work from 'front to back' to include or exclude differential diagnoses.

Common presenting symptoms

Start the ophthalmic history with open questions. This builds rapport with the patient by allowing them to describe the condition in their own words, and provides clues for more directed questions later.

The visual system has its own set of presenting symptoms, which prompt specific sets of questions. The most common are described here.

Altered vision

Vision may be altered by an intraocular disease that leads to a change in the optical or refractive properties of the eye and prevents incident light rays from being clearly focused on the retina. Alternatively, it may result from extraocular factors associated with damage to the visual pathway, which runs from the optic nerve to the occipital lobe (see Fig. 8.5).

Establish whether the change in vision is sudden or gradual, as these will have their own specific set of differential diagnoses (Box 8.1 and Fig. 8.7; Box 8.2 and Fig. 8.8).

Vision may be not just reduced but also distorted. This results from disruption to the normal structure of the macula, the central part of the retina. The most common cause is macular degeneration but it may also frequently stem from an epiretinal membrane, vitreous traction or central serous retinopathy.

Flashes and floaters result from disturbance of the vitreous and the retina, occurring most commonly in posterior vitreous detachment. This is usually found in older patients as the vitreous gradually degenerates and liquefies, causing it to peel off from the retina. The vitreous is attached to the retina in certain regions; in these regions the vitreous either detaches with traction, resulting in flashing lights, or detaches by tearing the retina, releasing retinal pigment cells. Patients will see either of these as floaters.

Haloes are coloured lights seen around bright lights. They occur with corneal oedema and are most commonly associated with angle-closure glaucoma.

When patients present with a change in vision, ask:
- Did the change in vision start suddenly or gradually?
- How is the vision affected (loss of vision, cloudy vision, floaters, distortion)?
- Is it one or both eyes that are affected?
- Is the whole or only part of the visual field affected?
- If partial, which part of the visual field is affected?

Pain

Ask:
- when the pain began
- whether anything started the pain
- about the character of the pain
- how severe the pain is
- if the pain is exacerbated or relieved by any factors
- whether the pain is associated with any other symptoms.

The cornea is one of the most highly innervated regions of the body. When the corneal nerves are activated, this leads to pain, the sensation of foreign body, reflex watering and photophobia. There are, however, many other causes of a painful eye. Box 8.3 summarises the history and examination findings associated with these.

Red eye

The eye is covered in a network of vessels in the conjunctiva, episclera and sclera. Ciliary vessels are also found around the cornea. Dilatation or haemorrhage of any of these vessels can lead to a red eye. Additionally, in uveitis, acute angle-closure glaucoma and corneal irritation the ciliary vessels around the cornea become more prominent (a 'ciliary flush'). The appearance is distinct from conjunctivitis, in which there is a relative blanching of vessels towards the cornea.

Ask:
- if the eye is painful or photophobic
- if vision is affected
- if there has been any recent trauma
- whether the eye is itchy
- whether there is any discharge
- whether there has been any recent contact lens wear or foreign body exposure.

Box 8.4 summarises the features of the common causes of a red eye on history and examination.

Double vision (diplopia)

Decipher whether the diplopia is monocular or binocular. Binocular diplopia is caused by an imbalance in eye movement. Monocular diplopia results from intraocular disease in one eye. There are several causes of double vision (Box 8.5 and Figs 8.9 and 8.10).

Ask:
- whether the double vision occurs in one or both eyes
- about the character of the double vision, and whether the images are seen side by side, one above the other or at an angle
- whether the double vision is associated with any recent trauma.

Test the eye movements (see Fig. 8.11), and use your knowledge of the function of the extraocular muscles (see Fig. 8.2) to work out which cranial nerve is affected in binocular diplopia.

Discharge

Increasing discharge from the eye results from either an increase in production or a decrease in drainage from the ocular surface. Irritation of corneal nerves activates cranial nerve V(I) and results in a reflex tearing response.

Tears normally drain through the punctum at the medial end of the lower eyelid into the nasolacrimal duct, which opens below the inferior turbinate into the nasal cavity. Blockage of tear drainage or abnormal lid position can also result in excessive discharge.

Ask:
- whether the discharge is clear or opaque
- whether there is associated pain, foreign body sensation or itchiness
- whether the patient has noticed other abnormalities, such as red eye.

There are many causes of eye discharge, and their clinical features are summarised in Box 8.6.

Swollen eyes

The orbit is an enclosed structure, except anteriorly. Any swelling inside the orbit can lead to proptosis or anterior displacement of the globe.

Ask if:
- the swelling is unilateral or bilateral
- the changes were acute or gradual
- the swelling is painful
- there is any itchiness or irritation
- the swelling is associated with any double vision.

Box 8.7 summarises the common causes of swollen eyes.

8.1 Common causes of an acute change in vision

Cause	Clinical features	Cause	Clinical features
Unilateral Giant cell arteritis	• Painless loss of vision • Age >50 years • Weight loss • Loss of appetite, fatigue • Jaw or tongue claudication • Temporal headache • Pale or swollen optic disc • RAPD	Vitreous haemorrhage	• Painless loss of vision • Risk in proliferative diabetic retinopathy • History of flashing lights or floaters may precede haemorrhage in posterior vitreous detachment • Poor fundus view on examination • Reduction or loss of the red reflex • Usually no RAPD if retina is intact
Central retinal vein occlusion	• Acute, painless loss of vision • May have RAPD if severe • Greater risk if hypertensive • Haemorrhages, exudates and tortuous retinal veins (Fig. 8.7A)	Wet age-related macular degeneration	• Sudden painless loss of central vision • Age >55 years • Increased risk in smokers • Haemorrhage at the macula (Fig. 8.7E)
Retinal detachment	• Painless loss of vision • Association with flashing lights or floaters • History of a curtain coming across vision • Myopic patients at greater risk • RAPD if macula is involved • Pale raised retina usually with a retinal tear (Fig. 8.7B)	Anterior ischaemic optic neuropathy	• Painless loss of upper or lower visual field • Increased risk in vasculopaths • Examination may reveal optic disc swelling
Central retinal arterial occlusion	• Acute, painless loss of vision • Carotid bruit may be heard • RAPD • Increased risk in vasculopaths • Examination: pale retina with a cherry red spot at the fovea (Fig. 8.7C)	Optic neuritis/ retrobulbar neuritis	• Visual reduction over hours • Usually aged 20–50 • Pain exacerbated by eye movement • RAPD • Reduced colour sensitivity • Swollen optic disc in optic neuritis (Fig. 8.7F) or normal appearances in retrobulbar neuritis
Corneal disease	• Usual association with pain • Foreign body sensation • Corneal opacity may be visible (e.g. Fig. 8.7D)	Amaurosis fugax	• Painless loss of vision for minutes • History of cardiovascular disease • May have associated atrial fibrillation or carotid bruit • Normal ocular examination
Bilateral Giant cell arteritis	• Painless loss of vision • Age >50 years • Weight loss • Loss of appetite, Fatigue • Jaw or tongue, claudication • Temporal headache • Pale or swollen optic disc	Cerebral infarct	• May have associated headache and/or neurological signs • Usually specific field defects dependent on how the visual pathway is affected (Fig. 8.5) • Normal fundus examination • If post chiasmal visual pathway affected, bilateral visual field abnormalities
Raised intracranial pressure	• Headache • Often asymmetric • Pulsatile tinnitus • Swollen optic discs	Migraine	• Gradually evolving usually bilateral visual loss • Vision loss is usually preceded by visual aura • Normal ocular examination • Ocular examination: normal • Vision usually returns to normal after hours

RAPD, *relative afferent pupillary defect (p. 162).*

8.2 Common causes of a gradual loss of vision

Cause	Clinical features	Cause	Clinical features
Refractive error	• No associated symptoms • Normal ocular examination • Vision can be improved by pinhole (Fig. 8.4D)	Diabetic maculopathy	• History of diabetes • Central vision reduced or distorted • Haemorrhages and exudates at the macula on examination (Fig. 8.17A)
Glaucoma	• Usually bilateral but asymmetric loss of visual field • Cupped optic discs on examination	Compressive optic neuropathy	• Gradual unilateral loss of vision • Pale optic disc on examination (Fig. 8.8D)
Cataract	• Gradual clouding of vision • May be associated with glare • Usually seen in the elderly • Examination: clouding of the pupil and altered red reflex (see Fig. 8.8A and B)	Retinitis pigmentosa	• Gradual bilateral symmetric loss of peripheral visual field • Nyctalopia (poor vision in dim light) • Family history • Examination: bone spicule fundus, attenuated blood vessels and waxy optic disc (Fig. 8.8E)

8.2 Common causes of a gradual loss of vision – *cont'd*

Cause	Clinical features	
Dry age-related macular degeneration	• Gradual loss of central vision • Usually bilateral • Examination: drusen, atrophy and pigmentation at the macula (Fig. 8.8C)	

8

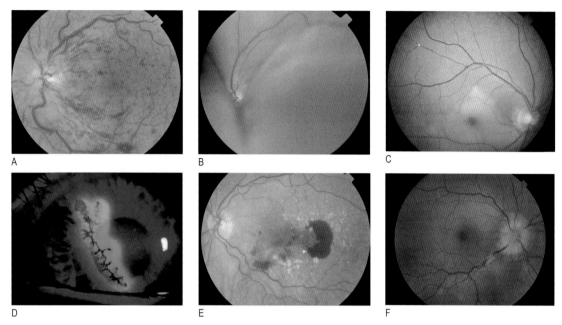

Fig. 8.7 Common causes of an acute change in vision. [A] Central retinal vein occlusion. [B] Retinal detachment. Elevation of the retina around the 'attached' optic disc; the retina may even be visible on viewing the red reflex. [C] Central retinal arterial occlusion. [D] Herpes simplex virus keratitis. [E] Wet age-related macular degeneration. [F] Swollen optic nerve head in acute optic neuritis.

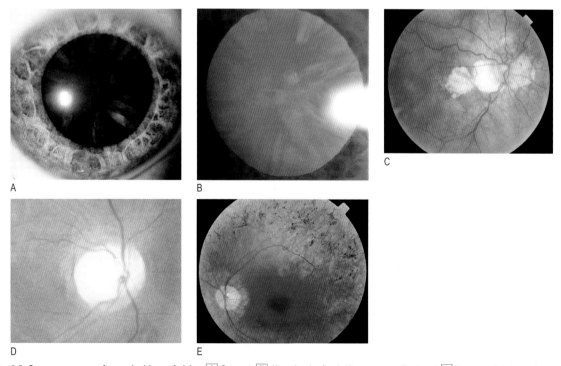

Fig. 8.8 Common causes of a gradual loss of vision. [A] Cataract. [B] Altered red reflex in the presence of cataract. [C] Dry age-related macular degeneration. [D] Compressive optic neuropathy. Optic nerve sheath meningioma causing optic disc pallor and increased disc cupping with sparing of the outer optic nerve rim. [E] Retinitis pigmentosa, with a triad of optic atrophy, attenuated retinal vessels and pigmentary changes. The latter typically start peripherally in association with a ring scotoma and symptoms of night blindness.

8.3 Causes of a painful eye

Cause	Clinical features	Cause	Clinical features
Blocked gland on lid	Pain on lid Tenderness to touch Ocular examination: redness and swelling of lid	Conjunctivitis	Increased clear or purulent discharge Ocular examination: red eye Vision is usually unaffected
Corneal foreign body	Foreign body sensation Watery eye Photophobia Ocular examination: foreign body visible or found under the eyelid	Uveitis	Floaters Blurry vision Photophobia Ocular examination: ciliary flush
Corneal infection	Foreign body sensation Photophobia Red eye Ulcer on cornea, which can be highlighted with fluorescein staining (see Fig. 8.7D) Ocular examination: white infiltrate may be visible	Optic neuritis	Reduction in vision Reduction in colour sensitivity Constant pain worsened by eye movement Ocular examination: swollen disc in optic neuritis (see Fig. 8.7F), normal disc in retrobulbar neuritis
Scleritis	Severe pain that keeps the patient awake at night Soreness of the eye to touch Association with recent infection, surgery or rheumatic disease Ocular examination: scleral injection	Orbital cellulitis	Constant ache around the eyes Reduced vision Double vision Association with a recent viral infection Ocular examination: conjunctival chemosis and injection, restricted eye movements; in severe cases, visual reduction with RAPD
Angle-closure glaucoma	Constant pain around the eye Acute reduction in vision Possibly, haloes seen around lights Association with nausea and vomiting Ocular examination: fixed mid-dilated pupil, hazy cornea and usually a cataract	Thyroid eye disease	Symptoms of hyperthyroidism (p. 197) Sore, gritty eyes Double vision Ocular examination: lid retraction, proptosis, restricted eye movements and conjunctival injection, conjunctival chemosis (see Fig. 10.4)

RAPD, *relative afferent pupillary defect (p. 162)*.

8.4 Common causes of a red eye

Causes	Clinical features	Causes	Clinical features
Allergic conjunctivitis	Itchy eyes Clear discharge Possibly, more frequent occurrence at certain times of year	Episcleritis	Focal or diffuse injection Possible association with a nodule No pain Vision not affected
Viral conjunctivitis	Watery discharge Possible itch Swollen conjunctiva Usually bilateral Ocular examination: gland swelling and follicles under the lid	Scleritis	Focal or diffuse injection Vision may be affected Association with recent infection, surgery or rheumatic disease Severe pain that keeps the patient awake at night Pain to touch
Bacterial conjunctivitis	Purulent discharge Pain	Dry eyes	Gritty or burning sensation Watery eyes Ocular examination: corneal fluorescein staining
Trauma	History of trauma Ocular examination: may reveal subconjunctival haemorrhage or injection	Subconjunctival haemorrhage	No pain Vision unaffected Ocular examination: mildly raised conjunctiva with a bleed
Acute angle-closure glaucoma	Acute-onset reduction in vision Pain Blurring of vision Haloes seen around lights Nausea Ocular examination: fixed, mid-dilated pupil with a hazy cornea	Corneal ulcer/ abrasion	Vision usually reduced Foreign body sensation Photophobia Watering Ocular examination: ulcer seen on fluorescein staining (see Fig. 8.7D) May be associated with a white corneal infiltrate
Acute anterior uveitis	Gradual onset of pain Photophobia Floaters Ocular examination: ciliary flush		

8.4 Common causes of a red eye – *cont'd*

Causes	Clinical features	Causes	Clinical features
Orbital cellulitis	Usual occurrence in young children Recent history of intercurrent viral illness Vision may be affected Possible double vision Ocular examination: reduced vision and colour vision, proptosis, eye movement restriction; in severe cases, RAPD	Thyroid eye disease	Chronic red eyes Sore, gritty sensation Foreign body sensation Double vision Ocular examination: lid retraction, proptosis, conjunctival injection and chemosis (see Fig. 10.4)

RAPD, *relative afferent pupillary defect (p. 162).*

8.5 Causes of double vision

Monocular

- High astigmatism
- Corneal opacity
- Abnormal lens
- Iris defect

Binocular

- Myasthenia gravis (p. 125)
- VI nerve palsy (Fig. 8.9)
- IV nerve palsy
- III nerve palsy (Fig. 8.10)
- Internuclear ophthalmoplegia
- Thyroid eye disease (see Fig. 10.4)
- Complex or combined palsy
- Severe orbital cellulitis or orbital inflammation

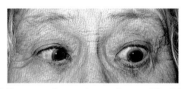

Fig. 8.9 Sixth nerve palsy causing weakness of the lateral rectus muscle. The patient is attempting to look to the left.

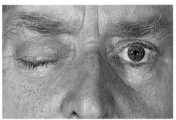

A

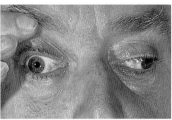

B

Fig. 8.10 Third nerve palsy. **A** Complete ptosis in right III nerve palsy. **B** The same patient looking down and to the left. The right eye is unable to adduct or depress due to a complete right III nerve palsy. It remains in slight abduction due to the unopposed action of the right lateral rectus muscle and an intact VI nerve. *From Forbes CD, Jackson WF. Color Atlas of Clinical Medicine. 3rd edn. Edinburgh: Mosby; 2003.*

Past ocular history

Ask the patient whether they have any known ophthalmic conditions. Enquire specifically about amblyopia, which is a reduction in vision in one eye from childhood, as this may limit best-corrected visual acuity. Check whether the patient normally wears glasses or contact lenses, and the last time they had their eyes checked for refractive correction. Ask about any previous eye operations that may also affect vision.

Past medical history

Focus on systemic diseases that can affect the eyes directly or as a side effect of treatment, in particular:

- a history of diabetes or hypertension, especially in the context of visual loss or double vision
- thyroid disease in the context of red, swollen eyes and double vision
- asthma, chronic obstructive pulmonary disease (COPD) or peripheral vascular disease if starting glaucoma medication.

Drug and allergy history

The eyes may be affected by medication given for other conditions (such as glaucoma exacerbated by conjunctival absorption of nebulised anticholinergic drugs in COPD). Medication given for the eyes (such as beta-blocker eye drops) can aggravate other conditions like asthma.

Ask about a history of hay fever and allergies if the patient has itchy eyes.

Family history

Several eye diseases have an inherited predisposition. Ask specifically about a history of glaucoma in first-order relatives. Genetic diseases affecting the eyes include retinitis pigmentosa (see Fig. 8.8E). Patients with thyroid eye disease may have a positive family history of autoimmune disease.

Social history

Visual impairment has a wide range of effects on daily life.

Ask about:

- Daily activities requiring good vision: reading, television, sport, hobbies and so on.
- Driving.
- Occupation: certain professions, including drivers of heavy goods vehicles and pilots, require specific visual acuity criteria.
- Smoking and alcohol use: this may affect vascular and optic nerve function within the eye.

8

8.6 Common causes of increased discharge from the eyes

Causes	Clinical features
Bacterial conjunctivitis	Red eye Yellow or green sticky discharge Vision usually unaffected
Viral conjunctivitis	Red eye Clear, watery discharge Possible itchy eye Vision usually unaffected Ocular examination: conjunctival chemosis and injection
Blocked tear duct	White eye Clear, colourless tearing Possible occluded punctum Possible malposition of the lid
Trichiasis/ foreign body	Foreign body sensation Clear discharge Possible positive fluorescein staining
Allergic conjunctivitis	Possible red eyes Possible itchy eyes Clear discharge Possible history of hay fever or atopy, or recent start of eye medication
Blepharitis	Mild injection of lids Deposits on lashes
Poor tear film/dry eyes	Constant tearing Watering increased in the wind Improvement with tear supplements Ocular examination: early break-up time (<3 seconds) with fluorescein staining of tear film

8.7 Common causes of periorbital swelling

	Causes	
Category	Unilateral	Bilateral
Infective	Orbital cellulitis	
Inflammatory	Granulomatous polyangiitis Idiopathic orbital inflammatory disease Vasculitis	
Neoplastic	Orbital tumours Lymphoma Metastases	
Systemic	Thyroid eye disease (asymmetric)	Thyroid eye disease
Vascular	Caroticocavernous fistula Orbital varices	
Pseudoproptosis	Ptosis	Severe viral conjunctivitis Myopia Lid retraction

The physical examination

General examination

Carefully and systematically examine:

- posture and gait
- head position
- facial asymmetry and dysmorphic features
- eyelid position and periocular skin
- position and symmetry of gaze (any squint/strabismus?).

Visual acuity

Assessment of visual acuity is mandatory in all ophthalmic patients. Each eye must be tested separately. The most commonly used method of testing distance visual acuity is using a Snellen chart, which displays a random selection of letters at diminishing font size in successive lines. Ask patients to wear their distance spectacles if they usually require them. Near/reading spectacles should be worn only when testing reading vision.

Examination sequence

- Use a backlit Snellen chart positioned at 6 metres and dim the room lighting.
- Cover one eye and ask the patient to read the chart from the top down until they cannot read any further. Repeat for the other eye.
- If the patient cannot see the largest font, reduce the test distance to 3 metres, then to 1 metre if necessary.
- If they still cannot see the largest font, document instead whether they can count fingers, see hand movement or just perceive the difference between light and dark.
- On the Snellen chart, lines of decreasing font size are numbered according to the distance in metres that a person with normal vision could read them. Express visual acuity as the distance at which text is read (usually 6 metres) over the number of the smallest font line read correctly on the chart. For example, 6/60 means that the patient sees at 6 metres the font size that is seen at 60 metres by a person with normal vision.
- If the patient cannot read down to line 6 (6/6), place a pinhole directly in front of the eye (with the patient keeping their usual spectacles on, if they wear them) to correct any residual refractive error (see Fig. 8.4D).
- If the visual acuity is not improved with a pinhole, this indicates the presence of eye disease not related to the refractive apparatus alone, such as retinal or optic nerve pathology.
- Note that 6/6 is regarded as normal vision; in the UK, 6/12 or better with both eyes is the requirement for driving.
- Assess near vision with a similar test using text of reducing font size held at a comfortable reading distance. It is important to consider the need for reading spectacles in patients over the age of 40 years because of presbyopia (age-related deterioration in near vision).

Orbit and periorbital examination

Examination sequence

- Observe the face and orbit for asymmetry and any obvious abnormality, including swelling, erythema or any other skin changes.
- Look for any abnormality in the position of the lids and ptosis (Box 8.8).
- Look for any asymmetry in the position of the eyeballs. Eyeball protrusion (proptosis) is best detected by looking down on the head from above.
- Palpate around the orbital rim and orbit, looking for any masses.
- Check eye movements (Fig. 8.11).
- Use an ophthalmoscope (Fig. 8.12) to look for optic disc swelling from compression.

Pupils

First inspect generally for squint and ptosis. Examine pupil shape and symmetry. Physiological anisocoria (unequal pupil size) is seen in 20% of the population.

Anisocoria

The eyes should be assessed to determine which is the abnormal pupil.

Examination sequence

- With the patient fixating at a point in the distance, increase and decrease the illumination and look for any change in the degree of anisocoria.

8.8 Causes of eyelid ptosis

Cause	Diagnosis	Associated distinguishing features
Neurogenic	Horner's syndrome	Ptosis, miosis, eye movement spared
	Cranial nerve III palsy	Dilated pupil, eye movements affected (see Fig. 8.10)
Myogenic	Myotonic dystrophy	Frontal balding, sustained handgrip
	Chronic progressive external ophthalmoplegia	Bilateral ptosis and impairment of eye movements, often without diplopia, sparing of pupil reflexes
	Oculopharyngeal dystrophy	History of swallowing abnormalities
Neuromuscular junction	Myasthenia gravis	History of variable muscular fatigue
Mechanical	Eyelid tumour	Evident on inspection
	Eyelid inflammation/ infection	Evident on inspection
	Trauma	Scarring/history of trauma
Degenerative	Levator aponeurosis degeneration	Often unilateral, eye movement normal
	Long-term contact lens wear	History of contact lens use

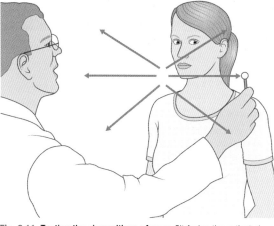

Fig. 8.11 Testing the six positions of gaze. Sit facing the patient, 1 metre away. Perform the test with both eyes open. Hold a pen torch or target in front of the patient and ask them if they see the target as double. Move the target to the six positions of gaze *(blue arrows)*.

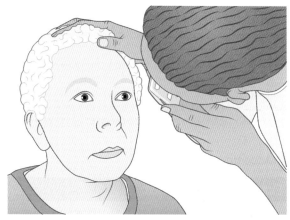

Fig. 8.12 Ophthalmoscopy. Ask the patient to focus on a distant target. To examine the left eye, use your left eye to look through the ophthalmoscope and left hand to hold it, index finger on the wheel. Hold the patient's head with your free hand. Gradually move in to visualise the optic disc. Rotate the wheel to obtain a clear, focused image.

If the degree of anisocoria is greater in brighter lighting, then it is the larger pupil that is abnormal; if it is more pronounced in dim lighting, the smaller pupil is the abnormal one. An equal degree of anisocoria in all levels of lighting indicates physiological anisocoria.

Direct and consensual light reflex

Examination sequence

- With the patient fixating on a point in the distance and in ambient lighting, shine a bright light from the temporal side into one eye and look for constriction of the ipsilateral pupil.
- To test the consensual reflex, assess the pupil response in the contralateral pupil when light is directed towards the ipsilateral pupil. Repeat for the other pupil.

8

8.9 Causes of anisocoria

Dilated pupil

- Cranial nerve III palsy
- Pharmacological treatment with a dilating agent (e.g. tropicamide or atropine)
- Physiological
- Post-surgical
- Adie's tonic pupil

Constricted pupil

- Horner's syndrome
- Mechanical, e.g. secondary to posterior synechiae in iritis or trauma
- Physiological
- Late-stage Adie's tonic pupil
- Pharmacological treatment with a constricting agent (e.g. pilocarpine)

Relative afferent pupillary defect

Relative afferent pupillary defect (RAPD) is an important clinical sign that occurs when disease of the retina or optic nerve reduces the response of the eye to a light stimulus. Testing for RAPD is an extension of the direct and consensual light responses.

Examination sequence

- Use a bright light source.
- Move the light briskly from one eye to the other, but place it on each eye for a minimum of 3 seconds.

In normal patients, this results in symmetrical constriction of both pupils. In RAPD, light in the affected eye causes weaker constriction (apparent dilatation) compared to light shone in the normal eye.

Accommodation

Examination sequence

- Ask the patient to look at a close fixation target (do not use a light source) after fixating on a distant target.
- There should be constriction of the pupil on near gaze.
- Failure to constrict to light but constriction on near gaze is referred to as light-near dissociation.

There are many causes of a dilated or constricted pupil (Box 8.9).

Pupillary examination will distinguish the various causes of anisocoria, as described here.

Horner's syndrome

Horner's syndrome is the clinical picture resulting from dysfunction of sympathetic nerve supply to the eye, which originates in the hypothalamus and emerges in the root of the neck before innervating the pupil (see Fig. 8.6B). Damage at any point in this pathway will result in Horner's syndrome. On examination, there is a constricted pupil (loss of sympathetic dilator tone) and a partial ptosis resulting from denervation of Müller's muscle in the upper eyelid. There may also be anhydrosis (loss of sweating) on the affected side. Diagnosis may be confirmed by administering cocaine eye drops, which will cause pupil dilatation in the unaffected pupil but no dilatation on the affected side. Causes of Horner's syndrome include demyelination, neck trauma/surgery, apical lung tumour (Pancoast tumour) and carotid artery dissection.

Adie's pupil

This is a mid-dilated pupil that responds poorly to both light and accommodation. With time, however, the affected pupil can become constricted. Adie's pupil is thought to result from parasympathetic pathway dysfunction in the orbit. It typically affects young women and is benign. When associated with diminished Achilles tendon reflexes, it is referred to as Holmes–Adie syndrome.

Argyll Robertson pupil

The pupil is small and irregular, and reacts to accommodation but not light. This is classically the result of neurosyphilis. There are other causes of light-near dissociation, however, including diabetes mellitus, severe optic nerve disease and midbrain lesions.

Visual fields

The normal visual field extends 160 degrees horizontally and 130 degrees vertically. Fixation is the very centre of the patient's visual field. The physiological blind spot is located 15 degrees temporal to the point of visual fixation and represents the entry of the optic nerve head into the eye.

The aim of the visual field examination is to test the patient's visual fields against your own (making the assumption that you have normal visual fields). The visual field can be tested using the fingers for gross examination. Finer examination can be performed using a small hatpin.

Examination sequence

- Check visual acuity and ensure that the patient has at least enough vision to count fingers.
- Sit directly facing the patient, about 1 metre away.
- With your eyes and the patient's eyes open, ask the patient to look at your face and comment on whether they have any difficulty seeing parts of your face.
- Ask the patient to keep looking straight at your face. Test each eye separately. Ask the patient to close or cover one eye and look directly across to your opposite eye; you should also close your other eye.
- Hold your hands out and bring an extended finger in from the periphery towards the centre of the visual field. For an accurate assessment of the patient's fields, it is vital that the testing finger is always kept in the plane exactly halfway between yourself and the patient. Wiggle your fingertip and ask the patient to point to it when they first see it (Fig. 8.13). If the patient fails to notice your finger when it is clearly visible to you, their field is reduced in that area.
- Test all four quadrants separately.
- More subtle visual field defects can be elicited using a small white hatpin or a white Neurotip. With the patient looking directly at your eye, bring the white target in from the periphery to the centre (again always in the plane halfway between you and the patient). Ask the patient to say when they first see the target.
- Undertake this for all four quadrants, testing each eye separately.
- To assess very early visual field loss, repeat the same test using a red hatpin or a red Neurotip (Fig. 8.14).

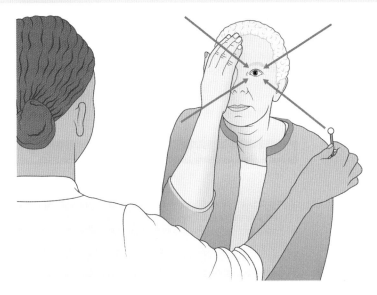

Fig. 8.13 Confrontation visual field testing. Sit facing the patient, 1 metre away. To compare your visual field (assumed normal) with the patient's, present a white target or wiggle your fingers at a point equidistant between yourself and the patient in the periphery. Bring the target inwards in the direction of the blue arrows, asking the patient to alert you when they first see it. Test each eye separately.

8

- It is important to show the patient the red target and ask them to report what colour they see. A dull or pale red suggests colour desaturation, which may indicate optic nerve dysfunction.
- When testing each quadrant with a red target, be sure to explain to the patient that they should say when they first see that the target is red and not when they first see it. The target may be visualised before they appreciate the red colour.
- To test the blind spot, place a red-tipped target equidistant between the patient and yourself at the visual fixation point.
- Move the target temporally until it disappears.
- Then move the target slowly up and down, as well as from side to side, until it reappears. This allows you to compare the patient's blind spot with yours.

Ocular alignment and eye movements

The eyes are normally parallel in all positions of gaze except for convergence. Any misalignment is referred to as a squint (strabismus). Squints are described as manifest (tropia) if present with both eyes open, or latent (phoria) if revealed only by covering one eye. In addition, they can be concomitant (where the angle of squint remains the same in all positions of gaze) or incomitant (where the angle of squint deviation is greatest in a single position of gaze). The latter is commonly the result of paralysis of particular extraocular muscles.

Detection of squint

Examination sequence

- Sit directly facing the patient, approximately 1 metre away and at a similar height.
- Check visual acuity as part of the examination.
- Look for any abnormal head posture such as head tilts (seen in cranial nerve IV palsy) or head turns (cranial nerve VI palsy). These signs may be subtle.
- Hold a pen torch directly in front of the patient and instruct them to look at the light. Observe the reflection of the light

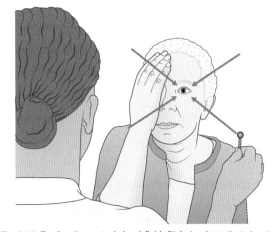

Fig. 8.14 Testing the central visual field. Sit facing the patient, 1 metre away. Present a red target at a point equidistant between yourself and the patient in the periphery, starting when you can first see the target as red. Bring the target inwards in the direction of the blue arrows, asking the patient to alert you when they first see the target as red. Test each eye separately.

on the cornea in relation to the pupil. The reflections should be symmetrical between the two eyes. Ask the patient if they see a single or double light. If they see double, this may indicate the presence of a squint, but not seeing double does not exclude a squint. If the reflection is on the nasal aspect of the pupil in one eye, this suggests that the eye is deviated outwards and is described as an exotropia.

- To confirm the presence of a squint, perform the cover/uncover test:
  - Ask the patient to look at the pen torch at all times and then cover one eye.
  - Look at the uncovered eye for any movement. It may be helpful to repeat this several times.
  - Inward movement of the uncovered eye suggests that it was positioned abnormally outwards and is described as an exotropia (divergent manifest squint).

- Conversely, if the eye moves outwards when the contralateral eye is covered, this suggests that it was abnormally positioned inwards and is described as an esotropia (convergent manifest squint).
  - Repeat the cover/uncover test for the other eye.
- Failure of an eye to move despite an obvious corneal light reflex may indicate that the eye has such poor vision that it cannot take up fixation or else it is restricted from moving.
- The alternating cover test involves covering the eyes alternately and quickly while the patient is fixated on the pen torch. Leave the cover on each eye for about 2 seconds but move between the eyes in less than 1 second. The movement is repeated multiple times. This test will help to elicit latent squint.

Ocular movements

Examination sequence

- In the same seating position, ask the patient to look at a target or pen-torch light about 50 cm away.
- Ask them to say if and when they experience diplopia.
- Starting from the primary position, move the target in the six positions of gaze (see Fig. 8.11) and up and down.
- If diplopia is present, ask whether this is horizontal, vertical or a combination of the two.
- Determine where the image separation is most pronounced.
- Look for nystagmus and determine whether the eye movement is smooth.

Interpretation of any limitation of excursion is made by reference to the functions of the extraocular muscles (see Fig. 8.2).

Oculocephalic (doll's-eye) reflex

This reflex is the ability of the eyes to remain fixated while the head is turned in the horizontal plane (Fig. 8.15). An impaired reflex indicates a brainstem abnormality.

Examination sequence

- With the patient supine, ask them to look at your face. Gently turn their head from side to side, noting the movement of the eyes.
- This can also be performed on a comatose patient.

Nystagmus

Nystagmus is continuous, uncontrolled movement of the eyes. Biphasic or jerk nystagmus is the most common type. It is characterised by slow drift in one direction, followed by fast correction/recovery in the opposite direction. The direction of the fast phase designates the direction of the nystagmus. If there are equal oscillations in both directions, it is called pendular nystagmus.

Nystagmus commonly indicates vestibular disease, and the examination sequence and differential diagnosis are covered on page 174.

Ophthalmoscopy

The direct ophthalmoscope is a useful tool for assessing both the anterior and the posterior segments of the eye. Pharmacological pupil dilatation is essential for a thorough fundus examination, though the optic disc can be examined sufficiently without dilatation.

Examination sequence

- Ask the patient to sit upright and look at a distant target.
- When using the direct ophthalmoscope to examine the patient's right eye, hold it in your right hand and use your right eye to examine. Hold it in your left hand and use your left eye to examine the patient's left eye.
- Place your free hand on the patient's forehead and brow, as this will steady the head and improve your proprioception when moving closer to the patient with the ophthalmoscope.
- Rotate the ophthalmoscope lens to +10. This will allow a magnified view of the anterior segment. You will be able to examine the eyelid margins, conjunctiva, cornea and iris. If epithelial defects are suspected, fluorescein can be administered and a cobalt blue filter used to reveal these.
- To examine the fundus, dial the lens back to 0.
- With your hand on the forehead and the brow, use the ophthalmoscope to see the red reflex (red light reflected off the retina) at a distance of about 10 cm. When the red reflex is in focus, look for opacities and determine whether they are static or mobile. Static opacities are usually due to cataract changes, while mobile opacities indicate vitreous opacities.
- Slowly move the ophthalmoscope closer to the patient almost to the point that your forehead touches your thumb, which is resting on the patient's forehead and brow (see Fig. 8.12).
- Turn the lens dial until the optic disc comes into focus; if it does not, focus on a blood vessel.
- The optic disc can usually be located easily; if not, follow a blood vessel centrally (in the direction opposite to its branches) to locate it.
- Examine the optic disc, paying particular attention to its shape, colour, edges and cup size.
- Follow each blood-vessel arcade and examine each of the retinal quadrants.
- To examine the macula, ask the patient to look directly at the light.

The normal retina looks different in Asian and Caucasian patients (Fig. 8.16).

Swelling of the optic disc is a very important clinical sign. Causes of unilateral and bilateral optic disc swelling, and their distinguishing features, are summarised in Box 8.10.

A variety of diseases that can damage the optic nerve cause an abnormally pale optic disc (see Fig. 8.8D). The differential diagnosis of optic disc pallor is summarised in Box 8.11.

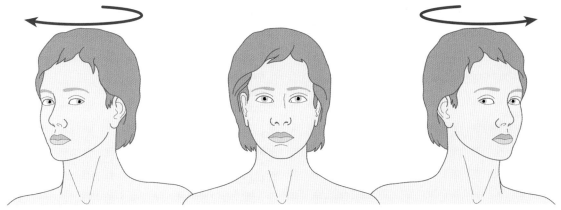

Fig. 8.15 Oculocephalic reflex. Move the head in the horizontal plane. Note that the eyes move in the opposite direction to head movement.

8

Retinopathies

Diabetes mellitus leads to a wide range of important abnormalities in the retina, which are summarised on Fig. 8.17.

The eye also provides an opportunity to view the effects of hypertension on the microvasculature. The retinal arteries are effectively arterioles. Chronic arteriosclerosis with vessel-wall thickening and hyalinisation appears as widening of the arterioles, arteriovenous nicking where arterioles cross venules, and a 'silver and copper wiring' light reflex.

More acute changes can also be seen in malignant hypertension. Various grading systems have been created to try to link retinal findings to end-organ damage. The retinal appearances in hypertension are illustrated in Fig. 8.18 and classified using the Modified Scheie classification:

• Grade 0: no changes.
• Grade 1: barely detectable arteriolar narrowing.
• Grade 2: obvious retinal arteriolar narrowing with focal irregularities.
• Grade 3: grade 2 plus retinal haemorrhages, exudates, cotton-wool spots or retinal oedema.
• Grade 4: grade 3 plus optic disc swelling.

Inherited retinopathies result from a wide range of genetic mutations. The most common inherited retinopathy is retinitis pigmentosa, which causes symptoms of nyctalopia (difficulty seeing in dim light) and tunnel vision. Examination reveals a pale optic disc, attenuated arterioles and bone-spicule retinal pigmentation (see Fig. 8.8E).

Investigations

Appropriate initial tests for a variety of common presenting eye problems are summarised in Box 8.12.

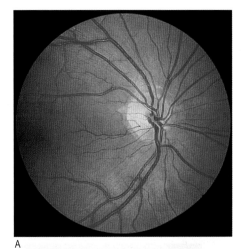

A

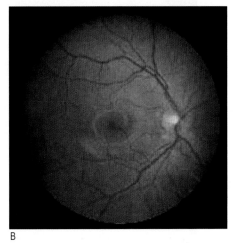

B

Fig. 8.16 The normal fundus. A Caucasian. B Asian.

8.10 Causes of optic disc swelling

Unilateral

- Optic neuritis
- Anterior ischaemic optic neuropathy
- Syphilis
- Lyme disease
- *Bartonella* infection
- Sarcoidosis
- Leukaemia
- Optic nerve glioma
- Secondary metastases

Bilateral

- Papilloedema
- Optic disc drusen
- Diabetic papillitis
- Pseudopapilloedema in hypermetropes
- Hypertensive papillopathy

8.11 Differential diagnosis of optic disc pallor

Inherited

- Congenital optic atrophy, including Leber's and Behr's

End-stage glaucoma

Trauma

Compressive

- Orbital neoplasm
- Thyroid eye disease
- Orbital cellulitis

Neurological

- End-stage papilloedema
- Devic's disease

Metabolic

- Nutritional deficiency
- Toxic amblyopia
- Ethambutol
- Sulphonamide
- Diabetes mellitus

Vascular

- Central retinal artery occlusion
- Giant cell arteritis

Inflammatory

- Meningitis
- Postoptic neuritis

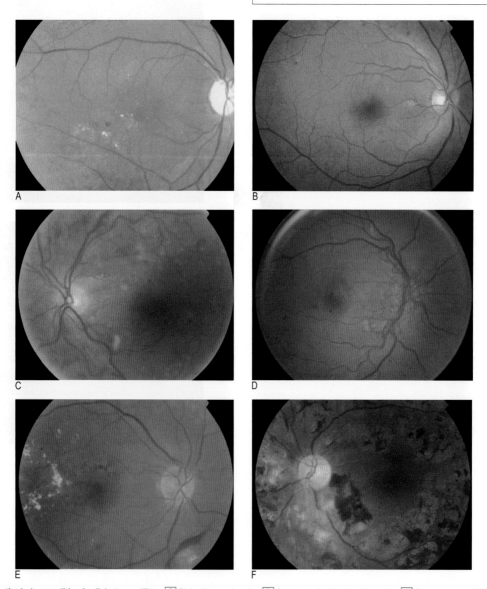

Fig. 8.17 Retinal abnormalities in diabetes mellitus. A Diabetic maculopathy. B Background diabetic retinopathy. C Severe non-proliferative diabetic retinopathy. D Proliferative diabetic retinopathy. E Proliferative diabetic retinopathy with a vitreous haemorrhage. F Previous panretinal laser photocoagulation in treated proliferative diabetic retinopathy.

8

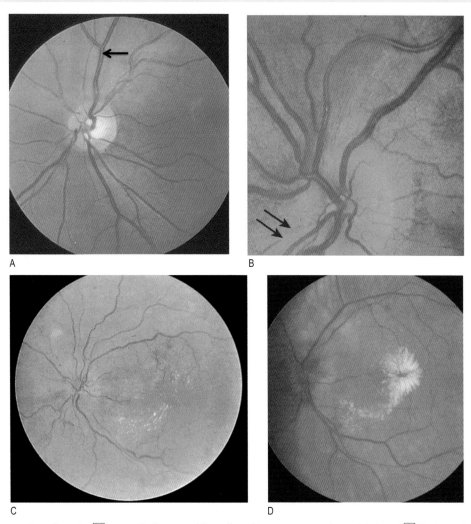

A

B

C

D

Fig. 8.18 Hypertensive retinopathy. A Increased reflectance, giving a silver wiring appearance to the arteriole *(arrow).* B Focal arteriolar narrowing *(double arrows)* seen in grade 2 disease. C Exudates and flame haemorrhages in grade 3 retinopathy. D Signs of malignant hypertension in grade 4 disease with a swollen optic disc and macular exudate.

8.12 Investigations

Investigation	Indication
Clinic tests	
Refraction	Refractive error, cataract and corneal disorders
Fluorescein staining	Corneal epithelial disease
Schirmer's test	Dry eyes, Sjögren's syndrome
Nasolacrimal duct washout	Watery eyes
Blood pressure	Hypertensive retinopathy, retinal vein occlusion
Bacterial culture and sensitivity	Bacterial conjunctivitis
Viral swab	Viral conjunctivitis
Blood tests	
Erythrocyte sedimentation rate, C-reactive protein	Vasculitis, including giant cell arteritis
Antinuclear antibody	Systemic lupus erythematosus
Rheumatoid factor	Scleritis
Fasting glucose	Diabetic retinopathy
Anti-acetylcholinesterase receptor antibody	Myasthenia gravis
Quantiferon	Uveitis
Serum angiotensin-converting enzyme	Uveitis
Human immunodeficiency virus serology	Vasculitis, uveitis
Syphilis serology	Unexplained pathology and uveitis/vasculitis
Thyroid function tests	Thyroid eye disease
Radiology	
Chest X-ray	Sarcoidosis/tuberculosis
Orbital ultrasound	Incomplete fundal view
Optical coherence tomography	Macular disease, glaucoma
Fundus fluorescein angiography	Diabetic retinopathy, retinal vein occlusion
Computed tomography brain and sinuses	Orbital cellulitis, thyroid eye disease, intracranial tumours, orbital compressive disease
Magnetic resonance imaging brain and orbits	Pituitary tumour, compressive lesion
Carotid Doppler ultrasound	Carotid artery stenosis in ocular ischaemic syndrome
Invasive tests	
Lumbar puncture	Idiopathic intracranial hypertension, inflammatory orbital neuropathies
Temporal artery biopsy	Giant cell arteritis

OSCE example 1: Gradual visual loss

Mrs Johnson, 55 years old, presents with a gradual reduction of vision over the last 6 months in both eyes. She says that she also has distortion in her vision when she is looking at straight lines. In addition, she feels constantly thirsty and is passing urine frequently.

Please examine this patient's eyes

- Introduce yourself and clean your hands.
- Perform a general inspection, looking for any signs of squint. Check the bedside for any clues that the patient wears glasses.
- Assess visual acuity using a Snellen chart at the appropriate distance.
- Examine the eyes, looking for any conjunctival injection, chemosis or swelling.
- Dim the room lights.
- Test the pupillary light reflexes.
- Ideally, dilate the pupils at this stage.
- Test the red reflex in each eye.
- Dial the fundoscope to +10 and examine the anterior portion of the eye, including the lens.
- Dial the fundoscope back to 0 and examine the fundus, looking at the disc and superior, nasal, inferior and temporal fundus.
- Finally, inspect the macula.
- Thank the patient and clean your hands.

Summarise your findings

Visual acuity is reduced to 6/18 in both eyes, and fundoscopy reveals multiple retinal haemorrhages and exudates, some close to the macula.

Suggest a diagnosis

The most likely diagnosis is diabetic maculopathy.

Suggest initial investigations

Urine dipstick, fasting blood glucose and blood pressure.

Advanced level comments

Diabetic macular oedema is the most common cause of reduced vision in diabetic patients. It may result in distortion of vision, making straight lines appear bent.

OSCE example 2: Double vision

Mr Penrose, 75 years old, presents with double vision that has increased rapidly over the last week. He says not only that objects appear side by side but also that the two images are separated vertically. He feels that his eyelid is drooping on his left side. He constantly has to lift his eyelid to see out of his left eye.

Please examine the patient's eye movements

- Introduce yourself and clean your hands.
- Perform a general inspection: look for ptosis and squint, and examine the bedside for any spectacles that may contain a prism.
- Inspect visual acuity for each eye.
- Dim the room lights.
- Test pupillary light reflexes.
- Test all eye movements for ophthalmoplegia.
- Examine the optic nerve using an ophthalmoscope.
- Examine cranial nerves I, V, VI, VII, VIII, IX, X, XI and XII.
- Thank the patient and clean your hands.

Summarise your findings

The patient has a partial ptosis on the left with a dilated pupil. Eye movements are diminished with impaired adduction and elevation of the eyeball. Double vision is confirmed on testing of eye movements.

Suggest a diagnosis

The most likely diagnosis is left incomplete III nerve palsy (complete palsy would cause total ptosis with relief of double vision).

Suggested investigations

Fasting glucose and cholesterol, blood pressure, erythrocyte sedimentation rate, and a magnetic resonance angiogram to check for an underlying cerebral artery aneurysm.

Advanced level comments

Palsies of the III nerve result in ptosis and diplopia. Microvascular damage to the III nerve usually spares the pupil. Compressive lesions such as aneurysm cause a dilated pupil, which responds poorly or is completely unresponsive to light.

Integrated examination sequence for ophthalmology

- Introduce yourself and clean your hands.
- Explain what you will be doing.
- Observe the patient as they walk into the room, looking for:
  - Facial asymmetry.
  - Proptosis.
  - Gait (may indicate a possible cerebrovascular accident).
- Check visual acuity in each eye for distance and near vision.
- Undertake an assessment of the visual fields:
  - Look for homonymous hemianopia, bitemporal hemianopia or any other obvious visual field defect.
- Check the pupils:
  - Assess direct and consensual reflex.
  - Test for a relative afferent pupillary defect. Note that the pupils should be checked only after visual acuity and visual field assessment has been undertaken, as the lights used to examine the pupils may dazzle the patient and interfere with accurate visual field and acuity assessment.
- Dilate both pupils using tropicamide 1% eye drops.
- Examine each eye using the direct ophthalmoscope:
  - Assess the ocular surface.
  - Look at the red reflex (opacity may indicate either a cataract or vitreous opacities such as debris or haemorrhage).
  - Focus on the optic disc: look at colour, shape and cupping, as well as swelling.
  - Examine the blood vessel arcades in each quadrant.
  - Examine the macula.
  - Ask patient to look up, down, right and left so that you can examine the peripheral retina.
- Examine extraocular movements if the patient presents with diplopia or if it is clinically indicated.

Iain Hathorn

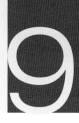

The ear, nose and throat

EAR

Anatomy and physiology

The ear is the specialised sensory organ of hearing and balance. It is divided anatomically into the external, middle and inner ear.

External ear

The external ear consists of the cartilaginous pinna, the external auditory canal (cartilage in the lateral one-third, bone in the medial two-thirds) and the lateral surface of the tympanic membrane (Fig. 9.1). Sound is collected and channelled by the pinna and transmitted via the external auditory canal to the tympanic membrane. The external auditory canal has an elongated S-shaped curve; hence it is important to retract the pinna when examining the ear to see the tympanic membrane

clearly. The outer portion of the canal has hair, and glands that produce ear wax, which forms a protective barrier.

Middle ear

The middle ear is an air-filled space that contains the three bony, articulated ossicles: the malleus, incus and stapes. The Eustachian tube opens into the middle ear inferiorly and allows equalisation of pressure and ventilation. Vibrations of the tympanic membrane are transmitted and amplified through the ossicular chain and focused on to the smaller oval window on which the stapes sits (Fig. 9.1B). The malleus is attached to the tympanic membrane and can be seen clearly on otoscopy (Fig. 9.2). The long process of the incus can also be visible occasionally. The tympanic membrane has a flaccid upper part (pars flaccida) and it is important to look carefully in this area, as this is where a

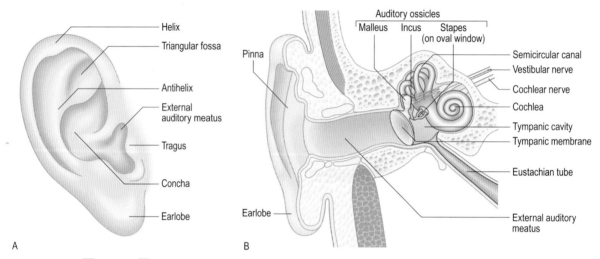

Fig. 9.1 The ear. A The pinna. B Cross-section of the outer, middle and inner ear.

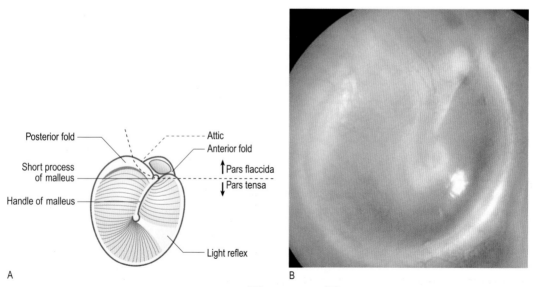

Fig. 9.2 Structures seen on otoscopic examination of the right ear. A Main structures. B Normal tympanic membrane.

cholesteatoma (an invasive collection of keratinising squamous epithelium) can form. The chorda tympani nerve runs through the middle ear carrying taste fibres from the anterior two-thirds of the tongue; these 'hitch a ride' with the facial nerve, which runs through the mastoid bone in the wall of the middle ear.

Inner ear

The inner ear contains the organs of hearing (cochlea) and balance (vestibular system). The vibration of the stapes footplate stimulates fluid within the cochlea. This results in the movement of hair cells in the cochlea, which are converted to electrical impulses along the vestibulocochlear nerve (VIII).

The vestibular system helps maintain balance, along with visual input and proprioception. The vestibular part of the inner ear contains:

- The lateral, superior and posterior semicircular canals: these lie at right angles to detect rotational motion of their fluid (endolymph) in three planes.
- The utricle and the saccule: their hair cells are embedded in a gel layer containing small crystals (otoliths), which are subject to gravity and enable detection of head tilt and linear acceleration.

The history

Common presenting symptoms

Pain and itching

Ask about:

- quality of the pain
- preceding trauma, upper respiratory tract infection (URTI)
- associated symptoms: dysphagia/voice change (suggesting possible referred pain from a throat lesion).

Otalgia (ear pain) associated with pruritus (itching) is often due to otitis externa. Acute otitis media is common in children and otalgia often follows an URTI. Other causes of otalgia are described in Box 9.1.

Ear discharge

Ask about:

- purulent, mucoid or blood-stained discharge (otorrhoea)
- associated pain.

A purulent discharge can be caused by otitis externa or acute otitis media with a perforation. A chronic offensive discharge may be a sign of cholesteatoma.

Blood-stained discharge may suggest the presence of granulation tissue from infection or can be a result of trauma, with or without an associated cerebrospinal fluid (CSF) leak.

Hearing loss

Ask about:

- sudden or gradual onset
- precipitating factors: trauma, URTI, noise exposure, antibiotics
- impact of the hearing loss on the patient's function.

Hearing loss can be due to disruption in the conduction mechanism or may have sensorineural causes, such as failure

9.1 Causes and features of earache (otalgia)

Cause	Clinical features
Otological	
Acute otitis externa	Pain worse on touching outer ear, tragus
	Swelling of ear canal
	Purulent discharge and itching
Acute otitis media	Severe pain, red, bulging tympanic membrane, purulent discharge if tympanic membrane perforation present
Perichondritis	Erythematous, swollen pinna
Trauma	Pinna haematoma, pinna laceration, haemotympanum (blood behind tympanic membrane); cerebrospinal fluid leak or facial nerve palsy may be present
Herpes zoster (Ramsay Hunt syndrome)	Vesicles in ear canal, facial nerve palsy may be present; vertigo is common
Malignancy	Mass in ear canal or on pinna
Non-otological	
Tonsillitis	Sore throat, tonsil inflammation
Peritonsillar abscess	Trismus, soft-palate swelling in peritonsillar abscess
Temporomandibular joint dysfunction	Tenderness, clicking of joint on jaw opening
Dental disease	Toothache, e.g. due to dental abscess
Cervical spine disease	Neck pain/tenderness
Cancer of the pharynx or larynx	Associated sore throat, hoarseness, dysphagia, weight loss, neck lump

9.2 Causes of hearing loss

Conductive[a]

- Wax
- Otitis externa
- Middle ear effusion
- Trauma to the tympanic membrane/ossicles
- Otosclerosis
- Chronic middle ear infection
- Tumours of the middle ear

Sensorineural[b]

- Genetic, e.g. Alport's syndrome
- Prenatal infection, e.g. rubella
- Birth injury
- Infection:
  - Meningitis
  - Measles
  - Mumps
- Trauma
- Ménière's disease
- Degenerative (presbyacusis)
- Occupation- or other noise-induced
- Acoustic neuroma
- Idiopathic

[a]Disruption to the mechanical transfer of sound in the outer ear, eardrum or ossicles. [b]Cochlear or central damage.

of the VIII nerve or cochlea (Box 9.2). Profound loss before speech acquisition affects speech development and quality.

Tinnitus

Tinnitus is an awareness of a noise in the absence of an external stimulus.

Ask about:

- quality of tinnitus: high-pitched, ringing, pulsatile
- intermittent or constant nature
- whether it is unilateral or bilateral
- associated hearing loss or other ear symptoms.

Tinnitus is usually associated with hearing loss. An acoustic neuroma (a tumour of the vestibulocochlear nerve, cranial nerve VIII) needs to be considered in unilateral tinnitus or tinnitus with an asymmetrical sensorineural hearing loss.

Vertigo

Vertigo is a sensation of movement relative to one's surroundings. Rotational movements are most common and patients often have associated nausea, vomiting and postural or gait instability. Vertigo can originate peripherally or, less often, centrally (brainstem, cerebellum). Patients will often say they are 'dizzy' when describing the illusion of movement: that is, vertigo. It is very important to clarify exactly what they mean by this. Lightheadedness is not a vestibular symptom, but unsteadiness may be.

Ask about:

- duration and frequency of episodes
- aggravating or provoking factors (position, head movement)
- associated 'fullness in the ear' during the episode (Ménière's disease)
- associated focal neurology (cerebrovascular event)
- fluctuating hearing loss or tinnitus

- associated headaches, nausea or aura (migraine)
- previous significant head injury; previous URTI.

The most common causes of vertigo include benign paroxysmal positional vertigo (attributed to debris within the posterior semicircular canal), vestibular neuritis (also known as vestibular neuronitis, a viral or postviral inflammatory disorder) and Ménière's disease (caused by excess endolymphatic fluid pressure). Other causes include migraine, cerebral ischaemia, drugs and head trauma. Discriminating features are described in Box 9.3.

Nystagmus

Nystagmus is an involuntary rhythmic oscillation of the eyes, which can be horizontal, vertical, rotatory or multidirectional. It may be continuous or paroxysmal, or evoked by manœuvres such as gaze or head position. The most common form, 'jerk nystagmus', consists of alternating phases of a slow drift in one direction with a corrective saccadic 'jerk' in the opposite direction. The direction of the fast jerk is used to define the direction of nystagmus (Box 9.4). Pendular nystagmus, in which there is a sinusoidal oscillation without a fast phase, is less common. Nystagmus may be caused by disorders of the vestibular, visual or cerebellar pathway.

9.3 Diagnosing vertigo

	Benign paroxysmal positional vertigo	Vestibular neuritis	Ménière's disease	Central vertigo (migraine, MS, brainstem ischaemia, drugs)
Duration	Seconds	Days	Hours	Hours – migraine Days and weeks – MS Long-term – cerebrovascular accident
Hearing loss	–	–	++	–
Tinnitus	–	–	++	–
Aural fullness	–	–	++	–
Episodic	Yes	Rarely	Recurrent vertigo; persistent tinnitus and progressive sensorineural deafness	Migraine – recurs Central nervous system damage – usually some recovery but often persistent
Triggers	Lying on affected ear	Possible presence of upper respiratory symptoms	None	Drugs (e.g. aminoglycosides) Cardiovascular disease

MS, *multiple sclerosis*.

9.4 Characteristics of nystagmus

Nystagmus type	Clinical pathology	Characteristics	
		Fast phase	Maximal on looking
Jerk: Peripheral	Semicircular canal, vestibular nerve	Unidirectional Not suppressed by optic fixation Patient too dizzy to walk Dix–Hallpike fatigues on repetition	Away from affected side
Central	Brainstem, cerebellum	Bidirectional (changes with direction of gaze) Suppressed by optic fixation Patient can walk (even with nystagmus) Dix–Hallpike persists	To either side
Dysconjugate (ataxic)	Interconnections of III, IV and VI nerves (medial longitudinal bundle)	Typically affects the abducting eye	To either side
Pendular	Eyes, e.g. congenital blindness	No fast phase	Straight ahead

Past medical history

Ask about:

- previous ear surgery, trauma
- recurrent ear infections
- systemic conditions associated with hearing loss (such as granulomatosis with polyangiitis)
- any significant previous illnesses such as meningitis, which can result in significant sensorineural hearing loss.

Drug history

The aminoglycoside antibiotics (such as gentamicin), aspirin, furosemide and some chemotherapy agents (cisplatin) are ototoxic.

Family history

Some causes of sensorineural hearing loss and otosclerosis are congenital. Otosclerosis causes a conductive hearing loss due to fixation of the stapes footplate.

Social history

The patient's occupation should be noted, as well as any significant previous exposure to loud noise.

The physical examination

Examination sequence

Inspection

- Pinna skin, shape, size, position, scars from previous surgery/trauma, deformity.

Palpation

- Gently pull on the pinna and push on the tragus to check for pain.
- Gently palpate over the mastoid bone behind the ear to assess for pain or swelling.

Otoscopy

- Use the largest otoscope speculum that will comfortably fit the meatus.
- Explain to the patient what you are going to do.
- Hold the otoscope in your right hand for examining the right ear (left hand to examine left ear). Rest the ulnar border of your hand against the patient's cheek to enable better control and to avoid trauma if the patient moves (Fig. 9.3).
- Gently pull the pinna upwards and backwards to straighten the cartilaginous external auditory canal. Use the left hand to retract the right pinna (Fig. 9.3).
- Inspect the external auditory canal through the speculum, noting wax, foreign bodies or discharge. You should identify the tympanic membrane and the light reflex anteroinferiorly (see Fig. 9.2).

Congenital deformities of the pinna, like microtia (Fig. 9.4A) or low-set ears, can be associated with other conditions such as hearing loss and Down's syndrome. Children can also have protruding ears that occasionally require corrective surgery (pinnaplasty). Trauma can result in a pinna haematoma (Fig. 9.4B) and subsequent 'cauliflower ear' due to cartilage necrosis if untreated. Trauma may also cause mastoid bruising ('Battle's sign'), suggesting a possible skull-base fracture. Lesions on the pinna are relatively common and can be related to sun exposure; they include actinic keratosis, and basal cell and squamous cell cancers (Fig. 9.4C).

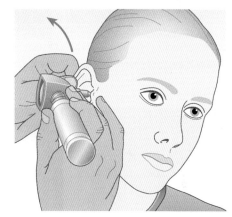

Fig. 9.3 **Examination of the ear using an otoscope.**

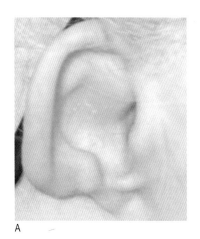
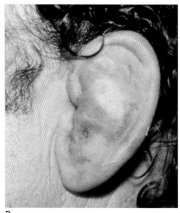
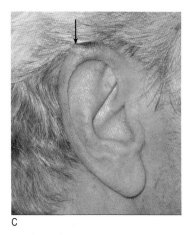

A   B   C

Fig. 9.4 **The pinna.** [A] Microtia. [B] Haematoma. [C] Squamous cancer *(arrow).*

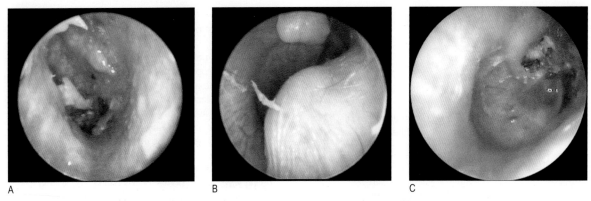

Fig. 9.5 Auditory canal abnormalities. [A] Otitis externa. [B] Exostosis of the external auditory meatus. [C] Cholesteatoma.

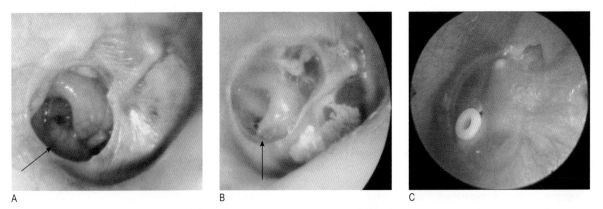

Fig. 9.6 Tympanic membrane abnormalities. [A] Tympanic membrane perforation *(arrow)*. [B] Retraction pocket of the pars tensa *(arrow)*. [C] Grommet in situ.

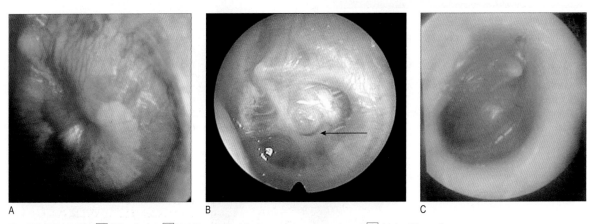

Fig. 9.7 Otitis media. [A] With effusion. [B] Fluid level behind the tympanic membrane *(arrow)*. [C] Acute otitis media.

If discharge is noted on otoscopy and the tympanic membrane is intact, otitis externa is the likely cause (Fig. 9.5A). The canal can reveal exostoses, abnormal bone growth due to cold water exposure, often seen in surfers (Fig. 9.5B).

Scarring on the tympanic membrane (tympanosclerosis) can be caused by previous grommet insertion or infections. Tympanic membrane perforations can be central or marginal, and the position and size of the perforation should be noted as a percentage (Fig. 9.6A). A severe retraction pocket of the pars tensa can mimic a perforation (Fig. 9.6B). A retraction of the pars flaccida can contain a cholesteatoma, which may cause

an offensive discharge and erode the bony ossicles, resulting in a conductive hearing loss (Fig. 9.5C). Fluid behind the tympanic membrane is called otitis media with effusion (OME or 'glue ear', Fig. 9.7A), and a fluid level may be seen (Fig. 9.7B). This commonly affects children and can be treated surgically with insertion of a ventilation tube or grommet (see Fig. 9.6C). If persistent OME is seen in adults, the postnasal space needs to be examined by a specialist to exclude a lesion in that site. Acute otitis media presents with pain; the tympanic membrane can become inflamed (Fig. 9.7C), and may bulge and eventually perforate.

Testing hearing

Whispered voice test

Examination sequence

- Stand behind the patient.
- Start testing with your mouth about 15 cm from the ear you are assessing.
- Mask hearing in the patient's other ear by rubbing the tragus ('masking').
- Ask the patient to repeat a combination of multisyllable numbers and words. Start with a normal speaking voice to confirm that the patient understands the test. Lower your voice to a clear whisper.
- Repeat the test but this time at arm's length from the patient's ear. People with normal hearing can repeat words whispered at 60 cm.

Tuning fork tests

A 512-Hz tuning fork can be used to help differentiate between conductive and sensorineural hearing loss.

Weber's test

Examination sequence

- Strike the prongs of the tuning fork against a hard surface to make it vibrate.
- Place the base of the vibrating tuning fork in the middle of the patient's forehead (Fig. 9.8).
- Ask the patient, 'Where do you hear the sound?'
- Record which side Weber's test lateralises to if not central.

In a patient with normal hearing, the noise is heard in the middle, or equally in both ears.

In conductive hearing loss the sound is heard louder in the affected ear. In unilateral sensorineural hearing loss it is heard louder in the unaffected ear. If there is symmetrical hearing loss it will be heard in the middle.

Rinne's test

Examination sequence

- Strike the prongs of the tuning fork against a hard surface to make it vibrate.
- Place the vibrating tuning fork on the mastoid process (Fig. 9.9A).
- Now place the still-vibrating base at the external auditory meatus and ask, 'Is it louder in front of your ear or behind?' (Fig. 9.9B).

With normal hearing, the sound is heard louder when the tuning fork is at the external auditory meatus. That is, air conduction (AC) is better than bone conduction (BC), recorded as AC>BC. This normal result is recorded as 'Rinne-positive'.

In conductive hearing loss, bone conduction is better than air conduction (BC>AC); thus the sound is heard louder when the tuning fork is on the mastoid process ('Rinne-negative'). A false-negative Rinne's test may occur if there is profound hearing loss on one side. This is due to sound being conducted through the bone of the skull to the other 'good' ear. Weber's

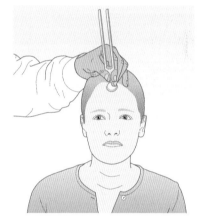

Fig. 9.8 Weber's test.

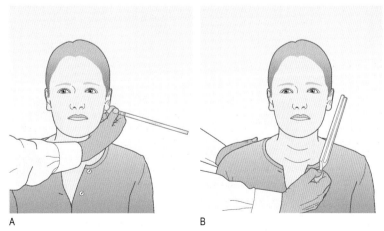

A   B

Fig. 9.9 Rinne's test. A Testing bone conduction. B Testing air conduction.

9

test is more sensitive and therefore the tuning fork will lateralise to the affected ear in conductive hearing loss before Rinne's test becomes abnormal (negative). In sensorineural hearing loss, Rinne's test will be positive, as air conduction is better than bone conduction.

Tuning fork test findings are summarised in Box 9.5.

Testing vestibular function

Testing for nystagmus

Examination sequence

- Patients should be tested with spectacles or contact lenses for best corrected vision.
- With the patient seated, ask them to fixate on a stationary target in a neutral gaze position and observe for spontaneous nystagmus.
- Hold your finger an arm's length away, level with the patient's eye, and ask the patient to focus on and follow the tip of your finger. Slowly move your finger from side to side and up and down and observe the eyes for any oscillations, avoiding extremes of gaze where physiological

9.5 Tuning fork tests		
	Weber test	Rinne test
Bilateral normal hearing	Central	AC>BC, bilateral
Bilateral symmetrical sensorineural loss	Central	AC>BC, bilateral
Unilateral or asymmetrical sensorineural loss LEFT	Louder right	AC>BC, bilateral[a]
Unilateral conductive loss LEFT	Louder left	BC>AC, left AC>BC, right
Bilateral conductive loss (worse on LEFT)	Louder left	BC>AC, bilateral

[a]Patients with a severe sensorineural loss may have BC>AC due to BC crossing to the other better-hearing cochlea that is not being tested (false-negative Rinne test).
AC, air conduction; BC, bone conduction.

nystagmus may occur. This assesses for gaze nystagmus and smooth pursuit.
- If any oscillations are present, note:
  - whether they are horizontal, vertical or rotatory
  - which direction of gaze causes the most marked nystagmus
  - in which direction the fast phase of jerk nystagmus occurs.

Discriminating characteristics of nystagmus are detailed in Box 9.4.

Dix–Hallpike positional test

Examination sequence

- Ask the patient to sit upright, close to the end of the couch.
- Turn the patient's head 45 degrees to one side (Fig. 9.10A).
- Rapidly lower the patient backwards so that their head is now 30 degrees below the horizontal. Keep supporting the head and ask the patient to keep their eyes open, even if they feel dizzy (Fig. 9.10B).
- Observe the eyes for nystagmus. If it is present, note latency (time to onset), direction, duration and fatigue (decrease on repeated manœuvres).
- Repeat the test, turning the patient's head to the other side (Fig. 9.10C).

Normal patients have no nystagmus or symptoms of vertigo. A positive Dix–Hallpike manœuvre is diagnostic for benign paroxysmal positional vertigo. There is a delay of 5–20 seconds before the patient experiences vertigo and before rotatory jerk nystagmus towards the lower ear (geotropic) occurs; this lasts for less than 30 seconds. The response fatigues on repeated testing due to adaptation. Immediate nystagmus without adaptation, and not necessarily with associated vertigo, can be caused by central pathology.

Head impulse test (or head thrust test)

Examination sequence

- Sit opposite the patient and ask them to focus on a target (usually your nose).

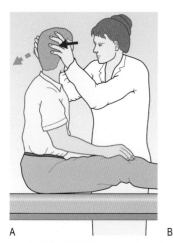
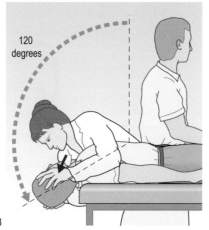
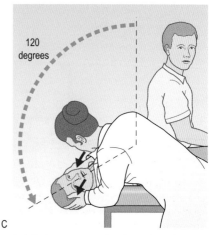

A   B   C

Fig. 9.10 Dix–Hallpike position test. The examiner looks for nystagmus (usually accompanied by vertigo). Both nystagmus and vertigo typically decrease (fatigue) on repeat testing. See text for details.

9.6 Investigations in ear disease

Investigation	Indication/comment
Swab from external auditory meatus	Otorrhoea, such as in otitis externa or otitis media with a tympanic membrane perforation; microscopy and culture can help guide treatment
Magnetic resonance imaging	Acoustic neuroma (Fig. 9.11) Asymmetrical sensorineural hearing loss or unilateral tinnitus
Audiometry	Hearing loss A single-frequency tone at different noise levels is presented to each ear in turn through headphones in a soundproof booth. The intensity of sound is reduced in 10-decibel steps until patients can no longer hear it. The hearing threshold is the quietest sound they can hear. Audiograms display air and bone conduction thresholds, and conductive and sensorineural hearing loss can therefore be differentiated (Fig. 9.12)
Impedance audiometry (tympanometry)	Conductive hearing loss (e.g. otitis media with effusion, ossicular discontinuity, otosclerosis) Eustachian tube dysfunction The compliance of the tympanic membrane is measured during changes in pressure in the ear canal; compliance should be maximal at atmospheric pressure

Vestibular testing:
  Caloric tests
 	
  Posturography
	Unilateral vestibular hypofunction
	Water at 30°C and then 44°C is irrigated into the external ear canal. Electronystagmography records nystagmus. The response is reduced in vestibular hypofunction
	Reveals whether patients rely on vision or proprioception more than usual
	Usually reserved for specialist balance clinics

9

- Hold the patient's head, placing a hand on each side of it.
- Rapidly turn the patient's head to one side in the horizontal plane (roughly 15 degrees) and watch for any corrective movement of the eyes. Repeat, turning the head towards the other side. The eyes remain fixed on the examiner's nose in a normal test. When the head is turned towards the affected side the eyes move with the head and there is then a corrective saccade.

This is a test of the vestibulo-ocular reflex. The presence of a corrective saccade is a positive test and indicates a deficiency in the vestibulo-ocular reflex. It is useful to identify unilateral peripheral vestibular hypofunction. You must be careful when performing this test in patients with neck problems because of the rapid movements of the head.

Unterberger's test

Examination sequence

- Ask the patient to march on the spot with their eyes closed. The patient will rotate to the side of the damaged labyrinth.

Fistula test

Examination sequence

- Compress the tragus repeatedly against the external auditory meatus to occlude it.

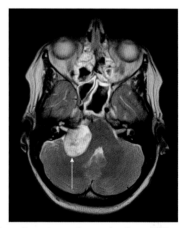

Fig. 9.11 Magnetic resonance image showing a right acoustic neuroma *(arrow)*.

If imbalance or vertigo with nystagmus is induced, it suggests an abnormal communication between the middle ear and vestibular system (such as erosion due to cholesteatoma).

Investigations

Initial investigations in ear disease are summarised in Box 9.6 and Figs 9.11–9.12.

NOSE AND SINUSES

Anatomy and physiology

The external nose consists of two nasal bones that provide support and stability to the nose. The nasal bones articulate with each other and with bones of the face: the frontal bone, the ethmoid bone and the maxilla. The nasal bones also attach to the nasal septum and the paired upper lateral cartilages of the nose. There are two further paired cartilages, the lower lateral cartilages, which form the nasal tip. Internally the nasal septum, which is bone posteriorly and cartilage anteriorly, separates the nose into two nasal cavities that join posteriorly in the postnasal space. There are three turbinates on each side of the nose, superior, middle and inferior, which warm and moisten nasal airflow (Figs 9.13 and 9.14A).

One important function of the nose is olfaction. The olfactory receptors are situated high in the nose in the olfactory cleft. Olfactory fibres from the nasal mucosa pass through the cribriform plate to the olfactory bulb in the anterior cranial fossa.

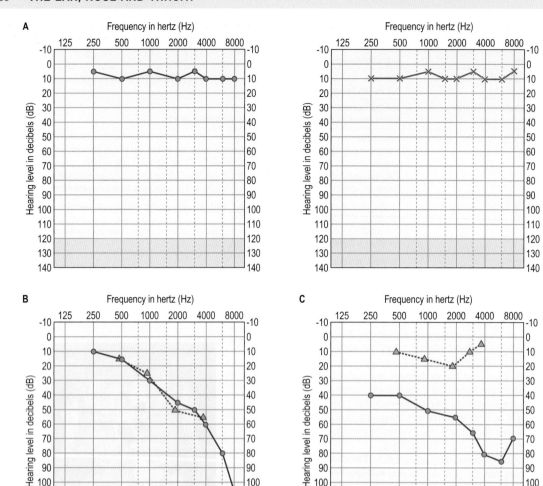

Fig. 9.12 Hearing test (audiogram). A Normal-hearing right and left ears. B Right sensorineural loss. C Right conductive hearing loss. (● Right air conduction, ✕ Left air conduction, △ Bone conduction)

The paranasal sinuses are air-filled spaces in the skull. There are paired frontal, sphenoid, maxillary and anterior and posterior ethmoid sinuses. The anterior nasal sinuses (frontal, maxillary and anterior ethmoid) drain into the middle meatus (between the middle turbinate and lateral wall of the nose). The posterior ethmoid and sphenoid sinuses drain into the sphenoethmoidal recess (between the superior turbinate and nasal septum).

The history

Common presenting symptoms

Nasal obstruction

Ask about:

- unilateral or bilateral obstruction
- associated symptoms (bleeding, swelling, pain).

Unilateral nasal obstruction may be caused by anatomical blockage, such as a deviated septum possibly secondary to trauma. Bilateral obstruction can be due to rhinitis (allergic or non-allergic), or chronic rhinosinusitis with or without polyps.

Nasal discharge

Ask about:

- unilateral or bilateral discharge (rhinorrhoea)
- purulent or clear nature
- anterior discharge or postnasal drip.

Clear, bilateral watery discharge suggests allergic or non-allergic rhinitis. Purulent discharge can point to acute bacterial rhinosinusitis or chronic rhinosinusitis. A unilateral, purulent discharge in a child raises the possibility of a foreign body in the nose. Following a head injury, unilateral clear rhinorrhoea suggests a possible CSF leak secondary to an anterior skull-base fracture.

Epistaxis (bleeding from inside the nose)

Ask about:

- unilateral or bilateral bleeding
- frequency and duration of episodes

- provoking factors such as trauma, sneezing, or blowing or picking nose
- bleeding from the front or back of the nose.

The nasal septum has a very rich blood supply, particularly in Little's area (anterior septum), which is a common site for bleeding.

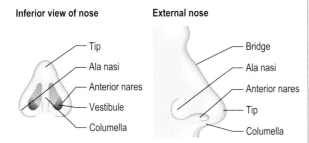

Inferior view of nose — Tip, Ala nasi, Anterior nares, Vestibule, Columella

External nose — Bridge, Ala nasi, Anterior nares, Tip, Columella

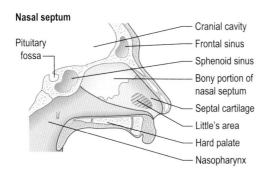

Nasal septum

Pituitary fossa — Cranial cavity, Frontal sinus, Sphenoid sinus, Bony portion of nasal septum, Septal cartilage, Little's area, Hard palate, Nasopharynx

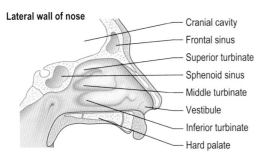

Lateral wall of nose — Cranial cavity, Frontal sinus, Superior turbinate, Sphenoid sinus, Middle turbinate, Vestibule, Inferior turbinate, Hard palate

Fig. 9.13 The nose and paranasal sinuses.

If bleeding is unilateral and associated with nasal obstruction and pain, the possibility of sinonasal malignancy should be considered. In adolescent males with unilateral nasal obstruction and epistaxis, the rare diagnosis of juvenile angiofibroma should be excluded on nasendoscopy by an ear, nose and throat specialist.

Sneezing

Ask about:

- associated itchy, red eyes
- whether symptoms occur all year round, only during certain seasons, or during contact with allergens.

Sneezing is a protective sudden expulsive effort triggered by local irritants in the nose and is most commonly due to allergy or viral URTIs.

Disturbance of smell

Ask about:

- complete loss of smell (anosmia)
- reduced sense of smell (hyposmia)
- unpleasant smells (cacosmia)
- associated nasal symptoms such as obstruction and rhinorrhoea, which may suggest rhinitis or nasal polyps
- recent head injury
- recent URTI.

A sudden onset of anosmia can occur following a significant head injury or viral URTI due to damage to the olfactory epithelium. Inflammation and swelling in the nasal mucosa as a result of rhinitis, chronic rhinosinusitis or nasal polyps usually cause hyposmia. Cacosmia is usually caused by infection in the nose or sinuses, or occasionally by a foreign body in the nose. Phantosmia describes olfactory hallucinations, which may occur in temporal lobe epilepsy.

Nasal and facial pain

Nasal pain is rare, except following trauma. Facial pain can be caused by a number of problems but is often incorrectly attributed to sinusitis. The key to identifying the cause of facial pain is an accurate history.

9

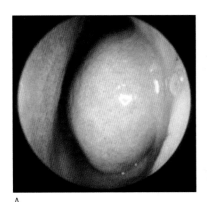

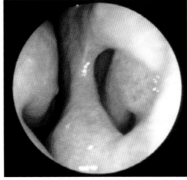

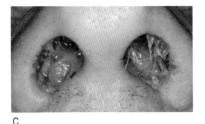

A   B   C

Fig. 9.14 Nasal abnormalities. A Turbinate hypertrophy. B Nasal septum perforation post-surgery. C Nasal polyps.

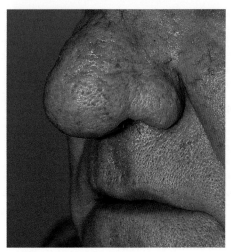

Fig. 9.15 Rhinophyma as a complication of rosacea.

Ask about:
- quality of pain: for example, throbbing, aching, sharp, stabbing, tight-band
- location of pain: unilateral or bilateral
- duration and frequency of pain
- associated nasal symptoms
- associated nausea, photophobia or aura (migraine)
- relieving and exacerbating factors.

The differential diagnosis of facial pain includes temporo-mandibular joint dysfunction, migraine, dental disease, chronic rhinosinusitis, trigeminal neuralgia (severe, sharp pain in a trigeminal distribution), tension headache (band-like, tight pain) and cluster headaches (unilateral nasal discharge, eye watering).

Nasal deformity

The most common cause of nasal deformity is trauma, resulting in swelling, bruising and deviation of the nose. The swelling following trauma will settle over a couple of weeks but residual deviation may remain if the nasal bones were fractured and displaced. It is important to establish the impact of the nasal injury on function (nasal breathing, sense of smell) and cosmetic appearance.

Nasal septal destruction or perforation can result in 'saddle deformity' of the nasal bridge. Causes include granulomatosis with polyangiitis, trauma, cocaine abuse, congenital syphilis and iatrogenic factors (septal surgery, Fig. 9.14B).

The nose can appear widened in acromegaly or with advanced nasal polyposis (Fig. 9.14C). Rhinophyma can also result from chronic acne rosacea of the nasal skin (Fig. 9.15).

Past medical history

Ask about:
- history of atopy
- asthma (around one-third of patients with allergic rhinitis have asthma)
- prior nasal trauma or surgery
- history of bronchial infection (cystic fibrosis or ciliary disorders may affect the nose and lower airways).

For patients with epistaxis it is important to identify any history of bleeding diathesis or hypertension.

Drug history

Ask about:
- use of anticoagulants, including warfarin, apixaban or rivaroxaban
- use of antiplatelet drugs (aspirin, clopidogrel).

Intranasal cocaine use can cause septal perforation, epistaxis, crusting and whistling.

Family history

A family history of atopy is relevant in rhinitis. In patients with epistaxis it is important to establish a family history of hereditary haemorrhagic telangiectasia or inherited bleeding disorders.

Social history

Occupation is relevant because exposure to inhaled allergens, occupational dusts and chemicals may exacerbate rhinitis. Exposure to hardwood dust is associated with an increased risk of sinonasal cancers. Atopic patients should be asked about pets.

Heavy alcohol intake, leading to liver disease, can affect coagulation and is relevant for epistaxis. Smoking impedes mucociliary clearance and can contribute to nasal problems.

The physical examination

Examination sequence

- Assess the external appearance of the nose, noting swelling, bruising, skin changes and deformity.
- Stand above the seated patient to assess any external deviation.
- Ask the patient to look straight ahead. Elevate the tip of their nose using your non-dominant thumb to align the nostrils with the rest of the nasal cavity.
- Look into each nostril and assess the anterior nasal septum (Fig. 9.16); note the mucosal covering, visible vessels in Little's area, crusting, ulceration and septal perforation. In trauma, a septal haematoma should be excluded.
- Using an otoscope with a large speculum in an adult, assess the inferior turbinates. Note any hypertrophy and swelling of the turbinate mucosa.
- You may see large polyps on anterior rhinoscopy. To distinguish between hypertrophied inferior turbinates and nasal polyps, you can lightly touch the swelling with a cotton bud (polyps lack sensation).
- Palpate the nasal bones to assess for bony or cartilaginous deformity.
- In trauma, palpate the infraorbital ridges to exclude a step deformity and also to check infraorbital sensation. Eye movements should be assessed to rule out restriction of movement related to 'orbital blowout'.
- Place a metal spatula under the nostrils and look for condensation marks to assess airway patency.
- Palpate for cervical lymphadenopathy (p. 32).
- Note that rigid nasendoscopy and tests of olfaction are confined to specialist clinics.

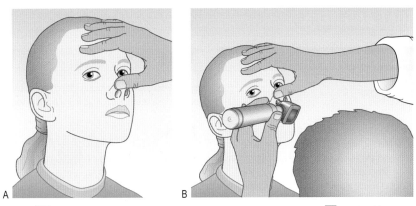

Fig. 9.16 Nasal examination. [A] Elevation of the tip of the nose to give a clear view of the anterior nares. [B] Anterior rhinoscopy using an otoscope with a large speculum.

9

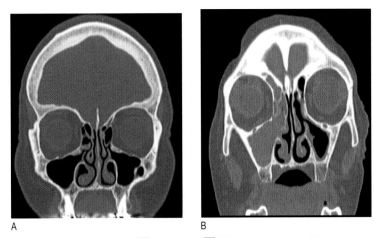

Fig. 9.17 Computed tomograms of the paranasal sinuses. [A] Normal scan. [B] Right-sided chronic sinusitis.

9.7 Investigations in nasal disease	
Investigation	**Indication/comment**
Plain X-ray	Not indicated for nasal bone fracture Only required if associated facial fracture is suspected
Nasal endoscopy	Inflammatory sinus disease, malignancy
Allergy tests	Skin-prick tests for common inhaled allergens, specific immunoglobulin E blood test (RAST)
Computed tomography	Inflammatory sinus disease, trauma and malignancy Demonstrates extent of sinus disease, provides evidence of invasion into local structures and shows detailed bony anatomy, enabling planning of endoscopic surgical procedures (see Fig. 9.17)
Tests of olfaction	Used in specialist clinics only Include the UPSIT smell test and Sniffin' Sticks
RAST, *radioallergosorbent test;* UPSIT, *University of Pennsylvania smell identification test.*	

The mucosa of the inferior turbinate on anterior rhinoscopy is pale, moist and hypertrophied in allergic rhinitis (see Fig. 9.14A). In chronic rhinitis the mucosa is swollen and red. Large polyps may be seen on anterior rhinoscopy as pale yellow/grey swellings (see Fig. 9.14C).

A septal haematoma will appear as a soft, red, fluctuant swelling of the anterior septum. The septal cartilage receives its blood supply from the overlying perichondrium; a septal haematoma interrupts this supply and can result in cartilage necrosis, septal perforation and 'saddle deformity'. It must therefore be identified and referred for early drainage.

Facial swelling is not usually seen in chronic sinusitis but can occur with dental abscesses and cancer of the maxillary antrum.

Investigations

Initial investigations are summarised in Box 9.7 and Fig. 9.17.

MOUTH, THROAT AND NECK

Anatomy and physiology

Mouth

The mouth extends from the lips anteriorly to the anterior tonsillar pillar posteriorly and is divided into the vestibule, between the buccal (cheek) mucosa and the teeth, and the oral cavity internal to the teeth. The oral cavity contains the anterior two-thirds of the tongue, the floor of the mouth, the hard palate and the inner surfaces of the gums and teeth (Fig. 9.18). The tongue anteriorly has filiform papillae containing taste buds, giving the tongue its velvet texture. The circumvallate papillae are groups of taste buds marking the boundary between the anterior two-thirds and posterior third of the tongue.

Saliva is secreted into the mouth from the parotid, submandibular and sublingual salivary glands (Fig. 9.19). The parotid gland is situated anterior to the ear and has a superficial and deep lobe relative to the facial nerve that runs through it. The parotid duct opens into the buccal mucosa opposite the second upper molar. The submandibular gland lies anterior and medial to the angle of the mandible and its duct opens into the floor of the mouth next to the frenulum of the tongue (see Fig. 9.18).

Throat

The pharynx is a shared upper aerodigestive channel that runs from the anterior tonsillar pillar to the laryngeal inlet. The larynx ('voice box') is responsible for phonation and also has a protective function to prevent aspiration. It consists of two external cartilages, the thyroid cartilage (Adam's apple) and the cricoid cartilage (prominence at the top of the trachea; see Fig. 10.1A). The membrane between the two is called the cricothyroid membrane; a cricothyroidotomy may be performed by an experienced clinician at this site as an emergency procedure to obtain an airway. The sensory supply to the larynx is via the superior and recurrent laryngeal branches of cranial nerve X (vagus). The motor supply is mainly from the recurrent laryngeal nerve, which loops round the aortic arch on the left side and the subclavian artery on the right.

Teeth

In children the 20 deciduous teeth erupt by 3 years. There are 32 secondary teeth, erupting from ages 6 to 16 or later (Fig. 9.20).

Neck

Anatomically the neck is divided into anterior and posterior triangles (Fig. 9.21). The anterior triangle is bounded by the midline, the anterior border of the sternocleidomastoid muscle and the body of the mandible. The posterior triangle of the neck is bounded by the posterior border of sternocleidomastoid, the trapezius muscle and the clavicle. The cervical lymph nodes drain the head and neck (see Fig. 3.26). Examination of these nodes is described on page 33 and shown in Fig. 3.27. Palpable lymphadenopathy is most commonly due to URTI but may be caused by atypical infection, inflammation, lymphoma or metastatic malignancy. The neck can also be subdivided further into different levels that are used to describe the location of enlarged lymph nodes in the neck (Fig. 9.22).

The history

Common presenting symptoms

Sore mouth

Ask about:
- how long pain has been present and any progression
- trauma to the mouth
- mouth ulcers
- problems with teeth or gums
- associated bleeding.

Aphthous ulcers are small, painful, superficial ulcers on the tongue, palate or buccal mucosa. They are common and usually heal spontaneously within a few days. Oral ulcers can be caused by trauma, vitamin or mineral deficiency, cancer, lichen planus or inflammatory bowel disease.

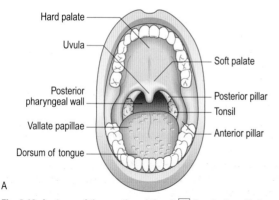

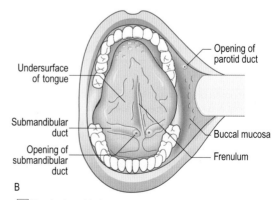

A   B

Fig. 9.18 Anatomy of the mouth and throat. A Examination with the mouth open. B Examination with the tongue touching the roof of the mouth.

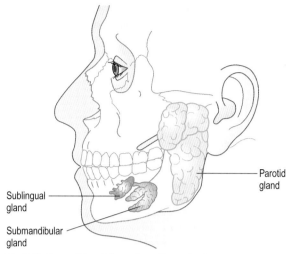

Fig. 9.19 The position of the major salivary glands.

Parotid gland

Sublingual gland

Submandibular gland

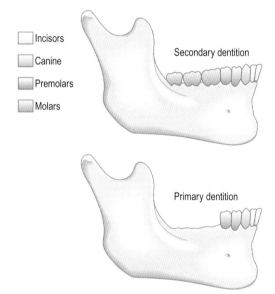

Incisors

Canine

Premolars

Molars

Secondary dentition

Primary dentition

Fig. 9.20 Primary and secondary dentition.

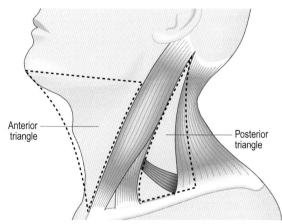

Anterior triangle

Posterior triangle

Fig. 9.21 Sites of swellings in the neck.

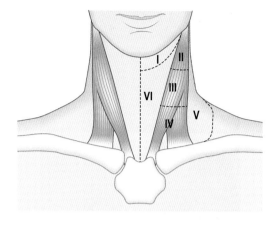

I   Submental and submandibular nodes
II   Upper third sternocleidomastoid (SCM) muscle
III Middle third SCM (between hyoid and cricoid)
IV   Lower third SCM (between cricoid and clavicle)
V   Posterior to SCM (posterior triangle)
VI   Midline from hyoid to manubrium

Fig. 9.22 Cervical lymph node levels.

9.8 The gums in systemic conditions	
Condition	**Description**
Phenytoin treatment	Firm and hypertrophied
Scurvy	Soft and haemorrhagic
Acute leukaemia	Hypertrophied and haemorrhagic
Cyanotic congenital heart disease	Spongy and haemorrhagic

A sore mouth can also be due to conditions of the gums, including inflammation (gingivitis) or systemic conditions (Box 9.8).

Infections, including candidiasis (caused by *Candida albicans*), herpes simplex and herpes zoster, as well as dental sepsis, can cause a painful mouth. Candidiasis may be secondary to poorly fitted dentures, the use of inhaled glucocorticoids or immunodeficiency. Herpes zoster of the maxillary division of the trigeminal nerve (see Fig. 7.9B) can cause unilateral painful vesicles on the palate.

Sore throat

Ask about:

- unilateral or bilateral pain
- otalgia (earache)
- difficulty opening the mouth (trismus, due to spasm of the jaw muscles)
- associated fever, malaise, anorexia, neck swelling
- associated red flag symptoms (dysphagia, odynophagia, hoarseness, weight loss).

Throat pain can radiate to the ear as a result of the dual innervation of the pharynx and external auditory meatus via the vagus nerve (referred pain). The most common cause of sore throat is pharyngitis (inflammation of the pharynx) and is usually viral. Acute tonsillitis may be viral or caused by streptococcal bacterial infection (Fig. 9.23A), and cannot be distinguished clinically.

9

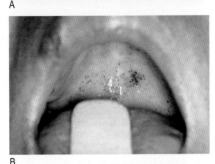

A

B

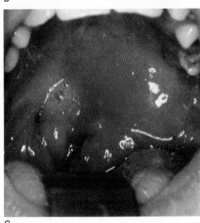

C

Fig. 9.23 Sore throat. [A] Acute tonsillitis. The presence of pus strongly suggests a bacterial (streptococcal) aetiology. [B] Glandular fever showing palatal petechiae. [C] A left peritonsillar abscess. *(A) From Bull TR. Color Atlas of ENT Diagnosis. 3rd edn. London: Mosby–Wolfe; 1995.*

Infectious mononucleosis caused by Epstein–Barr virus (glandular fever) results in tonsil erythema and swelling, a white pseudomembrane covering the tonsil, palatal petechiae (Fig. 9.23B), cervical lymphadenopathy and sometimes hepatosplenomegaly. A peritonsillar abscess (quinsy) can lead to unilateral throat pain, trismus, drooling of saliva, soft-palate swelling, deviation of the uvula to the opposite side (Fig. 9.23C) and 'hot-potato voice' (like you were trying to speak with a hot potato in your mouth).

It is important to establish whether there are any 'red flag' symptoms associated with sore throat. Progressive dysphagia or hoarseness associated with weight loss should raise suspicion of malignancy. A mass or ulcer on the tonsil associated with throat pain may be a tonsil squamous cancer. Human papillomavirus-related oropharyngeal cancer is the now most common primary head and neck malignancy in young, sexually active non-smokers.

Globus pharyngeus is a sensation of something in the throat in the context of a normal clinical examination. Patients classically describe the feeling of a lump in the throat, usually in the midline, which fluctuates from day to day and eases when swallowing. Anxiety, habitual throat clearing and acid reflux are thought to be contributory factors.

Stridor

Stridor is a high-pitched noise produced by turbulent airflow through a narrowed, partially obstructed upper airway and can indicate laryngeal or tracheobronchial (p. 79) obstruction. It most commonly occurs on inspiration but may also be expiratory or biphasic. The level of obstruction determines the type of stridor. Inspiratory stridor suggests narrowing at the level of the vocal cords, biphasic stridor suggests subglottic/tracheal obstruction, and stridor on expiration suggests tracheobronchial obstruction. Common causes of stridor include infection/inflammation, trauma, foreign bodies (particularly in children) and tumours. Stridor should always be urgently evaluated.

Ask about:

• sudden or gradual onset
• associated fever
• associated hoarseness.

Stertor differs from stridor. It is a low-pitched snoring or gasping sound audible during inspiration and is due to obstruction at the level of the nasopharynx or oropharynx. This can be as a result of enlarged inflamed tonsils, a peritonsillar abscess or tongue swelling (trauma, anaphylaxis).

Dysphonia

Ask about:

• how long dysphonia (hoarseness) has been present
• whether it is persistent or intermittent
• progression
• voice quality (croaky, breathy, weak)
• associated stridor, dysphagia, otalgia or weight loss.

If hoarseness has been present continuously for more than 3 weeks, urgent laryngoscopy is indicated to exclude laryngeal cancer. If voice quality is breathy and associated with a weak (bovine) cough (p. 78), a recurrent laryngeal nerve palsy due to lung or oesophageal cancer should be considered. Recurrent laryngeal nerve palsy may also be iatrogenic (thyroid surgery) or secondary to trauma or neurological conditions (Box 9.9).

Dysphagia

The approach to dysphagia is described on page 98.

Neck lump

Neck lumps are common; they may be reported by patients or found incidentally on physical examination. While many lumps are benign, there may be a more serious underlying diagnosis (Box 9.10).

Ask about:

• sudden or gradual onset
• progression
• associated pain
• associated hoarseness or dysphagia
• fever or other systemic symptoms (weight loss, night sweats).

9.9 Causes and features of dysphonia

Causes	Features
Neonate	
Congenital abnormality	Laryngomalacia most frequent cause More common in preterm neonates Associated stridor due to immature larynx folding in on inspiration
Neurological disorder	Examples include vocal cord palsy Unilateral causing weak, breathy cry Bilateral may cause stridor and airway obstruction
Child	
Infection:	
Croup (laryngotracheobronchitis)	Barking cough, stridor, hoarse voice
Laryngitis	Bacterial or viral
Voice abuse (screamer's nodules)	History of voice abuse
Adult	
Infection:	
Upper respiratory tract infection	Associated features of upper respiratory tract infection
Laryngitis	
Trauma	Mechanical or chemical injury Cigarette smoking Gastro-oesophageal reflux disease (reflux laryngitis)
Lung cancer	Vocal cord paralysis, breathy voice
Vocal cord nodules (singer's nodules)	Prolonged vocal strain Rough voice Reduced vocal range Vocal fatigue
Neurological disorder	Weak, wet or dysarthric voice
Cancer of the larynx	Rough voice, constant, progressive, often affects smokers Associated with dysphagia, odynophagia, otalgia
Functional cause	

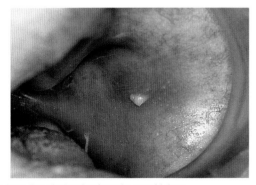

Fig. 9.24 Pus discharging from the parotid duct.

Sudden, painful, unilateral salivary gland swelling (sialadenopathy) is due to a stone obstructing the duct (sialolithiasis). Other causes of enlarged salivary glands are mumps (usually bilateral), sarcoidosis, human immunodeficiency virus-related cysts, bacterial infection (suppurative parotitis; Fig. 9.24) and cancer. The clinical features of important neck lumps are summarised in Box 9.10.

Past medical history

It is important to establish whether there are any previous dental problems or systemic disease, particularly those affecting the gastrointestinal tract, as the mouth is part of this. Neurological conditions may affect swallowing and cause drooling or dry mouth with secondary infection. Previous head and neck surgery and trauma should be noted.

Any prior intubations or admissions to intensive care should be recorded, as repeated or prolonged intubation can result in subglottic stenosis and stridor.

Drug history

Many drugs, including tricyclic antidepressants and anticholinergics, cause a dry mouth. Multiple, repeated courses of antibiotics increase the risk of oral candidiasis, as does any prolonged illness.

Social and family history

Risk factors for head and neck squamous cancer include alcohol and smoking. Oral cancer is more common in those who experience orogenital contact and in those who chew tobacco or betel nuts. Any history of head and neck cancer in the family should be established.

The physical examination

Mouth and throat

Examination sequence

- Listen to the patient's voice (rough, breathy, wet, muffled, nasal escape).
- Use a head light to leave both of your hands free to use instruments.

Inspection
- Ask the patient to remove any dentures.
- Look at their lips. Ask them to half-open their mouth and inspect the mucosa of the vestibule, buccal surfaces and buccogingival sulci for discoloration, inflammation or ulceration, then at bite closure. Inspect the parotid duct opening opposite the second upper molar for any pus or inflammation.
- Ask the patient to open their mouth fully and put the tip of their tongue behind their upper teeth. Check the mucosa of the floor of the mouth and the submandibular duct openings.
- Ask them to stick their tongue straight out, noting any deviation to either side (XII nerve dysfunction), mucosal change, ulceration, masses or fasciculation.
- Ask them to deviate their tongue to one side. Retract the opposite buccal mucosa with a tongue depressor to view the lateral border of the tongue. Repeat on the other side.
- Inspect the hard palate (Fig. 9.25) and note any cleft, abnormal arched palate or telangiectasia.
- Inspect the oropharynx. Ask the patient to say 'Aaah' and use a tongue depressor to improve visualisation.
- Assess the soft palate for any cleft, bifid uvula, swelling or lesions.

9

9.10 Causes and features of neck lumps

Location in neck	Diagnosis	Clinical features
Midline	Thyroglossal cyst	Smooth, round, cystic lump that moves when patient sticks out tongue
	Submental lymph nodes	Associated infection of lower lip, floor of mouth, tip of tongue or cheek skin
	Thyroid isthmus swelling	Lump moves on swallowing
	Dermoid cyst	Small, non-tender, mobile subcutaneous lump

Lateral
  Anterior triangle
	Thyroid lobe swellings:
	  Simple, physiological goitre
	  Multinodular goitre
	  Solitary nodule
	  Thyroid tumours: benign (adenoma) and malignant (papillary, follicular, medullary, anaplastic)
		Lump moves with swallowing but not on tongue protrusion

	Submandibular gland swelling:
	  Infection, stones, autoimmune disease
	  Benign or malignant tumours
		Swelling below the angle of the mandible. Can be felt bimanually. Involvement of more than one gland suggests a systemic condition. A lump within the gland suggests a tumour. Uniform enlargement with pain suggests infection or stones

	Parotid gland swelling: Mumps, parotitis, stones, autoimmune disease	Swelling in the preauricular area or just below the ear

	Parotid gland mass:
	  Benign
	  Malignant tumours
		Hard, fixed mass with facial nerve weakness suggests a malignant tumour of the parotid gland

	Branchial cyst	Smooth, non-tender, fluctuant mass. Not translucent. Slowly enlarging, may increase after upper respiratory tract infection

	Lymph nodes:
	  Malignant: lymphoma, metastatic cancer
	  Infection: bacterial infection of head and neck, viral infection (e.g. infectious mononucleosis), human immunodeficiency virus, tuberculosis
		Large, hard, fixed, matted, painless mass suggests malignancy
		Lymph nodes can be reactive to infection and are usually smooth, firm, mobile and tender

Posterior triangle	Lymph nodes:
	  Malignant
	  Benign
		See p. 32

	Carotid body tumour	Firm, rubbery, pulsatile neck mass, fixed vertically due to attachment to bifurcation of common carotid. A bruit may be present
	Carotid artery aneurysm	Rare, present as pulsatile neck mass
	Cystic hygroma	Soft, fluctuant, compressible and transilluminable mass, usually seen in children
	Cervical rib	Hard, bony mass
Supraclavicular fossa	Supraclavicular lymphadenopathy	Left supraclavicular (Virchow's) node may suggest gastric malignancy

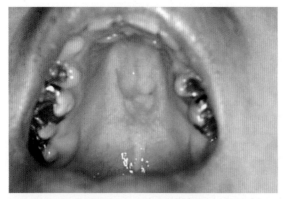

Fig. 9.25 Torus palatinus. This benign asymptomatic central palatal bony mass is more common in Asian populations. *From Scully C. Oral and Maxillofacial Medicine. 2nd edn. Edinburgh: Churchill Livingstone; 2008.*

- Inspect the tonsils, noting size, symmetry, colour and any pus or membrane.
- Touch the posterior pharyngeal wall gently with the tongue depressor to stimulate the gag reflex. Check for symmetrical movement of the soft palate.

Palpation

- If any lesion is seen in the mouth or salivary glands, palpate it (wearing gloves) with one hand outside on the patient's cheek or jaw and a finger of your other hand inside the mouth (bimanual palpation).
- Feel the lesion and identify its characteristics (p. 32).
- If the base of the tongue or the tonsils are asymmetrical, palpate it using a gloved finger.
- If the parotid gland is enlarged or abnormal on inspection, examine the facial nerve and check if the deep lobe (tonsil area) is displaced medially.
- Palpate the parotid and submandibular duct, feeling for stones.
- Palpate the cervical lymph nodes (p. 33).

Cracking of the lips can be the result of cold exposure ('chapped lips'), riboflavin deficiency, chronic atrophic candidiasis or iron deficiency (Fig. 9.26). Squamous and basal cell cancers occur on the lips and are associated with smoking and sun exposure.

The normal tongue appearance includes areas of smooth mucosa ('geographic tongue') or, conversely, excessive furring. A smooth red tongue with diffuse papillary atrophy occurs in iron or vitamin B_{12} deficiency. Tongue protrusion may be limited by neurological disease, painful mouth or a tight frenulum. Macroglossia (enlarged tongue) occurs in Down's syndrome, acromegaly (see Fig. 10.9), hypothyroidism and amyloidosis. Wasting and fasciculation of the tongue are features of motor neurone disease.

White plaques of candidiasis on the tongue or mucosa (Fig. 9.27A) come away easily when scraped but leukoplakia (a keratotic precancerous condition) does not and requires excision

biopsy (Fig. 9.27B). Cancers (usually squamous) may occur at any site in the mouth. Any painless persistent mass in the mouth should be assumed to be oral cancer and referred urgently for biopsy. Similarly, any mouth ulcer persisting for over 3 weeks requires biopsy to exclude cancer (Fig. 9.27C).

A stone may be felt in the submandibular (or, rarely, the parotid) duct. Rotten teeth (dental caries) are common in patients with poor oral hygiene (Fig. 9.27D).

Neck

The neck must be examined in all patients with mouth or throat symptoms, or a neck mass.

Examination sequence

- With the patient sitting down and their neck fully exposed (ties and scarves removed and shirt unbuttoned), look at their neck from in front. Inspect for scars, masses or pulsation.
- From behind, palpate the neck. Work systematically around the neck. Start in the midline and gently palpate the submental, submandibular and preauricular areas, assessing for the presence of any masses or swelling. Then palpate down the anterior border of the sternocleidomastoid muscle to the midline inferiorly.
- Palpate the midline structures of the neck from inferior to superior up to the submental area, noting any masses.
- If a midline mass is present, ask the patient to swallow (offer a glass of water if needed) and then instruct them to stick out their tongue while you palpate the mass. Movement superiorly on swallowing suggests a thyroid

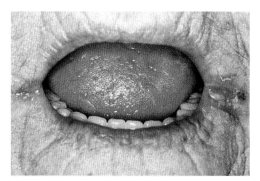

Fig. 9.26 Angular stomatitis.

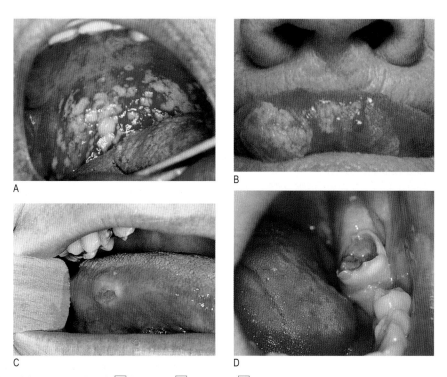

A

B

C

D

Fig. 9.27 Disorders of the tongue and teeth. [A] Oral thrush. [B] Leukoplakia. [C] Aphthous stomatitis causing a deep ulcer in a patient with inflammatory bowel disease. [D] Dental caries. *(B) From Bull TR. Color Atlas of ENT Diagnosis. 3rd edn. London: Mosby–Wolfe; 1995.*

swelling (p. 194), while movement on tongue protrusion suggests a thyroglossal cyst (Fig. 9.28).

- Palpate the posterior triangle of the neck, including the posterior border of sternocleidomastoid and anterior border of trapezius. Palpate for occipital lymph nodes posteriorly.
- For any mass, note the size, site, consistency, edge, fixation to deeper structures, tethering to the skin, warmth, fluctuance, pulsatility and transillumination (p. 32).

Investigations

Initial investigations are summarised in Box 9.11.

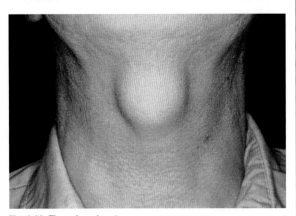

Fig. 9.28 Thyroglossal cyst.

9.11 Mouth, throat and neck investigations

Investigation	Indication/comment
Full blood count	Infective causes of mouth, throat or neck symptoms
Monospot	Infectious mononucleosis Hepatosplenomegaly can occur in infectious mononucleosis so liver function tests can be useful
Throat swab	Acute tonsillitis and pharyngitis Patients may carry *Streptococcus pyogenes* and have a viral infection (detected by PCR), so swab does not always help direct management PCR may help identify viral causes
Endoscopy and biopsy	Cancer of larynx and pharynx, changes in vocal cords Under general anaesthetic
Ultrasound ± fine-needle aspiration	Neck lumps, swellings
Computed tomography	Cancer and metastases Useful in staging

PCR, *polymerase chain reaction.*

OSCE example 1: Hoarseness

Mr Smith, 65 years old, presents with hoarseness.

Please take a history from the patient

- Introduce yourself and clean your hands.
- Invite the patient to describe the presenting symptoms, using open questioning.
- Take a detailed history of the presenting symptoms, asking specifically about onset, progression, fluctuation or constancy, provoking factors (work, singing, shouting) and weak or croaky voice. Enquire about associated cough, shortness of breath, throat pain, ear pain, dysphagia or weight loss.
- Ask about relevant past history, including previous neck surgery, neck trauma, prolonged intubation, reflux disease and significant systemic conditions, including neurological problems.
- Enquire about drug history: specifically, recent courses of antibiotics (laryngeal candidiasis), anticholinergics (causing dry throat) or angiotensin-converting enzyme inhibitors (causing chronic dry cough).
- Ask about social history, including profession (singer, teacher), smoking and alcohol consumption.
- Address any patient concerns.
- Thank the patient and clean your hands.

Summarise your findings

The patient is a heavy smoker and reports slowly progressive hoarseness associated with breathlessness and a dry cough.

Suggest a diagnosis

This history suggests recurrent laryngeal nerve damage from a bronchial carcinoma. The differential diagnosis would include laryngeal carcinoma.

Suggest initial investigations

Full ear, nose and throat examination, including oral cavity, throat and neck, with a chest X-ray to exclude a bronchial carcinoma at the left hilum causing recurrent laryngeal nerve palsy. Persistent hoarseness (>3 weeks) requires referral for laryngoscopy to exclude laryngeal malignancy.

OSCE example 2: Neck lump

Mrs Lewis, 55 years old, presents with a lump just under her left ear at the angle of her jaw.

Please examine her neck lump

- Introduce yourself and clean your hands.
- Inspect the neck for scars or swelling. If a neck lump is visible, describe its size, shape and site, as well as any skin changes. If it is in the midline, ask the patient to swallow and stick out their tongue.
- Ask if the lump is painful and if the patient minds you examining it.
- Palpate the lump to assess consistency, edge, fixation to deeper structures, tethering to the skin, warmth, fluctuance, pulsatility and transillumination.
- Palpate the anterior and posterior triangles of the neck, and the parotid region.
- Examine the oral cavity, throat, nose and ears (as potential primary sites of infection or malignancy that might be causing the neck mass).
- Assess facial nerve function if you suspect a parotid mass.
- Thank the patient and clean your hands.

Summarise your findings

Examination confirms a firm, non-tender, mobile lump about 1 cm in diameter behind the angle of the jaw on the left.

Suggest a diagnosis

The most likely diagnosis is a pleomorphic salivary adenoma in the tail of the parotid.

Suggest investigations

Ultrasound scan with or without fine-needle aspiration.

9

Integrated examination sequence for ear, nose and throat disease

- Position the patient: on an examination couch with the upper body at 45 degrees and neck fully exposed.
- Examine the ears:
  - Inspect: pinna skin, shape, size, position, deformity, scars.
  - Palpate: pinna, tragus, mastoid.
  - Otoscopy: external auditory canal (swelling, discharge), tympanic membrane (red, perforated).
  - If there is hearing loss: whispered voice test and tuning fork tests.
  - If there are balance symptoms: vestibular examination, including Dix–Hallpike.
- Examine the nose:
  - Inspect:
    - External nose (swelling, bruising, skin changes, deformity).
    - Anterior nasal septum (swelling, visible vessels, crusting ulceration, septal perforation). Exclude septal haematoma in nasal trauma.
    - Inferior turbinates (hypertrophy, swelling, polyps).
  - Palpate:
    - Nasal bones (bony or cartilaginous deformity).
    - Airway patency using metal spatula.
- Examine the mouth and throat:
  - Listen to the voice (rough, breathy, wet, muffled, nasal escape).
  - Remove any dentures.
  - Inspect:
    - Oral cavity, oropharynx.
    - Mucosal discoloration, inflammation, ulceration, masses, opening of parotid and submandibular ducts.
    - Hard palate for cleft, abnormal arched palate, telangiectasia.
    - Soft palate for cleft, bifid uvula, swelling or lesions.
    - Tonsils, noting size, symmetry, colour, pus or membrane.
  - Palpate:
    - Any lesion, identifying characteristics.
    - Base of tongue or tonsils if asymmetrical.
    - Parotid and submandibular ducts, feeling for stones.
- Examine the neck:
  - Inspect:
    - Scars, skin changes.
    - If there is midline swelling, ask the patient to swallow and stick out their tongue.
  - Palpate:
    - Anterior and posterior triangles of the neck and parotid region.
    - If there is a neck lump, note size, site, shape, consistency, edges, attachments, tenderness, warmth, pulsatility, transillumination.
    - If there is a parotid lump, assess the facial nerve.

Anna R Dover
Nicola Zammitt

10

The endocrine system

Endocrine glands synthesise hormones that are released into the circulation and act at distant sites. Diseases may result from excessive or inadequate hormone production, or target organ hypersensitivity or resistance to the hormone. The main endocrine glands are the pituitary, thyroid, adrenals, gonads (testes and ovaries), parathyroids and the endocrine pancreas. With the notable exception of the pancreatic islet cells (which release insulin) and the parathyroids, most endocrine glands are themselves controlled by hormones released from the pituitary.

Since hormones circulate throughout the body, symptoms and signs of endocrine disease are frequently non-specific, affecting many body systems (Box 10.1). Often, endocrine disease is picked up incidentally during biochemical testing or radiological imaging. Careful history taking and examination are required to recognise characteristic patterns of disease. Thyroid disease and diabetes mellitus are common and frequently familial; establishing a detailed family history is therefore important. Some less common endocrine disorders (such as multiple endocrine neoplasia) show an autosomal dominant pattern of inheritance.

10.1 Common clinical features in endocrine disease

Symptom, sign or problem	Differential diagnoses
Tiredness	Hypothyroidism, hyperthyroidism, diabetes mellitus, hypopituitarism
Weight gain	Hypothyroidism, PCOS, Cushing's syndrome
Weight loss	Hyperthyroidism, diabetes mellitus, adrenal insufficiency
Diarrhoea	Hyperthyroidism, gastrin-producing tumour, carcinoid
Diffuse neck swelling	Simple goitre, Graves' disease, Hashimoto's thyroiditis
Polyuria (excessive thirst)	Diabetes mellitus, diabetes insipidus, hyperparathyroidism, Conn's syndrome
Hirsutism	Idiopathic, PCOS, congenital adrenal hyperplasia, Cushing's syndrome
'Funny turns' or spells	Hypoglycaemia, phaeochromocytoma, neuroendocrine tumour
Sweating	Hyperthyroidism, hypogonadism, acromegaly, phaeochromocytoma
Flushing	Hypogonadism (especially menopause), carcinoid syndrome
Resistant hypertension	Conn's syndrome, Cushing's syndrome, phaeochromocytoma, acromegaly
Amenorrhoea/oligomenorrhoea	PCOS, hyperprolactinaemia, thyroid dysfunction
Erectile dysfunction	Primary or secondary hypogonadism, diabetes mellitus, non-endocrine systemic disease, medication-induced (e.g. beta-blockers, opiates)
Muscle weakness	Cushing's syndrome, hyperthyroidism, hyperparathyroidism, osteomalacia
Bone fragility and fractures	Hypogonadism, hyperthyroidism, Cushing's syndrome, primary hyperparathyroidism

PCOS, *polycystic ovary syndrome.*

THE THYROID

Anatomy and physiology

The thyroid is a butterfly-shaped gland that lies inferior to the cricoid cartilage, approximately 4 cm below the superior notch of the thyroid cartilage (Fig. 10.1A). The normal thyroid has a volume of <20 mL and is palpable in about 50% of women and 25% of men. It is comprised of a central isthmus approximately 1.5 cm wide, covering the second to fourth tracheal rings, and two lateral lobes that are usually no larger than the distal phalanx of the patient's thumb. The gland may extend into the superior mediastinum and can be partly or entirely retrosternal. Rarely, it can be located higher in the neck along the line of the thyroglossal duct, an embryological remnant of the descent of the thyroid from the base of the tongue to its final position. Thyroglossal cysts can also arise from the thyroglossal duct; they often occur at the level of the hyoid bone (Fig. 10.1A) and characteristically move upwards on tongue protrusion. The thyroid is attached to the pretracheal fascia and thus moves superiorly on swallowing or neck extension.

Thyrotoxicosis is a clinical state of increased metabolism caused by elevated circulating levels of thyroid hormones. Graves' disease is the most common cause (Fig. 10.2 and Box 10.2). It is an autoimmune disease with a familial component and is 5–10 times more common in women, usually presenting between 30 and 50 years of age. Other causes include toxic multinodular goitre, solitary toxic nodule, thyroiditis and excessive thyroid hormone ingestion.

Hypothyroidism is caused by reduced levels of thyroid hormones, usually due to autoimmune Hashimoto's thyroiditis, and affects women approximately six times more commonly than men. Most other causes are iatrogenic and include previous radioiodine therapy or surgery for Graves' disease.

The history

Common presenting symptoms

Neck swelling

Goitre is enlargement of the thyroid gland (Fig. 10.3). It is not necessarily associated with thyroid dysfunction and most patients

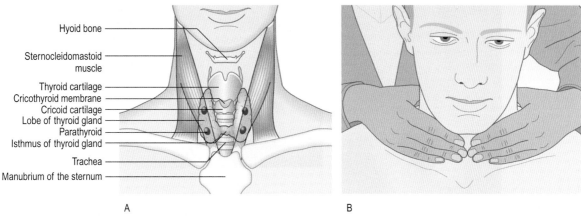

Fig. 10.1 The thyroid gland. [A] Anatomy of the gland and surrounding structures. [B] Palpating the thyroid gland from behind.

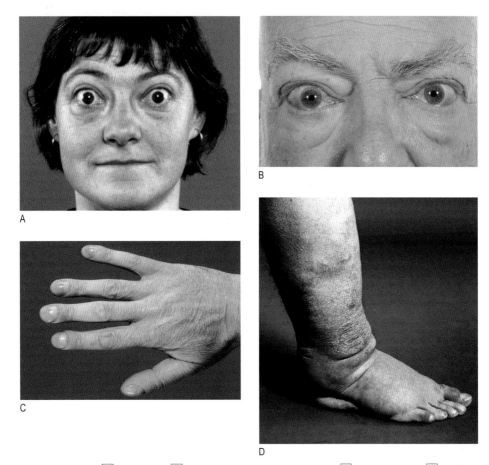

Fig. 10.2 Graves' hyperthyroidism. [A] Typical facies. [B] Severe inflammatory thyroid eye disease. [C] Thyroid acropachy. [D] Pretibial myxoedema.

with goitre are euthyroid. Large or retrosternal goitres may cause compressive symptoms, including stridor, breathlessness or dysphagia.

Thyroid nodules may be solitary (Fig. 10.3C) or may present as a dominant nodule within a multinodular gland. Palpable nodules (usually >2 cm in diameter) occur in up to 5% of women and less commonly in men, although up to 50% of patients have occult nodules; thus many are found incidentally on neck or chest imaging.

Neck pain

Neck pain is uncommon in thyroid disease and, if sudden in onset and associated with thyroid enlargement, may represent

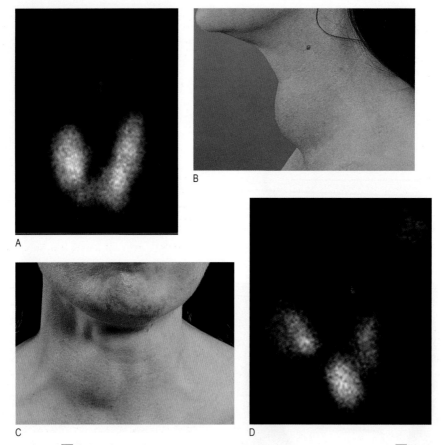

Fig. 10.3 Thyroid enlargement. [A] 99mTechnetium radionuclide scan demonstrating diffuse goitre due to Graves' disease. [B] Diffuse goitre due to Graves' disease. [C] Solitary toxic nodule. [D] 99mTechnetium radionuclide scan confirming multinodular goitre. *(A and D) Courtesy of Dr Dilip Patel.*

bleeding into an existing thyroid nodule. Pain can also occur in viral subacute (de Quervain's) thyroiditis.

History suggesting hyperthyroidism

Ask about:

- fatigue, poor sleep
- tremor, heat intolerance, excessive sweating (hyperhidrosis)
- pruritus (itch), onycholysis (loosening of the nails from the nail bed), hair loss
- irritability, anxiety, emotional lability
- dyspnoea, palpitations, ankle swelling
- weight loss, hyperphagia, faecal frequency, diarrhoea
- proximal muscle weakness (difficulty rising from sitting or bathing)
- oligomenorrhoea or amenorrhoea (infrequent or ceased menses, respectively)
- eye symptoms: 'grittiness', excessive tearing, retro-orbital pain, eyelid swelling or erythema, blurred vision or diplopia (these symptoms of ophthalmopathy occur in the setting of autoimmune thyroid disease).

History suggesting hypothyroidism

Ask about:

- fatigue, mental slowing, depression
- cold intolerance
- weight gain, constipation
- symptoms of carpal tunnel syndrome
- dry skin or hair.

10.2 Features suggestive of Graves' hyperthyroidism

History

- Female sex
- Prior episode of hyperthyroidism requiring treatment
- Family history of thyroid or other autoimmune disease
- Ocular symptoms ('grittiness', redness, pain, periorbital swelling)

Physical examination

- Vitiligo
- Thyroid acropachy
- Diffuse thyroid enlargement (can be nodular)
- Thyroid bruit
- Pretibial myxoedema
- Signs of Graves' ophthalmopathy (proptosis, redness, oedema)

Past medical, drug, family and social history

Ask about:

- prior neck irradiation (risk factor for thyroid malignancy)
- recent pregnancy (postpartum thyroiditis usually occurs in the first 12 months)
- drug therapy: antithyroid drugs or radioiodine therapy; amiodarone and lithium can cause thyroid dysfunction
- family history of thyroid or other autoimmune disease
- residence in an area of iodine deficiency, such as the Andes, Himalayas, Central Africa: can cause goitre and, rarely, hypothyroidism
- smoking (increases the risk of Graves' ophthalmopathy).

The physical examination

General examination

Look for signs of weight loss or gain (calculate the body mass index), and assess the patient's behaviour for signs of agitation, restlessness, apathy or slowed movements. Patients may have abnormal speech (pressure of speech suggests hyperthyroidism, while speech is often slow and deep in hypothyroidism). Hoarseness is suggestive of vocal cord paralysis and should raise suspicion of thyroid malignancy.

Features of hyperthyroidism and hypothyroidism on examination are summarised in Fig. 10.4.

Features of thyrotoxicosis include warm, moist skin, proximal muscle weakness (due to a catabolic energy state), tremor and brisk deep tendon reflexes. Hyperthyroidism may also be associated with tachycardia or atrial fibrillation, and a midsystolic cardiac flow murmur due to increased cardiac output.

Thyroid acropachy is an extrathyroidal manifestation of autoimmune thyroid disease. It is characterised by soft-tissue swelling and periosteal hypertrophy of the distal phalanges, and mimics finger clubbing (see Fig. 10.2C). It is often associated with dermopathy and ophthalmopathy. Pretibial myxoedema is a raised, discoloured (usually pink or brown), indurated appearance over the anterior shins; despite its name, it is specifically associated with Graves' disease and not hypothyroidism (see Fig. 10.2D).

Many clinical features of hypothyroidism are produced by myxoedema (non-pitting oedema caused by tissue infiltration by mucopolysaccharides, chondroitin and hyaluronic acid; Figs 10.4 and 10.5). Other common findings in hypothyroidism include goitre, cool, dry or coarse skin, bradycardia, delayed ankle reflexes and a slowing of movement.

Examination sequence

- Observe the facial appearance, noting signs of dry or coarse hair and periorbital puffiness (Fig. 10.5).
- Inspect the hands for vitiligo, thyroid acropachy, onycholysis and palmar erythema.
- Assess the pulse (tachycardia, atrial fibrillation, bradycardia) and blood pressure.
- Auscultate the heart for a midsystolic flow murmur (hyperthyroidism).
- Inspect the limbs for coarse, dry skin and pretibial myxoedema.
- Assess proximal muscle power and deep tendon (ankle) reflexes (p. 139).

Thyroid gland

Examination sequence

- Inspect the neck from the front, noting any asymmetry or scars. Inspect the thyroid from the side with the patient's neck slightly extended. Extending the neck will cause the thyroid (and trachea) to rise by a few centimetres and may make the gland more apparent. Give the patient a glass of water and ask them to take a sip and then swallow. The thyroid rises (with the trachea) on swallowing.
- Palpate the thyroid by placing your hands gently on the front of the neck with your index fingers just touching, while standing behind the patient (see Fig. 10.1B). The patient's neck should be slightly flexed to relax the

10

Hyperthyroidism

- Exophthalmos, ophthalmoplegia (in Graves' disease)
- Goitre (with bruit in Graves' disease)
- Tachycardia, angina, atrial fibrillation
- Systolic hypertension
- Oligomenorrhoea
- Diarrhoea
- Sweaty, tremulous, warm hands
- Proximal myopathy
- Pretibial myxoedema (in Graves' disease)
- Ankle swelling (in heart failure)

General
- Weight loss despite increased appetite
- Heat intolerance
- Anxiety, irritability
- Fast, fine tremor

Hypothyroidism

- Periorbital oedema
- Husky voice
- Goitre
- Bradycardia
- Carpal tunnel syndrome
- Menorrhagia
- Constipation

General
- Low metabolic rate, weight gain
- Dry skin and hair loss
- Sensitivity to cold
- Lethargy, mental impairment, depression

Fig. 10.4 Features of hyper- and hypothyroidism.

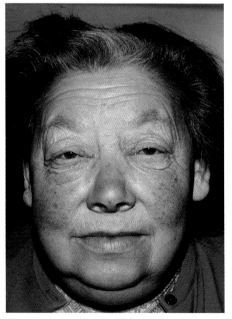

Fig. 10.5 Typical facies in hypothyroidism.

sternocleidomastoid muscles. Ask the patient to swallow again and feel the gland as it moves upwards.

- Note the size, shape and consistency of any goitre and feel for any thrill.
- Palpate for cervical lymphadenopathy (see Fig. 3.27).
- Percuss the manubrium to assess for dullness due to retrosternal extension of goitre.
- Auscultate with your stethoscope for a thyroid bruit. A thyroid bruit (sometimes associated with a palpable thrill) indicates abnormally high blood flow and is most commonly associated with Graves' disease. It may be confused with other sounds: bruits from the carotid artery or those transmitted from the aorta are louder along the line of the artery.

Early simple goitres are relatively symmetrical but may become nodular with time. In Graves' disease the surface of the thyroid is usually smooth and diffuse; in uninodular or multinodular goitre it is irregular (see Fig. 10.3). Diffuse tenderness is typical of viral thyroiditis. Localised tenderness may follow bleeding into a thyroid cyst. Fixation of the thyroid to surrounding structures (such that it does not move on swallowing) and associated cervical lymphadenopathy increase the likelihood of thyroid malignancy. Further investigation of thyroid disorders is summarised in Box 10.3.

Eyes

Examination sequence

- Look for periorbital puffiness or oedema, and lid retraction (this is present if the white sclera is visible above the iris in the primary position of gaze; see Fig. 10.2A).
- Examine for features of Graves' ophthalmopathy, including exophthalmos (look down from above and behind the patient), lid swelling or erythema, and conjunctival redness or swelling (chemosis).
- Assess for lid lag: ask the patient to follow your index finger as you move it from the upper to the lower part of the visual field. Lid lag means delay between the movement of the eyeball and descent of the upper eyelid, exposing the sclera above the iris.

10.3 Investigations in thyroid disease	
Investigation	**Indication/comment**
Biochemistry	
Thyroid function tests	To assess thyroid status
Immunology	
Antithyroid peroxidase antibodies	Non-specific, high in autoimmune thyroid disease
Antithyroid stimulating hormone receptor antibodies	Specific for Graves' disease
Imaging	
Ultrasound	Goitre, nodule
Thyroid scintigraphy (^{123}I, ^{99m}Tc)	To assess areas of hyper-/hypoactivity
Computed tomography	To assess goitre size and aid surgical planning
Invasive/other	
Fine-needle aspiration cytology	Thyroid nodule
Respiratory flow-volume loops	To assess tracheal compression from a large goitre

- Assess eye movements (see Fig. 8.11). Graves' ophthalmopathy is characteristically associated with restriction of upgaze.

Lid retraction (a staring appearance due to widening of the palpebral fissure) and lid lag (see earlier) are common eye signs associated with hyperthyroidism. Both are thought to be due to contraction of the levator muscles as a result of sympathetic hyperactivity. Periorbital puffiness (myxoedema) is sometimes seen in hypothyroidism.

Graves' ophthalmopathy occurs in around 20% of patients and is caused by an inflammatory infiltration of the soft tissues and extraocular muscles (see Fig. 10.2A,B). Features suggestive of active inflammation include spontaneous or gaze-evoked eye pain, and redness or swelling of the lids or conjunctiva. Proptosis (protrusion of the globe with respect to the orbit) may occur in both active and inactive Graves' ophthalmopathy and is often referred to as exophthalmos. Inflammation of the orbital soft tissues may lead to other more severe features, including corneal ulceration, diplopia, ophthalmoplegia and compressive optic neuropathy (see Fig. 8.8D).

THE PARATHYROIDS

Anatomy and physiology

There are usually four parathyroid glands situated posterior to the thyroid (see Fig. 10.1A). Each is about the size of a pea and produces parathyroid hormone, a peptide that increases circulating calcium levels.

The history

Common presenting symptoms

Parathyroid disease is commonly asymptomatic. In hyperparathyroidism the most common symptoms relate to hypercalcaemia:

polyuria, polydipsia, renal stones, peptic ulceration, tender areas of bone fracture or deformity ('Brown tumours': Fig. 10.6A), and delirium or psychiatric symptoms. In hypoparathyroidism, hypocalcaemia may cause hyper-reflexia or tetany (involuntary muscle contraction), most commonly in the hands or feet. Paraesthesiae of the hands and feet or around the mouth may occur. Hypoparathyroidism is most often caused by inadvertent damage to the glands during thyroid surgery but may also be caused by autoimmune disease. Patients with the rare autosomal dominant condition pseudohypoparathyroidism have end-organ resistance to parathyroid hormone and typically have short stature, a round face and shortening of the fourth and fifth metacarpal bones (Fig. 10.6B,C).

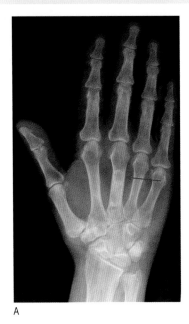

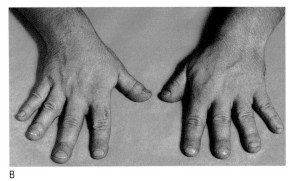

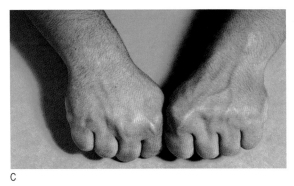

A

B

C

Fig. 10.6 Parathyroid disease. [A] Well-defined lucent lesion with surrounding sclerosis within the shaft of the third metacarpal of the right hand *(arrow)*, in keeping with a Brown tumour. [B] Pseudohypoparathyroidism: short fourth and fifth metacarpals. [C] These are best seen when the patient makes a fist. *(A) Courtesy of Dr Dilip Patel.*

Ask about:

- polyuria, polydipsia (hypercalcaemia)
- abdominal pain or constipation (hypercalcaemia)
- confusion or psychiatric symptoms (hypercalcaemia)
- bone pain (hypercalcaemia)
- muscle cramps, perioral or peripheral paraesthesia (hypocalcaemia).

Past medical, drug, family and social history

Ask about:

- recent neck surgery or irradiation
- past history of bone fractures
- past history of renal stones
- family history of hyperparathyroidism (which can be part of the autosomal dominant multiple endocrine neoplasia syndrome) or other endocrine disease (Addison's disease and type 1 diabetes can be associated with hypoparathyroidism as part of the autosomal recessive type 1 autoimmune polyglandular syndrome).

The physical examination

Examination sequence

- Hands: ask the patient to make a fist and assess the length of the metacarpals (in pseudohypoparathyroidism the metacarpals of the ring and little fingers are shortened; Fig. 10.6B,C).

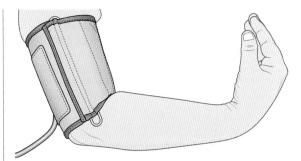

Fig. 10.7 Trousseau's sign.

- Examine the neck for scars. Parathyroid tumours are very rarely palpable.
- Measure the blood pressure and assess the state of hydration (p. 244). Inflating the blood pressure cuff in a patient with hypocalcaemia may precipitate carpal muscle contraction, producing a typical picture with the thumb adducted, the proximal interphalangeal and distal interphalangeal joints extended and the metacarpophalangeal joints flexed ('*main d'accoucheur*', hand of the obstetrician, or Trousseau's sign; Fig. 10.7).
- Test for muscle weakness and hyper-reflexia (p. 138).
- Look for evidence of recent fractures or bone deformity/ tenderness.
- Perform urinalysis (renal stones may result in haematuria).

10

THE PITUITARY

Anatomy and physiology

The pituitary gland is enclosed in the sella turcica at the base of the skull beneath the hypothalamus. It is bridged over by a fold of dura mater (diaphragma sellae) with the sphenoidal sinus below and the optic chiasm above. Lateral to the pituitary fossa are the cavernous sinuses, containing cranial nerves III, IV and VI and the internal carotid arteries. The gland comprises anterior and posterior lobes. The anterior lobe secretes adrenocorticotrophic hormone (ACTH), prolactin, growth hormone (GH), thyroid-stimulating hormone (TSH) and gonadotrophins (luteinising hormone (LH) and follicle-stimulating hormone (FSH)). The posterior lobe is an extension of the hypothalamus, and secretes vasopressin (antidiuretic hormone) and oxytocin.

The history

Common presenting symptoms

Pituitary tumours are common and are found incidentally in around 10% of patients undergoing head computed tomography (CT) or magnetic resonance imaging (MRI). Hypopituitarism can result from a space-occupying lesion or from a destructive or infiltrative process such as trauma, radiotherapy, sarcoidosis, tuberculosis or metastatic disease. Pituitary infarction or haemorrhage can result in acute hypopituitarism (referred to as pituitary apoplexy) and is a medical emergency; it is often associated with headache, vomiting, visual impairment and altered consciousness.

Non-functioning pituitary adenomas may be asymptomatic or may present with local effects, such as compression of the optic chiasm causing visual loss (typically bitemporal upper quadrantanopia or hemianopia; Fig. 10.8 and see Fig. 8.5)

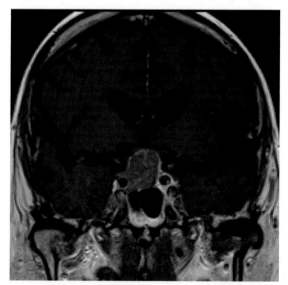

Fig. 10.8 Pituitary macroadenoma. The tumour extends into the suprasellar cistern and is compressing the optic chiasm. *Courtesy of Dr Dilip Patel.*

or headache due to expansion of the sella. Adenomas may produce hormones such as prolactin, GH or ACTH; the resulting symptoms and signs will depend on the excess hormone present.

Prolactinoma

Ask about:

- galactorrhoea (breast milk secretion)
- oligomenorrhoea, amenorrhoea or infertility (in women)
- reduced libido, erectile dysfunction and reduced shaving frequency (in men).

Acromegaly

GH excess prior to puberty presents as gigantism; after puberty, it causes acromegaly.

Ask about:

- headache
- excessive sweating
- changes in facial features (ask to see old photographs)
- an increase in shoe, ring or glove size
- associated medical conditions: arthropathy, carpal tunnel syndrome, hypertension, diabetes, colonic malignancy, sleep apnoea.

Hypopituitarism

Apart from headache due to stretching of the diaphragma sellae and visual abnormalities, clinical presentation depends on the deficiency of the specific anterior pituitary hormones involved. Individual or multiple hormones may be involved, so questioning in relation to deficiencies of the thyroid, adrenocortical and reproductive hormones is needed.

Family history

Enquire about family history since pituitary disease can occur as part of inherited multiple endocrine neoplasia or familial pituitary syndromes.

The physical examination

Acromegaly

Examination sequence

- Look at the face for coarsening of features, thick, greasy skin, prominent supraorbital ridges, enlargement of the nose, prognathism (protrusion of the mandible) and separation of the lower teeth (Fig. 10.9A,B).
- Examine the hands and feet for soft-tissue enlargement and tight-fitting rings or shoes, carpal tunnel syndrome and arthropathy (Fig. 10.9C,D).
- Assess the visual fields (p. 162).
- Check the blood pressure and perform urinalysis. Hypertension and diabetes mellitus are common associations.

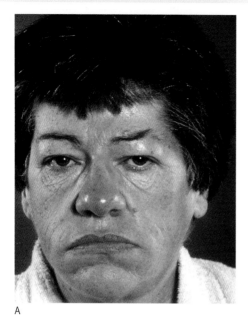

A

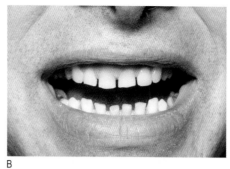

B

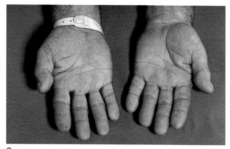

C

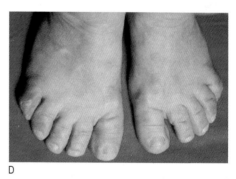

D

10

Fig. 10.9 **Acromegaly.** [A] Typical facies. [B] Prognathism and separation of the lower teeth. [C] Large, fleshy hands. [D] Widening of the feet.

Hypopituitarism

Examination sequence

Look for:
- extreme skin pallor (a combination of mild anaemia and melanocyte-stimulating hormone deficiency; Fig. 10.10A)
- absent axillary hair (Fig. 10.10B)
- reduced/absent secondary sexual hair and testicular atrophy (caused by gonadotrophin deficiency)
- visual field defects (most often bitemporal hemianopia), optic atrophy or cranial nerve defects (III, IV and VI), caused by a tumour compressing the optic chiasm, optic nerve or cavernous sinus.

THE ADRENALS

Anatomy and physiology

The adrenals are small, pyramidal organs lying immediately above the kidneys on their posteromedial surface. The adrenal medulla is part of the sympathetic nervous system and secretes catecholamines. The adrenal cortex secretes cortisol (a glucocorticoid), mineralocorticoids and androgens.

The history

Common presenting symptoms

Cushing's syndrome is caused by excess exogenous or endogenous glucocorticoid exposure. Most cases are iatro-

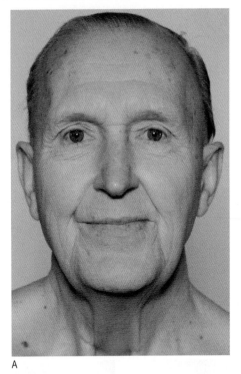
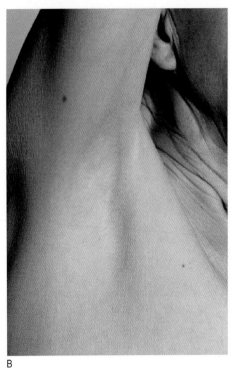

A   B

Fig. 10.10 Hypopituitarism. [A] Hypopituitarism caused by a pituitary adenoma (note the fine, pale skin). [B] Absent axillary hair.

genic and caused by side effects of glucocorticoid therapy. 'Endogenous' Cushing's usually results from an ACTH-secreting pituitary microadenoma, but other causes include a primary adrenal tumour or 'ectopic' ACTH secretion by a tumour. The catabolic effects of glucocorticoids cause widespread tissue breakdown (leading to proximal myopathy, fragility fractures, spontaneous bruising and skin thinning) and central accumulation of body fat (Fig. 10.11). Patients may develop hypertension or diabetes and are susceptible to infection. Hypertension can also result from overproduction of aldosterone (a mineralocorticoid) or catecholamines (Box 10.4).

Addison's disease is due to inadequate secretion of cortisol, usually secondary to autoimmune destruction of the adrenal cortex. Symptoms are usually non-specific (see later).

Adrenal adenomas usually present with features of hormone hypersecretion, as described later. Occasionally, they may be asymptomatic and are detected incidentally on abdominal CT or MRI scans. Functioning adrenal adenomas may present with refractory hypertension (Box 10.4).

Cushing's syndrome

Ask about:
- increase in weight, particularly if the weight is centrally distributed
- bruising, violaceous striae and skin thinning
- difficulty rising from a chair/bath (may indicate proximal myopathy).

Addison's disease

Ask about:
- weakness
- postural lightheadedness

- nausea, vomiting, diarrhoea, constipation, abdominal pain and weight loss
- muscle cramps.

Past medical and drug history

Enquire about recent or past exogenous glucocorticoid usage (route, dose, duration) as this may contribute to either iatrogenic Cushing's syndrome or suppression of the hypothalamic–pituitary–adrenal axis and resultant glucocorticoid insufficiency.

The physical examination

Cushing's syndrome

Examination sequence

- Look at the face and general appearance for central obesity; there may be a round, plethoric 'moon' face (Fig. 10.11A) or dorsocervical fat pad ('buffalo hump').
- Examine the skin for thinning and bruising (10.11D), striae (especially abdominal; Fig. 10.11C), acne, hirsutism and signs of infection or poor wound healing.
- Measure the blood pressure.
- Examine the legs for proximal muscle weakness and oedema.
- Perform ophthalmoscopy for cataracts and hypertensive retinal changes (see Fig. 8.18).
- Perform urinalysis for glycosuria.

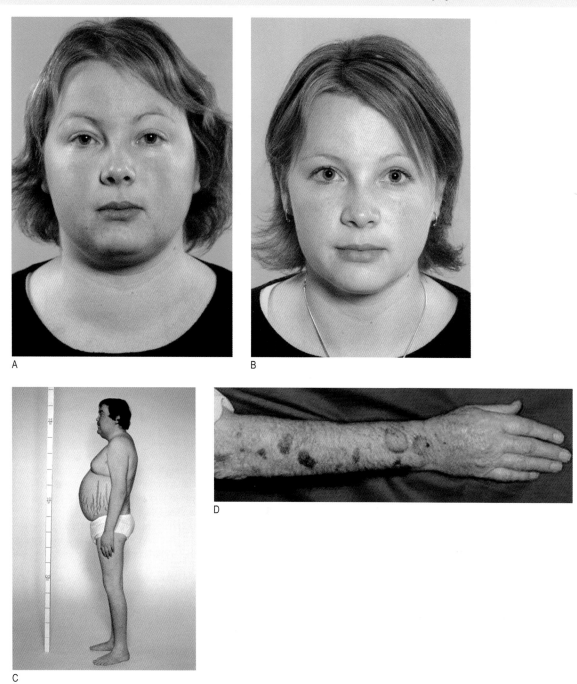

Fig. 10.11 Cushing's syndrome. A Cushingoid facies. B After curative pituitary surgery. C Typical features: facial rounding and plethora, central obesity, proximal muscle wasting and violaceous skin striae. D Skin thinning: purpura caused by wristwatch pressure.

10.4 Adrenal causes of endocrine hypertension		
Condition	**Hormone produced in excess**	**Associated features**
Conn's syndrome	Aldosterone	Hypokalaemia
Cushing's syndrome	Cortisol	Central obesity, proximal myopathy, fragility fractures, spontaneous bruising, skin thinning, violaceous striae, hypokalaemia
Phaeochromocytoma	Noradrenaline (norepinephrine), adrenaline (epinephrine)	Paroxysmal symptoms, including hypertension, palpitations, sweating

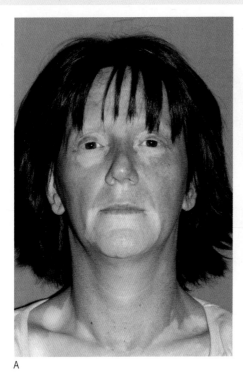

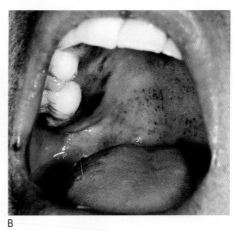

Fig. 10.12 **Addison's disease.** [A] Hyperpigmentation in a patient with coexistent vitiligo. [B] Buccal pigmentation.

Addison's disease

Examination sequence

- Look for signs of weight loss.
- Examine the skin for abnormal or excessive pigmentation. This is most prominent in sun-exposed areas or epithelia subject to trauma or pressure: skin creases, buccal mucosa (Fig. 10.12B) and recent scars. In primary adrenal insufficiency, the pituitary increases ACTH secretion in response to low cortisol levels. High levels of ACTH increase melanocyte-stimulating hormone, leading to increased skin pigmentation (most striking in white Caucasians). Vitiligo (depigmentation of areas of skin) occurs in 10–20% of Addison's disease cases (Fig. 10.12A).
- Measure the blood pressure and test for postural hypotension (p. 51), resulting from salt and water loss due to inadequate mineralocorticoid.

THE GONADS

Anatomy and physiology

The gonads (testes and ovaries) secrete sex hormones (testosterone and oestrogen) in response to gonadotrophin (FSH and LH) release by the pituitary. The reproductive system is covered in Chapter 11.

The history

Common presenting symptoms

Most commonly, men present with androgen deficiency, whereas women present with hyperandrogenism.

Hypogonadism can be primary (failure of the gonad itself) or secondary (where reduced gonadotrophin levels cause gonadal failure). Klinefelter's syndrome (47XXY) is the most common cause of primary hypogonadism in men (1:600 live male births; Fig. 10.13). Secondary hypogonadism may be caused by pituitary disease, extremes of weight, or drugs that suppress hypothalamic gonadotrophin releasing hormone release (such as anabolic steroids or opiates). Presenting symptoms in men include loss of libido, erectile dysfunction, loss of secondary sexual hair, reduction in testicular size and gynaecomastia (p. 214).

Hyperandrogenism in women usually presents with hirsutism (excessive male-pattern hair growth; Fig. 10.14), acne and/or oligomenorrhoea, and is commonly due to polycystic ovarian syndrome (PCOS; usually also associated with obesity). Other less common causes should be considered (such as congenital adrenal hyperplasia). Virilisation is suggested by male-pattern baldness, deepening of the voice, increased muscle bulk and clitoromegaly; if present in women with a short history of severe hirsutism, consider a testosterone-secreting tumour.

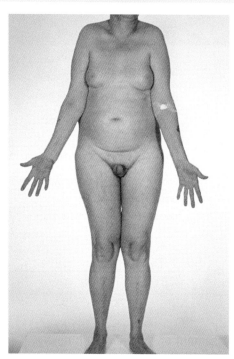

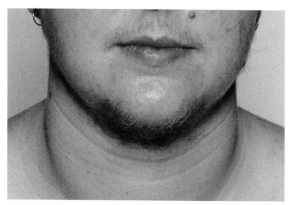

Fig. 10.14 Facial hirsutism.

10

Fig. 10.13 **Klinefelter's syndrome.** Tall stature, gynaecomastia, reduced pubic hair and small testes.

DIABETES

Anatomy and physiology

The pancreas lies behind the stomach on the posterior abdominal wall. Its endocrine functions include production of insulin (from beta cells), glucagon, gastrin and somatostatin. Its exocrine function is to produce alkaline secretions containing digestive enzymes.

Diabetes mellitus is characterised by hyperglycaemia caused by absolute or relative insulin deficiency.

Diabetes may be primary or secondary. Primary diabetes is divided into:

- type 1: severe insulin deficiency due to autoimmune destruction of the pancreatic islets. These patients are susceptible to acute decompensation due to hypoglycaemia or ketoacidosis, both of which require prompt treatment.
- type 2: commonly affects people who are obese and insulin-resistant, although impaired beta-cell function is also important. These patients may decompensate by developing a hyperosmolar hyperglycaemic state.

Secondary causes of diabetes and the associated history and examination features are described in Box 10.5.

The history

Common presenting symptoms

Diabetes mellitus commonly presents with a classical triad of symptoms:

- polyuria (and nocturia): due to osmotic diuresis caused by glycosuria

- thirst: due to the resulting loss of fluid
- weight loss: due to fluid depletion and breakdown of fat and muscle secondary to insulin deficiency.

Other common symptoms are tiredness, mood changes and blurred vision (due to glucose-induced changes in lens refraction). Bacterial and fungal skin infections are common because of the combination of hyperglycaemia, impaired immune resistance and tissue ischaemia. Itching of the genitalia (pruritus vulvae in women, balanitis in men) is due to *Candida* yeast infection (thrush).

Past medical, drug, family and social history

Ask about:

- Previous glucose intolerance or gestational diabetes, which are risk factors for progression to type 2 diabetes.
- Other autoimmune conditions such as thyroid disease (increased incidence of type 1 diabetes).
- Drug therapy: glucocorticoids can cause steroid-induced diabetes.
- Family history of diabetes or autoimmune disease. Monogenic diabetes is usually inherited in an autosomal dominant manner. Patients are often slim (unlike those with type 2 diabetes) but do not require insulin at diagnosis (unlike those with type 1 diabetes). Monogenic diabetes should be considered in people presenting with diabetes under the age of 30 who have an affected parent or a family history of early-onset diabetes in around 50% of first-degree relatives.
- Smoking habit: combines with diabetes to increase the risk of vascular complications.
- Alcohol: raises the possibility of pancreatic diabetes.

10.5 Causes of secondary diabetes[a]

Cause of diabetes	Examples	Clinical features
Pancreatic disease	Pancreatitis Trauma/pancreatectomy Neoplasia Cystic fibrosis Haemochromatosis	Abdominal pain Surgical scar Weight loss Chronic cough, purulent sputum Skin pigmentation ('bronze diabetes')
Endocrinopathies	Acromegaly, Cushing's syndrome	p. 202
Drugs	Glucocorticoids (e.g. prednisolone) Antipsychotics (e.g. olanzapine) Immunosuppressants (e.g. ciclosporin, tacrolimus)	Features of Cushing's syndrome (see Fig. 10.11) Gum hypertrophy may be seen with ciclosporin use
Pregnancy	Gestational diabetes may develop in the third trimester	Gravid uterus
Monogenic defects in beta-cell function	Glucokinase deficiency	Glucokinase deficiency is present from birth with stable mild hyperglycaemia
Genetic syndromes associated with diabetes	Down's syndrome Turner's syndrome	p. 36 p. 36

[a]Based on classification by the American Diabetes Association.

10.6 Routine history taking as part of the annual review in diabetes

Glycaemic control

- Ask about frequency of blood glucose testing and frequency and awareness of symptoms of hypoglycaemia
- When relevant, give guidance on driving and/or pre-pregnancy preparation

Injection sites

- Enquire about any lumpiness (lipohypertrophy), bruising or discomfort

Symptoms of macrovascular disease

- Ask whether there has been any angina, myocardial infarction, claudication, stroke or transient ischaemic attack since the last clinic review

Symptoms of microvascular disease

- Ask whether there has been any change in vision or any numbness or altered sensation in the feet

Feet

- Ask about neuropathy and peripheral vascular symptoms as above
- Enquire about any breaks in the skin, infections or ulcers

Autonomic neuropathy

- Enquire about erectile dysfunction in men
- Ask about postural hypotension, sweating, diarrhoea and vomiting in all patients

In established diabetes, vital aspects of the history (Box 10.6) and examination should be reviewed at least once a year.

The physical examination

The physical examination will differ, depending on whether this is a new presentation of diabetes or a patient with established diabetes attending for their annual review.

Assessment of a patient with newly diagnosed diabetes

Examination sequence

- Look for evidence of weight loss and dehydration. Unintentional weight loss is suggestive of insulin deficiency.
- Check for clinical features of acromegaly or Cushing's syndrome.
- Look for Kussmaul respiration (hyperventilation with a deep, sighing respiratory pattern) or the sweet smell of ketones, both of which suggest insulin deficiency and diabetic ketoacidosis.
- Skin: look for signs of infection such as cellulitis, boils, abscesses and fungal infections, paying particular attention to the feet (see later). Look for signs of insulin resistance such as acanthosis nigricans (Fig. 10.15A). Necrobiosis lipoidica, a yellow, indurated or ulcerated area surrounded by a red margin indicating collagen degeneration (Fig. 10.15B), may occur on the shins in type 1 diabetes and often causes chronic ulceration.
- Look for xanthelasmata and xanthomata (Fig. 10.15C; see Fig. 4.6); these are suggestive of dyslipidaemia, which may occur in type 2 diabetes.
- Measure the pulse and blood pressure, and examine the cardiovascular and peripheral vascular systems, with a particular emphasis on arterial pulses in the feet (p. 69).
- Examine the central nervous system, with a particular focus on sensation in the lower limbs (p. 143).
- Test visual acuity and perform fundoscopy (p. 164; see Fig. 8.16).
- Perform urinalysis for glycosuria.

Microvascular, neuropathic and macrovascular complications of hyperglycaemia can occur in patients with any type of diabetes mellitus, and may be present at diagnosis in patients with slow-onset type 2 disease.

Glycosuria is in keeping with diabetes; the presence of urinary (or blood) ketones suggests insulin deficiency and the possibility of diabetic ketoacidosis. Other investigations to consider are summarised in Box 10.7.

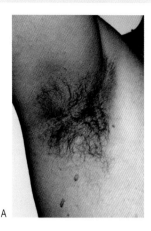

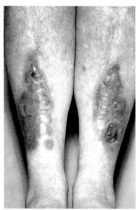

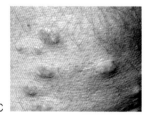

Fig. 10.15 Diabetes and the skin. [A] Acanthosis nigricans.
[B] Necrobiosis lipoidica. [C] Eruptive xanthomata.

10.7 Investigations in diabetes

Investigation	Indication/comment
Diagnostic investigations	
Fasting glucose, random glucose, oral glucose tolerance test	To make a diagnosis of diabetes. Patients will also monitor capillary blood glucose to adjust their treatment
HbA$_{1c}$	Can be used for diagnosis of type 2 diabetes and to assess glycaemic burden
Urine or blood ketone measurement	Ketones suggest insulin deficiency, which occurs in type 1 diabetes and in diabetes due to pancreatic pathology
Pancreatic antibodies (anti-GAD and islet cell)	To confirm a diagnosis of autoimmune diabetes
Annual review investigations	
HbA$_{1c}$	An important measure of glycaemic control over the preceding 3 months; predicts risk of complications
Urea and electrolytes	To assess for the presence of diabetic nephropathy
Lipid profile	To aid estimation of cardiovascular risk and guide treatment with lipid-lowering therapy
Thyroid function tests	To screen for the commonly associated hypothyroidism
Urine albumin:creatinine ratio	To assess for early signs of diabetic nephropathy (microalbuminuria)
Digital retinal photography or fundoscopy	To screen for diabetic retinopathy and/or maculopathy

GAD, *glutamic acid decarboxylase.*

Routine review of a patient with diabetes

Examination sequence

- Weigh the patient: weight gain in type 2 diabetes is likely to be associated with worsening insulin resistance while weight loss in type 1 diabetes often suggests poor glycaemic control and inadequate insulin dosage.
- For patients on insulin, examine insulin injection sites for evidence of lipohypertrophy (which may cause unpredictable insulin release), lipoatrophy (rare) or signs of infection (very rare).
- Measure the pulse and blood pressure.
- Test visual acuity and perform fundoscopy (p. 164; see Fig. 8.16).
- Examine the feet (see the next section).
- Perform routine biochemical screening (Box 10.7).

The diabetic foot

Up to 40% of people with diabetes have peripheral neuropathy and 40% have peripheral vascular disease, both of which contribute to a 15% lifetime risk of foot ulcers (Fig. 10.16).

Early recognition of the 'at-risk' foot is essential. There are two main presentations:

- Neuropathic: neuropathy predominates but the major arterial supply is intact.
- Neuroischaemic: reduced arterial supply produces ischaemia and exacerbates neuropathy.

Infection may complicate both presentations.

Examination sequence

- Look for hair loss and nail dystrophy.
- Examine the skin (including the interdigital clefts) for excessive callus, skin breaks, infections and ulcers. Look for any discoloration. Distal pallor can suggest early ischaemia, while purple/black discoloration suggests gangrene.
- Ask the patient to stand so that you can assess the foot arch; look for deformation of the joints of the feet.
- Feel the temperature of the feet.
- Examine the dorsalis pedis and posterior tibial pulses. If absent, arrange Doppler studies and evaluate the ankle:brachial pressure index (p. 69).
- Test for peripheral neuropathy: use a 10-g monofilament to apply a standard, reproducible stimulus. The technique

10.8 Risk assessment of the diabetic foot

Level of risk	Definition	Action required
Low	No sensory loss, peripheral vascular disease or other risk factors	Annual foot screening can be undertaken by any trained healthcare professional
Moderate	One risk factor present, e.g. absent pulses or reduced sensation	Annual foot screening should be undertaken by a podiatrist
High	Previous ulceration or amputation, or more than one risk factor present	Annual screening should be undertaken by a specialist podiatrist
Active foot disease	Ulceration, spreading infection, critical ischaemia or an unexplained red, hot, swollen foot	Prompt referral to a multidisciplinary diabetic foot team is required

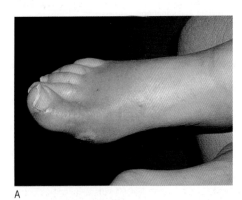

A

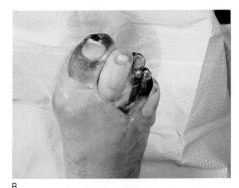

B

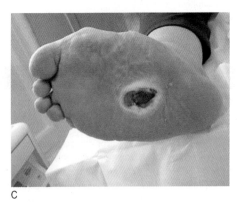

C

Fig. 10.16 Diabetic foot complications. A Infected foot ulcer with cellulitis and ascending lymphangitis. B Ischaemic foot: digital gangrene. C Charcot arthropathy with plantar ulcer.

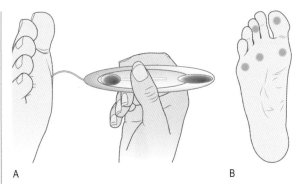

A   B

Fig. 10.17 Monofilament sensory testing of the diabetic foot.
A Apply sufficient force to allow the filament to bend. B Sites at highest risk (toes and metatarsal heads).

and the best sites to test are shown in Fig. 10.17. Avoid areas of untreated callus. Sensory loss typically occurs in a stocking distribution.

• Assess dorsal column function by testing vibration and proprioception.
• Undertake a foot risk assessment to guide management (Box 10.8).

Hair loss and nail dystrophy occur with ischaemia. Feet are warm in neuropathy and cold in ischaemia. Ischaemic ulcers are typically found distally: at the tips of toes (see Fig. 10.16B), for example. There may be skin fissures or tinea infection ('athlete's foot'). Loss of sensation to vibration (p. 143) and proprioception (p. 144) are early signs of diabetic peripheral neuropathy. Sensory neuropathy is present if the patient cannot feel the monofilament on the sites shown in Fig. 10.17. This suggests loss of protective pain sensation and is a good predictor of future ulceration.

With significant neuropathy, the foot arch may be excessive or collapsed (rocker-bottom sole). Both conditions cause abnormal pressures and increase the risk of plantar ulceration (see Fig. 10.16C), particularly in the forefoot. Charcot's arthropathy is disorganised foot architecture, acute inflammation, fracture and bone thinning in a patient with neuropathy. It presents acutely as a hot, red, swollen foot and is often difficult to distinguish clinically from infection.

OSCE example 1: Neck swelling

Miss Duncan, 27 years old, presents with a 6-month history of palpitations, weight loss and neck swelling.

Please examine her thyroid status

- Introduce yourself and clean your hands.
- Carry out a general inspection, observing dress, body habitus, agitation, restlessness, diaphoresis, anxiety, exophthalmos, goitre and neck scars.
- Inspect the hands for vitiligo, palmar erythema, thyroid acropachy and fine tremor (hands outstretched with paper over the dorsum).
- Palpate the pulse for bounding pulse, tachycardia and atrial fibrillation.
- Inspect the eyes for lid retraction (scleral show) and exophthalmos (look down from above and behind the patient).
- Test eye movements for ophthalmoplegia and lid lag.
- Examine the neck for scars, goitre, lymphadenopathy. Ask the patient to swallow to see the thyroid gland rise on swallowing.
- Palpate the thyroid (again on swallowing) and cervical lymph nodes; percuss manubrium for retrosternal goitre.
- Auscultate any goitre for bruit.
- Assess the patient for proximal myopathy (ask them to stand from sitting, with their arms crossed).
- Examine the shins for pretibial myxoedema and test for hyper-reflexia.
- Thank the patient and clean your hands.

Summarise your findings

The patient is thin, with a fine tremor, tachycardia, exophthalmos and lid lag. In the neck there is a smooth, non-tender goitre.

Suggest a diagnosis

These findings suggest autoimmune thyrotoxicosis (Graves' disease).

Suggest investigations

Thyroid function tests, thyroid receptor autoantibodies and thyroid scintigraphy.

Advanced level comments

Thyrotoxicosis may cause an elevated alkaline phosphatase and hypercalcaemia due to increased bone turnover and a normochromic normocytic anaemia.

10

OSCE example 2: Diabetic feet

Mr Birnam, 67 years old, has type 2 diabetes and presents with pain in his lower limbs.

Please examine his feet

- Introduce yourself and clean your hands.
- Carry out a general inspection of the lower limbs, looking for hair loss, nail dystrophy or discoloration.
- Inspect the skin for excessive callus, infections and ulcers.
- Inspect the joints. Ask the patient to stand so that you can assess the foot arch and look for deformation of the joints of the feet.
- Palpate the feet to assess the temperature of the skin.
- Palpate the dorsalis pedis and posterior tibial pulses.
- Test for peripheral neuropathy using a 10-g monofilament and tuning fork.
- Thank the patient and clean your hands.

Summarise your findings

The patient has pale, cool feet with absent dorsalis pedis pulses bilaterally. The skin is intact but there is loss of sensation in a stocking distribution in both feet.

Suggest a diagnosis

The most likely diagnosis is peripheral vascular disease and peripheral neuropathy secondary to diabetes.

Suggest investigations

Doppler studies to evaluate the ankle:brachial pressure index. Review of diabetes control.

Advanced level comments

With peripheral neuropathy, also take an alcohol history and check vitamin B_{12} levels to take other common causes of peripheral sensory loss into account. Peripheral neuropathy can be confirmed on nerve conduction studies. Offer an examination for other microvascular complications, such as retinopathy (fundoscopy) and nephropathy (test urine for microalbuminuria).

Oliver Young
Colin Duncan
Kirsty Dundas
Alexander Laird

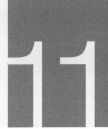

The reproductive system

BREAST

Anatomy and physiology

The breasts are modified sweat glands. The openings of the lactiferous ducts are on the apex of the nipple, which is erectile tissue. The nipple is in the fourth intercostal space in the mid-clavicular line, but accessory breast/nipple tissue may develop anywhere down the nipple line (axilla to groin) (Figs 11.1 and 11.2). The adult breast is divided into the nipple, the areola and four quadrants (upper outer to lower inner), with an axillary tail (of Spence) projecting from the upper outer quadrant (Fig. 11.3).

The size and shape of the breasts are influenced by age, hereditary factors, sexual maturity, phase of the menstrual cycle, parity, pregnancy, lactation and nutritional state. Fat and stroma surrounding the glandular tissue determine the size of the breast, except during lactation, when enlargement is mostly glandular. The breast responds to fluctuations in oestrogen and progesterone levels. Swelling and tenderness are common in the premenstrual phase. The glandular tissue reduces and fat increases with age, making the breasts softer and more pendulous. Lactating breasts are swollen and engorged with milk, and are best examined after breastfeeding.

The history

Benign and malignant conditions of the breast cause similar symptoms but benign changes are much more common. The most common presenting symptoms are a breast lump, breast pain, and skin and nipple changes. Men may present with gynaecomastia (breast swelling). Women are often worried that they have breast cancer, whatever breast symptom they have, and it is important to explore these concerns.

The history of the presenting symptoms is crucial. Find out the nature and duration of symptoms, any changes over time and any relationship to the menstrual cycle.

Ask about risk factors for breast cancer, in particular:

- previous personal history of breast cancer
- family history of breast or ovarian cancer and the age of those affected
- use of hormone replacement therapy
- previous mantle radiotherapy for Hodgkin's lymphoma.

Common presenting symptoms

Breast lump

Not all patients have symptoms. Women may present with an abnormality on screening mammography or concerns about their family history.

Ask:

- Is it a single lump or multiple lumps?
- Where is it?

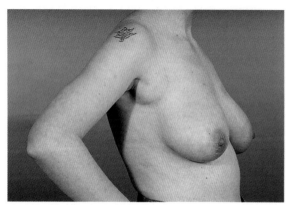

Fig. 11.1 Accessory breast tissue in the axilla.

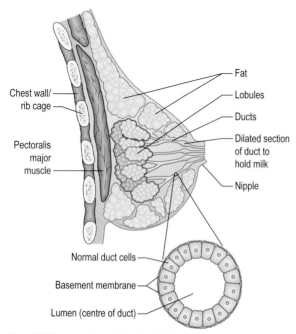

Fig. 11.2 Cross-section of the female breast.

Fat
Lobules
Ducts
Dilated section of duct to hold milk
Nipple
Chest wall/ rib cage
Pectoralis major muscle
Normal duct cells
Basement membrane
Lumen (centre of duct)

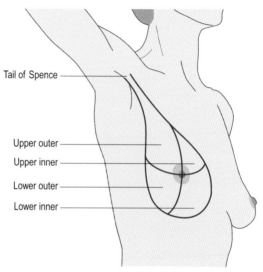

Fig. 11.3 Adult right breast.

Tail of Spence
Upper outer
Upper inner
Lower outer
Lower inner

- Is it tender?
- Is there any associated nipple discharge?
- Is there any variation in symptoms during the menstrual cycle?

Breast pain (mastalgia)

Ask if the pain varies during the menstrual cycle. Breast pain may be cyclical or non-cyclical and it is important to establish its timing and severity, and to distinguish it clearly from chest-wall pain. Cyclical mastalgia is common, worse in the latter half of the menstrual cycle and relieved by menstruation. Non-cyclical mastalgia does not vary with the menstrual cycle.

Skin changes

Women may report changes in the breast skin or these may be noted on examination. Possible skin changes include:

- Simple skin dimpling: the skin remains mobile over an underlying cancer (Fig. 11.4).
- Indrawing of the skin: the skin is fixed to the cancer.
- Lymphoedema of the breast: the skin is swollen between the hair follicles and looks like orange peel (*peau d'orange*; Fig. 11.5). The most common causes of lymphoedema are infection or tumour and it may be accompanied by redness, warmth and tenderness. Investigate any 'infection' that does not respond to one course of

antibiotics to exclude an inflammatory cancer. These are rare but aggressive tumours with a poor prognosis.

- Eczema of the nipple and areola: this may be part of a generalised skin disorder. If it affects the true nipple, it may be caused by Paget's disease of the nipple (Fig. 11.6), or invasion of the epidermis by an intraductal cancer.

Nipple changes

Women may report changes to the nipple or these may be noted on examination. Changes include:

- Nipple inversion: retraction of the nipple is common and often benign. It can be the first sign of malignancy, however, in which case it is usually asymmetrical (Fig. 11.7).
- Nipple discharge: a small amount of fluid may be expressed from multiple ducts by massaging the breast. It may be clear, yellow, white or green in colour. Investigate persistent single-duct discharge or blood-stained (macroscopic or microscopic) discharge to exclude duct ectasia, periductal mastitis, intraduct papilloma or intraduct cancer.
- Galactorrhoea: this is a milky discharge from multiple ducts in both breasts, most commonly caused by one of several drugs. Rarely, it is due to hyperprolactinaemia. Galactorrhoea may persist for some time after

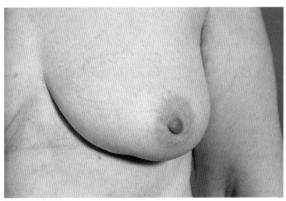

Fig. 11.4 **Skin dimpling due to underlying malignancy.**

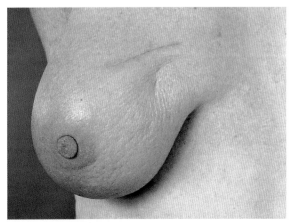

Fig. 11.5 *Peau d'orange* **of the breast.**

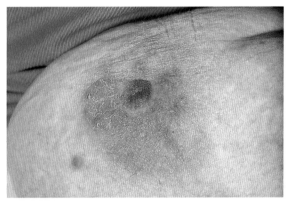

Fig. 11.6 **Paget's disease of the nipple.**

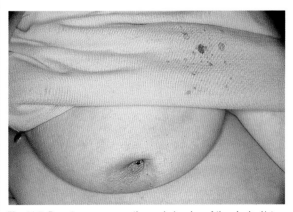

Fig. 11.7 **Breast cancer presenting as indrawing of the nipple.** Note the bloody discharge on the underclothing.

breastfeeding. It often causes hyperplasia of Montgomery's tubercles, the small rounded projections covering the areolar glands.

Gynaecomastia

Gynaecomastia is enlargement of the male breast and often occurs in pubertal boys. In chronic liver disease, gynaecomastia is caused by high levels of circulating oestrogens, which are not metabolised by the liver. Many drugs can cause breast enlargement (Box 11.1 and Fig. 11.8).

11.1 Causes of gynaecomastia	
Drugs	
• Cannabis	• Spironolactone
• Methadone	• Digoxin
• Oestrogens and other hormone-manipulating drugs used in treatment of prostate cancer	
Decreased androgen production	
• Klinefelter's syndrome	
Increased oestrogen levels	
• Chronic liver disease	• Some adrenal tumours
• Thyrotoxicosis	

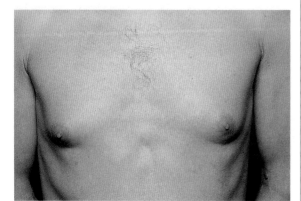

Fig. 11.8 Drug-induced gynaecomastia caused by cimetidine.

The physical examination

Always offer a chaperone and record that person's name; if the patient declines, note this. Male doctors should always have a chaperone. Ask the patient to undress to the waist and sit upright on a well-illuminated chair or on the side of a bed.

Examination sequence

- Ask the patient to rest her hands on her thighs to relax the pectoral muscles (Fig. 11.9A).
- Face the patient and look at the breasts for:
  - asymmetry
  - local swelling
  - skin changes
  - nipple changes.
- Ask the patient to press her hands firmly on her hips to contract the pectoral muscles and inspect again (Fig. 11.9B).
- Ask her to raise her arms above her head and then lean forward to expose the whole breast and exacerbate skin dimpling (Fig. 11.9C,D).
- Ask her to lie with her head on one pillow and her hand under her head on the side to be examined (Fig. 11.10).
- Hold your hand flat to her skin and palpate the breast tissue. Using two hands is often helpful. Breasts are often tender so pressing too firmly can be very uncomfortable.
- View the breast as a clock face. Examine each 'hour of the clock' from the outside towards the nipple, including under the nipple (Fig. 11.11). Examine all the breast tissue, comparing the texture of one breast with the other. The breast extends from the clavicle to the upper abdomen and from the midline to the anterior border of latissimus dorsi (posterior axillary fold). Define the characteristics of any mass (see Box 3.8).
- Elevate the breast with your hand to uncover dimpling overlying a tumour that may not be obvious on inspection.
- Is the mass fixed underneath? With the patient's hands on her hips, hold the mass between your thumb and forefinger. Ask her to contract and relax the pectoral muscles alternately by pushing into her hips. As the

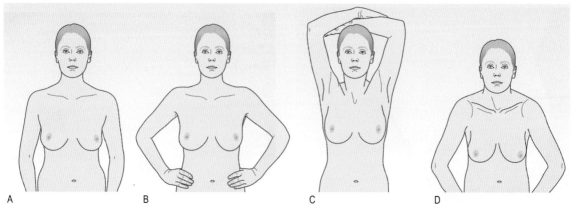

A   B   C   D

Fig. 11.9 Positions for inspecting the breasts. A Hands resting on the thighs. B Hands pressed on to the hips. C Arms above the head. D Leaning forward with the breasts pendulous.

pectoral muscle contracts, note whether the mass moves with it and if it is separate when the muscle is relaxed. Fixation suggests malignancy.
- Examine the axillary tail between your finger and thumb.
- Palpate the nipple by holding it gently between your index finger and thumb. Try to express any discharge. Massage the breast towards the nipple to uncover any discharge, noting the colour and consistency, and the number and position of the affected ducts. Test any discharge for blood using urine-testing sticks.
- Palpate the regional lymph nodes, including the supraclavicular group. Ask the patient to sit facing you, and support the full weight of her arm at the wrist with your opposite hand. Move the flat of your other hand high into the axilla and upwards over the chest to the apex.

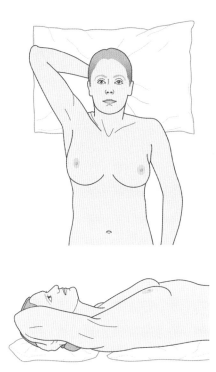

Fig. 11.10 Position for examination of the right breast.

This can be uncomfortable, so warn patients beforehand and check for any discomfort. Compress the contents of the axilla against the chest wall. Assess any palpable masses for:
- size
- consistency
- fixation.
- Examine the supraclavicular fossa, looking for any visual abnormality. Palpate the neck from behind and systematically review all cervical lymphatic chains (see Figs 3.27 and 9.22).

Cancers cause solid irregular masses. They are usually, but not always, painless, firm and hard, in contrast with the surrounding breast tissue. The cancer may extend directly into the overlying skin, pectoral fascia or pectoral muscle, causing the lump to feel fixed, or metastasise via regional lymph nodes or the systemic circulation.

In the UK, breast cancer affects 1 in 9 women. The incidence increases with age, but any mass is potentially malignant until proven otherwise. Cancer of the male breast is uncommon and may have a genetic basis. In contrast, fibroadenomas are smooth, mobile, discrete and rubbery lumps that are common in women under 35 years of age. These are benign overgrowths of the terminal duct lobules.

Fibrocystic changes are rubbery, bilateral and benign, and most prominent premenstrually, but investigate any new focal change in young women that persists after menstruation. These changes and irregular nodularity of the breast are common, especially in the upper outer quadrant in young women.

Breast cysts are smooth, fluid-filled sacs, most common in women aged 35–55 years. They are soft and fluctuant when the sac pressure is low but hard and painful if the pressure is high. Cysts may occur in clusters. A large majority are benign, but investigate any cyst where there is a residual mass following aspiration or which recurs after aspiration.

Breast abscesses occur as one of two types:
- Lactational abscesses in women who are breastfeeding. These are usually peripheral in the breast.
- Non-lactational abscesses, which occur as an extension of periductal mastitis, under the areola, often with nipple inversion. They usually affect young female smokers. Occasionally, a non-lactating abscess may discharge spontaneously through a fistula, classically at the edge of the areola (Fig. 11.12).

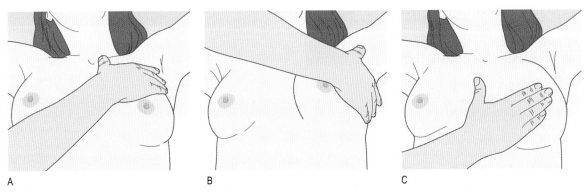

A   B   C

Fig. 11.11 Clinical examination of the breast. Palpating clockwise to cover all of the breast.

11.2 Investigation of breast lumps

Investigation	Indication/comment
Ultrasound	Lump
Mammography	Should not be used in women under 40 unless there is a strong suspicion of cancer
Magnetic resonance imaging	Dense breasts, ruptured implant, *BRCA1/2* mutation
Fine-needle aspiration	Should not be used to diagnose primary cancer but still useful for assessing lymph nodes
Core biopsy	To differentiate invasive or in situ cancer
Large-core vacuum-assisted core biopsy	Useful for large areas of diffuse change
Open surgical biopsy	Used as a last resort when multiple core biopsies have not provided a definite diagnosis

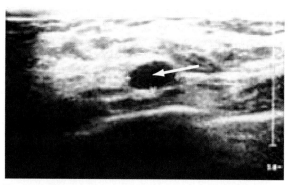

Fig. 11.13 Ultrasound of a breast cyst. A characteristic smooth-walled, hypoechoic lesion *(arrow)*.

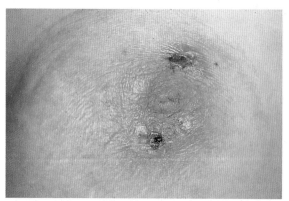

Fig. 11.12 Mammary duct fistula.

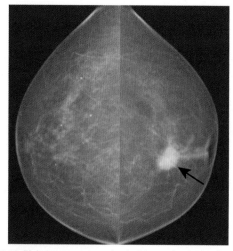

Fig. 11.14 Digital mammogram. A spiculate opacity characteristic of a cancer *(arrow)*.

Investigations

Accurate diagnosis of breast lesions depends on clinical assessment, backed up by mammography and/or breast ultrasound and pathological diagnosis; this should ideally be done by core biopsy, although fine-needle aspiration cytology can also be helpful in assessing axillary lymph nodes ('triple assessment') (Box 11.2 and Figs 11.13–11.14). Up to 5% of malignant lesions require excision biopsy for the diagnosis to be made. MRI is useful for investigating possible implant rupture or the extent of cancer in a mammographically dense breast, and for screening those with *BRCA1* or *BRCA2* gene mutations. In the UK, there are specific guidelines for the appropriate referral of patients with breast symptoms to specialist units.

FEMALE REPRODUCTIVE SYSTEM

Anatomy and physiology

The female reproductive organs are situated within the bony pelvis (Fig. 11.15). They cannot normally be felt on abdominal palpation. A vaginal examination is required for their routine assessment.

The vulva (Fig. 11.16) consists of fat pads, called labia majora, covered with hair. The labia minora are hairless skin flaps at each side of the vulval vestibule, which contains the urethral opening and the vaginal orifice. The clitoris is situated anteriorly where the labia minora meet and is usually obscured by the prepuce. Posteriorly the labia meet at the fourchette, and the perineum is the fibromuscular region posteriorly that separates it from the anus.

The vagina is a rugged tube 10–15 cm in length. There is an irregular mucosal ring two centimetres into the vagina that represents the remnants of the hymen (see Fig. 11.16). Bulging into the top of the vagina is the grape-sized fibrous uterine cervix, with the external cervical os on its surface (Fig. 11.17). The fornices are the areas of the top of the vagina next to the cervix (Fig. 11.18).

The uterus is a muscular pear-shaped structure, about the size of a large plum, situated in the midline and usually tilted anteriorly over the bladder (Fig. 11.19). Its internal cavity is lined by endometrium that proliferates, secretes and breaks down during the menstrual cycle. The Fallopian tubes run laterally from the uterine fundus towards the ovaries (see Fig. 11.17). Their distal finger-like fimbriae collect the oocyte after ovulation.

The ovaries are about the size of a walnut and sit behind and above the uterus close to the pelvic side wall. At mid-cycle, one ovary will have developed a fluid-filled preovulatory follicle measuring around 2 cm in diameter. The female reproductive tract is in close proximity to the bladder, ureter and lower gastrointestinal tract (see Fig. 11.19).

The history

Identify the woman's main symptoms, how these developed, their day-to-day impact, how she copes and her ideas, concerns and expectations of the encounter. Document any previous investigations and management. Check the history, even if an asymptomatic patient has come for a routine cervical smear.

Take a gynaecological history by asking about:

- (in pre- or perimenopausal women) last menstrual period (LMP) and whether it was normal; always consider that these patients might be pregnant
- past and present contraceptive use
- plans for fertility
- previous cervical smears, when taken, and any treatment required for abnormalities
- prior abdominal surgery, pelvic infection or sexually transmitted disease

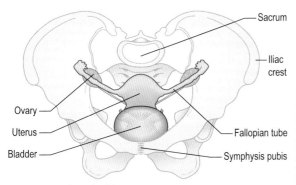

Fig. 11.15 Pelvis and pelvic organs.

- prior pregnancies and their outcomes
- current or previous hormone replacement therapy
- other medication with potential gynaecological effects (see later).

Common presenting symptoms

Abnormal vaginal bleeding

If women present with heavy periods, ask about:

- flooding: whether menstrual blood soaks through protection, increased requirements for sanitary protection
- passing of blood clots.

Women normally experience monthly menstruation from the menarche (average age 12) until the menopause (average age 51). Menstrual bleeding for 3–6 days normally occurs every 22–35 days (average 28). A menstrual cycle with bleeding for 4–5 days every 25–29 days is recorded as 4–5/25–29. Heavy menstrual bleeding (HMB, previously called menorrhagia) affects 20% of women over 35 and is defined as >80 mL blood loss during a period (average 35 mL). As this is not quantified in routine practice, HMB is subjective. Anaemia implies heavy bleeding.

Unexpected bleeding suggests endometrial or cervical pathology. Ask when the bleeding occurs:

- between periods (intermenstrual, IMB)
- after intercourse (postcoital, PCB)
- more than 1 year after the menopause (postmenopausal, PMB).

Approximately 4% of women experience PMB, which must be investigated as 10% have endometrial cancer.

Lack of periods (amenorrhoea) in the absence of pregnancy implies ovarian dysfunction and affects 5–7% of woman in their reproductive years. Distinguish between:

- Primary amenorrhoea: periods have not started by age 16. Both ovarian function and the structure of the reproductive tract should be investigated.
- Secondary amenorrhoea: there have been no periods for ≥6 months but there was previous menstruation.
- Oligomenorrhoea: the menstrual cycle is longer than 35 days.

In early pregnancy, 30% of women experience vaginal bleeding. Establish if this is associated with lower abdominal pain. Although the pregnancy may continue normally, bleeding is associated with miscarriage and ectopic pregnancy. Further investigation

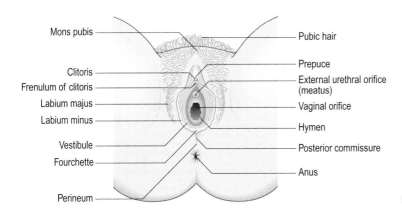

Fig. 11.16 External female genitalia.

is required, particularly if the bleeding is associated with lower abdominal pain.

Lower abdominal pain

Lower abdominal pain may arise from the reproductive organs or the urinary or gastrointestinal tract, or be musculoskeletal or

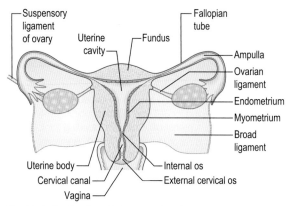

Fig. 11.17 Section through the pear-shaped, muscular uterus. The cervix, uterine body (corpus), fundus and Fallopian tubes, with the ligamentous attachments of the ovary. The uterine mucosa is the endometrium. The cervical canal has an internal and an external os.

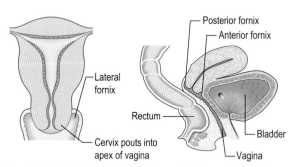

Fig. 11.18 Sagittal and coronal sections of the uterus. The vaginal fornices are shown.

neurological in origin (p. 96). Psychological and social factors may also contribute to a woman's experience of pain.

To differentiate between the possible causes of lower abdominal pain, ask about:

- site of the pain (unilateral, bilateral or midline)
- onset (sudden or gradual, cyclical/related to menstruation or not).

Ovarian pain is often unilateral and can be physiological (*Mittelschmertz* is discomfort associated with ovulation). Ovarian cyst accidents involving torsion (twisting on the vascular pedicle causing acute ischaemia), haemorrhage or rupture can lead to acute severe pain.

Primary dysmenorrhoea is pain arising from uterine contraction that is most intense just before and during peak menstruation. Secondary or progressive dysmenorrhoea, due to underlying pathology such as endometriosis or chronic infection, often manifests as pain that lasts beyond the normal menstrual cycle. Infection, pelvic adhesions and endometriosis can cause generalised pain (Box 11.3).

Dyspareunia is pain during intercourse. Ask if it is felt around the vaginal entrance (superficial) or within the pelvis (deep). Pain due to involuntary spasm of muscles at the vaginal entrance (vaginismus) may make intercourse impossible. Persistent deep dyspareunia suggests underlying pelvic pathology. Dyspareunia can be due to vaginal dryness following the menopause.

Iliac fossa pain in early pregnancy is commonly associated with a corpus luteum cyst of the ovary but may indicate a tubal ectopic pregnancy. Ruptured ectopic pregnancy results in generalised abdominal pain, peritonism, haemodynamic instability and referred pain in the shoulder.

Abdominal distension and bloating

Pelvic masses can cause non-specific symptoms like abdominal distension, bloating or urinary frequency due to pressure on the bladder. They may also be asymptomatic and picked up during routine abdominal or vaginal examination. Uterine masses include pregnancy and benign leiomyoma tumours (fibroids). Large ovarian cysts can also be midline and malignant ovarian cysts are associated with ascites.

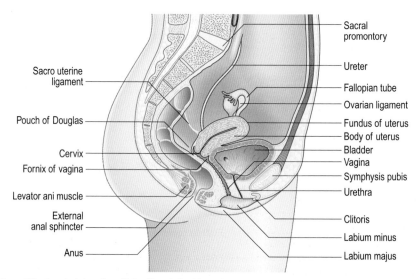

Fig. 11.19 Lateral view of the female internal genitalia. The relationship to the rectum and bladder.

11.3 Characteristics of pelvic pain

	Uterine pain	Ovarian pain	Adhesions or pelvic infection	Endometriosis
Site	Midline	Left or right iliac fossa	Generalised lower abdomen; more on one side	Variable
Onset	Builds up before period	Sudden, intermittent	Builds up, acute on chronic	Builds up, sudden
Character	Cramping	Gripping	Shooting, gripping	Shooting, cramping
Radiation	Lower back and upper thighs	Groin; if free fluid, to shoulder	–	–
Associated symptoms	Bleeding from vagina	Known cyst, pregnancy, irregular cycle	Discharge, fever, past surgery	Infertility
Timing	With menstruation	May be cyclical	Acute, may be cyclical	Builds up during period
Exacerbating factors	–	Positional	Movement, examination	Intercourse, cyclical
Severity	Variable in spasms	Intense	Intense in waves	Variable

Vaginal discharge

This may be normal and variable during the menstrual cycle. Prior to ovulation, it is clear and abundant, and stretches like egg white; after ovulation, it is thicker, does not stretch and is less abundant. Abnormal vaginal discharge occurs with infection. Ask about:

- consistency
- colour
- odour
- associated itch, pain or dysuria.

The most common non-sexually transmitted infection (caused by *Candida* species) gives a thick, white, curdy discharge often associated with marked vulval itching. Bacterial vaginosis is a common, non-sexually acquired infection, usually caused by *Gardnerella vaginalis*, producing a watery, fishy-smelling discharge. The pH of normal vaginal secretions is usually <4.5 but in bacterial vaginosis it is >5. Sexually transmitted infections (STIs) can cause discharge, vulval ulceration or pain, dysuria, lower abdominal pain and general malaise. They may also be asymptomatic.

Urinary incontinence

Inappropriate and involuntary voiding of urine severely affects 10% of women and its prevalence increases with age.

Stress incontinence occurs on exertion, coughing, laughing or sneezing and is associated with pelvic floor weakness.

Urge incontinence is an overwhelming desire to urinate when the bladder is not full, due to detrusor muscle dysfunction.

Prolapse

In 30% of women the pelvic contents bulge into the vagina (Fig. 11.20). Women feel something 'coming down', particularly when standing or straining. Uterine prolapse is associated with previous childbirth and is classified as:

- Grade 1: halfway to the hymen.
- Grade 2: at the hymen.
- Grade 3: beyond the hymen.
- Grade 4 (procidentia) : external to the vagina (Fig. 11.21).

The top of the vagina (vault) can also prolapse after a previous hysterectomy. More commonly the bulge relates to the vaginal wall. A cystocoele is a bulge on the anterior wall containing the bladder (see Fig. 11.20) and a rectocoele is a bulge on the posterior wall containing the rectum. An enterocoele is a bulge of the distal wall posteriorly containing small bowel and peritoneum.

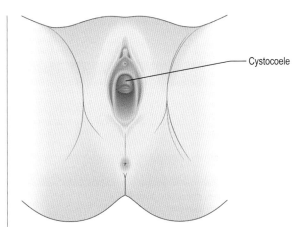

Fig. 11.20 Anterior vaginal wall prolapse.

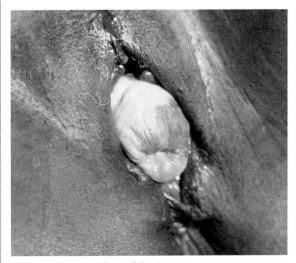

Fig. 11.21 External prolapse of the uterus.

Drug history

Tamoxifen has oestrogenic effects in postmenopausal women, antibiotics can cause vaginal candidiasis, antipsychotic drugs can cause hyperprolactinaemia, and antiepileptic or antituberculous drugs may reduce the effectiveness of oral contraceptives.

11

Family and social history

Family and social history, including smoking status and lifestyle, may also have an impact on gynaecological conditions. For example, obesity is associated with an increased risk of gynaecological malignancy.

Sexual history

Sometimes a sexual history is required but people often find it difficult talking about sexual matters. It is important for you to be at ease and ask questions in a straightforward manner. Explain why you need to enquire, use clear, unambiguous questions (Box 11.4) and be non-judgemental. The sexual partners of women with STIs should be informed and treated to prevent further transmission and reinfection of the treated person. Confidentiality is paramount, so do not give information to a third party. Do not perform a pelvic examination in someone who has not been sexually active.

The physical examination

A vaginal examination is required to perform a routine cervical smear. Otherwise the focus of gynaecological examination is to detect abnormalities that could explain the symptoms or alter treatment options (for example, body mass index (BMI) and blood pressure assessment affect the use of the contraceptive pill). Signs of gynaecological disease are not limited to the pelvis and a general as well as a pelvic examination is required (Box 11.5). You should offer a female chaperone and record this in the records. The examination area should be private, with the equipment and an adjustable light source available. The woman should have an empty bladder and remove her clothing from the waist down, along with any sanitary protection. Give her privacy to do this.

Passing a speculum

Explain what you are going to do and why it is necessary, and obtain verbal consent. Use a vaginal speculum to see the cervix and the vaginal walls, carry out a cervical smear and take swabs. Specula are metal or plastic and come in various sizes and lengths. Metal specula may be sterilised and reused; plastic specula are always disposable. A metal speculum is cold, so warm it under the hot tap. Most women find a speculum examination mildly uncomfortable, so always use a small amount of lubricating gel on the tip of each blade. Clean your hands and put on medical gloves. Ask the patient to lie on her back on the couch, covered with a modesty sheet to the waist, with her knees bent and apart (Fig. 11.22).

Examination sequence

- Look at the perineum for any deficiency associated with childbirth; note abnormal hair distribution and clitoromegaly (associated with hyperandrogenism). Note any skin abnormalities, discharge or swellings of the vulva, such as the Bartholin's glands on each side of the fourchette (Fig. 11.23).
- Ask the woman to cough while you look for any prolapse or incontinence.
- Gently part the labia using your left hand (Fig. 11.24). With your right hand, gently insert a lightly lubricated bivalve speculum (Figs 11.25–11.26A), with the blades vertical,

---

11.4 Taking a sexual history

- Are you currently in a sexual relationship?
- How long have you been with your partner?
- Have you had any (other) sexual partners in the last 12 months?
- How many were male? How many female?
- When did you last have sex with:
  - Your partner?
  - Anyone else?
- Do you use barrier contraception – sometimes, always or never?
- Have you ever had a sexually transmitted infection?
- Are you concerned about any sexual issues?

11.5 Focus of the gynaecological examination

Clinical feature	General examination	Pelvic examination
Abnormal bleeding	Anaemia Underweight (hypogonadotrophic hypogonadism) Galactorrhoea, visual field defects (hyperprolactinaemia) Hirsutism, obesity, acanthosis nigricans (PCOS)	Enlarged uterus (fibroids, pregnancy) Abnormal cervix Open cervical os (miscarriage) Vaginal atrophy (most common cause of PMB)
Pain	Abdominal tenderness	Uterine excitation (acute infection or peritonism) Fixed uterus (adhesions or endometriosis) Adnexal mass (ovarian cyst)
Vaginal discharge	Rash (associated with some STIs)	Clear from cervix (chlamydia) Purulent from cervix (gonorrhoea) Frothy with strawberry cervix (trichomoniasis)
Urinary incontinence	Obesity, chronic respiratory signs (stress incontinence) Neurological signs (urge incontinence)	Demonstrable stress incontinence Uterine or vaginal wall prolapse
Abdominal distension or bloating	Ascites, weight loss, lymphadenopathy, hepatomegaly (malignancy) Pleural effusion (some malignant or benign ovarian cysts)	Pelvic mass (uterine, ovarian or indiscriminate) Fixed uterus and adnexae Abnormal vulva (skin disease or malignancy)

PCOS, *polycystic ovary syndrome*; PMB, *postmenopausal bleeding*; STI, *sexually transmitted infection*.

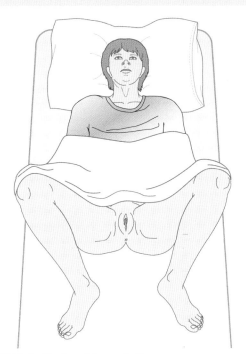

Fig. 11.22 Position for pelvic examination.

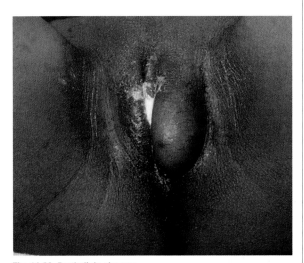

Fig. 11.23 Bartholin's abscess.

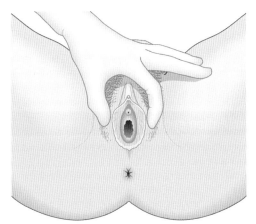

Fig. 11.24 Inspection of the vulva.

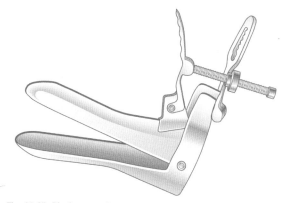

Fig. 11.25 Bivalve speculum.

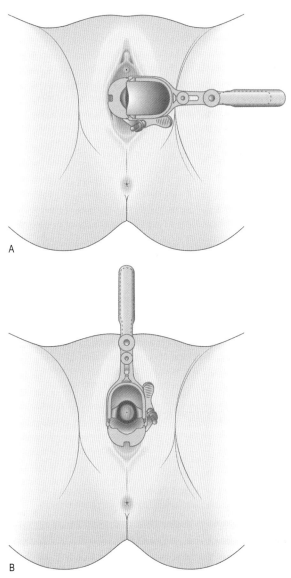

A

B

Fig. 11.26 Bivalve speculum examination. [A] Insertion of the speculum. [B] Visualisation of the cervix after rotation through 90 degrees.

11

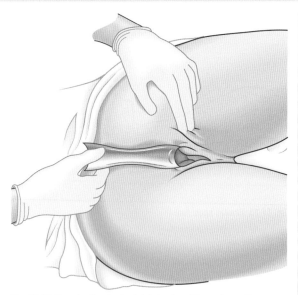

Fig. 11.27 Examination in the left lateral position using a Sims speculum.

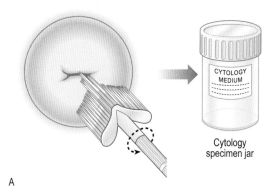

A

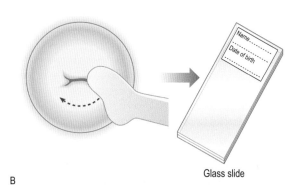

B

Fig. 11.28 Taking a cervical smear. A Liquid-based cytology. B Using a spatula.

fully into the vagina, rotating the speculum through 90 degrees so that the handles point anteriorly and the blades are now horizontal (Fig. 11.26B). A woman who has been pregnant may need a larger or longer speculum, or a bolster under the sacrum, if the cervix is very posterior. If the woman finds the examination difficult, ask her to try to insert the speculum herself.
- Slowly open the blades and see the cervix between them. If you cannot see it, reinsert the speculum at a more downward angle, as the cervix may be behind the posterior blade. Note any discharge or vaginal or cervical abnormalities.

To assess prolapse
- Ask the woman to lie on her left side and bring her knees up to her chest.
- Use a univalve Sims speculum, placing a small amount of lubricating jelly on the blade.
- Insert the blade to hold back the posterior wall.
- Ask the women to cough while you look for uterine descent and the bulge of a cystocoele (Fig. 11.27).
- Repeat, using the speculum to hold back the anterior vaginal wall to see a rectocoele or enterocoele.

Taking a cervical smear

There are two ways of taking a smear:
- using liquid-based cytology
- using a microscope slide.

Liquid-based cytology is increasingly common, as it allows for efficient processing and gives fewer inadequate smears.

Examination sequence
- Always label the cytological medium or slide and ask the questions required to fill in the request form before starting the examination, to avoid mixing specimens.
- Clearly visualise the entire cervix.

Liquid-based cytology
- Insert the centre of the plastic broom into the cervical os.
- Rotate the broom 5 times through 360 degrees (Fig. 11.28A).
- Push the broom 10 times against the bottom of the specimen container.
- Twirl 5 times through 360 degrees to dislodge the sample.
- Firmly close the lid.

Conventional smear
- Insert the longer blade of the spatula into the cervical os.
- Rotate the spatula through 360 degrees (Fig. 11.28B).
- Spread once across the glass slide.
- Place the slide immediately into fixative (methylated spirits) for 3–4 minutes.
- Remove it and leave it to dry in air.

Bimanual examination

Examination sequence
- Apply gloves and lubricate your right index and middle finger with gel.
- Gently insert them into the vagina and feel for the firm cervix. The uterus is usually anteverted (Fig. 11.29A) and you feel its firmness anterior to the cervix. If the uterus is retroverted and lying over the bowel (15%; Fig. 11.29B), feel the firmness posterior to the cervix.

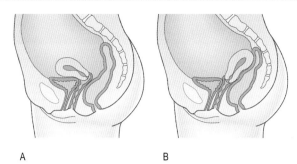

Fig. 11.29 Coronal section. [A] Anteverted uterus. [B] Retroverted uterus.

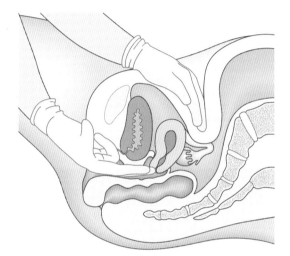

Fig. 11.30 Bimanual examination of the uterus. Use your vaginal fingers to push the cervix back and upwards, and feel the fundus with your abdominal hand.

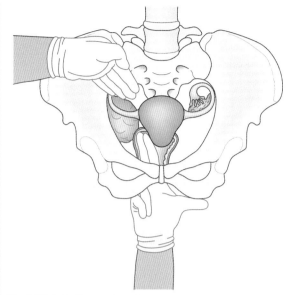

Fig. 11.31 Palpating an adnexal mass.

- Push your fingers into the posterior fornix and lift the uterus while pushing on the abdomen with your left hand.
- Place your left hand above the umbilicus and bring it down, palpating the uterus between both hands and note its size, regularity and any discomfort (Fig. 11.30).
- Move your vaginal fingers into the anterior fornix and palpate the anterior surface of the uterus, holding it in position with your abdominal hand.
- Move your fingers to the lateral fornix and, with your left hand above and lateral to the umbilicus, bring it down to assess any adnexal masses between your hands on each side (Fig. 11.31).
- If urinary leakage occurs when the patient coughs, try lifting the anterior vaginal wall with your fingers and asking her to cough again. This stops genuine stress incontinence.

The normal cervix os may be a slit after childbirth. Vaginal squamous epithelium and the endocervical columnar epithelium meet on the cervix. The position of this squamocolumnar junction varies considerably, so the cervix can look very different in individual women. If the transition zone is on the cervix, this is called an ectopy and looks red and friable; there may be small cysts called Nabothian follicles. The normal uterus should feel regular and be mobile and the size of a plum. The Fallopian tubes cannot be felt and normal ovaries are palpable only in very slim women.

Vulval changes include specific skin disease, infections such as herpes or thrush, and malignancy. Visual abnormalities of the cervix such as ulceration or bleeding suggest cervical pathology, including polyps or malignancy. Tender nodules in the posterior fornix suggest endometriosis, and both endometriosis and pelvic adhesions cause fixation of the uterus. Acute pain when touching the cervix (cervical excitation) suggests an acute pelvic condition such as infection, cyst accident or tubal rupture.

Fibroids can cause uterine irregularity and enlargement. The size is related to that of the uterus in pregnancy. A tangerine-sized uterus is 6 weeks, apple 8 weeks, orange 10 weeks and grapefruit 12 weeks. After 12 weeks the uterus can be palpated suprapubically on abdominal palpation. A large midline mass may be ovarian or uterine. Push the mass upwards with your left hand and feel the cervix with your right hand; if the mass moves without the cervix, this suggests it is ovarian.

Investigations

Common gynaecological investigations are summarised in Box 11.6. A woman of reproductive age should be considered potentially pregnant and a pregnancy test is routine. The mainstay of gynaecological investigation is a pelvic ultrasound scan, which can be carried out abdominally or transvaginally (Fig. 11.32). Endometrial biopsy is a common test, particularly for PMB, and is performed during vaginal examination using a suction catheter (pipelle, Fig. 11.33). When a couple present with subfertility, the key female investigations are serum progesterone 1 week before expected menses to confirm ovulation, and a test of tubal patency (Fig. 11.34).

11.6 Investigations in gynaecological disease

Clinical feature	Investigations	Diagnosis
Abnormal bleeding	Full blood count	Anaemia
	Ultrasound scan	Fibroids, endometrial polyp or pregnancy outcome and location
	Endometrial biopsy	Endometrial hyperplasia or carcinoma
	Hysteroscopy	Intrauterine polyps or fibroids
	Colposcopy	Cervical premalignant and malignant changes
	Gonadotrophins, sex steroids and prolactin	PCOS, premature ovarian insufficiency, hyperprolactinaemia or hypogonadotrophic hypogonadism
Pain	White blood count	Infection
	C-reactive protein	Acute inflammation
	High vaginal and endocervical swabs	Pelvic and vaginal infections, chlamydia or gonorrhoea
	Midstream specimen of urine	Urinary tract infection
	Ultrasound scan	Ovarian cysts, tubo-ovarian abscesses or intraperitoneal bleeding
	Laparoscopy	Pelvic adhesions and endometriosis
	Serial serum HCG	Ectopic pregnancy
Vaginal discharge	High vaginal and endocervical swabs	Pelvic and vaginal infections, chlamydia or gonorrhoea
Urinary incontinence	Midstream specimen of urine	Urinary tract infection
	Urodynamic studies	Degree of stress or urge incontinence
Abdominal distension or bloating	Ultrasound	Ovarian cysts, fibroids, pregnancy and ascites
	CT/MRI scan	Staging of pelvic malignancy
	Serum CA-125	Ovarian tumour marker
	Renal and liver function tests	Systemic effects of pelvic masses
	Direct or ultrasound-guided biopsy	Diagnosis of potential malignancy

CA-125, *cancer antigen 125;* CT, *computed tomography;* HCG, *human chorionic gonadotrophin;* MRI, *magnetic resonance imaging;* PCOS, *polycystic ovary syndrome.*

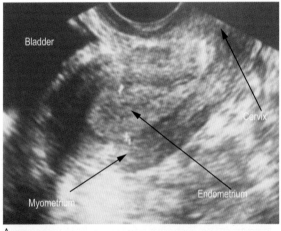

A

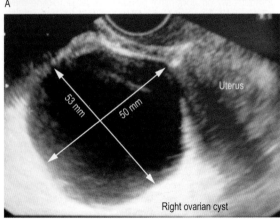

B

Fig. 11.32 Pelvic ultrasound. A Transvaginal scan of the uterus. B Scan showing an ovarian cyst.

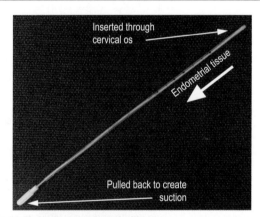

Fig. 11.33 Pipelle for endometrial biopsy.

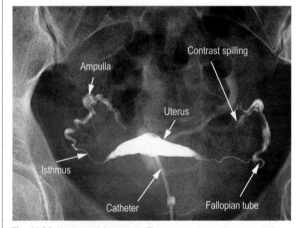

Fig. 11.34 Hysterosalpingogram. The scan assesses the uterus and bilateral tubal patency.

OBSTETRIC HISTORY AND EXAMINATION: THE BOOKING VISIT

In the UK, pregnant women are seen at approximately 10 antenatal visits; the visits may either be conducted by a midwife alone or be shared with an obstetrician. This plan is individualised depending on the age, past medical history and general health of the woman, as well as any complications that develop as the pregnancy proceeds.

The booking (first) visit takes place at 8–12 weeks' gestation.

The history

Take a full medical history and record details of any previous pregnancies (Boxes 11.7–11.8). Establish the date of the LMP (Box 11.9).

Past medical history

Ask about:
- all past medical and surgical events
- diseases that may be affected by pregnancy: for example, asthma may improve during pregnancy while inflammatory bowel disease may worsen postnatally
- diseases that cause increased risk in pregnancy such as diabetes.

Drug, alcohol and smoking history

Ask about:
- prescribed medications
- over-the-counter drugs and 'natural' remedies
- use of alcohol, tobacco and illegal drugs.

Find out at what gestation any drugs were taken. Advise all smokers to stop and all women to avoid alcohol. Check that pregnant women are taking 400 µg of folic acid daily until 12 weeks' gestation to reduce the incidence of neural tube defects (some higher-risk women need a higher dose).

Family history

To explore possible inherited conditions, take a full family history of both the pregnant woman and the father (Boxes 11.10 and 11.11).

Social history

Ask:
- who the patient's partner is
- how stable the relationship is

11.9 Definitions	
Term	**Definition**
LMP	First date of the last menstrual period
EDD	Estimated date of delivery: 40 weeks from LMP. Fewer than 5% of babies deliver on their due date; the majority deliver between 37 and 42 completed weeks – this period is called term. EDD is most accurately calculated from an ultrasound scan measurement of the fetal crown–rump length or head circumference done at the end of the first trimester
Parity	Number of previous births. Written in the format x+y, where x is the number of live births and any births over 24 weeks, and y is the number of all other pregnancies – babies born before 24 weeks with no signs of life, ectopic pregnancy, miscarriage and termination of pregnancy. Multiple pregnancy counts as one delivery – the number refers to pregnancies delivered and not to the number of fetuses/babies
Gestation	Number of weeks + days of pregnancy counted from LMP (although not conceived till ovulation approximately 2 weeks later or 14 days before the next period is due)
Trimester	The 40 weeks of pregnancy are divided into three trimesters of approximately 13 weeks each
Liquor or amniotic fluid	Fluid surrounding the fetus in utero
Oligohydramnios, polyhydramnios	Too little and excess amniotic fluid, respectively
Miscarriage	Expulsion of a fetus prior to viability
Live birth	Birth of a baby with signs of life
Still birth	Birth of a potentially viable baby without signs of life – in the UK, any that occur above 24 weeks; in Australia and other places, 20 weeks and above
Puerperium	The 6-week period after birth
Linea nigra	A dark line of discoloration in the midline of the abdominal skin
Striae gravidarum	Stretch marks – those from the current pregnancy appear white and those from any previous pregnancy are more silvery

11.7 Checklist for the obstetric history	
• Age	• Past obstetric history
• Parity	• Past medical and surgical history
• Menstrual history, last menstrual period, gestation, expected date of delivery	• Drug history
• Presenting symptom	• Family history
	• Social history

11.8 Information to be recorded for previous pregnancies
• Date and gestation of delivery
• Indication for and mode of delivery, e.g. spontaneous vaginal delivery, operative vaginal delivery (forceps or ventouse) or Caesarean section
• Singleton or multiple pregnancy
• Any pregnancy complications (take a full history)
• Duration of first and second stage of labour
• Weight and sex of the baby
• Health at birth, mode of infant feeding
• Postnatal information about mother and baby

11.10 Examples of single-gene disorders that can be detected antenatally	
Autosomal dominant	
• Huntington's chorea	• Myotonic dystrophy
Autosomal recessive	
• Cystic fibrosis	• Thalassaemia
• Sickle cell disease	
X-linked	
• Duchenne muscular dystrophy	• Haemophilia

11.11 Age-related risk of Down's syndrome (trisomy 21)	
Maternal age	**Risk**
20	1 in 1500
30	1 in 900
35	1 in 400
40	1 in 100
45	1 in 30

- if she is not in a relationship, who will give her support during and after the pregnancy
- whether the pregnancy was planned; if unplanned, find out how she feels about it.

Lower socioeconomic status is linked with increased perinatal and maternal mortality.

Encourage regular exercise and avoidance of certain foods, such as tuna (high mercury content), soft cheeses (risk of *Listeria*) and liver (high vitamin A content). Domestic violence can start or escalate in pregnancy and is associated with an increased risk of maternal death. All women must be seen alone (without their partner) on at least one antenatal visit to allow this to be explored.

Occupational history

Ask the patient about her occupation and whether she plans to continue it. Occupations involving exposure to ionising radiation pose specific risks to the fetus or mother, so her job plan may require modification for safety reasons. There is no definitive evidence of a link between heavy work and preterm labour or pre-eclampsia.

Examination sequence

- Calculate BMI (weight/height^2).
- Obtain a midstream specimen of urine for microscopy, culture and sensitivities.
- Measure blood pressure.
- Do not perform a routine full physical examination (including breast and vaginal examination) in healthy pregnant women. It is unnecessarily intrusive and has a low sensitivity for disease identification. However, you should perform a full examination of any woman with poor general health. Immigrant women newly arrived in the UK should have heart auscultation performed to exclude pre-existing cardiac disease.

Investigations

Routine investigations are required at the booking visit (Box 11.12).

ROUTINE ANTENATAL CHECK IN LATER PREGNANCY

The history

Ask about:
- any new symptoms
- symptoms relevant to ongoing conditions unrelated to pregnancy
- the mother's perception of fetal movements.

Fetal movements are initially felt at 16–20 weeks' gestation. Their frequency increases until about 32 weeks to an average of 30 movements per hour and this level remains unchanged until delivery. The 'classic' fetal movement is a kick but any perceived fetal activity counts as movement. Movements may decrease if the mother is given sedative drugs, and may be felt less well if the placenta is anterior. They also may decrease with intrauterine compromise, which may precede stillbirth.

Common presenting symptoms

Physiological symptoms

- Breast tenderness: often the earliest symptom of pregnancy and may occur even before a missed period.
- Mild dyspnoea: may be due to increased respiratory drive early in pregnancy or diaphragmatic compression by the growing uterus late in pregnancy.

- Heartburn: gradually increases in prevalence, affecting up to three-quarters of women by the third trimester. It results from relaxation of the gastro-oesophageal sphincter and acid reflux.
- Constipation, urinary frequency, nausea and vomiting (which usually resolve by 16–20 weeks).
- Aches and pains, especially backache, carpal tunnel syndrome and pubic symphyseal discomfort.

These physiological symptoms affect women to different degrees and will occasionally merit examination and investigation to exclude other problems. Secondary amenorrhoea is the most obvious symptom of early pregnancy.

Reduced fetal movements

This is a common emergency presentation or reason for referral to hospital by a midwife, and merits a full history, examination and fetal monitoring. It can be a sign of fetal compromise.

Vaginal bleeding in pregnancy

Vaginal bleeding in pregnancy before viability may herald a miscarriage; after 24 weeks, it is called an antepartum haemorrhage. It can be a sign of a placental abruption, where the placenta prematurely separates, or of a low-lying placenta. At term, light vaginal bleeding can also be a sign of labour. Vaginal bleeding is never considered normal in pregnancy and

11.12 Antenatal investigations

Investigation	Timing	Indication/comment
Mid-stream specimen urine (MSU) for culture	Booking; always sent	Detects asymptomatic bacteriuria (and group B streptococcus)
Urinalysis	Every visit	Trace or + proteinuria: send MSU, ask about symptoms of urinary tract infection ++ Proteinuria: consider pre-eclampsia or, rarely, underlying renal disorder Glycosuria: consider random blood glucose or glucose tolerance test
Full blood count	Booking, 28 weeks, 36 weeks	If haemoglobin is <105, treat; consider checking haematinics
Haemoglobin electrophoresis	Booking	To check for sickle cell disease and thalassaemias
Blood group and antibody screen	Booking, 28 weeks	More often if advised by laboratory
Hepatitis B	Booking	If the patient is a previous intravenous drug abuser or is known to be HIV- or hepatitis B-positive, also carry out hepatitis C screening
HIV	Booking	Unless the patient opts out
Syphilis	Booking	
Plasma glucose	Booking	
Carbon monoxide level	Every visit for smokers	Advice and referral for cessation, growth scans
Combined biochemical screening and nuchal translucency measurement for trisomy 21	11–14 weeks	Detects 80–90% of affected pregnancies
First-trimester ultrasound scan	6–13 weeks	Viability, gestational age ± 7 days, fetal number, some major anomalies, e.g. anencephaly
Detailed ultrasound scan	18–22 weeks	Detects 90% of major congenital abnormalities and placental site
Placental site	If low at 20 weeks, recheck later at about 34 weeks	If there is an anterior placenta in a woman who has had a previous Caesarean section, recheck the scan at 28 weeks to consider the risk of placenta acreta
Growth scan	After 24 weeks; can be as often as 2–4-weekly	Previous growth-restricted baby, other risk factors, measurement of a small-for-dates baby, reduced fetal movements
Presentation scan	After 36 weeks	If there is concern that presentation is not cephalic
Amniocentesis	15 weeks onwards	For fetal karyotype; 0.5–1% risk of miscarriage
Chorionic villus biopsy	10 weeks onwards	For fetal karyotype, single-gene disorder; 2% risk of miscarriage
Free fetal DNA maternal test (non-National Health Service)	End of first trimester	To detect trisomy: current guidance advocates use as a screening test only

HIV, *human immunodeficiency virus.*

11

always merits hospital review with a full history and examination. Painless bleeding is more typical of local causes, such a cervical polyp, or of a low-lying placenta, whereas painful bleeding is more in keeping with placental abruption. It is imperative always to consider venous access and send blood for blood count and cross-matching in any pregnant woman presenting with vaginal bleeding.

Abdominal pain

Abdominal pain is common in pregnancy. It can be caused by benign physiological issues such as constipation and is also a common presenting feature of labour when women are contracting in established labour or tightening in early labour. It can also be caused by polyhydramnios or placental abruption.

Any condition causing abdominal pain can present coincidentally in pregnancy, however. A common example is urinary tract infection; less common causes include appendicitis, ovarian cyst accidents or inflammatory bowel disease. It is critical to take a clear history in a pregnant woman with abdominal pain and to perform a full obstetric and abdominal examination, including renal angle palpation. This becomes more difficult as pregnancy progresses and the expanding uterus makes palpation of other organs and masses difficult. Ultrasound or MRI scanning may aid diagnosis.

Pre-eclampsia

Pre-eclampsia is a multifactorial syndrome comprised of high blood pressure, proteinuria and placental compromise, and is a significant cause of maternal and fetal morbidity. It is often asymptomatic and detected by blood pressure monitoring and urinalysis, although some women develop generalised headache and rapidly worsening peripheral oedema. A history focused on headache, worsening oedema and upper abdominal pain should be taken. The examination is that of a routine antenatal assessment but should also include a check for hyper-reflexia and ankle clonus.

Pruritus

Pruritus (itching) affects one-quarter of pregnant women. Rarely, it is associated with liver cholestasis, in which case it is generalised and there is no rash.

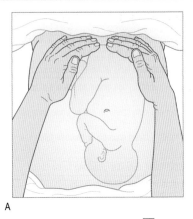 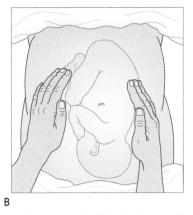 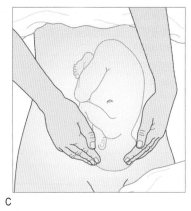

A B C

Fig. 11.35 Abdominal examination. [A] Palpate the fundal area to identify which pole of the fetus (breech or head) is occupying the fundus. [B] Slip your hands gently down the sides of the uterus to identify which side the firm back and knobbly limbs of the fetus are positioned on. [C] Turn to face the patient's feet and slide your hands gently on the lower part of the uterus.

Breathlessness

Mild breathlessness is physiological in pregnancy. Rarely, increased breathlessness is due to pulmonary oedema in pre-eclampsia or exacerbation of heart disease. If breathlessness is associated with chest pain, pulmonary embolism (p. 77) should be considered. The chest should be examined and oxygen saturation and respiratory rate measured. An electrocardiogram is helpful and the risks/benefits of radiological imaging should be assessed.

The physical examination

Examination sequence

- Before examining the patient, ask her to empty her bladder (perform urinalysis). She should lie with her head on a low pillow, with her abdomen exposed from the symphysis pubis to the xiphisternum.
- Examine women in late pregnancy in the left lateral position or semirecumbent, 15 degrees to the horizontal, to avoid vena caval compression, which can cause hypotension for the mother and hypoxia for the fetus.
- Measure blood pressure.
- Note her general demeanour. Is she at ease or distressed by physical pain?
- On inspection look for signs of pregnancy such as the linea nigra (a dark discoloration of the midline of the abdominal skin) and striae gravidarum (stretch marks).
- Look for any scars, particularly from a previous Caesarean section. Note the swelling of the uterus arising from the pelvis and any other swellings. You may also see fetal movements.

Uterine examination

- Ask the patient to report any tenderness and observe her facial and verbal responses constantly.
- Place the flat of your hand on the uterine swelling. Gently flex your fingers to palpate the upper and lateral edges of its firm mass. Note any tenderness, rebound or guarding outside the uterus. Palpate lightly to avoid triggering myometrial contraction, which makes fetal parts difficult to feel. Avoid deep palpation of any tender areas of the uterus. Note any contractions and any fetal movements.

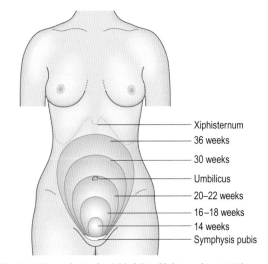

Xiphisternum
36 weeks
30 weeks
Umbilicus
20–22 weeks
16–18 weeks
14 weeks
Symphysis pubis

Fig. 11.36 Approximate fundal height with increasing gestation.

- Face the woman's head. Place both your hands on either side of the fundus and feel the fetal parts. Estimate if the liquor volume is normal. Assess how far from the surface the fetal parts are. If you can feel them only on deep palpation, this implies large amounts of fluid (Fig. 11.35A).
- With your right hand on the woman's left side, feel down both sides of the uterus. The side that is fuller suggests the location of the fetal back (Fig. 11.35B).
- Now face the woman's feet. Place your hands on either side of the uterus, with your left hand on the woman's left side, and feel the lower part of the uterus to try to identify the presenting part. Ballott the head by pushing it gently from one side to the other and feel its hardness move between your fingers (Fig. 11.35C).
- The size of the uterus increases as pregnancy advances (Fig. 11.36). At 20 weeks the uterine fundus is at the umbilicus; by 36 weeks it reaches the xiphisternum. The distance from the pubic symphysis to the top of the uterine fundus is the symphyseal fundal height (SFH). In a singleton pregnancy, if the baby is growing well, the SFH in centimetres approximates to the duration of pregnancy

in weeks. In multiple pregnancy the fundus will measure larger at each stage. After 20 weeks, measure the SFH in centimetres. With a tape measure, fix the end at the highest point on the fundus (not always in the midline) and measure to the top of the symphysis pubis. To avoid bias, place the blank side of the tape facing you, lift the tape and read the measurement on the other side.

- In late pregnancy or labour, you need to assess the fetal lie, fetal presentation and engagement of the head in the maternal pelvis. The lie describes the longitudinal axis of the fetus related to the longitudinal axis of the mother's uterus. Most fetuses have a longitudinal lie in the third trimester (Fig. 11.37).
- The presentation is the part of the fetus's body that is expected to deliver first. With a longitudinal lie, there is either a cephalic or a breech presentation. Finally, assess whether more than 50% of the presenting part has entered the bony pelvis. This is usually the head, which is then said to be engaged (Fig. 11.38).
- Percussion of the pregnant abdomen is unnecessary.
- Listen for the fetal heart if you cannot feel fetal movements. A hand-held Doppler machine can be used from 14 weeks. From 28 weeks, you can use a Pinard stethoscope over the anterior shoulder of the fetus. Face the mother's feet and place your ear against the smaller end. Take your hand away and keep the stethoscope in place using only your head. Listen for the fetal heart, which sounds distant, like a clock through a pillow.
- Do not perform a vaginal examination routinely in pregnancy unless there is a specific indication. Never perform a vaginal examination after 20 weeks unless the placental location is known not to be low, as there is a risk of severe bleeding if it is low.

Abdominal organs are displaced during pregnancy so swelling may be difficult to identify; for example, in the case of ovarian cysts or an inflamed appendix, the pain and tenderness may not be in the usual sites. The kidneys and liver cannot normally be palpated and listening for bowel sounds may be difficult in late pregnancy. In tall or thin patients, the SFH may be smaller than expected; in obese patients, it may be larger. Ultrasound scanning is now used routinely to assess fetal development (Figs 11.39–11.40).

After 25 weeks' gestation a difference of 3 or more between the number of completed weeks of pregnancy and the SFH in centimetres may suggest that the baby is small or large for dates. Investigate this with ultrasound. From 36 weeks a lie other

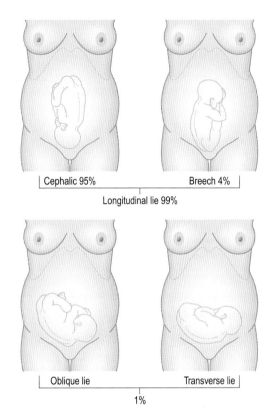

Cephalic 95%   Breech 4%

Longitudinal lie 99%

Oblique lie   Transverse lie

1%

Fig. 11.37 The lie and presentation of the fetus at term.

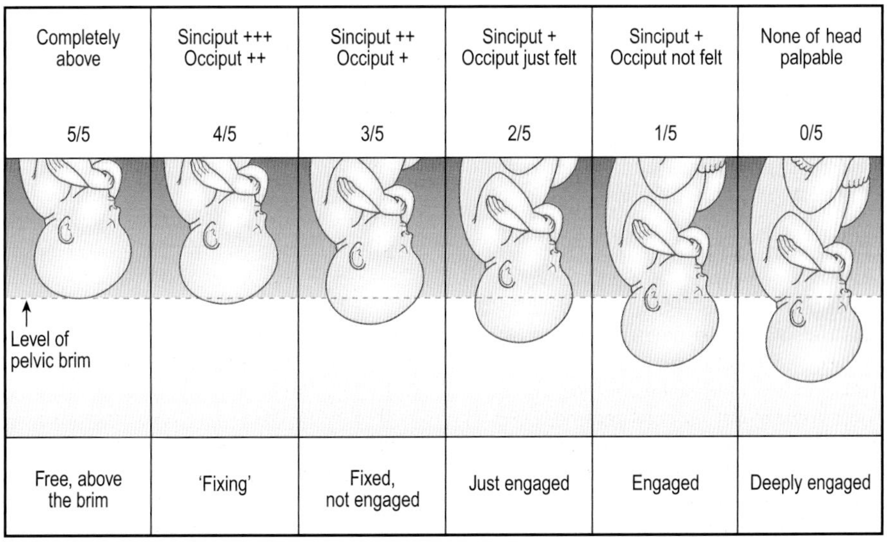

Completely above	Sinciput +++ Occiput ++	Sinciput ++ Occiput +	Sinciput + Occiput just felt	Sinciput + Occiput not felt	None of head palpable
5/5	4/5	3/5	2/5	1/5	0/5
Free, above the brim	'Fixing'	Fixed, not engaged	Just engaged	Engaged	Deeply engaged

Level of pelvic brim

Fig. 11.38 Descent of the fetal head.

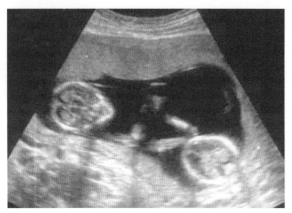

Fig. 11.39 Ultrasound scan at 12 weeks showing a twin pregnancy.

than longitudinal is abnormal and requires further investigation or treatment.

Investigations

Routine investigations are required at specific antenatal visits (Box 11.12).

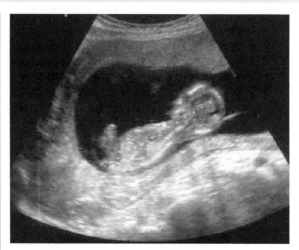

Fig. 11.40 Ultrasound scan at 13 weeks showing crown–rump measurement.

Perform dipstick urinalysis at each visit, looking for glycosuria or proteinuria. Protein of ≥1+ may indicate a urinary tract infection or pre-eclampsia. Glycosuria requires a formal test for gestational diabetes.

MALE REPRODUCTIVE SYSTEM

Anatomy and physiology

The male genitalia include the testes, epididymides and seminal vesicles, penis, scrotum and prostate gland (Fig. 11.41).

The testes develop intra-abdominally near the kidneys, and migrate through the inguinal canal into the scrotum by birth. They have their own blood, lymphatic and nerve supply, so testicular problems may cause abdominal pain and enlargement of the para-aortic lymph nodes. The scrotum is a pouch with thin, pigmented, wrinkled skin that helps to regulate the temperature of the testes (Fig. 11.42), as sperm production is most efficient below body temperature. The left testis lies lower than the right. Each testis is oval, 3.5–4 cm long and covered by the tunica albuginea, which forms the posterior wall of the tunica vaginalis. This is a prolongation of the peritoneal tube that forms as the testis descends during development. If it persists, it may be associated with an indirect inguinal hernia sac or a congenital hydrocoele. Along the posterior border of each testis is the epididymis.

The testes produce sperm and testosterone, starting at puberty (10–15 years of age; see Fig. 15.18). Sperm mature in the epididymis and pass down the vas deferens to the seminal vesicles. They are ejaculated from the urethra, together with prostatic and seminal vesicle fluid, at orgasm.

The penis has two cylinders of endothelium-lined spaces surrounded by smooth muscle, the corpora cavernosa (Fig. 11.43). These are bound with the bulbospongiosus surrounding the urethra, which expands into the glans penis. The penile skin is reflected over the glans, forming the prepuce (foreskin). Sexual arousal causes a parasympathetically mediated increased blood flow into the corpora cavernosa with erection to enable vaginal penetration. Continued stimulation causes sympathetic-mediated

contraction of the seminal vesicles and prostate, closure of the bladder neck and ejaculation. Following orgasm, reduction in blood inflow causes detumescence.

The prostate and seminal vesicles contribute to seminal fluid. After age 40 the prostate develops a trilobar structure because of benign enlargement. Two lateral lobes and a variable median lobe protrude into the bladder and may cause urethral and bladder outflow obstruction. Prostate cancer develops in the peripheral tissue of the lateral lobes and sometimes may be detected by digital rectal examination. Only the posterior aspect and the lateral lobes of the prostate can be felt by rectal examination (p. 111).

The history

Disorders of the male genitals may present as urinary symptoms, genital or pelvic pain, genital swellings, sexual dysfunction or infertility.

In addition to documenting the man's main genital or urinary problems, be sure to ask about:

- the timescale of their development
- how they affect lifestyle and any sexual activity
- sexual function, if appropriate
- past conceptions or problems with fertility
- general urological symptoms:
  - genital swelling
  - genital or pelvic pain
  - lower urinary tract symptoms
  - urethral discharge.

There may be associated systemic upset or clinical signs associated with urological disease; a full history and examination are therefore important.

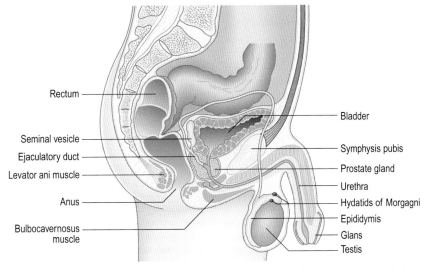

Fig. 11.41 Anatomy of the male genitalia. The male genitalia include the external organs, seminal vesicles and prostate gland.

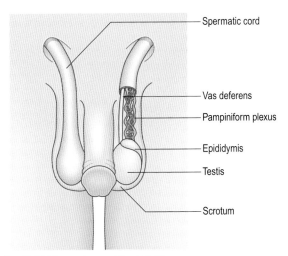

Fig. 11.42 The scrotum and its contents.

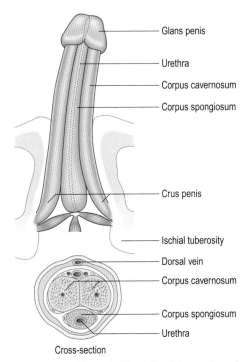

Cross-section

Fig. 11.43 Anatomy of the penis. The shaft and glans penis are formed from the corpus spongiosum and the corpus cavernosum.

Common presenting symptoms

Urinary symptoms

Urinary symptoms are a common presentation of genital or lower urinary tract dysfunction. Dysuria (see below), voiding symptoms and haematuria are covered in detail on pages 239 and 240.

Penile discharge or dysuria

Ask about:
- the duration of discharge or dysuria
- whether these are new or recurrent symptoms
- any other urinary symptoms
- the sexual history
- any systemic upset.

These symptoms usually represent urethritis that is the result of either a sexually transmitted infection (STI) or a urinary tract infection. They may precede and lead to epididymo-orchitis (see later) or prostatitis. Prostatitis is associated with pelvic, perineal or scrotal pain, fever and systemic upset in acute bacterial prostatitis, or may lead to chronic pain and urinary symptoms in chronic prostatitis.

Scrotal swelling or pain

Patients often present acutely with scrotal pain and swelling together; they may also, however, present with either symptom alone.

Ask about:
- duration of the swelling
- whether it is unilateral or bilateral
- association with pain
- onset of pain: sudden or gradual
- character and duration of the pain
- radiation of the pain
- any history of trauma

- any associated symptoms:
  - systemic upset (nausea, vomiting, fever or weight loss)
  - urinary symptoms
  - urethral discharge
- sexual history (see Box 11.4).

There are many causes of scrotal swelling or pain but a patient with sudden-onset unilateral scrotal pain should be considered to have testicular torsion until proven otherwise. Testicular torsion occurs most commonly between the ages of 10 and 30 years and is very rare over the age of 40. Pain is usually of acute onset and excruciating; it is not relieved by lying still. It is often associated with nausea and vomiting but not usually fever, lower urinary tract symptoms or urethral discharge.

Epididymo-orchitis is the most common differential diagnosis. The pain of epididymo-orchitis is often more insidious in onset compared to testicular torsion and the patient may report a dull ache initially. There may be associated fevers, dysuria or urethral discharge, suggesting underlying STI or urinary tract infection. The discomfort is often worse when standing or moving around and may be relieved when lying still. On examination, it is usually possible to distinguish the tender, inflamed epididymis from the adjacent testis. If testicular torsion cannot be excluded on history and examination, urgent testicular exploration is warranted, as torsion will cause loss of a testis if not relieved within 4–6 hours. While an ultrasound examination may be used to confirm a diagnosis of epididymo-orchitis, it should never be requested to assess for torsion.

Other scrotal swellings include hernia, varicocoele, hydrocoele, epididymal cyst and testicular tumour. These are usually painless, although vague or constant dull ache may be described (Fig. 11.44). Examination findings can usually differentiate these diagnoses (Box 11.13).

Penile skin lesions

Ask about:

- location, duration and progress of the lesion
- any pain
- any problem retracting the prepuce
- any associated systemic upset

- any urinary symptoms
- any history of dermatological disease
- sexual history.

The inability to retract the foreskin (phimosis) is a common symptom in the urology clinic. Phimosis may be normal; 95% of babies are born with a non-retractile prepuce but this usually resolves by the age of 16 years, when only 1% of boys have a persistent phimosis. This may produce balanitis (recurrent infection of the glans penis), posthitis (infection of the prepuce) or both (balanoposthitis).

If a tight foreskin is retracted and is not replaced, swelling and pain ensue, resulting in a paraphimosis due to the tight preputial band (Fig. 11.45).

Dermatological conditions and drug reactions may affect the genital skin. Painful genital ulcers are usually caused by herpes simplex; painless ulcers occur in reactive arthritis (p. 257), lichen simplex and (rarely) syphilis. Genital warts may also be present, as well as penile carcinoma.

Erectile dysfunction

Erectile dysfunction (ED) is the consistent or recurrent inability to attain and/or maintain a penile erection sufficient for penetrative intercourse.

Clarify from the history:

- Is the problem failure to gain or maintain an erection, painful erection, penile deformity on erection or a combination of these?
- How long has ED been a problem?
- Has the patient ever been able to gain a rigid erection?
- Does he ever have morning erections on waking?
- Is he able to gain an erection under any circumstances, such as masturbation?
- Do his problems prevent penetrative intercourse?
- Are there any other symptoms of sexual dysfunction, including reduced libido, problems achieving orgasm, premature ejaculation or failure to ejaculate?

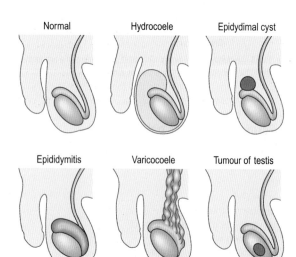

Fig. 11.44 Swellings of the scrotum.

11.13 Summary of examination findings in common scrotal pathologies
Inguinoscrotal: unable to 'get above'
Inguinoscrotal hernia
• May be reducible and have a cough impulse
• Does not transilluminate
• May be associated with bowel sounds on auscultation
Hydrocoele
• Is not reducible
• Transilluminates
• Not associated with bowel sounds
• It is possible to palpate the normal cord above some hydrocoeles
Scrotal mass: able to 'get above'
Epididymal cyst
• Firm, well circumscribed and separate from testicular body
• Transilluminates
Testicular tumour
• A hard, mass that may be well circumscribed or ill defined, arising from the testicular body
• Does not transilluminate
Varicocoele
• Described as feeling like a 'bag of worms' around the cord
• Present on standing or with a Valsalva manœuvre but usually resolves on lying flat

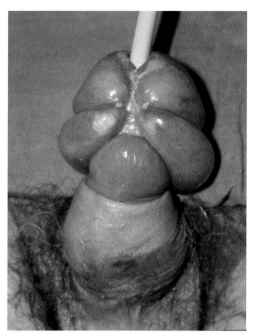

Fig. 11.45 Paraphimosis. Oedema of the foreskin behind an encircling constriction ring caused by the foreskin not being replaced – in this case, after catheterisation.

Consider possible precipitating events: for example, relationship difficulties or trauma. Assess cardiovascular, neurological and psychiatric comorbidities as well as taking a drug history.

If the patient has never had an erection, he may have primary ED due to an anatomical abnormality. Secondary ED is more common and may be psychological or organic in aetiology. Psychological ED may have a precipitating event and loss of erection occurs in some but not all situations; early-morning erections or erections with masturbation usually remain unaffected. Organic ED affects all erections and is often associated with medical comorbidities, including diabetes mellitus, cardiovascular disease, hypertension, peripheral vascular disease, endocrine disorder or neurological disorder. ED is a common early symptom of metabolic syndrome and should precipitate screening for cardiovascular disease and diabetes.

If erections are painful or associated with deformity, the likely diagnosis is Peyronie's disease. This is a fibrotic condition of the penile shaft, of unknown aetiology, producing painful curvature, narrowing or shortening of the corpora cavernosa with erection.

If the problem is a prolonged erection (priapism), establish the duration and whether it is painful. Particular attention should be paid to drug history, history of perineal trauma or past medical history of haematological, neurological or oncological disease. Painful (low-flow or ischaemic) priapism is a urological emergency, which requires urgent treatment to prevent permanent ED.

Past medical history

Ask about previous urological procedures, including neonatal surgery. Record relevant general surgical procedures, particularly pelvic operations that may contribute to lower urinary tract symptoms or ED. Cardiovascular, endocrine, neurological, renal and psychiatric disease may predispose or contribute to both urinary tract symptoms and ED.

Drug history

Ask about previous urological drug treatments and obtain a full list of all medications and drugs taken recreationally. In particular, note drugs such as:

- diuretics: contribute to urinary symptoms
- alpha-blockers: may cause retrograde ejaculation
- antihypertensive agents: may cause erectile dysfunction
- vasoactive drugs, such as alprostadil: may result in a prolonged erection
- antidepressants or antipsychotics: may affect sexual function.

Social history

Smoking, alcohol and recreational drugs can affect fertility and sexual function. Smoking is a significant risk factor for urological cancers.

11

The physical examination

Ensure privacy. Use a warm, well-lit room with a moveable light source. Explain what you are going to do and why it is necessary, and offer a chaperone. Record the chaperone's name; if the offer is refused, record the fact. Apply alcohol gel and put on gloves. Allow the patient privacy to undress.

Ask the patient to stand and expose the area from his lower abdomen to the top of his thighs, unless you are examining the inguinoscrotal area. In this case, ask him to lie on his back initially.

Skin

Examination sequence

- Look in turn at the groin, skin creases, perineum and scrotal skin for redness, swellings or ulcers. Note the hair distribution.
- If you see any swellings in the groin, palpate these and define them using 'SPACESPIT' (see Box 3.8).

There may be alopecia or an infestation. Patients who shave their pubic hair may have dermatitis or folliculitis (infection around the base of the hairs), causing an irritating red rash. Intertrigo (infected eczema) occurs in the skin creases, and lymphadenopathy may stem from local or general causes.

Scrotal oedema can be caused by systemic or local disease. Heart and liver dysfunction may lead to significant genital oedema, as may nephrotic syndrome and lymphoedema due to pelvic lymphadenopathy.

Penis

Examination sequence

- Look at the shaft and check the position of the urethral opening to exclude hypospadias (urethra opening partway along the shaft of the penis; see Fig. 15.11A).
- Palpate the shaft for fibrous plaques (usually on the dorsum). Palpate any other lesions to define them.
- Retract the prepuce and inspect the glans for red patches or vesicles.

- Always draw the foreskin forward after examination to avoid a paraphimosis.
- Take a urethral swab if your patient has a discharge or is having sexual health screening.

Normal enlarged follicles may mimic warts. Numerous uniform, pearly penile papules around the corona of the glans are normal.

Warts, sebaceous cysts, or a hard plaque of Peyronie's disease may occur on the shaft and phimosis, adhesions, inflammation or swellings on the foreskin or glans.

Scrotum

Examine the scrotum with the man standing. Then ask him to lie down if you find a swelling you cannot 'get above'. Ask the patient whether he has any genital pain. If he is cold or apprehensive, the dartos muscle contracts and you will not be able to palpate the scrotal contents properly.

Examination sequence

- Inspect the scrotum for redness, swelling or ulcers, lifting it to inspect the posterior surface.
- Note the position of the testes and any paratesticular swelling and tenderness.
- Palpate the scrotum gently, using both hands. Check that both testes are present. If they are not, examine the inguinal canal and perineum, checking for undescended or ectopic testes.
- Place the fingers of both your hands behind each testis in turn to immobilise it and use your index finger and thumb to palpate the body of the testis methodically. Feel the anterior surface and medial border with your thumb and the lateral border with your index finger (Fig. 11.46).
- Check the size and consistency of the testis. Note any nodules or irregularities. Measure the testicular size in centimetres from one to the other.
- Palpate the spermatic cord with your right hand. Gently pull the testis downward and place your fingers behind the neck of the scrotum. Feel the spermatic cord and within it the vas, like a thick piece of string.
- Decide whether a swelling arises in the scrotum or from the inguinal canal. If you can feel above the swelling, it originates from the scrotum; if you cannot, the swelling usually originates in the inguinal region (Fig. 11.47).
- Check any inguinoscrotal swelling for a cough impulse and auscultate for bowel sounds.

- Place the bright end of a torch against a scrotal swelling (transillumination; see Fig. 15.9). Fluid-filled cysts allow light transmission and the scrotum glows bright red. This is an inconsistent sign, which does not differentiate a hydrocoele from other causes of intrascrotal fluid such as a large epididymal cyst. With thick-walled cysts, transillumination may be absent.

The right testicle is usually closer to the inguinal canal than the left but the testes may be highly mobile (retractile). A normal testis is 5 cm long. The normal epididymis is barely palpable, except for its head (Fig. 11.48), which feels like a pea separate from the superior pole of the body of the testicle.

Sebaceous cysts are common in the scrotal skin. If you can get above a scrotal swelling, it is a true scrotal swelling. If not, it may be a varicocoele or inguinal hernia that has descended into the scrotum (see Fig. 11.44).

Varicocoele

A varicocoele is a dilatation of the veins of the pampiniform plexus and feels like a 'bag of worms' in the cord when the patient is standing and should disappear when he lies down. If it does not, consider a retroperitoneal mass, such as a renal cancer, compressing the testicular veins.

Hydrocoele

These are swellings caused by fluid in the tunica vaginalis. They are usually idiopathic but may be secondary to inflammatory conditions or tumours.

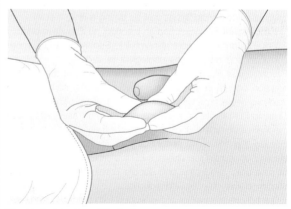

Fig. 11.46 Palpation of the testis.

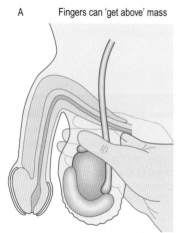
A   Fingers can 'get above' mass

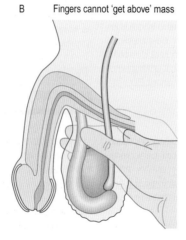
B   Fingers cannot 'get above' mass

Fig. 11.47 Testing for scrotal swellings. [A] It is possible to 'get above' a true scrotal swelling. [B] This is not possible if the swelling is caused by an inguinal hernia that has descended into the scrotum.

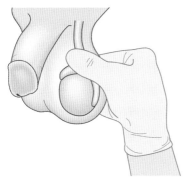

Fig. 11.48 **Palpation of the epididymis.** The epididymis is readily felt only at the top of the testis.

Epididymal cyst

Swellings of the epididymis that are felt to be completely separate from the body of the testis are epididymal cysts. They are isolated and adherent to the epididymis alone, they transilluminate and are never malignant. Painful swellings at the superior pole of the testis, or adjacent to the head of the epididymis, are usually due to torsion of a paramesonephric duct remnant, the hydatids of Morgagni.

Testicular tumour

Testicular tumours cause painless, hard swellings of the body of the testis. Around 15% of tumours may occur close to the rete testis and may give rise to epididymal swelling and pain.

Epididymitis

Inflammation of the epididymis produces painful epididymal swelling, most often caused by an STI in young men, or a coliform urinary infection in the elderly.

Testicular torsion

A retracted or high-lying testicle, accompanied by acute pain and swelling, occurs in testicular torsion (Fig. 11.49).

Single testis

This may be due to incomplete testicular descent of the 'missing' testis through the inguinal canal or an ectopic testis in the groin. Ask about previous surgery for a testicular tumour or testicular maldescent. Unilateral testicular atrophy may result from mumps infection, torsion, vascular compromise after inguinal hernia repair, or from a late orchidopexy for undescended testis.

Bilateral testicular atrophy

This suggests primary, or secondary, hypogonadism (p. 204) or primary testicular failure. Look for hormonal abnormalities or signs of anabolic steroid usage, and check the development of secondary sexual characteristics (see Fig. 15.19).

Prostate

Ask the patient to lie in the left lateral position.

Examination sequence

- Perform a rectal examination (p. 111).
- Palpate the prostate through the anterior rectal wall.

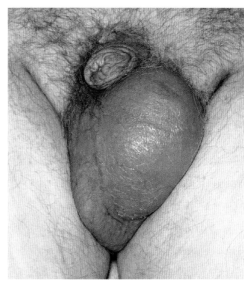

Fig. 11.49 **Left testicular torsion.** There is shortening of the cord with retraction of the testis and global swelling of the scrotal contents. Refer the patient urgently to a surgeon for scrotal exploration.

- Note any tenderness.
- Assess size, symmetry and consistency. Is it hard or boggy?
- Feel for any nodules.
- Withdraw your finger. Give the patient tissues to clean himself and privacy in which to get dressed.

The prostate is normally smooth, rubbery, non-tender and about the size of a walnut. It has defined margins with an indentation, or sulcus, between the two lateral lobes. Sometimes the seminal vesicles are felt above the prostate.

Tenderness or soft 'bogginess' suggests prostatitis or prostatic abscess.

Prostate cancer may cause a discrete nodule, a craggy mass or obliteration of the midline sulcus, and the prostate may feel fixed to the lateral pelvic side wall.

Investigations

The relevant urological investigations depend on the clinical problem revealed on history and examination. First-catch urine can be tested for both *Chlamydia trachomatis* and *Neisseria gonorrhoeae* from a single specimen using nucleic acid amplification tests, and this should be performed for all men presenting with urethritis or acute scrotal pain suspected to be due to epididymo-orchitis. Scrotal ultrasound is the gold standard for confirming the clinical diagnosis of scrotal swelling or pain, with the exception of testicular torsion.

When prostate cancer is suspected a prostate-specific antigen (PSA) blood test should be requested. PSA is raised in prostate cancer but also increases with age, prostatic volume, following prostatic trauma and in seminal or urinary tract infection. If the PSA is elevated, a transrectal ultrasound or MRI scan of the prostate may be considered to investigate for prostate carcinoma.

Early-morning testosterone should be measured in all patients with erectile dysfunction to assess for hypogonadism.

OSCE example 1: Breast examination

Ms McIntyre, 27 years old, presents with a 6-week history of a lump in her right breast.

Please examine her breast

- Introduce yourself and clean your hands.
- Obtain verbal consent for the examination from the patient.
- Offer a chaperone.
- Ask her to undress to the waist and sit on the edge of the bed.
- Inspect for asymmetry, skin or nipple changes, or obvious lumps.
- Ask her to put her hands on her hips and push in while you look for changes in the breast.
- Ask her to lie on the couch with her upper body at 45 degrees. Palpate her breasts, noting the characteristics of any lumps.
- Examine her axillae and supraclavicular fossae.
- Thank the patient and clean your hands.

Summarise your findings

There is a firm, mobile, non-tender lump about 2 cm in diameter at 11 o'clock in the right breast, 5 cm from the nipple. There are no overlying skin changes and the lump is not tethered. I could feel no lymphadenopathy in the neck or axilla.

Suggest a diagnosis

One possible diagnosis is breast cancer. The differential includes fibrocystic disease, a breast cyst or an abscess.

Suggest investigations

Triple assessment: clinical assessment, ultrasound scan and ultrasound-guided core biopsy.

OSCE example 2: Scrotal pain history

Mr Atkins, 20 years old, presents to the emergency department with scrotal pain.

Please take a focused history

- Introduce yourself and clean your hands.
- Obtain verbal consent to take a history from the patient.
- Ask an open question about why this person has come to the emergency department.
- Explore the symptoms offered at presentation – in this case, scrotal pain:
  - time of onset and duration
  - severity of pain
  - exacerbating/relieving factors
  - constant or intermittent nature
  - radiation to groin or loin
  - any precipitating event such as trauma
  - associated urinary symptoms, urethral discharge, swelling, fever, nausea or weight loss
  - sexual history
  - past medical history, including undescended testes
  - drug history
  - social history.

Summarise your findings

The patient reports a gradual onset of aching testicular and scrotal pain with some associated urethral discharge and fever.

Suggest a differential diagnosis

This history is most suggestive of epididymo-orchitis. The differential includes testicular torsion and testicular cancer.

Suggest initial investigations

Ultrasound may confirm epididymo-orchitis, but if testicular torsion cannot be excluded on history and examination, urgent testicular exploration is required.

Neeraj Dhaun
David Kluth

12

The renal system

Anatomy and physiology

The kidneys lie posteriorly in the abdomen, retroperitoneally on either side of the spine at the T12–L3 level, and are 11–14 cm long (Fig. 12.1). The right kidney lies 1.5 cm lower than the left because of the liver. The liver and spleen lie anterior to the kidneys. The kidneys move downwards during inspiration as the lungs expand.

Together, the kidneys receive approximately 25% of cardiac output. Each kidney contains about 1 million nephrons, each comprising a glomerulus, proximal tubule, loop of Henle, distal tubule and collecting duct (Fig. 12.2). Urine is formed by glomerular filtration, modified by complex processes of secretion and reabsorption in the tubules, and then enters the calyces and the renal pelvis.

The primary functions of the kidneys are:

- excretion of waste products of metabolism such as urea and creatinine
- maintenance of salt, water and electrolyte homeostasis
- regulation of blood pressure via the renin–angiotensin system
- endocrine functions related to erythropoiesis and vitamin D metabolism.

The renal capsule and ureter are innervated by T10–12/L1 nerve roots; pain from these structures is felt in these dermatomes.

The bladder acts as a reservoir. As it fills, it becomes ovoid, and rises out of the pelvis in the midline towards the umbilicus, behind the anterior abdominal wall. The bladder wall contains a layer of smooth muscle, the detrusor, which contracts under parasympathetic control, allowing urine to pass through the urethra (micturition). The conscious desire to micturate occurs when the bladder holds approximately 250–350 mL of urine. The male urethra runs from the bladder to the tip of the penis and has three parts: prostatic, membranous and spongiose (Fig. 12.3). The female urethra is much shorter, with the external meatus situated anterior to the vaginal orifice and behind the clitoris (Fig. 12.4). Two muscular rings acting as valves (sphincters) control micturition:

- The internal sphincter is at the bladder neck and is involuntary.
- The external sphincter surrounds the membranous urethra and is under voluntary control; it is innervated by the pudendal nerves (S2–4).

The anatomy and physiology of the prostate are covered in more detail on page 230.

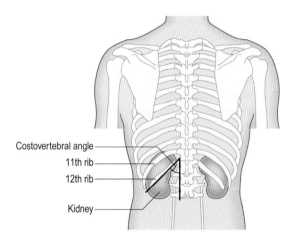

Fig. 12.1 **The surface anatomy of the kidneys from the back.**

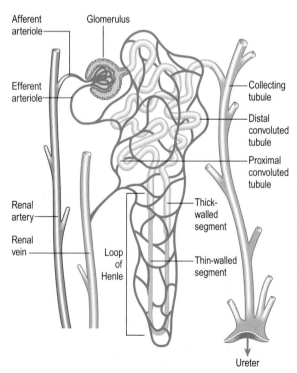

Fig. 12.2 **A single nephron.**

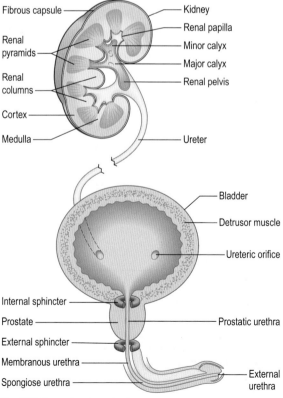

Fig. 12.3 **The male urinary tract.**

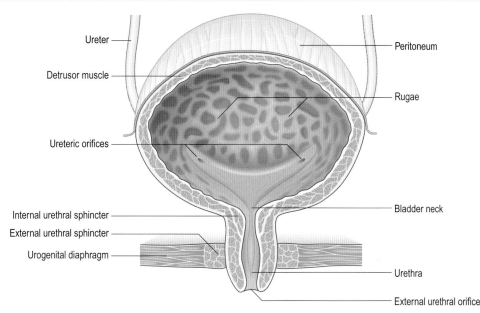

Fig. 12.4 **The female urinary tract.**

The history

Renal disease may be asymptomatic or present with non-specific symptoms such as lethargy or breathlessness. It is usually only after initial investigation that the history taking can be focused on the possible renal causes.

Common presenting symptoms

Dysuria

Dysuria (pain or discomfort during urination) is a common symptom of urinary tract infection (UTI). There is usually associated urinary frequency and urgency, and suprapubic discomfort (cystitis). Other causes include urethritis and acute prostatitis (which may be associated with severe perineal or rectal pain).

Ask about:

- Systemic upset with fever, and suprapubic discomfort. Pyelonephritis is suggested by a history of significant fever (>38.0°C), rigors, vomiting and flank pain. There may not always be symptoms of a preceding UTI.
- Symptoms of urine outflow obstruction (slow flow, hesitancy, incomplete emptying, dribbling, nocturia).
- History of sexual contacts.

Loin pain

Severe loin pain is usually due to ureteric obstruction; renal calculi are the most common cause. The pain often comes in waves and is described as 'colicky'. The patient is unable to find a comfortable position and will move around the bed (unlike a patient with peritonism, who lies still).

Ask about:

- Location of the pain: is it just in the loin (pelvic/upper ureter obstruction) or does it radiate into the testicle or labium (lower ureter obstruction)?
- Presence of fever, rigors and dysuria: these may suggest infection.
- Previous episodes of loin pain.

Loin pain may also occur due to bleeding from a renal or ureteric tumour, or due to infection. Non-renal causes of loin pain, such as a leaking aortic aneurysm (in older patients with vascular disease) and ectopic pregnancy (in women of child-bearing age), should be considered.

Voiding symptoms

Symptoms are usually due to either bladder storage or voiding-phase problems.

Ask about:

- Urgency, frequency, nocturia and urge incontinence (storage symptoms).
- Hesitancy, poor stream, straining to void and terminal dribbling (voiding symptoms). These symptoms may be followed by a sense of incomplete emptying.

Storage symptoms are usually associated with bladder, prostate or urethral problems, such as UTI, tumour, urethral calculi or obstruction from prostatic enlargement, or are caused by neurological disease such as multiple sclerosis.

Voiding symptoms are often the result of bladder outflow obstruction from prostatic enlargement (in men), urethral obstruction or genital prolapse (in women).

In women, incontinence is the most common symptom. Stress incontinence is urine leakage with increased abdominal pressure (such as when coughing or sneezing, or due to weakened pelvic floor muscles) and urge incontinence is the urge to pass urine followed by involuntary leakage. These symptoms can occur separately or together and increase with age. Overflow incontinence occurs without warning, often on changes in position, and is painless.

Polyuria, the passing of higher volumes of urine, has a number of causes, including excess water intake, osmotic diuresis (as in diabetes mellitus) and diabetes insipidus (inadequate secretion or action of vasopressin (antidiuretic hormone, ADH)).

Oliguria (passing of less than 500 mL of urine per day) and anuria (complete absence of urine) may be due to either very low fluid intake, mechanical obstruction or loss of kidney function (see later).

Labels in figure: Ureter, Detrusor muscle, Ureteric orifices, Internal urethral sphincter, External urethral sphincter, Urogenital diaphragm, Peritoneum, Rugae, Bladder neck, Urethra, External urethral orifice

Pneumaturia, passing gas bubbles in the urine, is suggestive of a fistula between the bladder and the colon, from a diverticular abscess, malignancy or inflammatory bowel disease.

Haematuria

The presence of blood in the urine is common. It may either be seen by the patient (visible haematuria) or be identified by urinalysis or microscopy (non-visible).

Visible haematuria

Visible haematuria will be described as pink, red or brown in colour. Ask about previous episodes, their time course and whether they were persistent or intermittent. Haematuria can arise anywhere along the renal tract from the glomerulus to the bladder (Fig. 12.5). Immunoglobulin A (IgA) nephropathy is the most common glomerular cause, which is often preceded by a non-specific upper respiratory tract infection. The haematuria associated with bladder tumours is usually painless and intermittent.

Ask about:

- Loin pain, as this may indicate ureteric obstruction due to blood, calculi or a tumour. Flank pain and haematuria may be features of renal cell carcinoma.
- Fever, dysuria, suprapubic pain and urinary frequency, which may indicate urinary infection.
- Family history of renal disease; polycystic kidney disease can present with visible haematuria due to cyst rupture.

Non-visible haematuria

Non-visible (or microscopic) haematuria is a dipstick urinalysis abnormality, with 1+ considered positive. It can indicate renal or urinary tract disease, especially if associated with proteinuria, hypertension or impaired renal function. The risk of malignancy increases with age; further evaluation is important in patients over 40 years, even in the absence of other symptoms. Non-visible haematuria in women of reproductive age is most commonly due to contamination by menstrual blood.

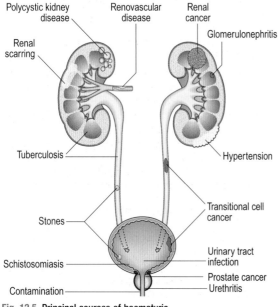

Fig. 12.5 Principal sources of haematuria.

Proteinuria and nephrotic syndrome

Proteinuria is the excretion of more than 150 mg per day of protein in the urine. It is usually asymptomatic but, if persistent, may indicate underlying renal disease.

Nephrotic syndrome is characterised by the combination of heavy proteinuria (>3.5 g/24 hours), hypoalbuminaemia and oedema. Nephrotic syndrome may come on over a few weeks (as in minimal change disease) and cause acute kidney injury (AKI), or it can evolve over many months (as in membranous nephropathy), giving a picture of chronic kidney disease (CKD). The most common cause of nephrotic syndrome is diabetes mellitus, although it can also be the result of other systemic diseases, including malignancy. Patients may notice that the urine is frothy due to the proteinuria. Hyperlipidaemia, hypercoagulability and an increased risk of infection may also develop.

Ask about:

- Weight loss, altered bowel habit, cough, back pain or chronic inflammatory conditions such as rheumatoid arthritis, inflammatory bowel disease or bronchiectasis (in particular if undertreated). The latter cause nephrotic syndrome as a result of renal AA amyloid deposition.
- Ankle swelling (pitting oedema). Younger patients may also notice facial swelling and puffy eyelids, especially first thing in the morning.
- Breathlessness (pleural effusions).
- Abdominal swelling (ascites).

Acute kidney injury

Acute kidney injury (AKI; Box 12.1) covers a range of presentations from relatively mild changes in kidney function to dialysis-requiring renal failure. The typical presentation is with a recently identified rise in serum creatinine. AKI may have prerenal, renal or postrenal causes (Box 12.2); there is an increased risk in patients with pre-existing CKD. The history should focus on differentiating between these.

Prerenal AKI

This is almost always due to volume depletion.

Ask about:

- fluid losses such as vomiting, diarrhoea or bleeding, and inadequate oral intake due to nausea or delirium

12.1 Definition of acute kidney injury		
RIFLE[a] AKIN[b]	Serum creatinine criteria	Urine output criteria
Risk AKIN stage 1	Increase >50%	<0.5 mL/kg/h for 6 hours
Injury AKIN stage 2	Increase >100%	<0.5 mL/kg/h for 12 hours
Failure AKIN stage 3	Increase >200% or serum creatinine >350 μmol/L (3.96 mg/dL)	<0.3 mL/kg/h for 24 hours or anuria for 12 hours
Loss	Renal replacement therapy for >4 weeks	–
End-stage kidney disease	Renal replacement therapy for >3 months	–

[a]Risk, Injury, Failure, Loss, End-stage kidney disease.
[b]Acute Kidney Injury Network.

12.2 Causes of acute kidney injury

Prerenal

- Hypovolaemia (e.g. blood loss, diarrhoea, vomiting, diuresis, inadequate oral intake)
- Relative hypovolaemia (e.g. heart failure, nephrotic syndrome)
- Sepsis
- Drugs (e.g. antihypertensives, diuretics, non-steroidal anti-inflammatory drugs)
- Renal artery stenosis or occlusion
- Hepatorenal syndrome

Intrarenal

- Glomerular disease (e.g. systemic vasculitis, systemic lupus erythematosus, immunoglobulin A nephropathy)
- Interstitial nephritis (drug-induced)
- Acute tubular necrosis/injury (may follow a prerenal cause)
- Multiple myeloma
- Rhabdomyolysis
- Intrarenal crystal deposition (e.g. urate nephropathy, ethylene glycol poisoning)
- Thrombotic microangiopathy (e.g. haemolytic uraemic syndrome, scleroderma renal crisis)
- Accelerated-phase hypertension
- Cholesterol emboli

Postrenal

- Renal stones (in papilla, ureter or bladder)
- Papillary necrosis
- Ureteric or bladder transitional cell carcinoma
- Intra-abdominal or pelvic malignancy (e.g. cervical carcinoma)
- Retroperitoneal fibrosis
- Blood clot
- Bladder outflow obstruction (e.g. prostatic enlargement)
- Neurogenic bladder
- Urethral stricture
- Posterior urethral valves
- Iatrogenic (e.g. ureteric damage at surgery, blocked urethral catheter)

- recent operations or investigations that may be associated with increased fluid losses or reduced intake (fasting, bowel preparation)
- any features of infection such as fever, sweats, productive cough or dysuria.

Establish whether there is an underlying condition that may predispose to a reduction in renal blood flow.
Ask about:

- history of heart failure or liver disease
- recent drug prescriptions such as those that block the renin–angiotensin system (for example, angiotensin-converting enzyme inhibitors), other antihypertensive agents, diuretics (such as furosemide or spironolactone) and non-steroidal anti-inflammatory drugs (NSAIDs). NSAIDs can also cause intrinsic renal disease.

Intrinsic AKI

The most common cause in the hospital setting will be acute tubular injury (ATI), which may lead to acute tubular necrosis (ATN). This usually follows renal hypoperfusion when any of the causes identified above results in ischaemia–reperfusion injury.

A less common cause is rhabdomyolysis, which is suggested by a history of prolonged immobilisation, such as following a fall. ATI normally recovers but this can take days to weeks. AKI can also be the first clinical presentation of a systemic disease that affects the kidney (such as myeloma, infective endocarditis, vasculitis or systemic lupus erythematosus).
Ask about:

- Recent illnesses or operations.
- Drug history and any recent changes in medications. Several commonly prescribed medications (such as antibiotics, NSAIDs, proton pump inhibitors) are recognised as causing an allergic interstitial nephritis but almost any drug can be implicated.
- Symptoms of systemic disease: weight loss, fever, night sweats, tiredness, arthralgia, myalgia, bony pain, numbness, weakness, rashes, cough and breathlessness.

Occasionally, AKI can be the result of a primary glomerulonephritis. IgA nephropathy is the most common cause in the northern and western hemispheres. This classically presents with visible haematuria following an upper respiratory tract infection, so-called 'synpharyngitic haematuria'.
Ask about:

- prior episodes
- loin pain and haematuria
- previous sore throat; a similar clinical illness can occur in postinfectious glomerulonephritis due to preceding beta-haemolytic streptococcal infection of the throat or skin.

Postrenal AKI

This is usually due to any cause of obstruction from the renal pelvis to the urethra. The most common cause is bladder outflow obstruction; in men, this is often due to prostatic hypertrophy, either benign or malignant.
Ask about:

- urinary urgency, frequency, nocturia and incontinence
- poor urine stream and terminal dribbling
- previous prostatic assessments, including prostate examination and measurements of prostate-specific antigen
- suprapubic pain
- leg weakness, perineal numbness or faecal incontinence (may indicate a spinal cord lesion).

In acute urinary retention there is usually a complete inability to pass urine and associated suprapubic discomfort. Chronic urinary retention is usually painless.

For ureteric disease to cause AKI, both kidneys need to be affected (or the patient has a single functioning kidney). Ureteric obstruction is most commonly due to malignancy, such as that of the bladder, cervix, ovary or uterus. These conditions are usually painless. The history should explore any previous diagnosis and recent operations and treatment, including radiotherapy.

Chronic kidney disease

Chronic kidney disease (CKD) is defined by degree of renal dysfunction and/or the presence of proteinuria (Boxes 12.3 and 12.4); these need to be present for at least 3 months. The diagnosis of CKD therefore requires preceding biochemical data to enable its distinction from AKI. Most patients with CKD have few symptoms until they have end-stage kidney disease.

12.3 Definition of chronic kidney disease (CKD)

CKD stage	eGFR (mL/min/1.73 m^2)	Description	Management
1	≥90	Kidney damage with normal or ↑ GFR	
2	60–89	Kidney damage with mild ↓ GFR	
3A	45–59	Moderate ↓ GFR	Observe; control blood pressure and risk factors
3B	30–44		
4	15–29	Severe ↓ GFR	Prepare for end-stage kidney disease
5	<15	End-stage kidney disease	Dialysis, transplantation or conservative care

p: the addition of p to a stage (e.g. 2p, 3Bp) means that there is significant proteinuria. Proteinuria is quantified on the basis of an albumin:creatinine (ACR) or protein:creatinine (PCR; see Box 12.4).
T: the addition of T to a stage (e.g. 4T) indicates that the patient has a renal transplant.
D: the addition of D to stage 5 CKD (i.e. 5D) indicates that the patient is on dialysis.

(e)GFR, (estimated) glomerular filtration rate.

12.4 Quantification of proteinuria using either urine albumin:creatinine ratio (ACR) or protein:creatinine ratio (PCR)

ACR (mg/mmol)	PCR (mg/mmol)	Interpretation
>2.5/3.5[a]	>15	Abnormal; adequate to define CKD stages 1 and 2; start ACE inhibitor or angiotensin-receptor blocker if diabetes is present
30	>50	Use ACE inhibitor or angiotensin-receptor blocker if blood pressure is elevated; suffix 'p' on CKD stage
70	100	Requires tight blood pressure control
>250	>300	Nephrotic-range proteinuria

[a]Values for males/females.
ACE, angiotensin-converting enzyme; CKD, chronic kidney disease.

The key in earlier stages is to ask about:

- underlying conditions that may explain the aetiology of CKD, including diabetes mellitus, vascular disease (evidence of previous myocardial infarction, stroke or peripheral vascular disease), hypertension, hyperlipidaemia, episodes of acute glomerulonephritis (such as IgA nephropathy) or nephrotic syndrome (such as membranous disease)
- previous incidental urine abnormalities such as proteinuria or non-visible haematuria that may suggest a preceding glomerular disease.

A number of genetic diseases can present with CKD, so a detailed family history is required (see later).

End-stage renal disease and uraemia

Occasionally, patients will present with symptoms of uraemia. This is most common in patients with known end-stage kidney disease, once the estimated GFR (eGFR) is <10 mL/min/1.73 m^2. The symptoms are often non-specific.

Ask about:

- anorexia, nausea and vomiting
- lethargy
- poor concentration

- pruritus
- breathlessness, which may occur due to fluid overload, worsening acidosis and/or anaemia
- peripheral oedema.

Less commonly, uraemia may present with features of pericarditis or peripheral neuropathy.

The patient with a renal transplant

Identifying the fact that a patient has had a kidney transplant is important early in the history. The main presenting problems are a decline in kidney function (usually identified by routine blood tests), infection or malignancy. The risks of the latter two are increased by immunosuppression. Infections in renal transplant patients may be masked by immunosuppression. It is important to consider lymphoma in the early years after a transplant.

Ask about:

- Date of transplant operation; organ rejection is more common in the first few weeks.
- Current and previous immunosuppression and any recent changes in treatment that may increase the risk of rejection; any intercurrent illness that may have contributed to AKI.
- Fever, weight loss, cough, breathlessness, dysuria and tenderness over the graft.

The dialysis patient

There are two main forms of dialysis: haemodialysis and peritoneal dialysis. Each group can have specific presentations. Haemodialysis is delivered via an arteriovenous fistula or tunnelled vascular access catheter. A fistula has an obvious thrill (p. 243) and the patient may complain that this has been lost. This is usually due to thrombosis and needs urgent attention from a vascular surgeon. The most common problem with vascular access catheters is infection. Peritoneal dialysis involves a tunnelled catheter and infection is also a common presentation. Ask about fever and rigors (and their relation to haemodialysis), abdominal pain and peritoneal dialysate fluid appearance (has it become 'cloudy'?)

Other presenting symptoms

Finally, hypertension, anaemia and electrolyte disorders are other common features of renal disease.

Past medical history

Ask the patient about their past medical history, including hypertension, vascular disease, diabetes mellitus, inflammatory diseases (such as rheumatoid arthritis, inflammatory bowel disease, chronic infections), urinary tract stones or surgery, and previous evidence of renal disease, which may include dialysis and renal transplantation.

Drug history

Enquire about long-term medication, any recent changes in treatment, recent courses of antibiotics and use of non-prescription medications such as NSAIDs and herbal remedies.

Family history

Document any family history of renal disease, hypertension, stroke, diabetes or deafness. If the parents are deceased, ask at what age and if the cause of death is known. The most common inherited renal conditions are autosomal dominant polycystic kidney disease (ADPKD) and Alport syndrome. ADPKD usually affects members in each generation, and both male and females are affected. However, around 10% of those affected have no preceding family history, possibly because family members died before the diagnosis was made. There is an association with berry aneurysms, so enquire about a history of subarachnoid haemorrhage in family members. Alport syndrome is caused by abnormalities in type IV collagen and can be associated with early-onset deafness. It is genetically heterogeneous but the X-linked form is most common. The typical presentation is with non-visible haematuria in childhood or more significant renal disease in the late teenage and early adult years.

Social history

Ask about smoking, alcohol intake and recreational drug use. Ask about the patient's social support (family, housing, social work input) and occupation. Enquire as to how independent they are in their activities of daily living and how their illness has affected their work.

The physical examination

The renal system can affect many aspects of the physical examination but this may also be relatively normal, even with significant disease.

General appearance

Advanced CKD is most likely to alter the general appearance. The patient may look unwell with pallor; the skin may have scratch marks from pruritus and in severe cases there may be drowsiness, myoclonic twitching (p. 136) or asterixis (p. 104). In marked uraemia the patient's skin may appear yellow but this a late feature. Hiccupping may occur. Breathlessness may represent fluid overload, or hyperventilation due to metabolic acidosis.

Hands

Examine the hands, looking for pallor of the palmar creases suggestive of anaemia. Inspect the nails, looking for Muehrcke's lines (Fig. 12.6), which may be a sign of hypoalbuminaemia (nephrotic syndrome), or the half-and-half (Lindsay's) nails of CKD (proximal half white, distal half red or brown; Fig. 12.7).

Dialysis access

Examine the arms for an arteriovenous fistula. This will look like prominent blood vessels on the forearm or upper arm (Fig. 12.8); there may be scars from previous fistulae on either arm. A functioning fistula will have a readily palpable fluid thrill (a continuous buzzing feel). A tunnelled venous access catheter may be seen exiting the anterior chest wall; the line can be followed under the skin and then entering the internal jugular vein (Fig. 12.9).

Face

Inspect the face for rashes, which may indicate underlying connective tissue disease: the butterfly rash of systemic lupus erythematosus, for example. Look for conjunctival pallor, as anaemia is common in CKD. An inflamed eye, seen with scleritis and/or uveitis, may occur in systemic vasculitis. Fundoscopy may reveal changes of diabetic or hypertensive retinopathy (see Figs 8.17–8.18). Most patients with CKD due to diabetes mellitus will

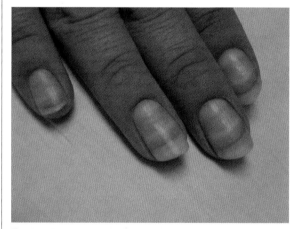

Fig. 12.6 Muehrcke's lines. *From Short N, Shah C. Muehrcke's lines. American Journal of Medicine 2010; 123(11):991–992, Elsevier.*

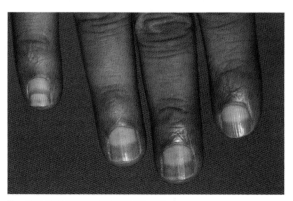

Fig. 12.7 Half-and-half (Lindsay's) nails.

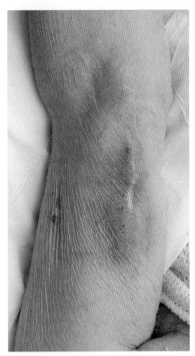

Fig. 12.8 Haemodialysis fistula.

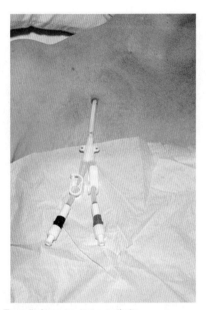

Fig. 12.9 Tunnelled venous access catheter.

have evidence of retinal disease. The presence of hypertensive retinopathy (such as arteriolar narrowing, arteriovenous nipping, cotton-wool exudates or blot haemorrhages) indicates chronic end-organ damage due to high blood pressure; more severe fundoscopy signs, such as flame haemorrhages and papilloedema, may indicate accelerated-phase hypertension, which can cause AKI. Inspection of the mouth may reveal gingival hyperplasia caused by calcineurin inhibitors (such as ciclosporin or tacrolimus). Uraemic fetor may be present.

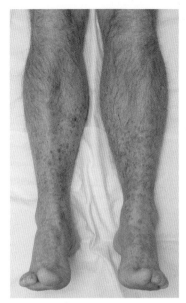

Fig. 12.10 Vasculitic rash.

Skin

Inspect the skin more generally for rashes, bruising, scratch marks and excoriations. A vasculitic rash will appear as purpura, most commonly on the legs (Fig. 12.10), and may be due to systemic vasculitis, Henoch–Schönlein purpura or cryoglobulinaemia, all of which can cause AKI and CKD. A drug rash increases the likelihood of an allergic interstitial nephritis.

Assessment of fluid balance

An accurate check on fluid balance is critical to assessing renal disease and can be completed as a single sequenced process.

General appearance

Does the patient look hypovolaemic or fluid-overloaded? In a dehydrated patient the eyes may appear sunken and the mucous membranes dry. Pinch the skin over the anterior chest wall (rather than forearms) to determine if there is reduced skin turgor (elasticity). These features, although relatively insensitive, are most common when there has been significant salt and water loss, as occurs with vomiting or diarrhoea. A patient with fluid overload may be breathless due to pulmonary oedema or pleural effusions, and there may be obvious signs of peripheral oedema.

Pulse and blood pressure

Measure pulse and blood pressure (avoiding an arm with an arteriovenous fistula). Hypertension is common in renal disease. Is there evidence of hypovolaemia (tachycardia, hypotension)? Ascertaining whether blood pressure falls when the patients stands or sits upright is a sensitive indicator of hypovolaemia.

Jugular venous pressure

Assess the jugular venous pressure (JVP; p. 52). The JVP may be elevated due to fluid overload or, rarely, due to cardiac tamponade from uraemic pericarditis.

Examination of the chest

Examine the chest for signs of pulmonary oedema and/or pleural effusion (p. 88); both are features of fluid overload. Auscultate the heart (p. 55), listening for a third heart sound, which provides further evidence of fluid overload. A fourth heart sound may indicate left ventricular stiffening due to hypertension. A flow murmur may be present in anaemia of chronic renal disease. Quiet heart sounds suggest a pericardial effusion. A pericardial rub may occur in uraemia.

Peripheral oedema

Examine for pitting oedema at the base of the spine (sacral oedema, common in bed-bound patients) and in the legs, starting at the ankles and noting the highest level at which oedema can be identified (such as mid-calf, knees, mid-thigh). In severe cases, oedema can extend into the scrotum or labia. Significant oedema is a hallmark of nephrotic syndrome.

Weight

Look for sequential measures of a patient's weight, as this will provide an accurate assessment of fluid loss or gain over the short term.

Fluid balance charts

The physical examination should be complemented, where possible, by measurement of fluid input (oral and intravenous) and output (urine volumes and other losses).

Abdominal examination

Examination sequence

Ask the patient to lie flat with their arms by their sides. Expose the abdomen fully down to the level of the anterior iliac spine.

Inspection

- Look for abdominal distension in the flanks (which may indicate ascites, a further marker of fluid overload, or large polycystic kidneys). Look for operative scars, such as those relating to a renal transplant in the left or right iliac

fossa, extending inferiorly to the midline (Fig. 12.11), and those of a previous nephrectomy in the left or right flank. A nephrectomy is often needed in patients with ADPKD to make space for a subsequent renal transplant. In addition, look for the presence of a peritoneal dialysis catheter.

Palpation

- Kneel beside the bed and use your right hand, keeping the palmar surface flat. Observe the patient's face for signs of discomfort throughout. Palpate each region in turn, beginning with light palpation followed by deeper palpation (p. 105 and Fig. 6.1C). Describe any masses you feel. Examine for abdominal aortic aneurysm (p. 66).
- Significantly enlarged kidneys are palpable as masses in the flanks. You should be able to 'get above' the mass. Identification of less obviously enlarged kidneys requires deeper palpation and a ballotting technique. Starting on the right side, your left hand should placed under the patient's back, with your index finger against the 12th rib in the paramedian position; the right pushes firmly down on the anterior abdominal wall. Ask the patient to take a deep breath in, and push up by flexing the fingers of your left hand (Fig. 12.12A). The kidney can be felt against the fingers of the right hand. The same procedure is followed on the left side with your left hand under the patient and your little finger against the 12th rib (Fig. 12.12B). The

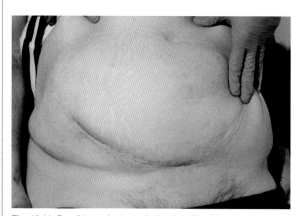

Fig. 12.11 Renal transplant scar in the right iliac fossa.

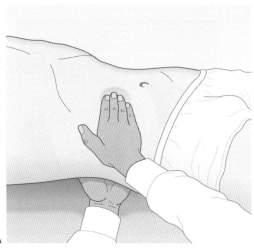

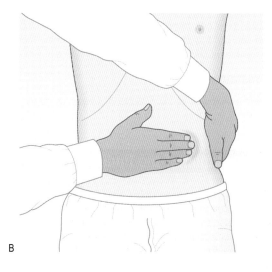

A   B

Fig. 12.12 Palpation of the kidney. A Right kidney. B Left kidney.

procedure is otherwise identical. ADPKD is the most common cause of palpable kidneys.

- A transplanted kidney may be palpated as a mass (usually 12–14 cm in length) in either iliac fossa, although the right is more common. Any tenderness should be noted, as this may indicate graft pyelonephritis or rejection.
- A palpable bladder may be felt as a soft, midline, suprapubic mass that you cannot 'get below'. In acute retention, palpation will worsen discomfort.
- When pyelonephritis is suspected, tenderness in the renal angle should be determined. If this is non-tender on palpation, you may sit the patient up and percuss with a closed fist over both renal angles.

Percussion

- Ascites should be assessed using the standard technique for shifting dullness (p. 109). Peritoneal dialysis fluid is also evident as a fluid level determined by percussion. To identify an enlarged bladder, you should percuss over the midline from a resonant area at the umbilicus, moving inferiorly to identify where the percussion note becomes dull. The percussion note should be resonant over enlarged kidneys.

Auscultation

- Listen for abdominal bruits over the epigastrium and over both renal arteries (p. 109). This may be a sign of renovascular disease or atheromatous disease in other arteries.

Targeted examination of other systems

The kidneys are involved in many multisystem diseases. Renal impairment itself may also affect other systems. The history will help direct the examination to these elements.

Joints

Examine for inflammation and swelling of joints, which can occur in systemic vasculitis. The presence of a chronic arthritis, such as rheumatoid disease, may lead to amyloid (a cause of nephrotic syndrome), and medication used to treat arthritis, such as NSAIDs, can cause AKI. Examine for areas of bony tenderness in the spine; this may be a feature of myeloma.

Nervous system

Examine for a peripheral neuropathy (sensory and/or motor), which can occur with vasculitic diseases. In diabetes mellitus the presence of neuropathy is common in those with CKD.

Prostate

Physical examination of the prostate is covered on pages 112 and 235.

Interpretation of the findings

Renal disorders may come to light because of patient symptoms or abnormalities on biochemical investigation. Clinical assessment will be dictated by the scenario; focus on the relevant positive and negative findings when describing the case.

In patients with an acute presentation the key element is to begin with a description of the patient's general appearance and fluid status. This should summarise whether they are clinically euvolaemic, hypovolaemic or fluid-overloaded. Are there any features of a multisystem disease (such as rash, joint swelling, eye inflammation), or any signs in the abdomen that suggest renal disease (such as enlarged kidneys, renal transplant, renal bruits, enlarged bladder) and that may point to a diagnosis. Urinalysis (see below) should be used to identify infection or intrinsic renal diseases such as glomerulonephritis or nephrotic syndrome.

In patients with CKD, fluid balance assessment should be presented in the same way. The examination findings should focus on whether there is evidence of an underlying disease that may explain CKD: for example, diabetes mellitus (retinopathy, neuropathy), hypertension (retinopathy), ADPKD (enlarged kidneys, previous surgery), renovascular disease (renal bruits) or previous renal transplantation. In addition, include any features of the adverse effects of CKD, such as anaemia, skin excoriations from pruritus or weight loss, in your presentation.

Investigations

Urinalysis

Urinalysis should be considered an essential part of the renal examination. Urine should be obtained as a mid-stream specimen so it can be optimally used for subsequent investigations (see later). Urine abnormalities may reflect:

- abnormally high levels of a substance in the blood exceeding the capacity for normal tubular reabsorption, such as glucose, ketones, conjugated bilirubin and urobilinogen
- altered kidney function: for example, proteinuria, failure to concentrate urine
- abnormal contents, such as blood arising at any point between the kidney and the urethra.

The urine dipstick test uses chemical reagents, which change colour when they are immersed and then removed from urine, to detect abnormalities. Urine test strips contain up to 10 of these chemical pads (Fig. 12.13); however, not all are used in

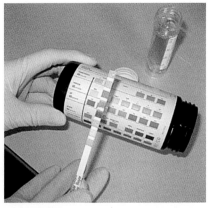

Fig. 12.13 Urine dipstick test. *From Pitkin J, Peattie AB, Magowan BA. Obstetrics and Gynaecology: An Illustrated Colour Text. Edinburgh: Churchill Livingstone; 2003.*

the assessment of renal disease. The key elements are described in Box 12.5.

Normal fresh urine is clear but varies in colour. Cloudy fresh urine is usually due to the presence of leucocytes (pyuria). Discoloration of the urine can occur due to drugs (such as rifampicin), foods (beetroot) or metabolites (bilirubin). Strong odours can be due to infections; some foods, like asparagus, impart a characteristic smell to the urine.

Investigation of renal function

Functional studies may be useful in patients with voiding symptoms (Box 12.6). In addition to urinalysis, there are a number of other blood and urine tests (Box 12.7), as well as imaging studies (Box 12.8), that may help in the assessment of the patient with renal disease.

12.5 Key elements of urine dipstick test

Investigation	Comment
Specific gravity	Reflects urine solute concentration. Varies between 1.002 and 1.035. Raised when kidneys actively reabsorb water, e.g. in fluid depletion or renal failure due to decreased perfusion. Abnormally low values indicate failure to concentrate urine
pH	Normally 4.5–8.0. In renal tubular acidosis, pH never falls <5.3 despite acidaemia
Glucose	Small amounts may be excreted by normal kidneys. Glycosuria may indicate poorly controlled diabetes mellitus. It may occur in intrinsic renal disease when tubular glucose reabsorption is impaired
Ketones	Test is specific for acetoacetate and does not detect other ketones, e.g. β-OH butyrate, acetone. Ketonuria occurs in diabetic ketoacidosis, starvation, alcohol use and very-low-carbohydrate diets
Protein	Varies between trace and 4+. The greater the degree of proteinuria, the more likely there is to be significant renal disease. Most patients with nephrotic syndrome will have 4+ protein. The presence of both blood (≥2+) and protein (≥2+), an 'active urinary sediment', often indicates intrinsic renal disease. As urinalysis is semiquantitative, confirmatory laboratory quantification should be undertaken using either a urine albumin : creatinine or protein : creatinine ratio (see Box 12.4)
Blood	≥1+ is positive for non-visible haematuria. The test does not differentiate between haemoglobin and myoglobin. If you suspect rhabdomyolysis, measure myoglobin with a specific laboratory test
Bilirubin and urobilinogen	Bilirubin is not normally present. Urobilinogen may be up to 33 μmol/L in health. Abnormalities of bilirubin and urobilinogen require investigation for possible haemolysis or hepatobiliary disease
Leucocyte esterase	Indicates the presence of neutrophils in urine. Seen in urinary tract infection or inflammation, stone disease and urothelial cancers
Nitrite	Most Gram-negative bacteria convert urinary nitrate to nitrite. A positive result indicates bacteriuria but a negative result does not exclude its presence

12.6 Functional assessment of the lower urinary tract

Frequency/volume chart

- Chart is used to monitor micturition patterns, including nocturia, and fluid intake
- The patient collects their urine, measures each void, and charts it against time over 3–5 days

Urine flow rate

- The patient voids into a special receptacle that measures the rate of urine passage
- A low flow does not differentiate between poor detrusor contractility and bladder outlet obstruction

Urodynamic tests

- Invasive tests, necessitating the insertion of bladder and rectal catheters to measure total bladder pressure and abdominal pressure, and to allow bladder filling
- Filling studies determine detrusor activity and compliance
- Low detrusor pressures with low urine flow suggest detrusor function problems
- High detrusor pressures with low flow suggest bladder outlet obstruction

12.7 Blood and urine investigations in renal and urological disease	
Investigation	**Indication/comment**
Serum urea/creatinine	Levels generally ↑ as GFR ↓, but values are affected by diet and muscle mass and do not measure renal function accurately
eGFR	Usually provided by the laboratory and is based on the serum creatinine. Usually reported as 'normal' if ≥60 mL/min/1.73 m^2 CKD is classified on the basis of the eGFR (see Box 12.3)
Creatinine clearance	A good measurement of GFR but requires a 24-hour urine collection and a blood sample
Plasma electrolytes	↑ Potassium (↓ excretion) in AKI and advanced CKD ↓ Bicarbonate (↓ H$^+$ excretion) common in AKI and CKD ↓ Calcium (impaired renal vitamin D$_3$ activation) and ↑ phosphate (↓ excretion) in CKD ↑ Urate common in CKD (may be associated with gout)
Plasma and urine osmolality	A measure of renal concentrating ability in unexplained hyponatraemia. If the plasma osmolality is low, the urine osmolality should be lower still (<150 mosmol/kg); in the absence of hypovolaemia, any other finding is consistent with syndrome of inappropriate ADH (vasopressin) secretion In patients with unexplained polyuria, test the concentrating ability of the kidneys by an overnight fluid deprivation test. In healthy people, urinary osmolality should rise to >600 mosmol/kg; any other finding suggests lack of ADH or renal tubular unresponsiveness to ADH
Alkaline phosphatase and parathyroid hormone	↑ in secondary hyperparathyroidism related to ↓ calcium and ↑ phosphate levels
Antinuclear factor and ANCA	Systemic lupus erythematosus and vasculitis may affect the kidney

ADH, *antidiuretic hormone (vasopressin)*; AKI, *acute kidney injury*; ANCA, *antineutrophil cytoplasmic antibody*; CKD, *chronic kidney disease*; (e)GFR, *(estimated) glomerular filtration rate.*

12.8 Imaging for the investigation of renal and urological disease	
Investigation	**Indication/comment**
Plain abdominal X-ray	Stones (>90% are radio-opaque), gas in the urinary collecting system
Ultrasound scan	Assesses kidney size/shape/position; evidence of obstruction; renal cysts or solid lesions; stones; ureteric urine flow; gross abnormality of bladder, postmicturition residual volume Used to guide kidney biopsy
Doppler ultrasound of renal vessels	Assesses renovascular disease, renal vein thrombosis Arterial resistive index may indicate obstruction
Computed tomography of the kidney ureter bladder (CTKUB)	Renal colic; renal, ureteric or bladder stones
CT urogram	Frank haematuria; renal or bladder malignancy
Angiography/CT or magnetic resonance angiography	Hypertension ± renal failure, renal artery stenosis Angioplasty and/or stenting
Isotope scan	Suspected renal scarring, e.g. reflux nephropathy; diagnosis of obstruction Assessment of GFR in each kidney – measures renal uptake and excretion of radiolabelled chemicals
Renal biopsy	Used to diagnose parenchymal renal disease

OSCE example 1: Renal history

Mrs Measham, 60 years old, is attending to discuss the results of her recent blood tests. She has presented with a 3-month history of tiredness and you know that her renal function was normal 1 year ago.

Investigations

Haemoglobin: 101 g/L (10.1 g g/dL) (normal range female 115–165 g/L (11.5–16.5 g/dL); male 130–180 g/L (13.0–18.0 g/dL))
White cell count: 8.9×10^9/L (normal range $4.0–11.0 \times 10^9$/L)
Platelet count: 510×10^9/L (normal range $150–400 \times 10^9$/L)
Potassium: 5.2 mmol/L (normal range 3.5–5.0 mmol/L)
Urea: 14.5 mmol/L (40.6 mg/dL; normal range 3.0–7.0 mmol/L (8.4–19.6 mg/dL))
Creatinine: 163 μmol/L (1.84 mg/dL; normal range 60–120 μmol/L (0.68–1.36 mg/dL))
Dipstick urinalysis: blood: 3+, protein 3+

Take a history from the patient

- Introduce yourself to the patient and clean your hands.
- Obtain consent to take a history.
- Establish that the patient was well until 3 months ago and that the main symptoms are tiredness and breathlessness on exertion.
- Ask about:
  - weight loss, appetite and bowel motions
  - peripheral oedema
  - haemoptysis
  - urinary symptoms: dysuria, nocturia, urgency, hesitancy, incontinence, loin pain
  - back pain, fevers and rigors.
- Confirm details of the past medical history.
- Document current medication and any relevant recent changes.
- Determine how symptoms are affecting the patient's lifestyle: both work and leisure.
- Establish the family history.
- Thank the patient and clean your hands.

Summarise your findings

The patient has presented with 3 months of lethargy and investigations reveal that he has anaemia in the context of renal impairment.

Suggest a differential diagnosis

The most likely diagnosis is an intrinsic renal disease, probably a glomerulonephritis, which may be part of a multisystem disorder. Infection is also possible.

Suggest additional investigations

Relevant further investigations might include erythrocyte sedimentation rate, C-reactive protein, vasculitis and myeloma screens, and iron stores. Renal ultrasound, chest X-ray and mid-stream urine for microscopy and culture could be considered. The patient would benefit from a referral to a nephrologist.

12

OSCE example 2: Renal examination

Mr Logan, 45 years old, is known to have adult polycystic kidney disease, and has a history of intermittent loin pain and hypertension.

Please examine the abdomen

- Introduce yourself and clean your hands.
- Obtain permission to examine the patient.
- Perform a peripheral examination, including hands, arms and face. Look for leuconychia, pallor, and an arteriovenous fistula for haemodialysis (if functioning, it will have a palpable thrill).
- Measure the blood pressure.
- Inspect the abdomen. Examine for scars from a previous nephrectomy (increasingly, these will be laparoscopic, rather than scars from an open nephrectomy), or from a current or previous renal transplant in the right or left iliac fossa, and a distended abdomen if polycystic kidneys are large.
- Ask if the abdomen is painful. Start with light palpation and then proceed more deeply across all abdominal regions. Assess for specific organomegaly, including liver, spleen, kidneys and bladder. Findings may include an irregular enlarged liver (polycystic liver), or palpable masses in one or both flanks (polycystic kidneys; it is key to distinguish these from the liver or spleen). Remember to ballott both kidneys.
- Percuss over any mass.
- Assess for shifting dullness due to ascites.
- Auscultate over the abdomen and over masses.

Summarise your findings

This man has bilateral flank masses, which are ballottable. I can get above the masses and the percussion note over them is resonant. These are most likely to represent bilaterally enlarged kidneys. The patient also has a functioning left arteriovenous fistula, most likely for haemodialysis.

Suggest a diagnosis

The most likely cause is autosomal dominant polycystic kidney disease.

Suggest initial investigations

An ultrasound scan would be the simplest test to show the presence of cysts. Magnetic resonance imaging would provide more detail about renal size.

Advanced level comments

In addition to hypertension and renal failure, complications of APCKD include cyst haemorrhage and infection, and subarachnoid haemorrhage due to a ruptured berry aneurysm.

Integrated examination sequence for renal disease

- Position the patient: start with patient at a 45-degree angle.
- Examine the general appearance:
  - Uraemic facies.
  - Myoclonus.
  - Scratch marks.
  - Dyspnoea, hyperventilation.
- Check the hands, arms and face:
  - Splinter haemorrhages.
  - Arteriovenous fistulae and scars.
  - Tunnelled vascular access catheter.
  - Pallor, eye inflammation.
  - Examine skin for vasculitic (purpuric) rash.
- Assess fluid balance:
  - Pulse, blood pressure, skin turgor and jugular venous pressure.
  - Heart sounds.
  - Chest examination: percussion and auscultation to assess for pleural effusions or pulmonary oedema.
  - Sacral and ankle oedema.
- Reposition the patient: supine with their arms at their sides.
- Perform an abdominal examination:
  - Inspection: peritoneal dialysis catheter, abdominal distension due to ascites or enlarged kidneys, scars from a renal transplant.
  - Palpation: ballott for enlarged kidneys, palpate the suprapubic area for the bladder, and any renal transplant in the right or left iliac fossa.
  - Percussion: shifting dullness for ascites, enlarged kidneys resonant to percussion, suprapubic dullness indicating bladder enlargement.
  - Auscultation: abdominal bruits.
- Other:
  - In men with a history of urinary outflow problems, perform a rectal examination of the prostate.
  - Perform dipstick urinalysis.

Jane Gibson
Ivan Brenkel

13

The musculoskeletal system

The history

Common presenting symptoms

Pain

In musculoskeletal pain, the acronym SOCRATES (see also Box 2.2, p. 12) prompts questions that reveal useful diagnostic clues.

Site

Fig. 13.1 illustrates the anatomy of a typical joint. Determine which component is painful: the joint (arthralgia), muscle (myalgia) or other soft tissue. Pain may be localised and suggest the diagnosis, such as a red, hot, tender first metatarsophalangeal joint in gout (Fig. 13.2), or swelling of several joints suggesting an inflammatory arthritis. Causes of arthralgia and myalgia are shown in Boxes 13.1 and 13.2.

Onset

Pain from traumatic injury is usually immediate and exacerbated by movement or haemarthrosis (bleeding into the joint). Inflammatory

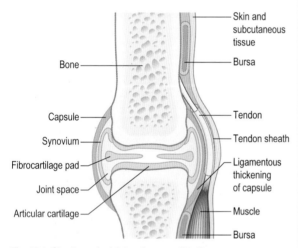

Fig. 13.1 Structure of a joint and surrounding tissues.

Labels: Bone; Capsule; Synovium; Fibrocartilage pad; Joint space; Articular cartilage; Skin and subcutaneous tissue; Bursa; Tendon; Tendon sheath; Ligamentous thickening of capsule; Muscle; Bursa

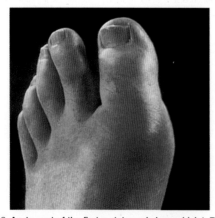

Fig. 13.2 Acute gout of the first metatarsophalangeal joint. This causes swelling, erythema, and extreme pain and tenderness (podagra). *From Colledge NR, Walker BR, Ralston SH, eds. Davidson's Principles and Practice of Medicine. 21st edn. Edinburgh: Churchill Livingstone; 2010.*

13.1 Common causes of arthralgia (joint pain)

Infective
- Viral, e.g. rubella, parvovirus B19, mumps, hepatitis B, chikungunya
- Bacterial, e.g. staphylococci, *Mycobacterium tuberculosis*, *Borrelia*
- Fungal

Postinfective
- Rheumatic fever
- Reactive arthritis

Inflammatory
- Rheumatoid arthritis
- Systemic lupus erythematosus
- Ankylosing spondylitis
- Systemic sclerosis

Degenerative
- Osteoarthritis

Tumour
- Primary, e.g. osteosarcoma, chondrosarcoma
- Metastatic, e.g. from lung, breast, prostate
- Systemic tumour effects, e.g. hypertrophic pulmonary osteoarthropathy

Crystal formation
- Gout, pseudogout

Trauma
- e.g. Road traffic accidents

Others
- Chronic pain disorders, e.g. fibromyalgia (usually diffuse pain)
- Benign joint hypermobility syndrome

13.2 Causes of muscle pain (myalgia)

Infective
- Viral: Coxsackie, cytomegalovirus, echovirus, dengue
- Bacterial: *Streptococcus pneumoniae*, *Mycoplasma*
- Parasitic: schistosomiasis, toxoplasmosis

Traumatic
- Tears
- Haematoma
- Rhabdomyolysis

Inflammatory
- Polymyalgia rheumatic
- Myositis
- Dermatomyositis

Drugs
- Alcohol withdrawal
- Statins
- Triptans

Metabolic
- Hypothyroidism
- Hyperthyroidism
- Addison's disease
- Vitamin D deficiency

Neuropathic

arthritis can develop over 24 hours, or more insidiously. Crystal arthritis (gout and pseudogout) causes acute, severe pain that develops quickly, often overnight. Joint sepsis causes pain that develops over 1–2 days.

Character

Bone pain is penetrating, deep or boring, and is characteristically worse at night. Localised pain suggests tumour, osteomyelitis (infection), osteonecrosis or osteoid osteoma (a benign bone tumour). Generalised bony conditions, such as osteomalacia, usually cause diffuse pain.

Fracture pain is sharp and stabbing, aggravated by attempted movement, and relieved by rest and splintage.

Muscle pain is often described as 'stiffness' or aching, and is aggravated by use of the affected muscle(s).

'Shooting' pain is often caused by impingement of a peripheral nerve or nerve root: for example, buttock pain, which 'shoots down the back of the leg', caused by lumbar disc protrusion.

Progressive joint pain in patients over 40 years of age is commonly caused by osteoarthritis.

Fibromyalgia, a chronic pain syndrome, causes widespread, constant pain with little diurnal variation, which is poorly controlled by conventional analgesic/anti-inflammatory drugs.

Radiation

Pain from nerve compression radiates to the distribution of that nerve or nerve root (see Fig. 7.23), such as lower leg pain in intervertebral disc prolapse, or hand pain in carpal tunnel syndrome. Neck pain radiates to the shoulder or scalp. Hip pain is usually felt in the groin but may radiate to the thigh or knee. Common patterns of radiation are summarised in Box 13.3.

Associated symptoms

For example, swelling and redness of a joint indicate inflammatory arthritis.

Timing (frequency, duration and periodicity of symptoms)

A history of several years of pain with a normal examination suggests fibromyalgia (Box 13.4). A history of several weeks of pain, early-morning stiffness and loss of function is likely to be an inflammatory arthritis. 'Flitting' pain starting in one joint and moving to others over a period of days is a feature of rheumatic

13.3 Common patterns of referred and radicular musculoskeletal pain	
Site where pain is perceived	Site of pathology
Occiput	C1, 2
Interscapular region	C3, 4
Tip of shoulder, upper outer aspect of arm	C5
Interscapular region or radial fingers and thumb	C6, 7
Ulnar side of forearm, ring and little fingers	C8
Medial aspect of upper arm	T1
Chest	Thoracic spine
Buttocks, knees, legs	Lumbar spine
Lateral aspect of upper arm	Shoulder
Forearm	Elbow
Anterior thigh, knee	Hip
Thigh, hip	Knee

fever and gonococcal arthritis. If intermittent, with resolution between episodes, it may be palindromic rheumatism.

Exacerbating/relieving factors

Pain from joints damaged by intra-articular derangement or osteoarthritic degeneration worsens with exercise. Pain from inflammatory arthritis worsens with rest. Pain from a septic joint is present both at rest and with movement.

Severity

Apart from trauma, the most severe joint pain occurs in septic and crystal arthritis. Disproportionately severe pain is seen acutely in compartment syndrome (increased pressure in a fascial compartment, compromising perfusion and viability of compartmental structures) and chronically in complex regional pain syndrome. Neurological involvement in diabetes mellitus, leprosy (Hansen's disease), syringomyelia and syphilis (tabes dorsalis) may impair joint sensation, reducing pain despite obvious pathology on examination. Grossly abnormal joints may even be pain-free (Charcot joints). Partial muscle tears are painful; complete rupture may be less so.

Patterns of joint involvement

Different patterns of joint involvement aid the differential diagnosis (Fig. 13.3). Are the small or large joints of the arms or legs affected? How many joints are involved? Involvement of one joint is called a monoarthritis; 2–4 joints, oligoarthritis; and more than 4, polyarthritis.

- Predominant involvement of the small joints of the hands and feet suggests an inflammatory arthritis, such as rheumatoid arthritis or systemic lupus erythematosus (SLE).

13

13.4 Clinical vignette: arthralgia and fatigue
A 34-year-old mother-of-two presents to her GP with a 1-year history of gradually worsening pain and persistent fatigue. The pain moves around and involves the back, neck, shoulders, elbows, hands and knees. All joints are described as swollen, particularly her hands, which swell 'all over'. Further history reveals poor sleep with the patient wakening every 2 hours and feeling unrefreshed in the morning. She has a difficult social background and a past history of depression and irritable bowel syndrome. Examination shows no skin or joint abnormality but there is widespread tenderness, particularly across her shoulders, in her neck and down her back (see figure). Blood tests are all normal. She is diagnosed with fibromyalgia.

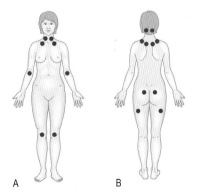

Typical tender points in fibromyalgia. **A** Anterior view. **B** Posterior view.

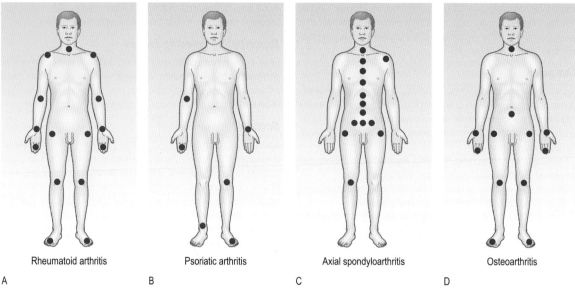

Fig. 13.3 Contrasting patterns of joint involvement in polyarthritis. [A] Rheumatoid arthritis (symmetrical, small and large joints, upper and lower limbs). [B] Psoriatic arthritis (asymmetrical, large > small joints, swelling of a whole digit – dactylitis, enthesitis). [C] Axial spondyloarthritis (spine and sacroiliac joints, asymmetrical peripheral arthritis, large > small joints, enthesitis). [D] Osteoarthritis (symmetrical, small and large joints, base of thumb, distal interphalangeal joints).

- Medium- or large-joint swelling is more likely to be degenerative (osteoarthritis) or a seronegative arthritis (such as psoriatic arthritis).
- Nodal osteoarthritis has a predilection for the distal interphalangeal (DIP) joints of the hands and the carpometacarpal (CMC) joint of the thumb.

Stiffness

Ask what the patient means by stiffness. Is it:
- restricted range of movement?
- difficulty moving, but with a normal range?
- painful movement?
- localised to a particular joint or more generalised?

There are characteristic differences between inflammatory and non-inflammatory presentations of joint stiffness.

Inflammatory arthritis causes early-morning stiffness that takes at least 30 minutes to wear off with activity.

Non-inflammatory, mechanical arthritis causes stiffness after rest that eases rapidly on movement.

Disease of the soft tissues, rather than the joint itself, may cause stiffness. In polymyalgia rheumatica, stiffness commonly affects the shoulder and pelvic areas.

Swelling

Ask about the site, extent and time course of the swelling.
The speed of onset of swelling is a clue to the diagnosis:
- Rapid (<30 minutes), severe swelling suggests a haemarthrosis (Fig. 13.4). This occurs when vascular structures such as bone or ligament are injured, and is worse in the presence of anticoagulants or bleeding disorders.
- Swelling over hours or days suggests traumatic effusion, such as with a meniscal tear or articular cartilage abrasion.
- Septic arthritis develops over a few hours with pain, marked swelling, tenderness, redness and extreme reluctance to move the joint actively or passively.

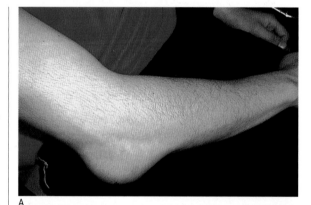

A

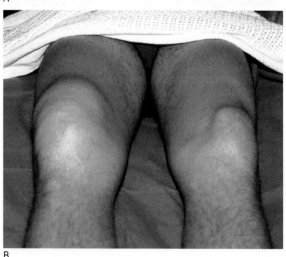

B

Fig. 13.4 Joint swelling. [A] Olecranon bursitis. [B] Right-knee haemarthrosis.

13.5 Extra-articular signs in rheumatic conditions

Condition	Extra-articular signs
Rheumatoid arthritis	Rheumatoid nodules, palmar erythema, episcleritis, dry eyes, interstitial lung disease, pleural ± pericardial effusion, small-vessel vasculitis, Raynaud's phenomenon, low-grade fever, weight loss, lymphadenopathy, splenomegaly, leg ulcers
Psoriatic arthritis	Psoriasis, nail pitting, onycholysis, enthesitis, dactylitis
Reactive arthritis	Urethritis, mouth and/or genital ulcers, conjunctivitis, iritis, enthesitis (inflammation of tendon or ligament attachments), e.g. Achilles enthesitis/plantar fasciitis, rash (keratoderma blenorrhagica)
Axial spondyloarthritis	Inflammatory bowel disease, psoriasis, enthesitis, iritis, aortic regurgitation, apical interstitial fibrosis
Septic arthritis	Fever, malaise, source of sepsis, e.g. skin, throat, gut
Gout	Tophi, signs of renal failure or alcoholic liver disease
Sjögren's syndrome	'Dry eyes' (keratoconjunctivitis sicca), xerostomia (reduced or absent saliva production), salivary gland enlargement, Raynaud's phenomenon, neuropathy
Systemic lupus erythematosus	Photosensitive rash, especially on face, mucocutaneous ulcers, alopecia, fever, pleural ± pericardial effusion, diaphragmatic paralysis, pulmonary fibrosis (rare), Raynaud's phenomenon, lymphopenia
Systemic sclerosis	Skin tightening (scleroderma, see Fig. 3.30C), telangiectasia, Raynaud's phenomenon, calcific deposits in fingers, dilated nail-fold capillaries, pulmonary fibrosis
Adult-onset Still's disease	Rash, fever, hepatomegaly, splenomegaly
Other	Erythema nodosum of shins in sarcoidosis, viral rashes, drug rashes

Concurrent glucocorticoid or non-steroidal anti-inflammatory drug therapy modifies these features.
- Crystal-induced arthritis (gout or pseudogout) can mimic septic arthritis. It commonly starts overnight or early in the morning due to the rise in serum urate following the evening meal.

Erythema and warmth

Erythema (redness) occurs in infective, traumatic and crystal-induced conditions, and mild erythema may be present in inflammatory arthritis. All affected joints will be warm. Erythema associated with DIP joint swelling helps to distinguish DIP joint psoriatic arthritis from the Heberden's nodes of osteoarthritis.

Weakness

Weakness suggests joint, neurological or muscle disease. The problem may be focal or generalised.

Joint disorders cause weakness, either through inhibition of function by pain, or by disruption of the joint or its supporting structures.

Nerve entrapment may be the cause: for example, carpal tunnel syndrome at the wrist.

Muscle disorders can produce widespread weakness associated with pain and fatigue, such as in myositis, and with a rash, as in dermatomyositis.

Proximal muscle weakness can occur in endocrine disorders: for example, hypothyroidism or excess of glucocorticoids.

Locking and triggering

'Locking' is an incomplete range of movement at a joint because of an anatomical block. It may be associated with pain. Patients use 'locking' to describe various problems, so clarify exactly what they mean.

True locking is a block to the normal range of movement caused by mechanical obstruction, such as a loose body or torn meniscus, within the joint. The patient is characteristically able to 'unlock' the joint by trick manœuvres.

Pseudolocking is a loss of the range of movement due to pain.

13.6 Clinical vignette: joint pain and rash

A 32-year-old lady is seen in the outpatient clinic with fatigue and intermittent pain and swelling in her hands, which she has had for the last year. She noticed a rash across her cheeks and on her arms while she was on holiday in Spain recently and this seems to have sparked off painful mouth ulcers and worsening joint pain. She has no other relevant history. Examination shows a 'butterfly' rash across the cheeks and nose, several mouth ulcers and two swollen metacarpophalangeal joints. Blood tests reveal anaemia, lymphopenia, positive antinuclear antibody and raised anti-double-stranded DNA antibodies.

A diagnosis of systemic lupus erythematosus is made.

Triggering is a block to extension of a finger, which then 'gives' suddenly when extending from a flexed position. In adults it usually affects the ring or middle fingers and results from nodular tendon thickening or fibrous thickening of the flexor sheath due to chronic low-grade trauma, which may be occupational or associated with inflammatory arthritis. Triggering can be congenital, in which case it usually affects the thumb.

Extra-articular symptoms

Patients may present with extra-articular features of disease (Box 13.5) that they may not connect with musculoskeletal problems.

Ask about:
- Rashes: occur with psoriasis, vasculitis and erythema nodosum. Ask whether they are photosensitive (SLE, Box 13.6).
- Weight loss, low-grade fever and malaise: associated with rheumatoid arthritis and SLE. High-spiking fevers in the evening, accompanied by a rash, occur in adult-onset Still's disease.
- Headache, jaw pain on chewing (claudication) and scalp tenderness: features of temporal arteritis.

Connective tissue disease may present with multiple extra-articular features:
- Raynaud's phenomenon.
- Sicca symptoms (dryness of mouth and eyes).

- Rashes.
- Gastrointestinal problems, including dysphagia and mouth ulcers.
- Respiratory problems, including dyspnoea from interstitial lung disease, or pleural pain or effusions associated with rheumatoid arthritis or connective tissue disease.
- Back pain and stiffness or arthritis associated with abdominal pain, diarrhoea, bloody stool and mouth ulcers: may suggest arthritis associated with inflammatory bowel disease.

Past medical history

Note past episodes of musculoskeletal involvement, extra-articular diseases as listed in the previous section, fractures and possible complicating comorbidities such as diabetes or obesity.

Drug history

Many drugs have side effects that may either worsen or precipitate musculoskeletal conditions (Box 13.7).

Family history

Inflammatory arthritis is more common if a first-degree relative is affected. Osteoarthritis, osteoporosis and gout are heritable in a variable polygenic fashion. Spondyloarthritis is more common in patients with human leucocyte antigen B27. A single-gene defect (monogenic inheritance) is found in hereditary sensorimotor neuropathy (Charcot–Marie–Tooth disease), osteogenesis imperfecta, Ehlers–Danlos syndrome, Marfan's syndrome and the muscular dystrophies.

Social, environmental and occupational histories

Identify functional difficulties, including the ability to use pens, tools and cutlery. How does the condition affect the patient's activities of daily living, such as washing, dressing and toileting? Can they use the stairs and do they need walking aids? Ask about functional independence, especially cooking, housework and shopping.

Ask about current and previous occupations. Is the patient working full- or part-time, on sick leave or receiving benefits? Has the patient had to take time off work because of the condition and is their job at risk? Litigation may be pending following injury

and in occupational disorders, such as repetitive strain disorder, hand vibration syndrome and fatigue fractures.

Smoking is a risk factor for rheumatoid arthritis and possibly other inflammatory arthritides. High alcohol intake contributes to gout and falls that may result in fracture. It can also cause myopathy, neuropathy and rhabdomyolysis.

Some conditions are seen in certain ethnic groups; for example, sickle cell disease may present with bone and joint pain in African patients. Osteomalacia is more common in Asian patients. Bone and joint tuberculosis is more common in African and Asian patients.

A sexual history may be relevant (p. 16), since sexually transmitted disease is associated with musculoskeletal problems, such as reactive arthritis, gonococcal arthritis, human immunodeficiency virus infection and hepatitis B.

The physical examination

Practise examining as many joints as possible to become familiar with normal appearances and ranges of movement.

General principles

Firstly, examine the patient's overall appearance for features such as pallor, rash, skin tightening and hair changes.

Look – feel – move

Follow a process of observation, palpation and movement for each joint or group of joints in turn.

Look at the skin, subcutaneous tissues and bony outline of each area. Before palpating, ask the patient which area is painful or tender. Feel for warmth, swelling, stability and deformity. Assess if deformity is reducible or fixed. Assess active before passive movement. Do not cause the patient additional pain. Compare one limb with the opposite side. Always expose the joint above and below the affected one. In suspected systemic disease, examine all joints and systems fully.

Use standard terminology to describe position and movement. Describe movements from the neutral position:

- flexion: bending at a joint from the neutral position
- extension: straightening a joint back to the neutral position
- hyperextension: moving beyond the normal neutral position (indicating a torn ligament or underlying ligamentous laxity, such as benign joint hypermobility syndrome)
- adduction: moving towards the midline of the body (finger adduction is movement towards the axis of the limb)
- abduction: moving away from the midline.

To describe altered limb position due to joint/bone deformity, use:

- valgus: the distal part deviates away from the midline
- varus: the distal part deviates towards the midline.

In the wrist and hand, use:

- radial deviation: the distal part deviates towards the radial side
- ulnar deviation: the distal part deviates towards the ulnar side.

13.7 Drugs associated with adverse musculoskeletal effects	
Drug	Possible adverse musculoskeletal effects
Glucocorticoids	Osteoporosis, myopathy, osteonecrosis, infection
Statins	Myalgia, myositis, myopathy
Angiotensin-converting enzyme inhibitors	Myalgia, arthralgia, positive antinuclear antibody
Antiepileptics	Osteomalacia, arthralgia
Immunosuppressants	Infections
Quinolones	Tendinopathy, tendon rupture

General examination

Skin, nail and soft tissues

The skin and related structures are common sites of associated lesions. The skin changes of psoriasis may be hidden, in the umbilicus, natal cleft or scalp (p. 286), for example. The rash of SLE is found across the cheeks and bridge of nose. Nail pitting and onycholysis occur in psoriasis (p. 24).

Small, dark-red spots due to capillary infarcts occur in rheumatoid arthritis, SLE and systemic vasculitis. Common sites are the nail folds (Fig. 13.5, often seen in rheumatoid arthritis), and the lower legs in systemic vasculitis (p. 288).

In systemic sclerosis, the thickened, tight skin produces a characteristic facial appearance (see Fig. 3.30C). In the hands, flexion contractures, calcium deposits in the finger pulps (Fig. 13.6) and tissue ischaemia leading to ulceration may occur. The telangiectasias of systemic sclerosis are purplish, blanch with pressure and are most common on the hands and face. In the fingers, the pallor of Raynaud's phenomenon, pulp atrophy or ulceration may be evident.

Reactive arthritis is associated with conjunctivitis, urethritis, circinate balanitis (painless superficial ulcers on the prepuce and glans) and superficial mouth ulcers.

Nodules

The firm, non-tender, subcutaneous nodules of rheumatoid arthritis most commonly occur on the extensor surface of the forearm (Fig. 13.7), sites of pressure or friction such as the sacrum or Achilles tendon, or in the lungs. Multiple small nodules can occur in the hands. Rheumatoid nodules are strongly associated with a positive anti-cyclic citrullinated peptide (anti-CCP) antibody or rheumatoid factor.

Bony nodules in osteoarthritis affect the lateral aspects of the DIP joints (Heberden's nodes) or the proximal interphalangeal (PIP) joints (Bouchard's nodes, Fig. 13.8). They are smaller and harder than rheumatoid nodules.

Gouty tophi are firm, irregular subcutaneous crystal collections (monosodium urate monohydrate). Common sites are the olecranon bursa, helix of the ear and extensor aspects of the fingers (Fig. 13.9), hands, knees and toes. If superficial, they may appear white, and may ulcerate, discharge crystals and become secondarily infected.

Eyes

Redness of the eyes may be due to conjunctivitis in reactive arthritis or 'dry eyes' in Sjögren's syndrome, rheumatoid arthritis and other connective tissue disorders. Scleritis and episcleritis occur in rheumatoid arthritis and psoriatic arthritis. An acutely painful, very red eye due to iritis occurs in axial spondyloarthritis (p. 262). The sclerae are blue in certain types of osteogenesis imperfecta (see Fig. 3.30A) and in the scleromalacia of longstanding rheumatoid arthritis.

General features

Weight loss, muscle loss, fever and lymphadenopathy are all features of systemic involvement in inflammatory arthritis and connective tissue disease.

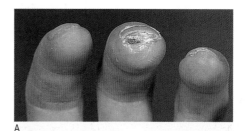
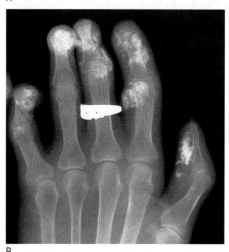

Fig. 13.6 Systemic sclerosis in the hand. [A] Calcium deposits ulcerating through the skin. [B] X-ray showing calcium deposits. *(A) From Forbes CD, Jackson WF. Color Atlas of Clinical Medicine. 3rd edn. Edinburgh: Mosby; 2003.*

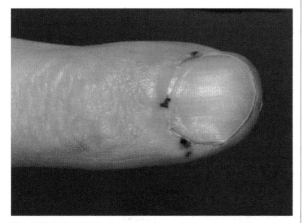

Fig. 13.5 Nail-fold infarcts caused by small-vessel vasculitis.

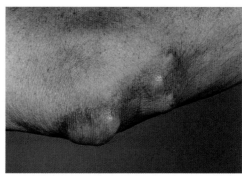

Fig. 13.7 Rheumatoid nodules at the olecranon and ulnar border.

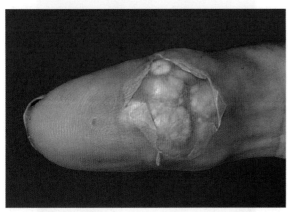

Fig. 13.8 Osteoarthritis of the hand. Heberden's (single arrow) and Bouchard's (double arrow) nodes.

Fig. 13.9 Gouty tophi.

Joints: the GALS screen

GALS (gait, arms, legs, spine) is a rapid screen for musculoskeletal and neurological deficits, and for functional ability; it helps to identify joints that require more detailed examination, as described later.

Initial questions

- Do you have any pain or stiffness in your muscles, joints or back?
- Do you have difficulty dressing yourself?
- Do you have difficulty walking up and down the stairs?

If all three replies are negative, the patient is unlikely to have a significant musculoskeletal problem; otherwise, perform the GALS screen.

Examination sequence

Ask the patient to undress to their underwear and stand in front of you. Demonstrate actions to the patient rather than simply telling them what to do. Any asymmetry, reduced range of movement, pain or deformity demands a detailed examination.

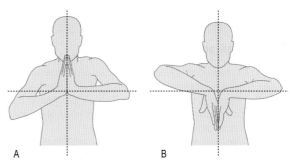

Fig. 13.10 Assessing the wrist. A Extension. B Flexion. There is a reduced range of movement at the right wrist.

Gait

- Ask the patient to walk ahead in a straight line, then turn and walk back towards you. Look for smoothness and symmetry of the gait.

Arms

- Stand in front of the patient.
- Inspect the dorsum of the hands and check for full extension at the metacarpophalangeal (MCP), PIP and DIP joints.
- Gently squeeze across the MCP joints. Tenderness suggests inflammation, as in rheumatoid arthritis.
- Ask the patient to:
  - Clench their fists and then open their hands flat.
  - Squeeze your index and middle fingers.
  - Touch each of their fingertips with the thumb.
  - Make a 'prayer sign', with their elbows as high as possible. Then reverse this with the backs of their hands together and elbows low (Fig. 13.10).
  - Put their arms straight out in front of their body.
  - Bend their arms up to touch their shoulders.
  - Place their elbows by the side of their body, bent at 90 degrees. Turn their palms up and down.
  - Put their hands behind their head, with their elbows back.
  - Put their hands behind their back.

Legs

- Ask the patient to lie supine on the couch.
- Palpate each knee for warmth, swelling and patellar tap.
- Flex each hip and knee with your hand on the patient's knee. Feel for crepitus in the patellofemoral joint and knee.
- If there is no contraindication, perform Thomas's test for fixed flexion deformity on both hips (see Fig. 13.35).
- Flex the patient's knee and hip to 90 degrees, and passively rotate each hip internally and externally.
- Look at the feet for any abnormality. Examine the soles, looking for calluses and ulcers, indicating abnormal load bearing.
- Gently squeeze across the metatarsal heads for tenderness.

Spine

- Stand behind the patient. Assess the straightness of the spine, muscle bulk and symmetry in the trunk, legs, ankle and foot.
- Stand beside the patient. Ask them to bend down and try to touch their toes, while you look for abnormal spinal curvature or limited hip flexion.

13.8 The Beighton scoring system to assess hypermobility	
Ask the patient to	**Score**
Bring the thumb to touch the forearm, with the wrist flexed	1 point each side
Extend the little finger > 90 degrees, with the hand in a neutral position	1 point each side
Extend the elbow > 10 degrees	1 point each side
Extend the knee > 10 degrees	1 point each side
Touch the floor, with the palms of hands and the knees straight	1 point
A score of ≥4 indicates hypermobility	

Reproduced from Beighton P, Solomon L, Soskolne CL. Annals of the Rheumatic Diseases 1973; 32(5):413, with permission from BMJ Publishing Group.

- Stand behind the patient, hold their pelvis, and ask them to turn from side to side without moving their feet.
- Ask them to slide their hand down the lateral aspect of their leg towards their knee.
- Stand in front of the patient. Ask them to put their ear to each shoulder in turn.
- Ask the patient to look down to the floor and then up to the ceiling.
- Ask them to open their jaw wide and move it from side to side.

Hypermobility

Some patients have a greater than normal range of joint movement. If this is severe, patients may present with recurrent dislocations or sensations of instability. Milder cases may develop arthralgia or be symptom-free. Mild hypermobility is normal but Marfan's, Ehlers–Danlos and benign joint hypermobility syndromes (Box 13.8) cause significant hypermobility.

Detailed examination of the musculoskeletal system

The GALS screen provides a rapid but limited assessment. This section describes the detailed examination required for thorough evaluation.

Gait

Gait is the cyclical pattern of musculoskeletal motion that carries the body forwards. Normal gait is smooth, symmetrical and ergonomically economical, with each leg 50% out of phase with the other. It has two phases: stance and swing. The stance phase is from foot-strike to toe-off, when the foot is on the ground and load-bearing. The swing phase is from toe-off to foot-strike, when the foot clears the ground. When both feet are on the ground, this is double stance.

A limp is an abnormal gait due to pain, structural change or spasticity.

Examination sequence

- Ask the patient to walk barefoot in a straight line. Then repeat in shoes.
- Observe the patient from behind, in front and from the side.

- Evaluate what happens at each level (foot, ankle, knee, hip and pelvis, trunk and spine) during both stance and swing phases.

Pain

An antalgic gait is one altered to reduce pain. Pain in a lower limb is usually aggravated by weight bearing, so minimal time is spent in the stance phase on that side. This results in a 'dot–dash' mode of walking. If the source of pain is in the spine, axial rotatory movements are minimised, resulting in a slow gait with small paces. Patients with hip pain may lean towards the affected side, as this decreases the compression force on the hip joint.

Structural change

Patients with limb-length discrepancy may limp or walk on tiptoe on the shorter side, with compensatory hip and knee flexion on the longer side. Assess for limb-length discrepancy (see Fig. 13.36). Other structural changes producing an abnormal gait include joint fusion, bone malunion and contracture.

Weakness

This may be due to nerve or muscle pathology or altered muscle tone. In a normal gait the hip abductors of the stance leg raise the contralateral hemipelvis. In Trendelenburg gait, abductor function is poor when weight-bearing on the affected side, so the contralateral hemipelvis falls (see Fig. 13.37).

Common causes of a Trendelenburg gait are:
- painful hip joint problems, as in osteoarthritis
- weak hip abductors, as in poliomyelitis or after hip replacement
- structural hip joint problems, as in congenital dislocation.

A high-stepping gait occurs in foot drop due to common peroneal nerve palsy. The knee is raised high to allow clearance of the weak foot.

Increased tone

This occurs with upper motor neurone lesions, such as cerebrovascular accident (stroke) or cerebral palsy. The gait depends on the specific lesion, contractures and compensatory mechanisms (see Fig. 7.17).

Spine

The spine is divided into the cervical, thoracic, lumbar and sacral segments (Fig. 13.11). Most spinal diseases affect multiple segments, causing altered posture or function of the whole spine. Spinal disease may occur without local symptoms, presenting with referred pain, neurological symptoms or signs in the trunk or limbs. Common causes of spinal pain are shown in Box 13.9.

Definitions

Scoliosis is lateral curvature of the spine (Fig. 13.12A).

Kyphosis is curvature of the spine in the sagittal (anterior–posterior) plane, with the apex posterior (Fig. 13.12B). The thoracic spine normally has a mild kyphosis.

Lordosis is curvature of the spine in the sagittal plane, with the apex anterior (Fig. 13.12C).

Gibbus is a spinal deformity caused by an anterior wedge deformity of a single vertebra, producing localised angular flexion (Fig. 13.12D).

13

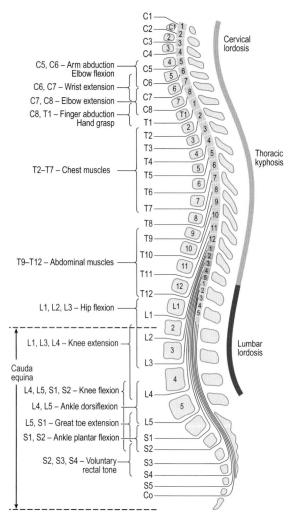

Fig. 13.11 The normal spinal curves and root innervations.

C1
C2
C3
C4
C5, C6 – Arm abduction
Elbow flexion
C6, C7 – Wrist extension
C7, C8 – Elbow extension
C8, T1 – Finger abduction
Hand grasp

T2–T7 – Chest muscles

T9–T12 – Abdominal muscles

L1, L2, L3 – Hip flexion

L1, L3, L4 – Knee extension

Cauda
equina

L4, L5, S1, S2 – Knee flexion
L4, L5 – Ankle dorsiflexion
L5, S1 – Great toe extension
S1, S2 – Ankle plantar flexion

S2, S3, S4 – Voluntary
rectal tone

Cervical
lordosis

Thoracic
kyphosis

Lumbar
lordosis

13.9 Common spinal problems

- Mechanical back pain
- Prolapsed intervertebral disc
- Spinal stenosis
- Ankylosing spondylitis
- Compensatory scoliosis from leg-length discrepancy
- Cervical myelopathy
- Pathological pain/deformity, e.g. osteomyelitis, tumour, myeloma
- Osteoporotic vertebral fracture resulting in kyphosis (or rarely lordosis), especially in the thoracic spine with loss of height
- Cervical rib
- Scoliosis
- Spinal instability, e.g. spondylolisthesis

Cervical spine

Anatomy and physiology

Head nodding occurs at the atlanto-occipital joint, and rotational neck movements mainly at the atlantoaxial joint. Flexion, extension and lateral flexion occur mainly at the mid-cervical level. The neural canal contains the spinal cord and the emerging nerve roots, which pass through exit foramina bounded by the facet joints

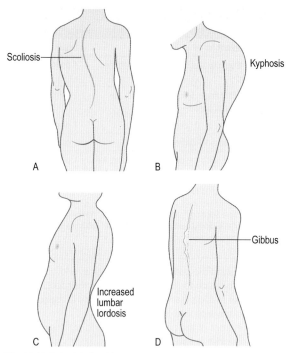

Fig. 13.12 Spinal deformities.

posteriorly and the intervertebral discs and neurocentral joints anteriorly. The nerve roots, particularly in the lower cervical spine, may be compressed or irritated by lateral disc protrusion or by osteophytes arising from the facet or neurocentral joints. Central disc protrusions may press directly on the cord (see Fig. 7.30).

The history

The most common symptoms are pain and difficulty turning the head and neck. Neck pain is usually felt posteriorly but may be referred to the head, shoulder, arm or interscapular region. Cervical disc lesions cause radicular pain in one arm or the other, roughly following the dermatomes of the affected nerve roots (see Box 13.3). If the spinal cord is compromised (cervical myelopathy), upper motor neurone leg weakness, altered sensation and sphincter disturbance may occur.

The physical examination

Be particularly careful when examining patients with rheumatoid arthritis, as atlantoaxial instability can lead to spinal cord damage when the neck is flexed.

In patients with neck injury, never move the neck. Splint it and check for abnormal posture. Check neurological function in the limbs and X-ray to assess bony injury.

Examination sequence ▶

Ask the patient to remove enough clothing for you to see their neck and upper thorax, then to sit on a chair.

Look

- Face the patient. Observe the posture of their head and neck. Note any abnormality (Box 13.10), such as loss of lordosis (usually due to muscle spasm).

Feel

- Feel the midline spinous processes from the occiput to T1 (usually the most prominent).

13.10 Causes of abnormal neck posture
Loss of lordosis or flexion deformity
• Acute lesions, rheumatoid arthritis, trauma
Increased lordosis
• Ankylosing spondylitis
Torticollis (wry neck)
• Sternocleidomastoid contracture, trauma
• Pharyngeal/parapharyngeal infection
Lateral flexion
• Erosion of lateral mass of atlas in rheumatoid arthritis

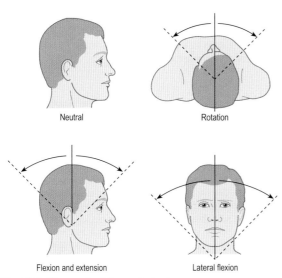

Neutral | Rotation

Flexion and extension | Lateral flexion

Fig. 13.13 Movements of the cervical spine.

• Feel the paraspinal soft tissues.
• Feel the supraclavicular fossae for cervical ribs or enlarged lymph nodes.
• Feel the anterior neck structures, including the thyroid.
• Note any tenderness in the spine, trapezius, interscapular and paraspinal muscles.

Move

Assess active movements (Fig. 13.13).
 Ask the patient to:
• Look down to the floor so that you can assess forward flexion. The normal range is 0 (neutral) to 80 degrees. Record a decreased range as the chin–chest distance.
• Look upwards at the ceiling as far back as possible, to assess extension. The normal range is 0 (neutral) to 50 degrees. Thus the total flexion–extension arc is normally approximately 130 degrees.
• Put their ear on to their shoulder, so that you can assess lateral flexion. The normal range is 0 (neutral) to 45 degrees.
• Look over their right/left shoulder. The normal range of lateral rotation is 0 (neutral) to 80 degrees.
 If active movements are reduced, gently perform passive movements. Establish if the end of the range has a sudden or a gradual resistance and whether it is pain or stiffness that restricts movement. Pain or paraesthesiae in the arm on passive neck movement suggests nerve root involvement.

13.11 Causes of thoracic spine pain
Adolescents and young adults
• Scheuermann's disease   • Disc protrusion (rare)
• Axial spondyloarthritis
Middle-aged and elderly
• Degenerative change   • Osteoporotic fracture
Any age
• Tumour   • Infection

Thoracic spine

Anatomy and physiology

This segment of the spine is the least mobile and maintains a physiological kyphosis throughout life. Movement is mainly rotational with a very limited amount of flexion, extension and lateral flexion.

The history

Presenting symptoms in the thoracic spine are localised spinal pain (Box 13.11), pain radiating round the chest wall or, less frequently, signs of cord compression: upper motor neurone leg weakness (paraparesis), sensory loss, and loss of bladder or bowel control. Disc lesions are rare but may cause pain radiating around the chest that mimics cardiac or pleural disease. Osteoporotic vertebral fractures may present with acute pain, or painless loss of height with increased kyphosis.
 Vertebral collapse due to malignancy may cause cord compression. Infection causes acute pain, often with systemic upset or fever. With poorly localised thoracic pain, consider intrathoracic causes, such as myocardial ischaemia or infarction, oesophageal or pleural pain, and aortic aneurysm.

The physical examination

Examination sequence

Ask the patient to undress to expose their neck, chest and back.

Look
• With the patient standing, inspect their posture from behind and from the side and the front, noting any deformity, such as a rib hump or abnormal curvature (see Fig. 13.12).

Feel
• Feel the midline spinous processes from T1 to T12. Feel for increased prominence of one or more posterior spinal processes, implying anterior wedge-shaped collapse of the vertebral body.
• Feel the paraspinal soft tissues for tenderness.

Move
• Ask the patient to sit with their arms crossed. Ask them to twist round both ways and look behind.

Lumbar spine

Anatomy and physiology

The surface markings are the spinous process of L4, which is level with the pelvic brim, and the 'dimples of Venus', which overlie the sacroiliac joints. The normal lordosis may be lost in disorders such as ankylosing spondylitis and lumbar disc protrusion.

13

The principal movements are flexion, extension, lateral flexion and rotation. In flexion, the upper segments move first, followed by the lower segments, to produce a smooth lumbar curve. However, even with a rigid lumbar spine, patients may be able to touch their toes if their hips are mobile.

In the adult, the spinal cord ends at L2. Below this, only the spinal nerve roots may be injured by disc protrusion.

The history

Low back pain is extremely common. Most is 'mechanical', and caused by degenerative changes in discs and facet joints (spondylosis).

Analyse the symptoms using 'SOCRATES'. For back pain, ask specifically about:

- occupational or recreational activity that may strain the back
- red flag features suggesting significant spinal pathology (Box 13.12)
- prior treatment with glucocorticoids.

Radicular pain caused by sciatic nerve root compression radiates down the posterior aspect of the leg to the lower leg or ankle (sciatica). Groin and thigh pain in the absence of hip abnormality suggests referred pain from L1–2.

Consider abdominal and retroperitoneal pathology, such as abdominal aortic aneurysm.

Mechanical low back pain is common after standing for too long or sitting in a poor position. Symptoms worsen as the day progresses and improve after resting or on rising in the morning.

Insidious onset of back or buttock ache and stiffness in an adolescent or young adult suggests inflammatory disease of the sacroiliac joints and lumbar spine (axial spondyloarthritis, Box 13.13). Symptoms are worse in the morning or after inactivity, and ease with movement. Morning stiffness is more marked than in osteoarthritis, lasting at least 30 minutes. Other clues to the diagnosis are peripheral joint involvement, extra-articular features or a positive family history.

Acute onset of low back pain in a young adult, often associated with bending or lifting, is typical of acute disc protrusion (slipped disc). Coughing or straining to open the bowels exacerbates the pain. There may be symptoms of lumbar or sacral nerve root compression. Cauda equina syndrome occurs when a central disc prolapse, or other space-occupying lesion, compresses the cauda equina. There are features of sensory and motor disturbance, including diminished perianal sensation and bladder function disturbance. The motor disturbance may be profound, as in paraplegia. Cauda equina syndrome and spinal cord compression are neurosurgical emergencies.

13.12 'Red flag' and 'yellow flag' features for acute low back pain

'Red flag' features
Features that may indicate serious pathology and require urgent referral

History
- Age <20 years or >55 years
- Recent significant trauma (fracture)
- Pain:
  - Thoracic (dissecting aneurysm)
  - Non-mechanical (infection/ tumour/pathological fracture)
- Fever (infection)
- Difficulty in micturition
- Faecal incontinence
- Motor weakness
- Sensory changes in the perineum (saddle anaesthesia)
- Sexual dysfunction, e.g. erectile/ejaculatory failure
- Gait change (cauda equina syndrome)
- Bilateral 'sciatica'

Past medical history
- Cancer (metastases)
- Previous glucocorticoid use (osteoporotic collapse)

System review
- Weight loss/malaise without obvious cause, e.g. cancer

'Yellow flag' features
Psychosocial factors associated with greater likelihood of long-term chronicity and disability
- A history of anxiety, depression, chronic pain, irritable bowel syndrome, chronic fatigue, social withdrawal
- A belief that the diagnosis is severe, e.g. cancer. Faulty beliefs can lead to 'catastrophisation' and avoidance of activity
- Lack of belief that the patient can improve leads to an expectation that only passive, rather than active, treatment will be effective
- Ongoing litigation or compensation claims, e.g. work, road traffic accident

---

13.13 Clinical vignette: back pain

A 34-year-old man attends his general practitioner's surgery with back pain. He first developed pain in his late teens but it improved for a few years. He has had persistent pain in his lower back and sometimes his buttocks for 5 years now. It wakes him from sleep and he can be very stiff in the mornings, although this eases as the morning progresses. There is no radiation to the leg. He is stiff after sitting or driving. He has always put it down to his occupation. He has used ibuprofen to good effect but has had diarrhoea and abdominal pain recently, which he attributes to this drug. Examination in the outpatient clinic shows a thin man with reduced lumbar mobility (modified Schober's index, reduced at 2 cm; see Fig. 13.15), pain on sacroiliac joint compression, and tenderness at his Achilles insertion. Investigations show him to have a raised C-reactive protein, an anaemia of chronic disease, a positive human leucocyte antigen B27 and a raised faecal calprotectin, suggesting inflammatory bowel disease. Magnetic resonance imaging confirms bilateral sacroiliitis and inflammatory changes in the lumbar spine.

A diagnosis of axial spondyloarthritis is made.

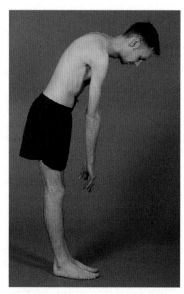

Ankylosing spondylitis. The patient trying to touch his toes.

Acute back pain in the middle-aged, elderly or those with risk factors, such as glucocorticoid therapy, may be due to osteoporotic fracture. This is eased by lying, exacerbated by spinal flexion and not usually associated with neurological symptoms.

Acute onset of severe progressive pain, especially when associated with malaise, weight loss or night sweats, may indicate pyogenic or tuberculous infection of the lumbar spine or sacroiliac joint. The infection may involve the intervertebral discs and adjacent vertebrae, and may track into the psoas muscle sheath, presenting as a painful flexed hip or a groin swelling.

Consider malignant disease involving a vertebral body in patients with unremitting spinal pain of recent onset that disturbs sleep. Other clues are a previous history of cancer, and systemic symptoms or weight loss.

Chronic intermittent pain in the lumbar spine is typical of degenerative disc disease. There is stiffness in the morning or after immobility. Pain and stiffness are relieved by gentle activity but recur with, or after, excessive activity.

Diffuse pain in the buttocks or thighs brought on by standing too long or walking is the presenting symptom of lumbosacral spinal stenosis. This can be difficult to distinguish from intermittent claudication (p. 64). The pain may be accompanied by tingling and numbness. Typically, it is relieved by rest or spinal flexion. Stooping or holding on to a supermarket trolley may increase exercise tolerance.

The physical examination

Examination sequence ▶

Ask the patient to stand with their back fully exposed.

Look
- Look for obvious deformity (decreased/increased lordosis, scoliosis) and soft-tissue abnormalities such as a hairy patch or lipoma that might overlie a congenital abnormality: for example, spina bifida.

Feel
- Palpate the spinous processes and paraspinal tissues. Note overall alignment and focal tenderness.
- After warning the patient, lightly percuss the spine with your closed fist and note any tenderness.

Move (Fig. 13.14)
- Flexion: ask the patient to try to touch their toes with their legs straight. Record how far down the legs they can reach. Some of this movement depends on hip flexion. Usually, the upper segments flex before the lower ones, and this progression should be smooth.
- Extension: ask the patient to straighten up and lean back as far as possible (normal 10–20 degrees from a neutral erect posture).
- Lateral flexion: ask them to reach down to each side, touching the outside of their leg as far down as possible while keeping their legs straight.

Special tests

Schober's test for forward flexion

Examination sequence ▶

- Mark the skin in the midline at the level of the posterior iliac spines (L5) (Fig. 13.15; mark A).
- Use a tape measure to draw two more marks: one 10 cm above (mark B) and one 5 cm below this (mark C).

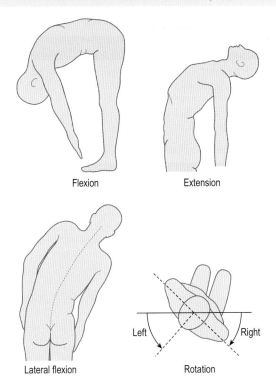

Fig. 13.14 Movements of the lumbar and dorsal spine.

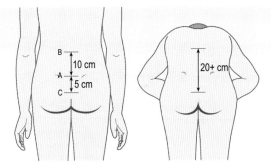

Fig. 13.15 Schober's test. When the patient bends forward maximally with the knees straight, distance BC should increase by at least 5 cm.

- Place the end of the tape measure on the upper mark (B). Ask the patient to touch their toes. The distance from B to C should increase from 15 to more than 20 cm.

Root compression tests

Intervertebral disc prolapse causing nerve root pressure occurs most often in the lower lumbar region, leading to compression of the corresponding nerve roots.

The femoral nerve (L2–4) lies anterior to the pubic ramus, so straight-leg raising or other forms of hip flexion do not increase its root tension. Problems with the femoral nerve roots may cause quadriceps weakness and/or diminished knee jerk on that side.

The sciatic nerve (L4–5; S1–3) runs behind the pelvis. Straight-leg raise tests L4, L5 and S1 nerve-root tension (L3/4, L4/5 and L5/S1 disc prolapse, respectively).

13

Sciatic nerve stretch test (L4–S1)

Examination sequence

- With the patient lying supine, lift their foot to flex the hip passively, keeping the knee straight.
- When a limit is reached, raise the leg to just less than this level, and dorsiflex the foot to test for nerve root tension (Fig. 13.16).

Femoral nerve stretch test (L2–4)

Examination sequence

- With the patient lying on their front (prone), flex their knee and extend the hip (Fig. 13.17). This stretches the femoral nerve. A positive result is pain felt in the back, or in the front of the thigh. This test can, if necessary, be performed with the patient lying on their side (with the test side uppermost).

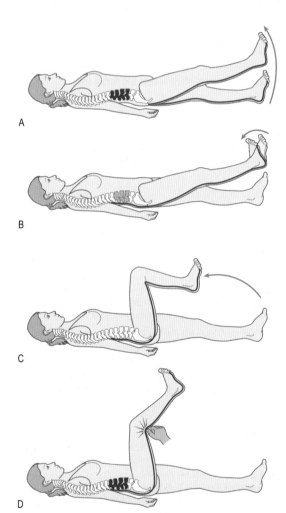

Fig. 13.16 Stretch test: sciatic nerve. [A] Straight-leg raising limited by the tension of the root over a prolapsed disc. [B] Tension is increased by dorsiflexion of the foot (Bragard's test). [C] Root tension is relieved by flexion at the knee. [D] Pressure over the centre of the popliteal fossa bears on the posterior tibial nerve, which is 'bowstringing' across the fossa, causing pain locally and radiation into the back.

Flip test for functional overlay

Examination sequence

- Ask the patient to sit on the end of the couch with their hips and knees flexed to 90 degrees (Fig. 13.18A).
- Examine the knee reflexes.
- Extend the patient's knee, as if to examine the ankle jerk. If achieved, this puts the straight leg at 90 degrees of hip flexion (Fig. 13.18B) and excludes sciatic nerve root compression; patients with root compression will lie back ('flip').

Sacroiliac joints

In general, examination of the sacroiliac joints is unreliable.

Examination sequence

- Lay the patient supine, flex the hip to 90 degrees and press down on the knee to transfer pressure through to the sacroiliac joints. This may cause pain in the buttock or lower back if the sacroiliac joint is inflamed.

Upper limb

The prime function of the upper limb is to position the hand appropriately in space. This requires shoulder, elbow and wrist

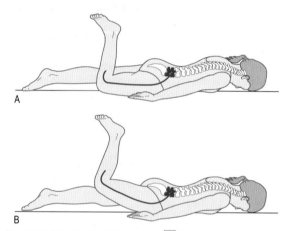

Fig. 13.17 Stretch test: femoral nerve. [A] Pain may be triggered by knee flexion alone. [B] Pain may be triggered by knee flexion in combination with hip extension.

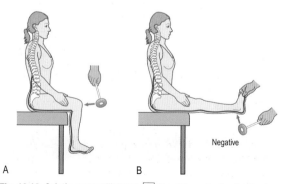

Fig. 13.18 Sciatic nerve: 'flip' test. [A] Divert the patient's attention to the tendon reflexes. [B] The patient with physical nerve root compression cannot permit full extension of the leg.

movements. The hand may function in both precision and power modes. The intrinsic muscles of the hand allow grip and fine manipulative movements, and the forearm muscles provide power and stability.

Distinguish between systemic and local conditions. Systemic conditions, such as rheumatoid arthritis, usually cause pathology at several sites. Differentiate local conditions from referred or radicular pain. Establish whether the condition is inflammatory or not from the pattern of diurnal stiffness and pain.

Hand and wrist

Motor and sensory innervation of the hand is shown in Fig. 7.27. The wrist joint has metacarpocarpal, intercarpal, ulnocarpal and radiocarpal components. There is a wide range of possible movements, including flexion, extension, adduction (deviation towards the ulnar side), abduction (deviation towards the radial side) and the composite movement of circumduction (the hand moves in a conical fashion on the wrist). Always name the affected finger (index, middle, ring and little) in documentation to avoid confusion. The PIP and DIP joints are hinge joints and allow only flexion and extension. The MCP joints allow flexion and extension, and some abduction/adduction, which is greatest when the MCP joints are extended.

The history

The patient will often localise symptoms of pain, stiffness, loss of function, contractures, disfigurement and trauma. If symptoms are vague or diffuse, consider referred pain or a compressive neuropathy, such as carpal tunnel syndrome (see Box 7.11). If PIP or MCP joint swelling is prominent, consider inflammatory arthritis.

Painful, swollen and stiff hand joints are common and important presenting symptoms, and scoring systems (Box 13.14) are used to define the presence of rheumatoid arthritis.

The physical examination

Examination sequence

Seat the patient facing you, with their arms and shoulders exposed. Start by examining the hand and fingers, and move proximally.

Look

- Erythema suggests acute inflammation caused by soft-tissue infection, septic arthritis, tendon sheath infection or crystal arthritis. Palmar erythema is associated with rheumatoid arthritis.
- Swelling of MCP joints due to synovitis produces loss of interknuckle indentation on the dorsum of the hand, especially when the MCP and interphalangeal joints are fully flexed (loss of the normal 'hill–valley–hill' aspect; Fig. 13.19A). 'Spindling' (swelling at the joint, tapering proximally and distally; Fig. 13.19B) is seen when the PIP joints are affected.
- Deformity of phalangeal fractures may produce rotation. Ask the patient to flex the fingers together (Fig. 13.20) and then in turn. Normally, with the MCP and interphalangeal joints flexed, the fingers should not cross, and should point to the scaphoid tubercle in the wrist.
- The fingers are long in Marfan's syndrome (arachnodactyly, see Fig. 3.21B).
- Boutonnière (or buttonhook) deformity is a fixed flexion deformity at the PIP joint with hyperextension at the DIP

13.14 American College of Rheumatology/European League Against Rheumatism classification criteria for rheumatoid arthritis, 2010	
Criteria	**Score**
Duration of symptoms (as reported by patient)	
<6 weeks	0
>6 weeks	1
Joint distribution (0–5)	
1 large joint[a]	0
2–10 large joints	1
1–3 small joints[b] (large joints not counted)	2
4–10 small joints (large joints not counted)	3
>10 joints (at least 1 small joint)	5
Serology (0–3)	
Negative RF and negative ACPA	0
Low positive RF or low positive ACPA	2
High positive RF or high positive ACPA	3
Acute-phase reactants	
Normal CRP and normal ESR	0
Abnormal CRP or abnormal ESR	1

Patients must have at least 1 swollen joint not better explained by another disease.
A score of ≥6 classifies the patient as having definite rheumatoid arthritis. A score of 4–5 is probable rheumatoid arthritis, i.e. a patient may have clinical rheumatoid arthritis but not fulfil all criteria.

[a]Large joints: shoulders, elbows, hips, knees and ankles
[b]Small joints: all metacarpophalangeal and proximal interphalangeal joints, thumb interphalangeal joint, wrists and 2nd–5th metatarsophalangeal joints.
ACPA, anti-cyclic citrullinated peptide antibody; CRP, C-reactive protein; ESR, erythrocyte sedimentation rate; RF, rheumatoid factor.
Reproduced from Aletaha D, Neogi T, Silman AJ, et al. Rheumatoid arthritis classification criteria: an American College of Rheumatology/European League Against Rheumatism collaborative initiative. Arthritis & Rheumatism 2010; 62(9): 2569–2581, with permission from John Wiley and Sons.

13

joint. 'Swan neck' deformity is hyperextension at the PIP joint with flexion at the DIP joint (Fig. 13.21).
- At the DIP joints (Fig. 13.21) a 'mallet' finger is a flexion deformity that is passively correctable. This is usually caused by minor trauma disrupting terminal extensor expansion at the base of the distal phalanx, with or without bony avulsion.
- There may be subluxation and ulnar deviation at the MCP joints in rheumatoid arthritis (Fig. 13.22).
- Bony expansion of DIP, PIP joints of the fingers and CMC joint of the thumb is typical of osteoarthritis (see Fig. 13.8).
- Anterior (or volar) displacement (partial dislocation) of the wrist may be seen in rheumatoid arthritis.

Extra-articular signs

- Dupuytren's contracture affects the palmar fascia, resulting in fixed flexion of the MCP and PIP joints of the little and ring fingers (see Fig. 3.5).
- Wasting of the interossei occurs in inflammatory arthritis and ulnar nerve palsy. Carpal tunnel syndrome causes wasting of the thenar eminence. T1 nerve root lesions (Fig. 13.23) cause wasting of all small hand muscles.
- Look for nail-fold infarcts, telangiectasia, palmar erythema, psoriasis, scars of carpal tunnel decompression, tendon transfer or MCP joint replacement.
- Nail changes, such as pitting and onycholysis (raising of the nail from its bed), occur in psoriatic arthritis (Fig. 3.7A).

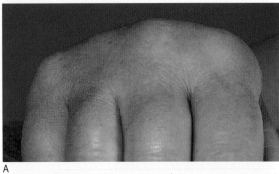

A

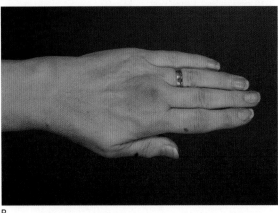

B

Fig. 13.19 Swelling of the metacarpophalangeal (MCP) and proximal interphalangeal (PIP) joints. [A] Ask the patient to make a fist. Look at it straight on to detect any loss of the 'hill–valley–hill' aspect. [B] Swelling and erythema of the middle finger MCP joint and index and middle finger PIP joints. Note also small muscle wasting.

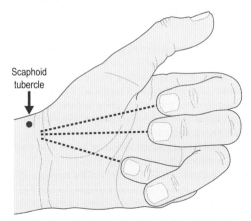

Fig. 13.20 Flexion of the fingers showing rotational deformity of the ring finger.

Feel

- Hard swellings are bony; soft swellings suggest synovitis.
- Palpate above and below the interphalangeal joints with your thumb and index finger to detect sponginess.
- Test the MCP joints by examining for sponginess and squeeze gently across them for pain.
- Palpate the flexor tendon sheaths in the hand and fingers to detect swelling or tenderness. Ask the patient to flex and then extend their fingers to establish whether there is triggering.

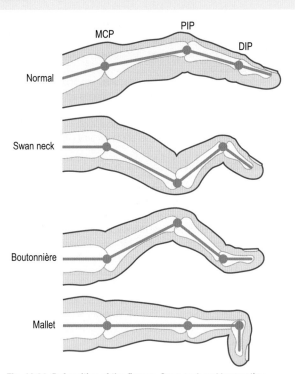

Fig. 13.21 Deformities of the fingers. Swan neck and boutonnière deformities occur in rheumatoid arthritis. Mallet finger occurs with trauma. DIP, distal interphalangeal; MCP, metacarpophalangeal; PIP, proximal interphalangeal.

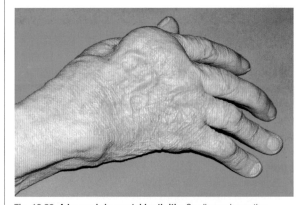

Fig. 13.22 Advanced rheumatoid arthritis. Small muscle wasting, subluxation and ulnar deviation at the metacarpophalangeal joints, boutonnière deformities at the ring and little fingers, and swelling and deformity of the wrist.

- De Quervain's tenosynovitis causes swelling, tenderness and crepitus (a creaking sensation that may even be audible) of the tendon sheaths of abductor pollicis longus and extensor pollicis brevis. Symptoms are aggravated by movements at the wrist and thumb.
- Crepitus may also occur with movement of the radiocarpal joints in osteoarthritis, most commonly secondary to old scaphoid or distal radial fractures.

Move
Active movements
- Ask the patient to make a fist and then extend their fingers fully.

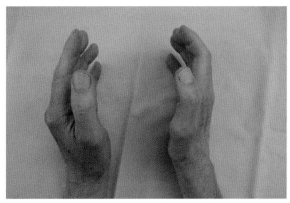

Fig. 13.23 T1 root lesion (cervical rib) affecting the right hand.
Wasting of the thenar eminence and interossei, and flexed posture of the fingers due to lumbrical denervation.

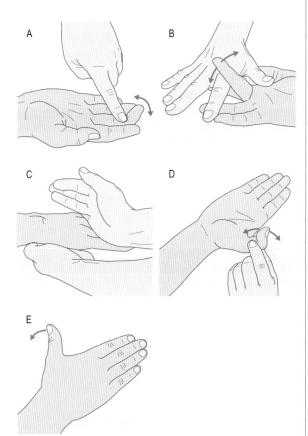

Fig. 13.24 Testing the flexors and extensors of the fingers and thumb. A Flexor digitorum profundus. B Flexor digitorum superficialis. C Extensor digitorum. D Flexor pollicis longus. E Extensor pollicis longus.

- Flexor digitorum profundus: ask the patient to flex the DIP joint while you hold the PIP joint in extension (Fig. 13.24A).
- Flexor digitorum superficialis: hold the patient's other fingers fully extended (to eliminate the action of flexor digitorum profundus, as it can also flex the PIP joint) and ask the patient to flex the PIP joint in question (Fig. 13.24B).
- Extensor digitorum: ask the patient to extend their fingers with the wrist in the neutral position (Fig. 13.24C).

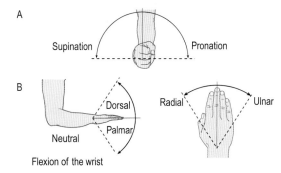

Fig. 13.25 Terms used to describe upper limb movements.

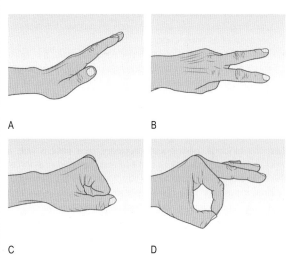

Fig. 13.26 Rapid assessment of the motor functions of the radial, ulnar and median nerves. A Paper (radial). B Scissors (ulnar). C Stone (median). D OK (median – anterior interosseus).

- Flexor and extensor pollicis longus: hold the proximal phalanx of the patient's thumb firmly and ask them to flex and extend the interphalangeal joint (Fig. 13.24D).
- Extensor pollicis longus: ask the patient to place their palm on a flat surface and to extend their thumb like a hitch-hiker (Fig. 13.24E). Pain occurs in de Quervain's disease.
- Insert your index and middle finger from the thumb side into the patient's palm and ask them to squeeze them as hard as possible to test grip.
- Ask the patient to put the palms of their hands together and extend the wrists fully – the 'prayer sign' (normal is 90 degrees of extension, see Fig. 13.10A).
- Ask the patient to put the backs of their hands together and flex the wrists fully – the 'reverse prayer sign' (normal is 90 degrees of flexion, see Fig. 13.10B).
- Check pronation and supination, flexion and extension, and ulnar and radial deviation (Fig. 13.25).

Passive movements
- Move each of the patient's fingers through flexion and extension and notice any loss of range of movement.
- Fully flex and extend the patient's wrist and note the range of movement and end-feel. Check radial and ulnar deviation.

Radial, ulnar and median nerve motor function
- Use 'Paper – scissors – stone – OK' as an aide-mémoire (Fig. 13.26).

13

- Radial nerve (wrist and finger extensors): ask the patient to extend the wrist and fingers fully ('paper sign').
- Ulnar nerve (hypothenar muscles, interossei, two medial lumbricals, adductor pollicis, flexor carpi ulnaris and the ulnar half of flexor digitorum profundus): ask the patient to make the 'scissors sign'.
- Median nerve (thenar muscles that abduct and oppose the thumb, the lateral two lumbricals, the medial half of flexor digitorum profundus, flexor digitorum superficialis, flexor carpi radialis, palmaris longus and pronator teres): ask the patient to clench the fist fully ('stone sign'). The best test of median nerve motor function is the ability to abduct the thumb away from the palm because of inconstant crossover in the nerve supply to the thenar eminence muscles other than abductor pollicis brevis. However, clenching the fist fully also depends on median function because of its flexor supply.
- Anterior interosseous nerve (flexor pollicis longus, the index finger flexor digitorum profundus and pronator quadratus): ask the patient to make the 'OK' sign. This depends on the function of both flexor pollicis longus and index finger flexor digitorum profundus.

Examining the wrist and hand with a wound

Test the tendons, nerves and circulation in a patient with a wrist or hand wound. The wound site and the hand position at the time of injury indicate which structures may be damaged. Normal movement may still be possible, however, even with 90% division of a tendon, so surgical exploration is needed for correct diagnosis and treatment. Sensory aspects of nerve injury are covered on page 142.

Elbow

Anatomy and physiology

The elbow joint has humeroulnar, radiocapitellar and superior radioulnar articulations. The medial and lateral epicondyles are the flexor and extensor origins, respectively, for the forearm muscles. These two prominences and the tip of the olecranon are easily palpated. They form an equilateral triangle when the elbow is flexed to 90 degrees, and lie in a straight line when the elbow is fully extended. A subcutaneous bursa overlies the olecranon and may become inflamed or infected (bursitis). Elbow pain may be localised or referred from the neck. Inflammatory arthritis and epicondylitis commonly cause elbow pain.

The physical examination

Examination sequence

Look
- Look at the overall alignment of the extended elbow. There is normally a valgus angle of 11–13 degrees with the elbow fully extended (the 'carrying angle').
- Look for:
  - the swelling of synovitis between the lateral epicondyle and olecranon, resulting in a block to full extension
  - the rash of psoriasis, olecranon bursitis, tophi or nodules
  - rheumatoid nodules on the proximal extensor surface of the forearm (see Fig. 13.7).

Feel
- Palpate the bony contours of the lateral and medial epicondyles and olecranon tip.
- Feel for sponginess, suggesting synovitis, on either side of the olecranon when the elbow is fully extended.
- Feel for focal tenderness over the lateral or medial epicondyle (see 'Special tests').
- Feel for olecranon bursa swelling, and nodules or tophi.
- Feel for rheumatoid nodules on the proximal extensor surface of the forearm.

Move
- Assess the extension–flexion arc: ask the patient to touch their shoulder on the same side and then straighten the elbow as far as possible. The normal range of movement is 0–145 degrees; a range of less than 30–110 degrees will cause functional problems.
- Assess supination and pronation: ask the patient to put their elbows by the sides of their body and flex them to 90 degrees. Now ask them to turn the palms upwards (supination: normal range 0–90 degrees) and then downwards (pronation: normal range 0–85 degrees).

Special tests

Tennis elbow (lateral epicondylitis)

Examination sequence

- Ask the patient to flex their elbow to 90 degrees and pronate and flex the hand/wrist fully.
- Support the patient's elbow. Ask them to extend their wrist against your resistance.
- Pain is produced at the lateral epicondyle and may be referred down the extensor aspect of the arm.

Golfer's elbow (medial epicondylitis)

Examination sequence

- Ask the patient to flex their elbow to 90 degrees and supinate the hand/wrist fully.
- Support the patient's elbow. Ask them to flex their wrist against your resistance.
- Pain is produced at the medial epicondyle and may be referred down the flexor aspect of the arm.

Shoulder

Anatomy and physiology

The shoulder joint consists of the glenohumeral joint, acromioclavicular joint and subacromial space. Movement also occurs between the scapula and the chest wall. The rotator cuff muscles are supraspinatus, subscapularis, teres minor and infraspinatus. They and their tendinous insertions help stability and movement, especially abduction at the glenohumeral joint.

The history

Pain is common (Boxes 13.15 and 13.16) and frequently referred to the upper arm. Glenohumeral pain may occur over the anterolateral aspect of the upper arm. Pain felt at the shoulder may be referred from the cervical spine or diaphragmatic and subdiaphragmatic peritoneum via the phrenic nerve. The most common cause of referred pain is cervical spondylosis, where disc-space narrowing and osteophytes cause nerve root impingement and inflammation.

13.15 Causes of shoulder girdle pain

Rotator cuff

- Degeneration
- Tendon rupture
- Calcific tendonitis

Subacromial bursa

- Calcific bursitis
- Polyarthritis

Capsule

- Adhesive capsulitis

Head of humerus

- Tumour
- Osteonecrosis
- Fracture/dislocation

Joints

- Glenohumeral, sternoclavicular:
  - Inflammatory arthritis, osteoarthritis, dislocation, infection
- Acromioclavicular:
  - Subluxation, osteoarthritis

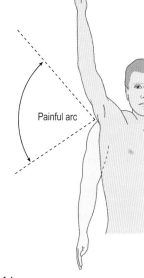

Fig. 13.27 Painful arc.

13

13.16 Common conditions affecting the shoulder

Non-trauma

- Rotator cuff syndromes, e.g. supraspinatus, infraspinatus tendonitis
- Impingement syndromes (involving the rotator cuff and subacromial bursa)
- Adhesive capsulitis ('frozen shoulder')
- Calcific tendonitis
- Bicipital tendonitis
- Inflammatory arthritis
- Polymyalgia rheumatica

Trauma

- Rotator cuff tear
- Glenohumeral dislocation
- Acromioclavicular dislocation
- Fracture of the clavicle
- Fracture of the head or neck of the humerus

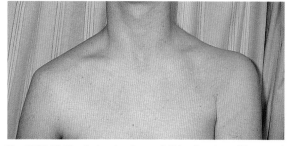

Fig. 13.28 **Right anterior glenohumeral dislocation.** Loss of the normal shoulder contour.

Stiffness and limitation of movement around the shoulder, caused by adhesive capsulitis of the glenohumeral joint, is common after immobilisation or disuse following injury or stroke. This is a 'frozen shoulder'. However, movement can still occur between the scapula and chest wall.

Some rotator cuff disorders, especially impingement syndromes and tears, present with a painful arc where abduction of the arm between 60 and 120 degrees causes discomfort (Fig. 13.27).

The physical examination

Examination sequence

Ask the patient to sit or stand and expose their shoulder completely.

Look

Examine from the front and back, and in the axilla, for:

- Deformity: the deformities of anterior glenohumeral and complete acromioclavicular joint dislocation are obvious (Fig. 13.28), but the shoulder contour in posterior glenohumeral dislocation may appear abnormal only when you stand above the seated patient and look down on the shoulder.
- Swelling.

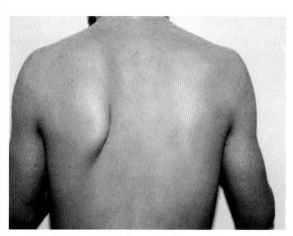

Fig. 13.29 **'Winging' of the left scapula.** This caused by paralysis of the nerve to serratus anterior.

- Muscle wasting, especially of the deltoid, supraspinatus and infraspinatus. Wasting of supraspinatus or infraspinatus indicates a chronic tear of their tendons.
- Size and position of the scapula: that is, whether it is elevated, depressed or 'winged' (Fig. 13.29).

Feel

- Feel from the sternoclavicular joint along the clavicle to the acromioclavicular joint.
- Palpate the acromion and coracoid (2 cm inferior and medial to the clavicle tip) processes, the scapula spine and the biceps tendon in the bicipital groove.
- Extend the shoulder to bring supraspinatus anterior to the acromion process. Palpate the supraspinatus tendon.

Move

Active movements (Fig. 13.30)

- Ask the patient to flex and extend their shoulder as far as possible.
- Abduction: ask the patient to lift their arm away from their side.
  - Palpate the inferior pole of the scapula between your thumb and index finger to detect scapular rotation and determine how much movement occurs at the glenohumeral joint. The first 0–15 degrees of abduction are produced by supraspinatus. The middle fibres of the deltoid are responsible for the next 15–90 degrees. Past 90 degrees the scapula needs to be rotated to achieve abduction, which is carried out by the trapezius and serratus anterior muscles (Fig. 13.31). If the glenohumeral joint is excessively stiff, movement of the scapula over the chest wall will predominate. If there is any limitation or pain (painful arc) associated with abduction, test the rotator cuff.
- Internal rotation: with the patient's arm by their side and the elbow flexed at 90 degrees, ask them to put their hand behind their back and feel as high up the spine as possible. Document the highest spinous process that they can reach with the thumb.
- External rotation: in the same position, with the elbow tucked against their side, ask them to rotate their hand outwards.
- Deltoid: ask the patient to abduct their arm out from their side, parallel to the floor, and resist while you push down on the humerus. Compare each side.

Rotator cuff muscles

To test the component muscles of the rotator cuff, the effect of other muscles crossing the shoulder needs to be neutralised.

- Internal rotation of the shoulder – subscapularis and pectoralis major:
  - To isolate subscapularis, place the patient's hand behind their back. If they cannot lift it off their back, it suggests a tear (Gerber test).
  - Pain on forced internal rotation suggests tendonitis.
- Abduction of the arm – supraspinatus:
  - With the patient's arm by their side, test abduction. Loss of power suggests a tear.
  - Pain on forced abduction at 60 degrees suggests tendonitis.
- External rotation – infraspinatus and teres minor:
  - Test external rotation with the arm in the neutral position and at 30 degrees to reduce the contribution of deltoid. Loss of power suggests a tear.
  - Pain on forced external rotation suggests tendonitis.
  - No movement or fixed internal rotation suggests a frozen shoulder.

Bicipital tendonitis

- Palpate the long head of biceps in its groove on the head of the humerus, noting any tenderness. Ask the patient to supinate their forearm and then flex the arm against resistance. Pain occurs in bicipital tendonitis. A rupture of the long head of biceps causes the muscle to bunch distally (the Popeye sign).

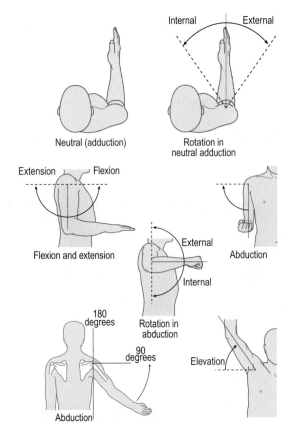

Fig. 13.30 Movements of the shoulder.

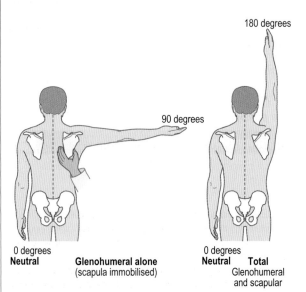

Fig. 13.31 Contribution of the glenohumeral joint and scapula to shoulder abduction.

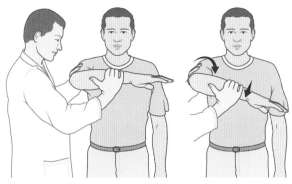

Fig. 13.32 Hawkins–Kennedy test for shoulder impingement.

Impingement (painful arc)

- Passively and fully abduct the patient's arm.
- Ask them to lower (adduct) it slowly.
  Pain occurring between 60 and 120 degrees of abduction occurs in painful arc.
- If the patient cannot initiate abduction, place your hand over their scapula to confirm there is no scapular movement.
- Passively abduct the internally rotated arm to 30–45 degrees.
- Ask them to continue to abduct their arm.
  Pain on active movement, especially against resistance, suggests impingement.

Special tests for impingement

Neer test

The patient sits in a relaxed position, with the elbow fully extended. Scapular rotation is prevented with one hand while the other abducts the arm in internal rotation. This causes the greater tuberosity to impinge against the acromion. A positive test is indicated by pain.

Hawkins–Kennedy test (Fig. 13.32)

The patient is examined sitting or standing, with their shoulder flexed at 90 degrees and their elbow flexed to 90 degrees, supported by the examiner to ensure maximal relaxation. The examiner forcefully rotates the arm internally. Reproduction of the patient's pain is a positive sign.

Lower limb

█ Hip

Anatomy

The hip is a ball-and-socket joint and allows flexion, extension, abduction, adduction, internal/external rotation and the combined movement of circumduction.

The history

Pain is usually felt in the groin but can be referred to the anterior thigh, the knee or the buttock. Hip pain is usually aggravated by activity, but osteonecrosis and tumours may be painful at rest and at night. Lateral hip or thigh pain, aggravated when lying on that side, suggests trochanteric pain syndrome. Fracture of the neck of the femur is common following relatively minor trauma in postmenopausal women and those aged over 70 years. The classical appearance is a shortened, externally rotated leg

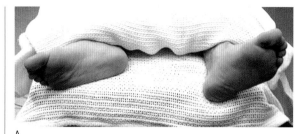

A

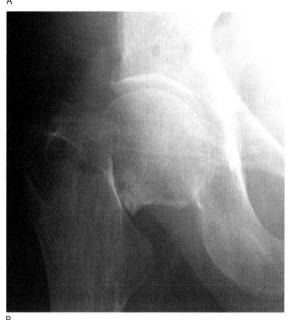

B

Fig. 13.33 Fracture of the neck of the right femur. [A] Shortening and external rotation of the leg. [B] X-ray showing translation and angulation.

(Fig. 13.33); the fracture also may be minimally displaced or impacted, however, and the patient may even be able to weight-bear.

Distinguish pain arising from the hip from:

- lumbar nerve root irritation (p. 263)
- spinal or arterial claudication (p. 64)
- abdominal causes such as hernia (p. 110).

Ask how the pain restricts activities. Record walking ability in terms of the time and distance the patient manages outside and on stairs, and note whether walking aids are used.

The physical examination

Examination sequence

Patients should undress to their underwear and remove socks and shoes. You should be able to see the iliac crests.

Look

- Assess gait.
- Carry out a general inspection: ask the patient to stand.
- From the front, check if:
  - stance is straight
  - shoulders lie parallel to the ground and symmetrically over the pelvis (this may mask a hip deformity or true shortening of one leg)

13

- hips, knees, ankles or feet are deformed
- muscles are wasted (from neuromuscular disease or disuse secondary to arthritis).
- From the side, look for:
  - a stoop or increased lumbar lordosis (both may result from limited hip extension)
  - scars, sinuses or skin changes around the hip.
- From behind, assess:
  - whether the spine is straight or curved laterally (scoliosis)
  - the relative positions of the shoulders and pelvis
  - any difference in leg lengths
  - for any gluteal atrophy.

Feel

- Palpate for tenderness over the greater trochanter, suggesting trochanteric pain syndrome.
- Feel the anterior superior iliac crest for enthesitis.
  This is a good time to check for leg shortening (see 'Special tests').

Move

With the patient supine on the couch, check that the pelvic brim is perpendicular to the spine.
- Check the range of flexion of each hip in turn.
- Abduction and adduction: stabilise the pelvis by placing your left hand on the opposite iliac crest. With your right hand, abduct the patient's leg until you feel the pelvis start to tilt (normal 45 degrees). Test adduction by crossing one of the patient's legs over the other and continuing to move it medially (normal 25 degrees) (Fig. 13.34A).
- Internal and external rotation: with the patient's leg in full extension, roll it on the couch and watch the foot to indicate the range of rotation. Test with the knee (and hip) flexed at 90 degrees. Move the foot medially to test external rotation and laterally to test internal rotation (normal 45 degrees for each movement) (Fig. 13.34B).
- Extension: ask the patient to lie prone on the couch. Place your left hand on the pelvis to detect any movement. Lift each of the patient's legs in turn to assess the range of extension (normal range 0–20 degrees) (Fig. 13.34C).

Thomas test

This reveals fixed flexion deformity (incomplete extension) that may be masked by compensatory movement at the lumbar spine or pelvis and increased lumbar lordosis.
- Place your left hand under the patient's back (to detect any masking of hip limitation by movement of the pelvis and lumbar spine).
- Passively flex both legs (hips and knees) as far as possible (Fig. 13.35A).
- Keep the non-test hip maximally flexed and by feeling with your left hand confirm that the lordotic curve of the spine remains eliminated.
- Ask the patient to extend the test hip. Incomplete extension in this position indicates a fixed flexion deformity at the hip (Fig. 13.35B).
- If the contralateral hip is not flexed sufficiently, the lumbar lordosis will not be eliminated and fixed flexion deformity of the ipsilateral knee confuses the issue. In this case, perform the test with the patient lying on their side.
- Do not perform the test if the patient has a hip replacement on the non-test side, as forced flexion may cause dislocation.

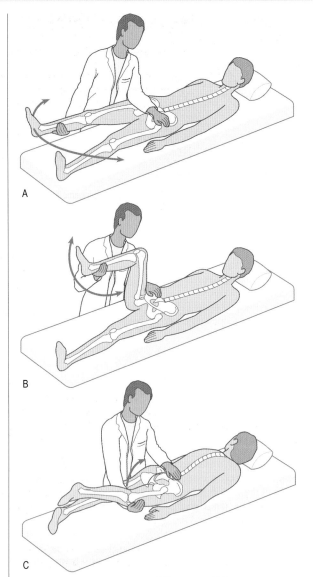

Fig. 13.34 **Testing hip movement.** A Abduction. B Flexion. C Extension.

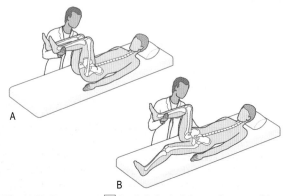

Fig. 13.35 **Thomas test.** A Passively flex both legs as far as possible. B Extend the test leg. Limitation indicates fixed flexion deformity.

13.17 Causes of true lower limb shortening

Hip

- Fractures, e.g. neck of femur
- Following total hip arthroplasty
- Slipped upper femoral epiphysis
- Perthes' disease (juvenile osteochondritis)
- Unreduced hip dislocation
- Septic arthritis
- Loss of articular cartilage (arthritis, joint infection)
- Congenital coxa vara
- Missed congenital dislocation of the hip

Femur and tibia

- Growth disturbance secondary to:
  - Poliomyelitis
  - Cerebral palsy
  - Fractures
  - Osteomyelitis
  - Septic arthritis
  - Growth-plate injury
  - Congenital causes

Special tests

Shortening

Shortening occurs in hip and other lower limb conditions (Box 13.17). Apparent shortening is present if the affected limb appears shortened, usually because of an adduction or flexion deformity at the hip.

Examination sequence

- Ask the patient to lie supine and stretch both legs out as far as possible equally, to eliminate any soft-tissue contracture/abnormal posture.
- Measure with a tape:
  - from umbilicus to medial malleolus: the apparent length
  - from anterior superior iliac spine to medial malleolus: the 'true length' (Fig. 13.36).
- Confirm any limb length discrepancy by 'block testing':
  - Ask the patient to stand with both feet flat on the ground.
  - Raise the shorter leg, using a series of blocks of graduated thickness until both iliac crests feel level.

Trendelenburg's sign

Examination sequence

- Stand in front of the patient.
- Palpate both iliac crests and ask the patient to stand on one leg for 30 seconds.
- Repeat with the other leg.
- Watch and feel the iliac crests to see which moves up or down.
- Normally, the iliac crest on the side with the foot off the ground should rise. The test is abnormal if the unsupported hemipelvis falls below the horizontal (Fig. 13.37). This may be caused by gluteal weakness or inhibition from hip pain, such as in osteoarthritis, or structural abnormality of the hip joint, such as in coxa vara or developmental hip dysplasia.

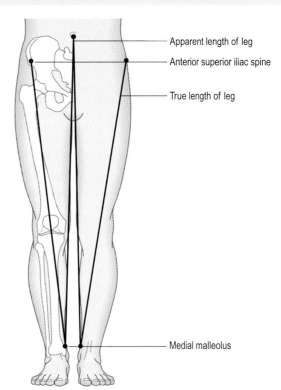

Fig. 13.36 True and apparent lengths of the lower limbs.

Apparent length of leg
Anterior superior iliac spine
True length of leg
Medial malleolus

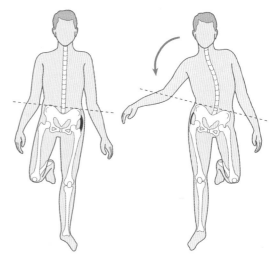

Fig. 13.37 Trendelenburg's sign. Powerful gluteal muscles maintain the position when standing on the left leg. Weakness of the right gluteal muscles results in pelvic tilt when standing on the right leg.

Knee

Anatomy

The knee is a complex hinge joint with tibiofemoral and patellofemoral components. It has a synovial capsule that extends under the quadriceps muscle (the suprapatellar pouch), reaching 5 cm above the superior edge of the patella. The joint is largely subcutaneous, allowing easy palpation of the patella, tibial tuberosity, patellar tendon, tibial plateau margin and femoral condyles. The knee depends on its muscular and ligamentous structures for stability (Fig. 13.38).

13

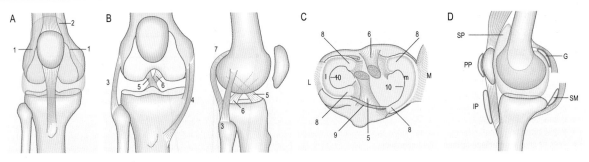

Key

G	Bursa under the medial head of gastrocnemius	1	Extensions of synovial sheath on either side of patella	7	Posterior ligament
IP	Infrapatellar bursa	2	Extension of synovial sheath at upper pole of patella	8	Horns of lateral (l) and medial (m) menisci
L	Lateral tibiofemoral articulation	3	Lateral ligament	9	Connection of anterior horns
M	Medial tibiofemoral articulation	4	Medial ligament	10	Unattached margin of meniscus
PP	Prepatellar bursa	5	Anterior cruciate ligament		
SM	Semimembranosus bursa	6	Posterior cruciate ligament		
SP	Suprapatellar pouch (or bursa)				

Fig. 13.38 Structure of the right knee. [A] Anterior view, showing the common synovial sheath. [B] Anterior and lateral views, showing the ligaments. [C] Plan view of the menisci. [D] Bursae.

13.18 Bone conditions associated with pathological fracture

- Osteoporosis
- Osteomalacia
- Primary or secondary tumour
- Osteogenesis imperfecta
- Renal osteodystrophy
- Parathyroid bone disease
- Paget's disease

The hamstring muscles flex the knee. Extension involves the quadriceps muscles, quadriceps tendon, patella, patellar tendon and tibial tuberosity. Any disruption of this 'extensor apparatus' prevents straight-leg raising or produces an extensor lag (a difference between active and passive ranges of extension).

The medial and lateral collateral ligaments resist valgus and varus stress, respectively. The anterior cruciate ligament (ACL) prevents anterior subluxation of the tibia on the femur, and the posterior cruciate ligament resists posterior translation. The medial and lateral menisci are crescentic fibrocartilaginous structures that lie between the tibial plateaux and the femoral condyles. There are several important bursae around the knee:

- anteriorly: the suprapatellar, prepatellar (between the patella and the overlying skin) and infrapatellar bursae (between the skin and the tibial tuberosity/patellar ligament)
- posteriorly: several bursae in the popliteal fossa (Fig. 13.38D).

The history

Pain

Generalised knee pain is likely to be due to pathology in the tibiofemoral joint (Box 13.18). Anterior knee pain, particularly after prolonged sitting or going downstairs, suggests patellofemoral joint pathology. Medial or lateral pain could come from the collateral ligaments or meniscal tears.

Pain in the knee may be referred from the hip.

Take a detailed history of the mechanism of any injury. The direction of impact, load and deformation predict what structures are injured.

Swelling

The normal volume of synovial fluid is 1–2 mL and is clinically undetectable. An effusion indicates intra-articular pathology. Haemarthrosis (bleeding into the knee) is caused by injury to a vascular structure within the joint, such as a torn cruciate ligament or an intra-articular fracture. The menisci are predominantly avascular and do not cause a haemarthrosis, unless torn at their periphery, or in conjunction with some other internal derangement.

Locking

Two common causes in the knee are a loose body, such as from osteochondritis dissecans, osteoarthritis or synovial chondromatosis, and a meniscal tear. Bucket-handle and anterior beak meniscal tears are especially associated with locking. Posterior horn tears commonly cause pain and limit movement in the last few degrees of flexion. Meniscal tears also cause local joint-line tenderness. Congenital discoid meniscus may present with locking and clunking.

Instability ('giving way')

Any of the four main ligaments may rupture from trauma or become incompetent with degenerative disease. The patella is prone to dislocate laterally because the normal knee has a valgus angle.

The physical examination

Examination sequence

Observe the patient walking and standing, as for gait. Note posture and deformities such as genu valgum (knock knee) or genu varum (bow legs).

Look

Ask the patient to lie supine on the couch. Expose both legs fully and look for:

- Scars, sinuses, erythema or rashes.
- Muscle wasting: quadriceps wasting is almost invariable with inflammation, internal derangement or chronic pain, and develops within days. Measure the thigh girth in both legs 20 cm above the tibial tuberosity.

- Leg length discrepancy.
- Flexion deformity: if the patient lies with one knee flexed, this may be caused by a hip, knee or combined problem.
- Swelling: look for an enlarged prepatellar bursa ('housemaid's knee') and any knee joint effusion. Large effusions form a horseshoe-shaped swelling above the knee. Swelling extending beyond the joint margins suggests infection, major injury or rarely tumour.
- Baker's cyst: bursa enlargement in the popliteal fossa.

Feel

- Warmth: compare both sides.
- Effusion.
- Patellar tap:
  - With the patient's knee extended, empty the suprapatellar pouch by sliding your left hand down the thigh until you reach the upper edge of the patella.
  - Keep your hand there and, with the fingertips of your right hand, press briskly and firmly over the patella (Fig. 13.39).
  - In a moderate-sized effusion you will feel a tapping sensation as the patella strikes the femur.
- 'Bulge' or 'ripple' test (Fig. 13.40):
  - Extend the patient's knee and, with the quadriceps muscles relaxed, empty the medial compartment into the suprapatellar bursa and lateral side by stroking the medial side of the knee (Fig. 13.40A).
  - Empty the suprapatellar bursa by sliding your hand down the thigh to the patella (Fig. 13.40B).
  - Without lifting your hand off the knee, extend your fingers (or thumb) to stroke the lateral side of the knee (Fig. 13.40C).
  - The test is positive if a ripple or bulge of fluid appears on the medial side of the knee. It is useful for detecting small amounts of fluid but may be falsely negative if a tense effusion is present.
- Synovitis: with the patient's knee extended and the quadriceps relaxed, feel for sponginess on both sides of the quadriceps tendon.
- Joint lines: feel the medial and lateral joint lines. If there is tenderness, localise this as accurately as possible. In adolescents, localised tibial tuberosity tenderness suggests Osgood–Schlatter disease, a traction osteochondritis.

Move
Active flexion and extension
- With the patient supine, ask them to flex their knee up to their chest and then extend the leg back down to lie on the couch (normal range 0–140 degrees).
- Feel for crepitus between the patella and femoral condyles, suggesting chondromalacia patellae (more common in younger female patients) or osteoarthritis.
- Record the range of movement: if there is a fixed flexion deformity of 15 degrees and flexion is possible to 110 degrees, record this as a range of movement of 15–110 degrees.
- Ask the patient to lift their leg and note any extensor lag.

Passive flexion and extension
- Normally the knee can extend so that the femur and tibia are in longitudinal alignment. Record full extension as 0 degrees. A restriction to full extension occurs with meniscal tears, osteoarthritis and inflammatory arthritis. To assess hyperextension, lift both of the patient's legs by the feet. Hyperextension (genu recurvatum) is present if the knee extends beyond the neutral position. Up to 10 degrees is normal.
- Test the extreme range of knee flexion with the patient face down on the couch, which makes comparison with the contralateral side easy. A block to full flexion is often caused by a tear of the posterior horn of the menisci.

Ligament testing
Collateral ligament
With the knee fully extended, abduction or adduction should not be possible. If either ligament is lax or ruptured, movement can occur. If the ligament is strained (partially torn) but intact, pain will be produced but the joint will not open.

Examination sequence

- With the patient's knee fully extended, hold their ankle between your elbow and side. Use both hands to apply a valgus and then varus force to the knee.
- Use your thumbs to feel the joint line and assess the degree to which the joint space opens. Major opening of the joint indicates collateral and cruciate injury (Fig. 13.41A).
- If the knee is stable, repeat the process with the knee flexed to 30 degrees to assess minor collateral laxity. In this position the cruciate ligaments are not taut.

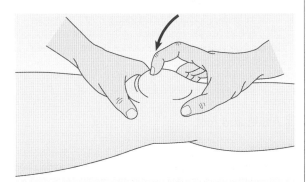

Fig. 13.39 Testing for effusion by the patellar tap.

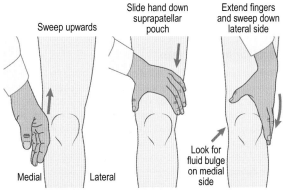

Sweep upwards · Slide hand down suprapatellar pouch · Extend fingers and sweep down lateral side · Medial · Lateral · Look for fluid bulge on medial side

Fig. 13.40 Bulge or ripple test to detect small knee effusions.

13

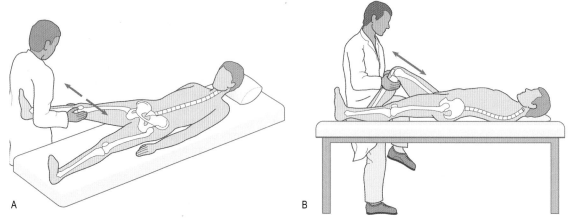

Fig. 13.41 **Testing the ligaments of the knee.** A Collateral ligaments. B Cruciate ligaments.

Anterior cruciate ligament

Examination sequence

Anterior drawer test

- Flex the patient's knee to 90 degrees and maintain this position using your thigh to immobilise the patient's foot.
- Check that the hamstring muscles are relaxed and look for posterior sag (posterior subluxation of the tibia on the femur). This causes a false-positive anterior drawer sign that should not be interpreted as ACL laxity.
- With your hands behind the upper tibia and both thumbs over the tibial tuberosity, pull the tibia anteriorly (Fig. 13.41B). Significant movement (compared with the opposite knee) indicates that the ACL is lax. Movement of >1.5 cm suggests ACL rupture. There is often an associated medial ligament injury.

Lachmann test

- Flex the knee at 20–30 degrees with the patient supine. Place one hand behind the tibia and grasp the patient's thigh with your other hand. Pull the tibia forward to assess the amount of anterior motion of the tibia in comparison to the femur. An intact ACL should prevent forward translational movement ('firm endpoint'), while a deficient ACL will allow increased forward translation without a decisive 'endpoint'.

Posterior drawer test

- Push backwards on the tibia. Posterior movement of the tibia suggests posterior cruciate ligament laxity.

Tests for meniscal tears

Meniscal tears in younger, sporty patients usually result from a twisting injury to the weight-bearing leg. In middle-aged patients, degenerative, horizontal cleavage of the menisci is common, with no history of trauma. Meniscal injuries commonly cause effusions, especially on weight bearing or after exercise. Associated joint-line tenderness is common.

A simple test for a meniscal tear is to extend the patient's knee rapidly from 30 degrees flexion to full extension. If the patient experiences medial or lateral pain, this suggests a tear, and formal testing should take place.

Meniscal provocation test (McMurray test)

Examination sequence

Ask the patient to lie supine on the couch. Test the medial and lateral menisci in turn.

Medial meniscus

- Passively flex the patient's knee to its full extent.
- Externally rotate the patient's foot and abduct the upper leg at the hip, keeping the foot towards the midline (that is, creating a varus stress at the knee).
- Extend the patient's knee smoothly. In medial meniscus tears a click or clunk may be felt or heard, accompanied by discomfort.

Lateral meniscus

- Passively flex the patient's knee to its full extent.
- Internally rotate the patient's foot and adduct the leg at the hip (that is, creating a valgus stress at the knee).
- Extend the patient's knee smoothly. In lateral meniscus tears a click or clunk may be felt or heard, accompanied by discomfort.

Patella

Examination sequence

- Look for prepatellar bursa swelling.
- Feel around the patella for tenderness suggestive of enthesitis or tendonitis.

Patellar apprehension test

- With the patient's knee fully extended, push the patella laterally and flex the knee slowly. If the patient actively resists flexion, this suggests previous patellar dislocation or instability.

Other tests for patellofemoral pathology are unreliable and may be positive in normal individuals.

▍ Ankle and foot

Anatomy

The ankle is a hinge joint. The talus articulates with a three-sided mortise made up of the tibial plafond and the medial and lateral malleoli. This allows dorsiflexion and plantar flexion, although

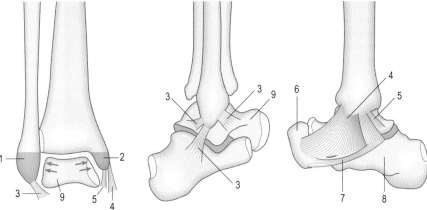

1. Lateral malleolus
2. Medial malleolus
3. Lateral (external) ligament
4. Medial ligament
5. Deep fibres of medial ligament
6. Navicular
7. Spring ligament
8. Calcaneus
9. Talus

Fig. 13.42 **Ankle ligaments.**

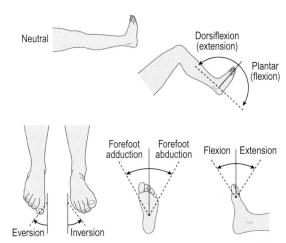

Fig. 13.43 **Terminology used for movements of the ankle and foot.**

some axial rotation can occur at the plantar-flexed ankle. The bony mortise is the major factor contributing to stability, but the lateral, medial (deltoid) and inferior tibiofibular ligaments are also important (Fig. 13.42).

Movements of the ankle and foot are summarised in Fig. 13.43. Foot movements are inversion and eversion, principally occurring at the mid-tarsal (talonavicular/calcaneocuboid) and subtalar (talocalcaneal) joints.

The history

A 'twisted' ankle is very common, and is usually related to a sporting injury or stepping off a kerb or stair awkwardly. Establish the exact mechanism of injury and the precise site of pain. Frequently there has been a forced inversion injury stressing the lateral ligament. A sprain occurs when some fibres are torn but the ligament remains structurally intact. A complete ligament tear allows excessive talar movement in the ankle mortise with instability.

Achilles tendon rupture is associated with sudden plantar flexion at the ankle. It is common in middle-aged patients doing unaccustomed activity such as squash, and is associated with some medications such as oral glucocorticoids and fluoroquinolone antibiotics. Sudden pain occurs above the heel and there is often a sensation or noise of a crack. Patients may feel as if they have been kicked or even shot.

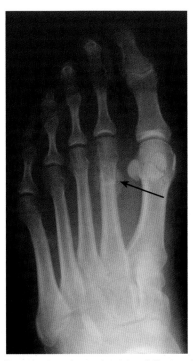

Fig. 13.44 **Stress fracture of second metatarsal.** Fracture site and callus *(arrow)*.

Forefoot pain, often localised to the second metatarsal, after excessive activity such as trekking, marching or dancing, suggests a stress fracture (Fig. 13.44). Symptoms are relieved by rest and aggravated by weight bearing.

Non-traumatic conditions

Anterior metatarsalgia with forefoot pain is common, especially in middle-aged women. Acute joint pain with swelling suggests an inflammatory arthropathy such as rheumatoid arthritis or gout. In severe cases the metatarsal heads become prominent and walking feels like walking on pebbles or broken glass.

Plantar surface heel pain that is worse in the foot-strike phase of walking may be caused by plantar fasciitis and tends to affect middle-aged patients and those with seronegative arthritides.

Posterior heel pain may be caused by Achilles tendonitis or enthesitis.

13

Spontaneous lancinating pain in the forefoot radiating to contiguous sides of adjacent toes occurs with Morton's neuroma. A common site is the interdigital cleft between the third and fourth toes. This occurs predominantly in women aged 25–45 years and is aggravated by wearing tight shoes.

The physical examination

Examination sequence

Ask patients to remove their socks and shoes.

Look

- Examine the soles of the shoes for abnormal patterns of wear.
- Assess gait. Look for:
  - increased height of step, indicating 'foot drop'
  - ankle movement (dorsiflexion/plantar flexion)
  - position of the foot as it strikes the ground (supinated/pronated)
  - hallux rigidus – loss of movement at the metatarsophalangeal (MTP) joints.
- From behind and with the patient standing:
  - Observe how the heel is aligned (valgus/varus).
- From the side:
  - Observe the position of the midfoot, looking particularly at the medial longitudinal arch. This may be flattened (pes planus – flat foot) or exaggerated (pes cavus).
  - If the arch is flattened, ask the patient to stand on tiptoe. This restores the arch in a mobile deformity but not in a structural one.
- A 'splay foot' has widening at the level of the metatarsal heads, often associated with MTP joint synovitis.
- Examine the ankle and foot for scars, sinuses, swelling, bruising, callosities (an area of thickened skin at a site of repeated pressure), nail changes, oedema, deformity and position.
- Look for deformities of the toes such as hallux valgus (Fig. 13.45) or overriding toes.
- Observe any bunion (a soft-tissue bursal swelling) over the first metatarsal head that may be inflamed or infected.

Feel

- Feel for focal tenderness and heat.
- In an acute ankle injury, palpate the proximal fibula, both malleoli, the lateral ligament and the base of the fifth metatarsal.
- Gently compress the forefoot. Assess the lesser toe MTP joints for swelling and tenderness suggestive of inflammatory arthritis.

Move (see Fig. 13.43)
Active movements
- Assess plantar flexion/dorsiflexion at the ankle, inversion/eversion of the foot and flexion/extension of the toes.

Passive movements
- Grip the patient's heel from below with the cup of your left hand, with your thumb and index finger on the malleoli.
- Put the foot through its arc of movement (normal range 15 degrees dorsiflexion to 45 degrees plantar flexion).
- If dorsiflexion is restricted, assess the contribution of gastrocnemius (which functions across both knee and ankle joints) by measuring ankle dorsiflexion with the knee extended and flexed. If more dorsiflexion is possible with the knee flexed, this suggests a gastrocnemius contracture.

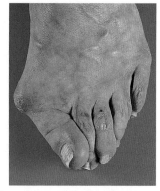

Fig. 13.45 Hallux valgus overriding the second toe.

Passive foot inversion/eversion
- Examine the subtalar joint in isolation by placing the foot into dorsiflexion to stabilise the talus in the ankle mortise.
- Move the heel into inversion (normal 20 degrees) and eversion (normal 10 degrees).
- Examine the combined mid-tarsal joints by fixing the heel with your left hand and moving the forefoot with your right hand into dorsiflexion, plantar flexion, adduction, abduction, supination and pronation.

Passive hallux and lesser toe movements
- Assess flexion and extension at MTP and interphalangeal joints. Pain and stiffness at the first MTP joint suggest hallux rigidus.
- If there is toe deformity, assess impingement on the other toes. Claw toes result from dorsiflexion at MTP joints and plantar flexion at PIP and DIP joints. Hammer toes are due to dorsiflexion at MTP and DIP joints, and plantar flexion at PIP joints. Mallet toes describe plantar flexion at DIP joints.

Special tests
Achilles tendon

Examination sequence

- Ask the patient to kneel with both knees on a chair.
- Palpate the gastrocnemius muscle and the Achilles tendon for focal tenderness and soft-tissue swelling. Achilles tendon rupture is often palpable as a discrete gap in the tendon about 5 cm above the calcaneal insertion (Fig. 13.46A).

Thomson's (Simmond's) test

Examination sequence

- Squeeze the calf just distal to the level of maximum circumference. If the Achilles tendon is intact, plantar flexion of the foot will occur (Fig. 13.46B).

Mulder's sign for Morton's neuroma

Examination sequence

- Squeeze the metatarsal heads together with one hand, at the same time putting pressure on the interdigital space with your other hand. The pain of the neuroma will be localised to the plantar surface of the interdigital space and may be accompanied by a 'clunk' as the neuroma slides between the metatarsal heads. Paraesthesia will radiate into the affected toes.

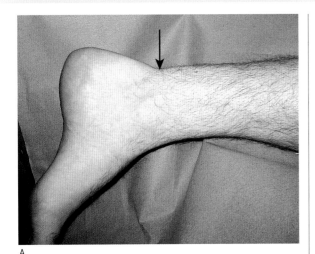

A

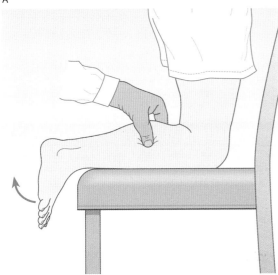

B

Fig. 13.46 Ruptured Achilles tendon. [A] Site of a palpable defect in the Achilles tendon *(arrow).* [B] Thomson's test. Failure of the foot to plantar-flex when the calf is squeezed is pathognomonic of an acute rupture of the Achilles tendon.

Fractures, dislocations and trauma

A fracture is a breach in the structural integrity of a bone. This may arise in:

- normal bone from excessive force
- normal bone from repetitive load-bearing activity (stress fracture)
- bone of abnormal structure (pathological fracture, see Box 13.18) with minimal or no trauma.

The epidemiology of fractures varies geographically. There is an epidemic of osteoporotic fractures because of increasing elderly populations. Although any osteoporotic bone can fracture, common sites are the distal radius (Fig. 13.47), neck of femur (see Fig. 13.33), proximal humerus and spinal vertebrae.

Fractures resulting from road traffic accidents and falls are decreasing because of legislative and preventive measures such as seat belts, air bags and improved roads. A fracture may occur in the context of severe trauma.

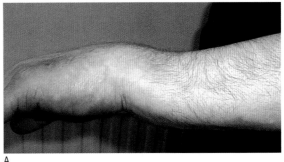

A

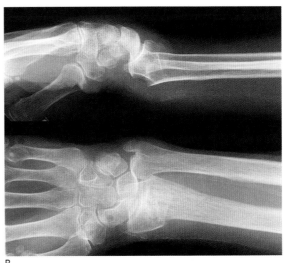

B

Fig. 13.47 Colles' fracture. [A] Clinical appearance of a dinner-fork deformity. [B] X-ray appearance.

The history

Establish the mechanism of injury. For example, a patient who has fallen from a height on to their heels may have obvious fractures of the calcaneal bones in their ankles but is also at risk of fractures of the proximal femur, pelvis and vertebral column.

The physical examination

Use the 'Look – feel – move' approach. Observe patients closely to see if they move the affected part and are able to weight-bear.

Examination sequence

Look
- See if the skin is intact. If there is a breach in the skin and the wound communicates with the fracture, the fracture is open or compound; otherwise it is closed.
- Look for associated bruising, deformity, swelling or wound infection (Fig. 13.48).

Feel
- Gently feel for local tenderness.
- Feel distal to the suspected fracture to establish if sensation and pulses are present.

13

Move

- Establish whether the patient can move joints distal and proximal to the fracture.
- Do not move a fracture site to see if crepitus is present; this causes additional pain and bleeding.

Describe the fracture according to Box 13.19. For each suspected fracture, X-ray two views (at least) at perpendicular planes of the affected bone, and include the joints above and below.

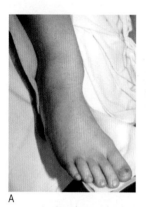 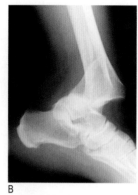

A   B

Fig. 13.48 Ankle deformity. A Clinical appearance. B Lateral X-ray view showing tibiotalar fracture dislocation.

13.19 Describing a fracture

- What bone(s) is/are involved?
- Is the fracture open (compound) or closed?
- Is the fracture complete or incomplete?
- Where is the bone fractured (intra-articular/epiphysis/physis/metaphysis/diaphysis)?
- What is the fracture's configuration (transverse/oblique/spiral/comminuted (multifragmentary)/butterfly fragment)?
- What components of deformity are present?
  - Translation is the shift of the distal fragment in relation to the proximal bone. The direction is defined by the movement of the distal fragment, e.g. dorsal or volar, and is measured as a percentage.
  - Angulation is defined by the movement of the distal fragment, measured in degrees.
  - Rotation is measured in degrees along the longitudinal axis of the bone, e.g. for spiral fracture of the tibia or phalanges.
  - Shortening: proximal migration of the distal fragment can cause shortening in an oblique fracture. Shortening may also occur if there has been impaction at the fracture site, e.g. a Colles' fracture of the distal radius.
- Is there distal nerve or vascular deficit?
- What is the state of the tissues associated with the fracture (soft tissues and joints, e.g. fracture blisters, dislocation)?

Investigations

Common investigations in patients with musculoskeletal disease are summarised in Box 13.20.

13.20 Common musculoskeletal investigations

Investigation	Indication/comment
Urinalysis	
Protein	Glomerular disease, e.g. SLE, vasculitis
	Secondary amyloid in RA and other chronic arthropathies
	Drug adverse effects, e.g. myocrisin, penicillamine
Blood	Glomerular disease, e.g. SLE, vasculitis
Haematological	
Full blood count	Anaemia in inflammatory arthritis, blood loss after trauma
	Neutrophilia in sepsis and very acute inflammation, e.g. acute gout
	Leucopenia in SLE, Felty's syndrome and adverse effects of antirheumatic drug therapy
Erythrocyte sedimentation rate/plasma viscosity	Non-specific indicator of inflammation or sepsis
C-reactive protein	Acute-phase protein
Biochemical	
Urea and creatinine	↑ in renal impairment, e.g. secondary amyloid in RA or adverse drug effect
Uric acid	May be ↑ in gout. Levels may be normal during an acute attack
Calcium	↓ in osteomalacia; normal in osteoporosis
Alkaline phosphatase	↑ in Paget's disease, metastases, osteomalacia and immediately after fractures
Angiotensin-converting enzyme	↑ in sarcoidosis
Urinary albumin : creatinine ratio	Glomerular disease, e.g. vasculitis, SLE
Serological	
Immunoglobulin M rheumatoid factor	↑ titres in 60–70% of cases of RA; occasionally, low titres in other connective diseases. Present in up to 15% of normal population. Superseded by anti-cyclic citrullinated peptide antibodies
Anti-cyclic citrullinated peptide antibody (ACPA)	Present in 60–70% of cases of RA and up to 10 years before onset of disease. Highly specific for RA. Occasionally found in Sjögren's syndrome
Antinuclear factors	↑ titres in most cases of SLE; low titres in other connective tissue diseases and RA
Anti-Ro, Anti-La	Sjögren's syndrome

13.20 Common musculoskeletal investigations – *cont'd*

Investigation	Indication/comment
Anti-double-stranded DNA	SLE
Anti-Sm	SLE
Anti-ribonucleoprotein	Mixed connective tissue disease
Antineutrophil cytoplasmic antibodies	Granulomatosis with polyangiitis, polyarteritis nodosa, Churg–Strauss vasculitis
Other	
Schirmer tear test, salivary flow test	Keratoconjunctivitis sicca (dry eyes), Sjögren's syndrome
Imaging	
Plain radiography (X-ray)	Fractures, erosions in RA and psoriatic arthritis, osteophytes and joint-space loss in osteoarthritis, bone changes in Paget's disease, pseudofractures (Looser's zones) in osteomalacia
Ultrasonography	Detection of effusion, synovitis, cartilage breaks, enthesitis and erosions in inflammatory arthritis. Double contour sign in gout
	Detection of bursae, tendon pathology and osteophytes
Magnetic resonance imaging	Joint and bone structure; soft-tissue imaging
Computed tomography	High-resolution scans of thorax for pulmonary fibrosis
Dual-energy X-ray absorptiometry	Gold standard for determining osteoporosis. Usual scans are of lumbar spine, hip and lateral vertebral assessment for fractures
Isotope bone scan	Increased uptake in Paget's disease, bone tumour, infection, fracture. Infrequently used due to high radiation dose.
Joint aspiration/biopsy	
Synovial fluid microscopy	Inflammatory cells, e.g. ↑ neutrophils in bacterial infection
Polarised light microscopy	Positively birefringent rhomboidal crystals – calcium pyrophosphate (pseudogout)
	Negatively birefringent needle-shaped crystals – monosodium urate monohydrate (gout)
Bacteriological culture	Organism may be isolated from synovial aspirates
Biopsy and histology	Synovitis – RA and other inflammatory arthritides

RA, *rheumatoid arthritis;* SLE, *systemic lupus erythematosus.*

13

OSCE example 1: Right shoulder pain

Mr Hunt, 38 years old, has a 2-month history of right shoulder pain with no history of trauma.

Please examine the shoulder

- Introduce yourself and clean your hands.
- Expose both of the patient's shoulders and arms.
- Comment on acromioclavicular deformity and muscle wasting; look for winging of the scapula.
- Compare the right shoulder to the normal left shoulder.
- Perform active and passive movements. In particular, look for frozen shoulder, which is diagnosed by limitation of external rotation and flexion.
- Finally, examine the arm, looking for conditions such as biceps rupture.
- If all movements of the shoulder are normal, conduct a full examination of the neck.
- Thank the patient and clean your hands.

Summarise your findings

The patient reports pain between 120 and 60 degrees of abduction when lowering the abducted shoulder. Pain is reproduced on abduction against resistance.

Suggest a differential diagnosis

The most common cause of these symptoms is impingement syndrome, which can be confirmed by carrying out special tests (Neer and Hawkins–Kennedy). Differentials include frozen shoulder, calcific tendonitis, acromioclavicular joint pain, arthritis (osteoarthritis, rheumatoid arthritis or post-traumatic), long head of biceps rupture and referred pain from the neck.

Suggested investigations

X-ray will reveal degenerative changes in osteoarthritis or tendon calcification. Ultrasound may demonstrate effusions, calcific deposits and tendon damage/rupture.

OSCE example 2: Painful hands

Mrs Hill, 46 years old, presents with an 8-week history of insidious onset of pain, stiffness and swelling of her hands. She smokes 15 cigarettes per day.

Please examine her hands

- Introduce yourself and clean your hands.
- Look:
  - In this case there is swelling of two MCP joints on the right, and one PIP joint on the left.
  - Normal nails and skin (therefore psoriatic arthropathy is unlikely).
- Feel:
  - Ask first what is sore and seek permission to examine gently.
  - Tender, soft swelling of the MCP and PIP joints in the hands and left elbow.
  - In feet: tender across her MTP joints on squeeze test but no palpable swelling.
- Move:
  - Painful MCP joints in right hand on active and passive flexion, reducing handgrip and fine movements.

Summarise your findings

The patient has tender, soft swelling of two MCP joints and one PIP joint. There is pain on active and passive movement of the affected joints, resulting in limitation of hand function.

Suggest a differential diagnosis

The pattern of joint involvement, patient's gender, duration of symptoms and history of smoking support a clinical diagnosis of rheumatoid arthritis. The differential diagnosis of psoriatic arthropathy is less likely because of her normal nails and lack of the typical skin changes of psoriasis.

Suggest initial investigations

Full blood count, renal function tests, calcium, phosphate and liver function tests to assess for anaemia of chronic disease and to determine suitability for disease-modifying antirheumatic drugs; C-reactive protein to assess the degree of systemic inflammation; anti-CCP antibody to confirm whether seropositive rheumatoid arthritis is present; application of the 2010 American College of Rheumatology/European League Against Rheumatism criteria (see Box 13.14) for classification of rheumatoid arthritis; hand and foot X-rays to detect any bony erosions; chest X-ray to look for rheumatoid lung disease.

Integrated examination sequence for the locomotor system

- Ask the patient to undress to their underwear.
- Ask the GALS (gait, arms, legs, spine) questions and perform the GALS screen.
- Identify which joints require more detailed examination:
  - What is the pattern of joint involvement?
  - Is it likely to be inflammatory or degenerative?
- Examine gait and spine in more detail first, if appropriate, then position the patient on the couch for detailed joint examination.
- Assess the general appearance:
  - Look for pallor, rashes, skin tightness, evidence of weight or muscle loss, obvious deformities.
  - Check the surroundings for a temperature chart, walking aids and splints, if appropriate.
- Examine the relevant joint, or all joints if systemic disease suspected:
  - Ask about tenderness before examining the patient.
  - Look at the skin, nails, subcutaneous tissues, muscles and bony outlines.
  - Feel for warmth, swelling, tenderness, and reducibility of deformities.
  - Move:
    - Active movements first: demonstrate to the patient then ask them to perform the movements. Is there pain or crepitus on movement?
    - Passive movements second: determine the patient's range of movement. Measure with a goniometer. What is the end-feel like? Describe the deformities.
- If systemic disease is suspected, go on to examine all other systems fully.
- Consider what investigations are required:
  - Basic blood tests.
  - Inflammatory markers.
  - Immunology.
  - Ultrasound.
  - X-rays.
  - Special tests.
  - Joint aspiration for synovial fluid analysis or culture.

Michael J Tidman

The skin, hair and nails

Dermatological conditions are very common (10–15% of general practice consultations) and present to doctors in all specialties. In the UK, 50% are lesions ('lumps and bumps'), including skin cancers, and most of the remainder are acute and chronic inflammatory disorders ('rashes'), including infections, with genetic conditions accounting for a small minority.

Dermatological diagnosis can be challenging: not only is there a vast number of distinct skin diseases, but also each may present with a great variety of morphologies and patterns determined by intrinsic genetic factors, with the diagnostic waters muddied still further by external influences such as rubbing and scratching, infection, and well-meaning attempts at topical and systemic treatment. Even in one individual, lesions with the same pathology can have a very variable appearance (for example, melanocytic naevi, seborrhoeic keratoses and basal cell carcinomas).

Many skin findings will have no medical significance, but it is important to be able to examine the skin properly in order to identify tumours and rashes, and also to recognise cutaneous signs of underlying systemic conditions. The adage that the skin is a window into the inner workings of the body is entirely true, and an examination of the integument will often provide the discerning clinician with important clues about internal disease processes, as well as with information about the physical and psychological wellbeing of an individual.

Anatomy and physiology

Skin

The skin is the largest of the human organs, with a complex anatomy (Fig. 14.1) and a number of essential functions (Box 14.1). It has three layers, the most superficial of which is the epidermis, a stratified squamous epithelium, containing melanocytes (pigment-producing cells) within its basal layer, and Langerhans cells (antigen-presenting immune cells) throughout.

The dermis is the middle and most anatomically complex layer, containing vascular channels, sensory nerve endings, numerous cell types (including fibroblasts, macrophages, adipocytes and smooth muscle), hair follicles and glandular structures (eccrine, sebaceous and apocrine), all enmeshed in collagen and elastic tissue within a matrix comprising glycosaminoglycan, proteoglycan and glycoprotein.

The deep subcutis contains adipose and connective tissue.

Dermatoses (diseases of the skin) may affect all three layers and, to a greater or lesser extent, the various functions of the skin.

14.1 Functions of the skin

- Protection against physical injury and injurious substances, including ultraviolet radiation
- Anatomical barrier against pathogens
- Immunological defence
- Retention of moisture
- Thermoregulation
- Calorie reserve
- Appreciation of sensation (touch, temperature, pain)
- Vitamin D production
- Absorption – particularly fetal and neonatal skin
- Psychosexual and social interaction

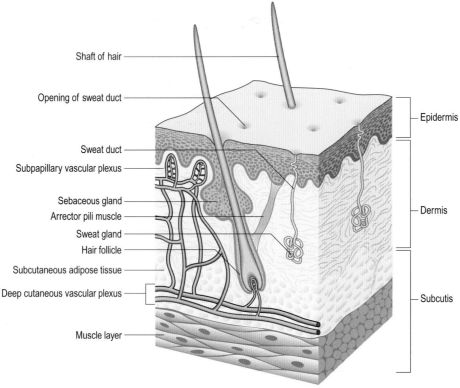

Shaft of hair

Opening of sweat duct

Sweat duct

Subpapillary vascular plexus

Sebaceous gland

Arrector pili muscle

Sweat gland

Hair follicle

Subcutaneous adipose tissue

Deep cutaneous vascular plexus

Muscle layer

Epidermis

Dermis

Subcutis

Fig. 14.1 Structures of the skin.

Hair

Hair plays a role in the protective, thermoregulatory and sensory functions of skin, and also in psychosexual and social interactions. There are two main types of hair in adults:

- vellus hair, which is short and fine, and covers most of the body surface
- terminal hair, which is longer and thicker, and is found on trunk and limbs, as well as scalp, eyebrows, eyelashes, and pubic, axillary and beard areas.

Abnormalities in hair distribution can occur when there is transitioning between vellus and terminal hair types (for example, hirsutism in women) or vice versa (androgenic alopecia). Hairs undergo regular asynchronous cycles of growth and thus, in health, mass shedding of hair is unusual. Hair loss can occur as a result of disorders of hair cycling, conditions resulting in damage to hair follicles (such as purposeful removal in trichotillomania), or structural (fragile) hair disorders.

Nails

The nail is a plate of densely packed, hardened, keratinised cells produced by the nail matrix. It serves to protect the fingertip and aid grasp and fingertip sensitivity. The white lunula at the base of the nail is the visible distal aspect of the nail matrix (Fig. 14.2). Fingernail regrowth takes approximately 6 months, and toenail regrowth 12–18 months.

The history

The possible diagnoses in dermatological conditions are broad and some diseases have pathognomonic features. Thus, in order to ensure that your history taking is focused and relevant, it may be appropriate to ask to glimpse the lesion or rash before embarking on detailed enquiry.

Common presenting symptoms

These include:
- a rash: scaly, blistering or itchy
- a lump or lesion

- pruritus (itch)
- hair loss or excess hair (hirsutism, hypertrichosis)
- nail changes.

Ask:
- When did the lesion appear or the rash begin?
- Where is the rash/lesion?
- Has the rash spread, or the lesion changed, since its onset?
- Is the lesion tender or painful? Is the rash itchy? Is the itch intense enough to cause bleeding by scratching or to disturb sleep, as in atopic eczema and lichen simplex? Are there blisters?
- Do the symptoms vary with time? For example, the pruritus of scabies is usually worse at night, and acne and atopic eczema may show a premenstrual exacerbation.
- Were there any preceding symptoms, such as a sore throat in psoriasis, a severe illness in telogen effluvium, or a new oral medication in drug eruptions?
- Are there any aggravating or relieving factors? For example, exercise or exposure to heat may precipitate cholinergic urticaria.
- What, if any, has been the effect of topical or oral medications? Self-medication with oral antihistamines may ameliorate urticaria, and topical glucocorticoids may help inflammatory reactions.
- Are there any associated constitutional symptoms, such as joint pain (psoriasis), muscle pain and weakness (dermatomyositis), fever, fatigue or weight loss?
- Very importantly, what is the impact of the rash on the individual's quality of life?

Past medical and drug history

Ask about general health and previous medical or skin conditions; a history of asthma, hay fever or childhood eczema suggests atopy. Coeliac disease is associated with dermatitis herpetiformis.

Take a full drug history, including any recent oral or topical prescribed or over-the-counter medication. Enquire about allergies not just to medicines but also to animals or foods.

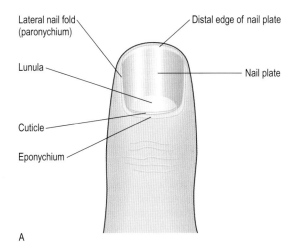

A

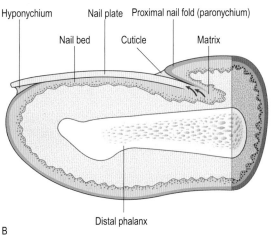

B

Fig. 14.2 Structure of the nail. A Dorsal view. B Cross-section.

Family and social history

Enquire about occupation and hobbies, as exposure to chemicals may cause contact dermatitis. If a rash consistently improves when a patient is away from work, the possibility of industrial dermatitis should be considered. Ask about alcohol consumption and confirm smoking status.

Document foreign travel and sun exposure if actinic damage, tropical infections or photosensitive eruptions are being considered. The risk of squamous cell and basal cell cancers increases with total lifetime sun exposure, and intense sun exposures leading to blistering burns are a risk factor for melanoma. The susceptibility of an individual to sun-induced damage can be determined by defining their skin type using the Fitzpatrick scale (Box 14.2).

Ask about a family history of atopy and skin conditions.

The history of a skin disorder alone rarely enables a definite diagnosis, with perhaps the occasional exception: an itchy eruption that resembles a nettle rash, the individual components of which last less than 24 hours, is very likely to be urticaria; and an intensely itchy eruption that affects all body areas except the head (in adults) and is worse in bed at night should be considered to be scabies until proved otherwise.

The physical examination

Proper assessment of the skin involves all the human senses, with the exception of taste. Once we have listened to the patient's history, we look at the rash or lesion, touch the skin, and occasionally use our sense of smell to diagnose infection and metabolic disorders such as trimethylaminuria (fish odour syndrome).

Examination of the skin should be performed under conditions of privacy in an adequately lit, warm room with, when appropriate, a chaperone present (p. 20). The patient should ideally be undressed to their underwear. Routinely, the hair, nails and oral cavity (p. 187) should be examined, and the regional lymph nodes (p. 33) palpated. Assess skin type using the Fitzpatrick scale (Box 14.2).

In documenting the appearance of a lesion or rash, use the correct descriptive terminology (Box 14.3); doing so often helps crystallise the diagnostic thought processes.

Distribution of a rash

The distribution of a dermatosis can be very informative. Is the eruption symmetrical? If so, it is likely to have a constitutional basis, and if not, it may well have an extrinsic cause. This golden rule has occasional exceptions (such as lichen simplex)

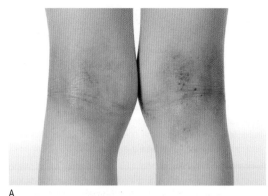

A

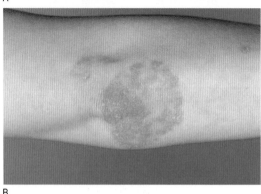

B

Fig. 14.3 Distribution of rash. [A] Atopic eczema localising to the flexural aspect of the knees. [B] Psoriasis involving the extensor aspect of the elbow.

but holds true in the majority of instances. Its application will almost always prevent the common misdiagnosis of 'bilateral cellulitis' (bacterial infection) of the legs, which in actuality is usually lipodermatosclerosis or varicose eczema; bacteria are not known for their sense of symmetry!

The pattern of a rash may immediately suggest a diagnosis: for example, the antecubital and popliteal fossae in atopic eczema (Fig. 14.3A); the extensor limb surfaces, scalp, nails and umbilicus in psoriasis (Fig. 14.3B); the flexural aspects of the wrists and the oral mucous membranes in lichen planus; the scalp, alar grooves and nasolabial folds in seborrhoeic dermatitis; and the sparing of covered areas in photosensitive eruptions. Does the rash follow a dermatome (as with shingles), or Langer's lines of skin tension (as with pityriasis rosea), or Blaschko (developmental) lines (as with certain genetic disorders)? The localisation of an eruption to fresh scars or tattoos may be a manifestation of sarcoidosis, and the anatomical location may provide a clue to diagnosis, such as the tendency of erythema nodosum, pretibial myxoedema and necrobiosis lipoidica (Fig. 14.4) to involve the shins.

Morphology of a rash

The morphology (shape and pattern) of a rash is equally important. Violaceous, polygonal, flat-topped papules, topped by a lacy patterning (Wickham striae), are typical of lichen planus (Fig. 14.5). The Koebner (isomorphic) phenomenon, where a dermatosis is induced by superficial epidermal injury, results in linear configurations (Fig. 14.6A), and occurs *par excellence* in

14.3 Descriptive terminology

Term	Definition	Term	Definition
Abscess	A collection of pus, often associated with signs and symptoms of inflammation (includes boils and carbuncles)	Macule	A flat (impalpable) colour change
		Milium	A keratin cyst
Angioedema	Deep swelling (oedema) of the dermis and subcutis	Naevus	A localised developmental defect (vascular, melanocytic, epidermal or connective tissue)
Annular	Ring-like	Nodule	A large papule (>0.5 cm)
Arcuate	Curved	Nummular	Coin-shaped
Atrophy	Thinning of one or more layers of the skin	Onycholysis	Separation of the nail plate from the nail bed
Blister	A liquid-filled lesion (vesicles and bullae)	Papilloma	A benign growth projecting from the skin surface
Bulla	A large blister (>0.5 cm)	Papule	An elevated (palpable) lesion, arbitrarily <0.5 cm in diameter
Burrow	A track left by a burrowing scabies mite	Patch	A large macule
Callus (callosity)	A thickened area of skin that is a response to repeated friction or pressure	Pedunculated	Having a stalk
Circinate	Circular	Petechiae	Pinhead-sized macular purpura
Comedo	A blackhead	Pigmentation	A change in skin colour
Crust (scab)	A hard, adherent surface change caused by leakage and drying of blood, serum or pus	Plaque	A papule or nodule that in cross-sectional profile is plateau-shaped
Cyst	A fluid-filled papular lesion that fluctuates and transilluminates	Poikiloderma	A combination of atrophy, hyperpigmentation and telangiectasia
Discoid	Disc-like	Purpura	Non-blanchable redness (also called petechiae)
Ecchymosis (bruise)	A deep bleed in the skin	Pustule	A papular lesion containing turbid purulent material (pus)
Erosion	A superficial loss of skin, involving the epidermis; scarring is not normally a result	Reticulate	Net-like
Erythema	Redness of the skin that blanches on pressure	Scale	A flake on the skin surface, composed of stratum corneum cells (corneocytes), shed together rather than individually
Erythroderma	Any inflammatory skin disease that affects >80% of the body surface	Scar	The fibrous tissue resulting from the healing of a wound, ulcer or certain inflammatory conditions
Exanthem	A rash	Serpiginous	Snake-like
Excoriation	A scratch mark	Stria(e)	A stretch mark
Fissure	A split, usually extending from the skin surface through the epidermis to the dermis	Targetoid	Target-like
		Telangiectasia	Dilated blood vessels
Freckle	An area of hyperpigmentation that increases in the summer months and decreases during winter	Ulcer	A deep loss of skin, extending into the dermis or deeper; usually results in scarring
Furuncle	A boil	Umbilication	A depression at the centre of a lesion
Gyrate	Wave-like	Verrucous	Wart-like
Haematoma	A swelling caused by a collection of blood	Vesicle	A small blister (<0.5 cm)
Horn	A hyperkeratotic projection from the skin surface	Wheal	A transient (<24 hours), itchy, elevated area of skin resulting from dermal oedema that characterises urticaria
Hyperkeratosis	Thickening of the stratum corneum		
Ichthyosis	Very dry skin	Xerosis	Mild/moderate dryness of the skin
Keratosis	A lesion characterised by hyperkeratosis		
Lentigo	An area of fixed hyperpigmentation		
Lichenification	Thickening of the epidermis, resulting in accentuation of skin markings; usually indicative of a chronic eczematous process		

psoriasis, lichen planus, viral warts and molluscum contagiosum. Linear or angular markings (erythema or scarring) raise the likelihood of artefactual (self-inflicted) damage to the skin. The presence of blisters limits the diagnostic possibilities to a relatively small number of autoimmune (such as dermatitis herpetiformis, pemphigoid (Fig. 14.6B) and pemphigus), reactive (including erythema multiforme, Stevens–Johnson syndrome and toxic epidermal necrolysis), infective (such as bullous impetigo and herpes simplex infection) and inherited (for example, epidermolysis bullosa) disorders. An annular (ring-like) morphology may be seen in granuloma annulare (Fig. 14.6C), subacute cutaneous lupus erythematosus, and fungal infections ('ringworm').

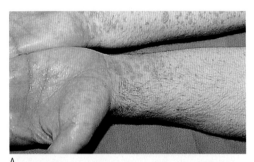

Fig. 14.4 Necrobiosis lipoidica diabeticorum.

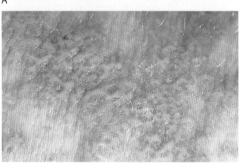

A

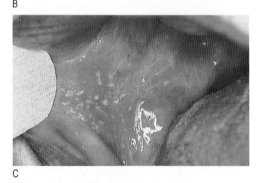

B

C

Fig. 14.5 Lichen planus. A Discrete flat-topped papules on the wrist. B Wickham striae, visible on close inspection. C A white lacy network of striae on the buccal mucosa.

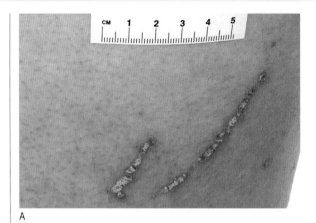

A

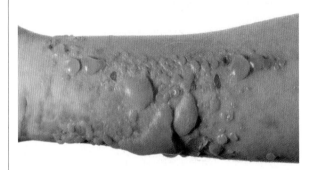

B

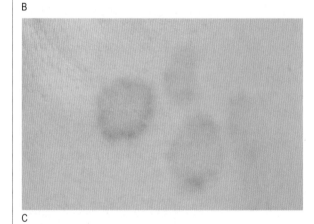

C

Fig. 14.6 Rash morphology. A Koebner response. B Pemphigoid. C Granuloma annulare.

The vascular contribution to the colour of a rash can be pivotal in diagnosis since erythematous and purpuric eruptions usually have very different underlying causes. It is not sufficient to describe a rash as 'red' or 'pink'; it is essential to demonstrate whether or not a rash blanches on direct pressure or when the skin is stretched. Blanchable redness (erythema) indicates that the red blood cells causing the colour remain within blood vessels; non-blanchable redness (purpura) is the result of erythrocyte extravasation and entrapment in the collagen and elastic fibres of the dermis.

The tint of the erythema may be helpful: a violaceous hue distinguishes lichen planus; a beefy-red or salmon-pink colour often typifies psoriasis; and a heliotrope (pink–purple) colour is a feature of dermatomyositis, especially on the eyelids.

Macular purpura may be the result of thrombocytopenia or capillary fragility, but palpable purpura (often painful) usually indicates vasculitis (Fig. 14.7A) and necessitates exclusion of vasculitic inflammation in other organs. Purpura elicitable by pinching the skin ('pinch purpura') may be indicative of AL (light-chain) amyloidosis (Fig. 14.7B).

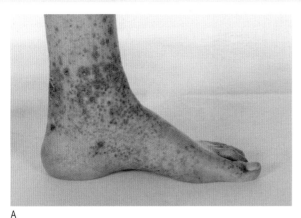

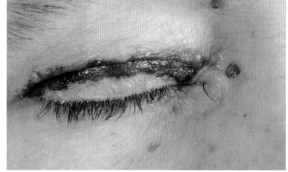

Fig. 14.7 Purpura. A Cutaneous vasculitis. B AL (light-chain) amyloidosis.

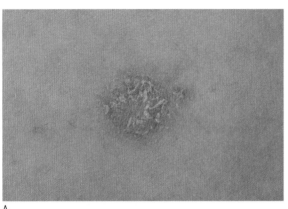

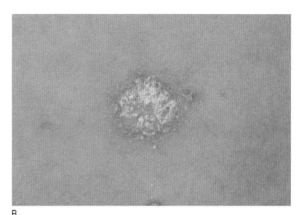

14

Fig. 14.8 Clinical signs in the diagnosis of skin disease. A Psoriasis before rubbing the surface. B After surface rubbing. C Lichen planus showing light reflection from small early lesions.

There are also a number of subtle clinical signs that can be of great diagnostic help in common rashes, such as the distinctive silver-coloured scale that appears when psoriasis is scratched with a wooden orange stick (Fig. 14.8AB), the urtication that develops when the pigmented lesions of urticaria pigmentosa (a form of cutaneous mastocytosis) are rubbed (Darier's sign), the separation of epidermis on applying a shearing force in pemphigus (Nikolsky's sign), and the very earliest lesions of lichen planus glinting in reflected light like stars in the night sky (Fig. 14.8C).

Scratch marks (excoriations) indicate an itchy rash. In any pruritic eruption it is prudent to look specifically for the burrows of scabies (Fig. 14.9) on the hands and feet, as well as testing for dermographism and examining for lymphadenopathy (p. 33), as urticaria and lymphoma are also important causes of itch.

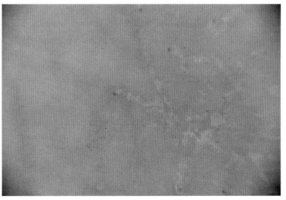

Fig. 14.9 Scabies burrows.

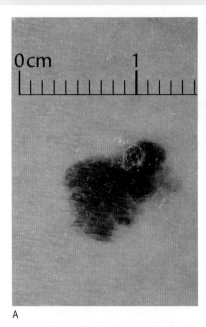

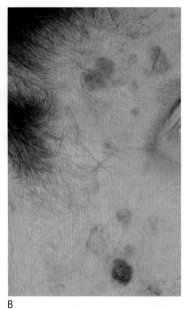

A   B

Fig. 14.10 Lesion morphology. A Malignant melanoma. B Seborrhoeic keratosis.

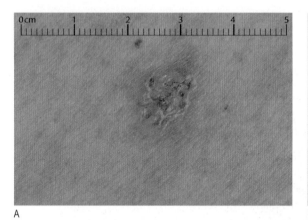

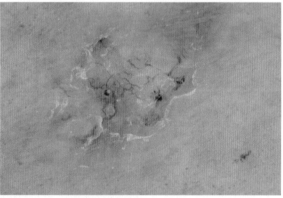

A   B

Fig. 14.11 Basal cell carcinoma. A Viewed with the naked eye. B Dermatoscopy highlights distinctive telangiectasia.

Morphology of lesions

Lesions should be measured and described according to their anatomical location, colour, symmetry, surface texture, consistency, demarcation of margin, and whether they are freely mobile or attached to underlying tissue (p. 32). Remember to examine the regional lymph nodes. If a pigmented lesion demonstrates a variable outline and colour variation, the possibility of malignant melanoma must be considered (Fig. 14.10A). It is reassuring to see hair growing out of pigmented lesions, as this usually indicates a benign process such as a melanocytic naevus. An irregularly roughened, jagged surface texture is often indicative of sunlight-induced damage (actinic keratosis), whereas the surface of a seborrhoeic keratosis (Fig. 14.10B) has a smoother feel. The consistency of a lesion is often of diagnostic help: for example, the firm, button-like quality of a dermatofibroma is very characteristic; neurofibromas are rather soft; calcium deposits are hard; and cysts fluctuate and transilluminate. Basal cell carcinoma, the most common malignant tumour, is usually smooth (but may ulcerate); on inspection, it exhibits a milky, pearlescent colour (which may glint) and irregular telangiectasia (Fig. 14.11).

Hair and nail signs

General physical examination should always include the hair and nails. Is there excess hair, either in a masculine distribution (hirsutism) or not (hypertrichosis), or hair loss (alopecia)? Hirsutism may be a marker for hyperandrogenism, and hypertrichosis may be seen in malnutrition states, malignancy and porphyria cutanea tarda. Discrete, coin-sized areas of hair loss, with small 'exclamation mark' hairs at the periphery, are characteristic of alopecia areata (Fig. 14.12), an autoimmune disorder that may coexist with other autoimmune disorders. Diffuse, pronounced hair shedding (telogen effluvium) may be a physiological response to severe illness, major surgical operations or childbirth, and may be accompanied by transverse grooves on the finger nails, which gradually grow out normally (Beau's lines; see Fig. 3.7B).

Common abnormalities of the nails associated with underlying disease are covered on page 24 and in Box 3.4 and Fig. 3.7.

Some rare diseases produce specific nail appearances, such as the 'ragged cuticles' and abnormal capillary nail-bed loops associated with dermatomyositis (Fig. 14.13AB), and the progressive thickening and opacification of nails in yellow nail syndrome (Fig. 14.13C).

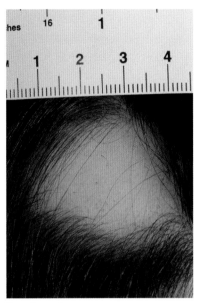

Fig. 14.12 **Alopecia areata.**

Supplementary examination techniques

It is often necessary to complement naked-eye observation of the skin with assisted examination techniques, such as dermatoscopy, diascopy and Wood's lamp.

Dermatoscopy

A dermatoscope consists of a powerful light source (polarised or non-polarised) and a magnifying lens, and enables considerably more cutaneous anatomical detail to be seen (Fig. 14.14).

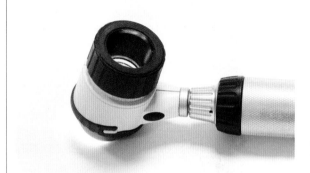

Fig. 14.14 **Dermatoscope.**

14

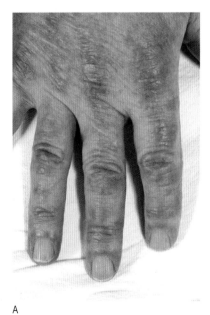

A

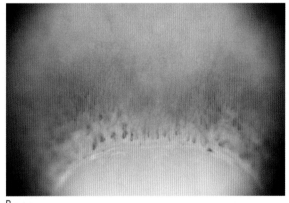

B

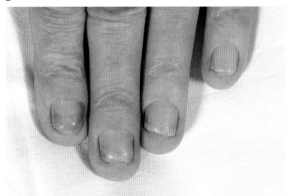

C

Fig. 14.13 **Nail appearances in systemic diseases.** A The typical linear pattern of dermatomyositis with Gottren's papules on the dorsum of the hand. B Nail-fold telangiectasia in dermatomyositis, viewed through the dermatoscope. C Yellow nail syndrome in a patient with lymphoedema and pleural effusions.

Dermatoscopy is particularly useful in the assessment of pigmented lesions but is also often of great help in assessing other skin tumours, hair disorders and certain infections (scabies, viral warts and molluscum contagiosum).

Diascopy

The pressure of a glass slide on the skin will compress the cutaneous blood vessels and blanch the area of contact. If blood is still visible through the glass, it is because red blood cells have extravasated (purpura). When granulomatous disorders (such as sarcoidosis or granuloma annulare) are diascoped, they typically manifest a green–brown ('apple jelly') colour.

Wood's lamp

Examination of the skin using an ultraviolet light (Wood's lamp) is useful in two clinical situations: it enhances the contrast between normal skin and under- or overpigmented epidermis (making conditions such as vitiligo and melasma easier to see); and it can identify certain infections by inducing the causative organisms to fluoresce (such as erythrasma, pityriasis versicolor and some ringworm infections).

Investigations

After clinical examination, specific investigative techniques may be necessary in some cases to enable a precise diagnosis.

Skin biopsy

This involves a sample of skin being removed, under local anaesthesia, and subjected to histological or immunohistochemical examination in the laboratory. However, clinicopathological correlation is usually necessary.

Mycology

A fungal infection can be confirmed (or refuted) by scraping scale from the surface of a rash with a scalpel blade, clipping samples of nail or plucking hair, and undertaking microscopic examination and culture.

Patch testing

Patch testing (Fig. 14.15) is performed to establish whether a contact allergy is the cause of an individual's rash. It involves applying putative allergens to the patient's skin, leaving the test patches undisturbed for 2 days, removing them and then reading the final result after 4 days. A positive result is indicated by an inflammatory reaction at the site of the patch.

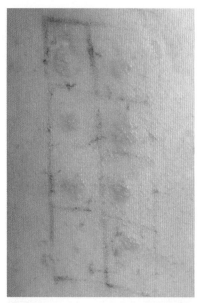

Fig. 14.15 Patch testing.

OSCE example 1: Pruritus

Mr Thomson, 45 years old, presents with a 4-month history of intense itch disturbing his sleep.

Please examine his skin

- Introduce yourself to the patient and clean your hands.
- Ask him to undress to underwear.
- Carry out a general inspection, observing for scratch marks (and whether they are symmetrical), colour and dryness of the skin, presence of a rash, pallor, jaundice, exophthalmos or goitre.
- Palpate the pulse for tachycardia and atrial fibrillation.
- Examine the hands and insteps for scabietic burrows, fine tremor, thyroid acropachy and koilonychia.
- Examine the abdomen for an enlarged liver or spleen.
- Examine the mouth for a smooth tongue or angular cheilitis.
- Test for dermographism.
- Examine for lymphadenopathy.
- Thank the patient and clean your hands.

Suggest a differential diagnosis

Intense pruritus may be caused by dermatoses such as scabies and dermatitis herpetiformis, but also by systemic disorders such as polycythaemia, iron deficiency, liver or renal dysfunction, hyper- or hypothyroidism, and lymphoma.

Suggest investigations

Full blood count, renal, liver and thyroid function tests, ferritin level and chest X-ray.

OSCE example 2: Pigmented lesion

Ms Forsythe, 55 years old, presents with a 6-week history of a changing pigmented lesion on her right calf.

Please examine her skin

- Introduce yourself to the patient and clean your hands.
- Ask her to undress to underwear.
- Carry out a general inspection of the skin, estimating her Fitzpatrick skin type, and observing for signs of actinic damage and for other lesions that might require close assessment.
- Observe the lesion on her calf for size, symmetry, regularity of margins, variation of pigmentation and ulceration.
- Palpate the lesion.
- Examine for enlargement of regional lymph nodes.
- Examine the abdomen for an enlarged liver.
- Undertake a similar examination of any other suspicious lesions.
- Thank the patient and clean your hands.

Suggest a differential diagnosis

Any changing lesion should raise suspicion of malignant melanoma, although melanocytic naevi, seborrhoeic keratoses, dermatofibromas, haemangiomas and pigmented basal cell carcinomas can cause diagnostic confusion.

Suggested investigations

If, after examination, there is still suspicion regarding the malignant potential of the lesion, it should be excised for histological examination.

Integrated examination sequence for the skin

- Prepare the patient:
  - Arrange for privacy.
  - Arrange for a chaperone, if necessary.
  - Remove sufficient clothing.
  - Remove makeup and wigs, if face and scalp are being examined.
- Carry out a general examination of the skin:
  - Look for excoriations, xerosis (dry skin), actinic damage and suspicious lesions, for example.
- Carry out a specific examination of a rash:
  - Extent.
  - Distribution: symmetry, pattern.
  - Morphology.
  - Colour.
  - Erythema/purpura.
  - Specific features, e.g. scale, signs of infection/infestation.
  - Mouth, hair and nails.
  - Regional lymph nodes.
- Carry out a specific examination of a lesion:
  - Site, size, colour.
  - Symmetry.
  - Surface texture.
  - Consistency.
  - Mobility.
  - Pattern of vasculature.
  - Regional lymph nodes.

14

Section 3

Applying history and examination skills in specific situations

Ben Stenson
Steve Cunningham

15

Babies and children

BABIES

A baby is a neonate for its first 4 weeks and an infant for its first year. Neonates are classified by gestational age or birthweight (Box 15.1).

The history

Ask the mother and look in the maternal notes for relevant history:

Maternal history

- Is there a family history of significant illness (e.g. diabetes, hereditary illnesses)?
- What were the outcomes of any previous pregnancies?

Pregnancy history

- How was maternal health?
- Did the mother take medications or other drugs?
- What did antenatal screening tests show?

Birth history

- What was the birthweight, gestation at birth and mode of delivery?
- Was there prolonged rupture of the fetal membranes or maternal pyrexia?
- Was there a non-reassuring fetal status during delivery or meconium staining of the amniotic fluid?
- Was resuscitation required after birth?
- What were the Apgar scores (Box 15.2) and the results of umbilical cord blood gas tests?

Infant's progress

- Has the infant passed meconium and urine since birth?
- In later infancy, what are the specific signs and systems and developmental progress, depending on the presenting problem?

15.1 Classification of newborn infants
Birthweight
• Extremely low: <1000 g
• Very low: <1500 g
• Low: <2500 g
• Normal: ≥2500 g
Gestational age
• Extremely preterm: <28 weeks
• Preterm: <37 weeks (<259th day)
• Term: 37–42 weeks
• Post-term: >42 weeks (>294th day)

Presenting problems and definitions

Infants cannot report symptoms, so you must recognise the presenting problems and signs of illness, which are non-specific in young infants. Always take the concerns of parents seriously.

Pallor

Always investigate pallor in a newborn, as it implies anaemia or poor perfusion. Newborn infants have higher haemoglobin levels than older children and are not normally pale. Haemoglobin levels of <120 g/L (<12 g/dL) in the perinatal period are low. Preterm infants look red because they lack subcutaneous fat.

Respiratory distress

Respiratory distress is tachypnoea (respiratory rate) >60 breaths per minute with intercostal and subcostal indrawing, sternal recession, nasal flaring and the use of accessory muscles.

Cyanosis

Bluish discoloration of the lips and mucous membranes due to hypoxia is difficult to see in newborn infants unless oxygen saturation (SpO_2) is <80% (normal is >95%). Causes include congenital heart disease and respiratory disease, and cyanosis always needs investigation (p. 28).

Acrocyanosis

Acrocyanosis is a bluish-purple discoloration of the hands and feet and is a normal finding, provided the newborn is centrally pink.

Jaundice

Many newborns develop jaundice in the days after birth. Look for yellow sclerae in newborns with coloured skin or you may miss it. Examine the baby in bright normal light. Normal physiological jaundice cannot be distinguished clinically from jaundice from a pathological cause. Do not use clinical estimates instead of measurements to evaluate jaundice.

15.2 Apgar score			
Clinical score	**0**	**1**	**2**
Heart rate	Absent	<100 bpm	>100 bpm
Respiratory effort	Absent	Slow and irregular	Good: strong
Muscle tone	Flaccid	Some flexion of arms and legs	Active movement
Reflex irritability	No responses	Grimace	Vigorous crying, sneeze or cough
Colour	Blue, pale	Pink body, blue extremities	Pink all over

Add scores for each line; maximum score is 10.
bpm, *beats per minute.*
Reproduced with permission of International Anesthesia Research Society from Current researches in Anesthesia & Analgesia Apgar V 1953; 32(4), permission conveyed through Copyright Clearance Center, Inc.

Jitteriness

Jitteriness is high-frequency tremor of the limbs, and is common in term infants in the first few days. It is stilled by stimulating the infant and is not associated with other disturbance. If jitteriness is excessive, exclude hypoglycaemia, polycythaemia and neonatal abstinence syndrome (drug withdrawal). Infrequent jerks in light sleep are common and normal; regular clonic jerks are abnormal.

Dysmorphism

Identifying abnormal body structure (dysmorphism) is subjective because of human variability. Individual features may be minor and isolated, or may signify a major problem requiring investigation and management. A recognisable pattern of several dysmorphic features may indicate a 'dysmorphic syndrome' such as Down's syndrome (p. 36). Use caution and sensitivity when discussing possible dysmorphism with parents of a newborn child.

Hypotonia

Hypotonia (reduced tone) may be obvious when you handle an infant. Term infants' muscle tone normally produces a flexed posture at the hips, knees and elbows. Hypotonic infants may lack this flexion. Hypotonia can occur with hypoxia, hypoglycaemia or sepsis, or may be due to a specific brain, nerve or muscle problem. Preterm infants have lower tone than term infants and are less flexed.

Apgar score

This first clinical assessment of a neonate is made immediately after birth. Tone, colour, breathing, heart rate and response to stimulation are each scored 0, 1 or 2 (Box 15.2), giving a maximum total of 10. Healthy neonates commonly score 8–10 at 1 and 5 minutes. The score predicts the need for, and efficacy of, resuscitation. A low score should increase with time; a decreasing score is a cause for concern. Persistently low scores at 10 minutes predict death or later disability. Neonates with scores of less than 8 at 5 minutes require continued evaluation until it is clear they are healthy.

The physical examination of newborns

Timing and efficacy of the routine neonatal examination

Examine a newborn with the parents present. There is no ideal time. If it is performed on day 1, some forms of congenital heart disease may be missed because signs have not developed. If it is delayed, some babies will present before the examination with illness that may have been detectable earlier. Around 9% of neonates have an identifiable congenital abnormality but most are not serious. Always record your examination comprehensively to avoid problems if illness or physical abnormality is identified later. Fewer than half of all cases of congenital heart disease or congenital cataract are detected by newborn examination.

General examination

Examine babies and infants in a warm place on a firm bed or examination table. Have a system to avoid omitting anything, but avoid an overly rigid approach as you may be unable to perform key elements if you unsettle the baby. Do things that may disturb the baby later in the examination.

Examination sequence

- Observe whether the baby looks well and is well grown.
- Look for:
  - cyanosis
  - respiratory distress
  - pallor
  - plethora (suggesting polycythaemia).
- Note posture and behaviour.
- Note any dysmorphic features.
- Auscultate the heart and palpate the abdomen if the baby is quiet.
- If the baby cries, does the cry sound normal?

Skin

Normal findings

The skin may look normal, dry, wrinkled or vernix-covered in healthy babies. There may be meconium staining of the skin and nails.

Prominent capillaries commonly cause pink areas called 'stork's beak marks' at the nape of the neck, eyelids and glabella (Fig. 15.1). Facial marks fade spontaneously over months; those on the neck often persist. Milia (fine white spots) and acne neonatorum (larger cream-coloured spots) are collected glandular secretions and disappear within 2–4 weeks. Erythema toxicum is a common fleeting, blanching, idiopathic maculopapular rash of no consequence, affecting the trunk, face and limbs in the first few days after birth.

Abnormal findings

Document any trauma such as scalp cuts or bruising.

Dense capillary haemangiomas (port wine stains) will not fade. Referral to a dermatologist is advisable, as laser treatment may help in some cases. Around the eye they may indicate Sturge–Weber syndrome (a facial port wine stain with an underlying brain lesion, associated with risk of later seizures, cerebral calcification and reduced cognitive function). Melanocytic naevi require follow-up and treatment by a plastic surgeon or dermatologist. A Mongolian blue spot (Fig. 15.2) is an area of bluish discoloration over the buttocks, back and thighs. Easily mistaken for bruising, it usually fades in the first year.

15

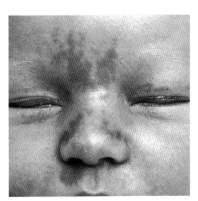

Fig. 15.1 Stork's beak mark.

Fig. 15.2 Mongolian blue spot.

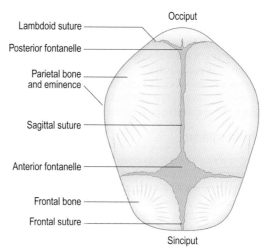

Fig. 15.3 The fetal skull from above.

Labels on figure: Occiput, Lambdoid suture, Posterior fontanelle, Parietal bone and eminence, Sagittal suture, Anterior fontanelle, Frontal bone, Frontal suture, Sinciput

15.3 Neonatal head shapes	
Head shape	**Description**
Microcephalic (small-headed)	Small cranial vault
Megalencephalic (large-headed)	Large cranial vault
Hydrocephalic (water-headed)	Large cranial vault due to enlarged ventricles
Brachycephalic (short-headed)	Flat head around the occiput
Dolichocephalic (long-headed)	Head that looks long relative to its width
Plagiocephalic (oblique-headed)	Asymmetrical skull

Subcutaneous fat necrosis causes palpable firm plaques, often with some erythema under the skin. If extensive, there can be associated hypercalcaemia that may require treatment. Blisters or bullae are usually pathological.

Head

Examination sequence

- Note the baby's head shape (Box 15.3) and any swellings.
- Feel the anterior fontanelle (Fig. 15.3). Is it sunken, flat or bulging?
- Palpate the cranial sutures.

Normal findings

Transient elongation of the head is common from moulding during birth. Caput succedaneum is soft-tissue swelling over the vertex due to pressure in labour. Overriding cranial sutures have a palpable step.

Abnormal findings

Cephalhaematoma is a firm, immobile, usually parietal swelling caused by a localised haemorrhage under the cranial periosteum. It may be bilateral, and periosteal reaction at the margins causes a raised edge. No treatment is required. Do not confuse this with the boggy, mobile, poorly localised swelling of subgaleal haemorrhage (beneath the flat sheet of fibrous tissue that caps the skull), which can conceal a large blood loss and is life-threatening if unrecognised.

Separated cranial sutures with an obvious gap indicate raised intracranial pressure. Rarely, the cranial sutures are prematurely fused (synostosis), producing ridging, and the head shape is usually abnormal. Abnormal head size requires detailed investigation, including neuroimaging.

Eyes

Examination sequence

- Inspect the eyebrows, lashes, lids and eyeballs.
- Gently retract the lower eyelid and check the sclera for jaundice.
- Test ocular movements and vestibular function:
  - Turn the newborn's head to one side; watch as the eyes move in the opposite direction. These are called doll's-eye movements and disappear in infancy (see Fig. 8.15).
  - Hold the infant upright at arm's length and move in a horizontal arc. The infant should look in the direction of movement and have optokinetic nystagmus. This response becomes damped by 3 months.

Normal findings

Harmless yellow crusting without inflammation is common after birth in infants with narrow lacrimal ducts.

Term infants usually fix visually.

Abnormal findings

Eye infection gives a red eye and purulent secretions. An abnormal pupil shape is usually a coloboma (a defect in the iris inferiorly that gives the pupil a keyhole appearance, Fig. 15.4). This can also affect deeper structures, including the optic nerve, and lead to visual impairment. It can be associated with syndromes, as can microphthalmia (small eyeballs). Large eyeballs that feel hard when palpated through the lids suggest congenital glaucoma (buphthalmos).

Ophthalmoscopy

Examination sequence

- Hold the baby in your arms. Turn your body from side to side so that the baby will open their eyes.

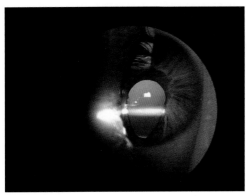

Fig. 15.4 Coloboma.

- Look at each pupil from about 20 cm through the ophthalmoscope. You should see the red reflex of reflected light from the retina.

Normal findings

Puffy eyes in the first days after birth impede the examination. If this happens, always examine again later because failure to detect and treat a cataract will cause permanent amblyopia.

Abnormal findings

An absent red reflex suggests cataract; refer to an ophthalmologist.

Nose

Examination sequence

- Exclude obstructed nostrils (choanal atresia) by blocking each nostril in turn with your finger to check that the infant breathes easily through the other.

Mouth

Examination sequence

- Gently press down on the lower jaw so that the baby will open their mouth. Do not use a wooden tongue depressor, as this may cause trauma or infection.
- Shine a torch into the mouth and look at the tongue and palate.
- Palpate the palate using your fingertip.

Normal findings

Epstein's pearls are small, white mucosal cysts on the palate that disappear spontaneously.

White coating on the tongue that is easily scraped off with a swab is usually curdled milk.

Abnormal findings

Ankyloglossia (tongue tie) is when the lingual frenulum joining the underside of the tongue to the floor of the mouth is abnormally short, which may interfere with feeding. A white coating on the tongue, which is not easily removed and may bleed when scraped, is caused by *Candida albicans* (thrush). Macroglossia (a large protruding tongue) occurs in Beckwith–Wiedemann syndrome. A normal-sized tongue protrudes through a small mouth in Down's syndrome (glossoptosis).

Cleft palate may involve the soft palate or both hard and soft palates. It can be midline, unilateral or bilateral and may also involve the gum (alveolus). Cleft lip can appear in isolation or in association with it. Refer affected infants early to a specialist multidisciplinary team. Micrognathia (a small jaw) is sometimes associated with cleft palate in the Pierre Robin syndrome, with posterior displacement of the tongue and upper airway obstruction.

A ranula is a mucous cyst on the floor of the mouth that is related to the sublingual or submandibular salivary ducts. Congenital ranulas may resolve spontaneously but sometimes require surgery.

Teeth usually begin to erupt at around 6 months but can be present at birth.

Ears

Examination sequence

- Note the size, shape and position.
- The helix should attach above an imaginary line through the inner corners of the eyes.
- Check that the external auditory meatus looks normal.

Normal findings

The helix can be temporarily folded due to local pressure in utero. Preauricular skin tags do not require investigation.

Abnormal findings

Abnormal ear shape and position is a feature of some syndromes.

Neck

Examination sequence

- Inspect the neck for asymmetry, sinuses and swellings.
- Palpate any masses. Use 'SPACESPIT' (see Box 3.8) to interpret your findings.
- Transilluminate swellings. Cystic swellings glow, as the light is transmitted through clear liquid. Solid or blood-filled swellings do not.

Normal findings

One-third of normal neonates have palpable cervical, inguinal or axillary lymph nodes. Neck asymmetry is often due to fetal posture and usually resolves.

Abnormal findings

A lump in the sternocleidomastoid muscle (sternomastoid 'tumour') is caused by a fibrosed haematoma with resultant muscle shortening. This may produce torticollis, with the head turned in the contralateral direction.

Cardiovascular examination

Examination sequence

- Observe the baby for pallor, cyanosis and sweating.
- Count the respiratory rate.
- Palpate for the apex beat with your palm in the mid-clavicular line in the fourth or fifth intercostal space.
- Note if the heart beat moves your hand up and down (parasternal heave) or if you feel a vibration (thrill).
- Count the heart rate for 15 seconds and multiply by 4.

15

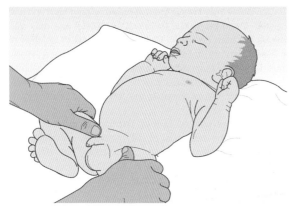

Fig. 15.5 Palpating the femoral pulses. The pulse can be difficult to feel at first. Use a point halfway between the pubic tubercle and the anterior superior iliac spine as a guide.

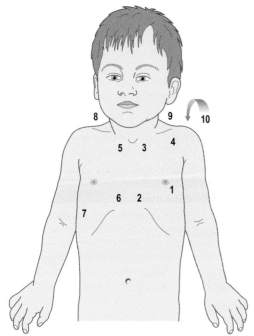

Fig. 15.6 Auscultation positions in infants and children.
Recommended order of auscultation: **1,** apex; **2,** left lower sternal edge; **3,** left upper sternal edge; **4,** left infraclavicular; **5,** right upper sternal edge; **6,** right lower sternal edge; **7,** right mid-axillary line; **8,** right side of neck; **9,** left side of neck; **10,** posteriorly.

- Feel the femoral pulses by placing your thumbs or fingertips over the mid-inguinal points while abducting the hips (Fig. 15.5).
- Auscultate the heart. Start at the apex using the stethoscope bell (best for low-pitched sounds). Then use the diaphragm in all positions for high-pitched sounds and murmurs (Fig. 15.6).
- Describe the heart sounds S_1 and S_2, any additional heart sounds and the presence of murmurs. The fast heart rate of a newborn makes it difficult to time additional sounds. Take time to tune into the different rate of the harsh breath sounds of a newborn, as they are easily confused with a murmur.

15.4 Normal ranges for heart and respiratory rate in the newborn		
Sign	Preterm neonate	Term neonate
Heart rate (beats per minute)	120–160	100–140
Respiratory rate (breaths per minute)	40–60	30–50

- Do not measure the blood pressure of healthy babies. In ill babies, cuff measurements overestimate the values when compared with invasive measurements. The cuff width should be at least two-thirds of the distance from the elbow to the shoulder tip.
- Palpate the abdomen for hepatomegaly (see later).

Normal findings

In the early newborn period the femoral pulses may feel normal in an infant who later presents with coarctation because an open ductus arteriosus can maintain flow to the descending aorta. Routine measurement of postductal oxygen saturation is increasingly popular as an additional newborn screening test for congenital heart disease. Lower limb SpO_2 should be 95% or higher.

Heart rates between 80 and 160 beats per minute (bpm) can be normal in the newborn, depending on the arousal state (Box 15.4).

Abnormal findings

Infants with heart failure typically look pale and sweaty, and have respiratory distress (p. 298).

If the apex beat is displaced laterally, there may be cardiomegaly, or mediastinal shift due to contralateral pneumothorax or pleural effusion.

Weak or absent femoral pulses suggest coarctation of the aorta. Radiofemoral delay is not identifiable in the newborn.

Patent ductus arteriosus may cause a short systolic murmur in the early days of life because the pulmonary and systemic blood pressures are similar, which limits shunting through the duct. The murmur progressively lengthens over subsequent weeks or months to become the continuous 'machinery' murmur recognised later in childhood.

Transient murmurs are heard in up to 2% of neonates but only a minority have a structural heart problem. An echocardiogram is needed to make a structural diagnosis.

Respiratory examination

Examination sequence

- Note chest shape and symmetry of chest movement.
- Count the respiratory rate (for 15 seconds and multiply by 4).
- Listen for additional noises with breathing.
- Look for signs of respiratory distress: tachypnoea; suprasternal, intercostal and subcostal recession; flaring of the nostrils.
- Remember that percussion of the newborn's chest is not helpful.
- Use the diaphragm to auscultate anteriorly, laterally and posteriorly, comparing the sides. Breath sounds in the healthy newborn have a bronchial quality compared with older individuals (p. 88).

Normal findings

Male and female newborn infants at term have small buds of palpable breast tissue. Small amounts of fluid are sometimes discharged from the nipple in the early days after birth.

Abnormal findings

Stridor indicates large airway obstruction and is predominantly inspiratory (p. 79). Stridor and indrawing beginning on days 2–3 of life in an otherwise well baby may be due to laryngomalacia (softness of the larynx). Causes of respiratory distress include retained lung fluid, infection, immaturity, aspiration, congenital anomaly, pneumothorax, heart failure and metabolic acidosis.

Abdominal examination

Examination sequence

- Remove the nappy.
- Inspect the abdomen, including the umbilicus and groins, noting any swellings.
- From the infant's right side, gently palpate with the flat of your warm right hand. Palpate superficially before feeling for deeper structures.
- Palpate for splenomegaly. In the neonate the spleen enlarges down the left flank, not towards the right iliac fossa.
- Palpate for hepatomegaly:
  - Place your right hand flat across the abdomen beneath the right costal margin.
  - Feel the liver edge against the side of your index finger.
  - If you feel more than the liver edge, measure the distance in the mid-clavicular line from the costal margin to the liver edge. Describe it in fingerbreadths or measure it with a tape in centimetres.
- Check that the anus is present, patent and normally positioned.
- Digital rectal examination is usually unnecessary and could cause an anal fissure. Indications include suspected rectal atresia or stenosis and delayed passage of meconium. Put on gloves and lubricate your little finger. Gently press your fingertip against the anus until you feel the muscle resistance relax and insert your finger up to your distal interphalangeal joint.

Normal findings

Abdominal distension from a feed or swallowed air is common.

You may see the contour of individual bowel loops through the thin anterior abdominal wall in the newborn, particularly with intestinal obstruction.

The umbilical cord stump usually separates after 4–5 days. A granuloma may appear later as a moist, pink lump in the base of the umbilicus. A small amount of bleeding from the umbilicus is common in the neonate.

The liver edge is often palpable in healthy infants.

In the neonate the kidneys are often palpable, especially if ballotted (see Fig. 12.12).

Abnormal findings

In excessive umbilical bleeding, check that the infant received vitamin K and consider factor XIII deficiency. Spreading erythema around the umbilicus suggests infective omphalitis and requires urgent treatment.

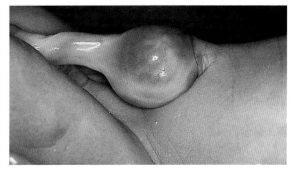

Fig. 15.7 Small exomphalos with loops of bowel in the umbilicus. *From Lissauer T, Clayden G. Illustrated Textbook of Paediatrics. 2nd edn. Edinburgh: Mosby; 2001.*

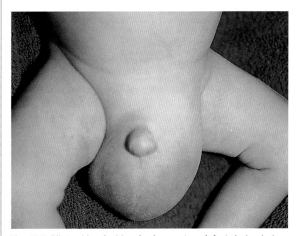

Fig. 15.8 Bilateral inguinal hernias in a preterm infant. An inguinal hernia is primarily a groin swelling; only when it is large does it extend into the scrotum. *From Lissauer T, Clayden G. Illustrated Textbook of Paediatrics. 2nd edn. Edinburgh: Mosby; 2001.*

Umbilical hernias are common; they are easily reduced, have a very low risk of complications and close spontaneously in infancy. An omphalocoele, or exomphalos (Fig. 15.7), is a herniation through the umbilicus containing intestines and other viscera, covered by a membrane that includes the umbilical cord. It may be associated with other malformations or chromosomal abnormality. Gastroschisis is a defect in the anterior abdominal wall with intestines herniated through it, without a covering membrane. The most common site is above and to the right of the umbilicus.

Inguinal hernias are common in the newborn, especially in boys and preterm infants (Fig. 15.8).

Meconium in the nappy does not guarantee that the baby has a patent anus because meconium can be passed through a rectovaginal fistula.

Perineum

Examination sequence

Female

- Abduct the legs and gently separate the labia.
- In preterm infants the labia minora appear prominent, giving a masculinised appearance that resolves spontaneously over a few weeks. Milky vaginal secretions

15

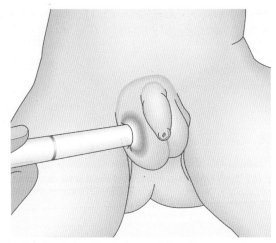

Fig. 15.9 How to transilluminate a scrotal swelling.

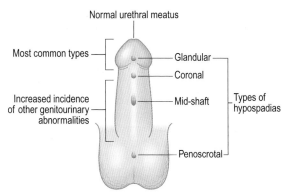

Fig. 15.10 Varieties of hypospadias.

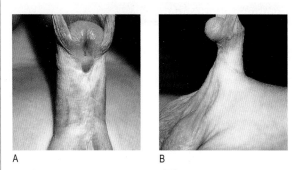

A   B

Fig. 15.11 Hypospadias and chordee. [A] Penile shaft hypospadias. [B] Lateral view showing the ventral curvature of the penis (chordee). *From Lissauer T, Clayden G. Illustrated Textbook of Paediatrics. 2nd edn. Edinburgh: Mosby; 2001.*

are normal. Later in the first week, there is sometimes slight vaginal bleeding (pseudomenses) as the infant uterus 'withdraws' from maternal hormones. Vaginal skin tags are common and do not require treatment.

Male

- Do not attempt to retract the foreskin. It is normal for it to be adherent in babies.
- Check that the urethral meatus is at the tip of the penis.
- Note the shape of the penis.
- Palpate the testes.
- If you cannot feel the testes in the scrotum, assess for undescended, ectopic or retractile testes. Palpate the abdomen for smooth lumps, moving your fingers down over the inguinal canal to the scrotum and perineum.
- A retractile testis just below the inguinal canal may be gently milked into the scrotum. Re-examine at 6 weeks if there is any doubt about the position of the testes.
- Transilluminate any large scrotal swellings using a torch to see if the light is transmitted through the swelling. This suggests a hydrocoele but can be misleading, because a hernia of thin-walled bowel may transilluminate (Fig. 15.9).
- An inguinal hernia usually produces a groin swelling but, if large, this may extend into the scrotum. Try to reduce it by gently pushing the contents upwards from the scrotum through the inguinal canal into the abdomen.

Normal findings

The testes are smooth and soft, and measure 0.7×1 cm across. The right testis usually descends later than the left and sits higher in the scrotum.

Abnormal findings

A hydrocoele is a collection of fluid beneath the tunica vaginalis of the testis and/or the spermatic cord (p. 234). Most resolve spontaneously in infancy.

In hypospadias the meatal opening is on the ventral aspect of the glans, the ventral shaft of the penis, the scrotum or more posteriorly on the perineum (Figs 15.10 and 15.11A). In epispadias, which is rare, it is on the dorsum of the penis. Chordee is curvature of the penis and is commonly associated with hypospadias and tethering of the foreskin (Fig. 15.11B).

Spine and sacrum

Examination sequence

- Turn the baby over.
- Inspect and palpate the entire vertebral column from neck to sacrum for neural tube defects.

Normal findings

Sacral dimples are common and unimportant, provided the dimple base has normal skin and they are single, <5 mm in diameter and <2.5 cm from the anus.

Abnormal findings

Pigmented patches may indicate spina bifida occulta. Dimples above the natal cleft, away from the midline, or hairy or pigmented patches with a base that cannot be visualised require further investigation.

Neurological examination

This includes tone, posture, movement and primitive reflexes.

General neurological assessment

Examination sequence

- Look for asymmetry in posture and movement, and for muscle wasting.
- To assess tone, pick the baby up and note if they are stiff or floppy. Note any difference between each side.

- Power is difficult to assess and depends on the state of arousal. Look for strong symmetrical limb and trunk movements and grasp.
- Tendon reflexes are of value only in assessing infants with neurological or muscular abnormalities.
- Check sensation by seeing whether the baby withdraws from gentle stimuli. Do not inflict painful stimuli or use a pin or needle.
- Check eyesight by carrying the alert baby to a dark corner. This normally causes the eyes to open wide. In a bright area the baby will screw up their eyes.

Ideally, electronic audiological screening should also be performed in the newborn period.

Normal findings

Movements should be equal on both sides.

Tone varies and may be floppy after a feed.

Reflexes are brisk in term infants, often with a few beats of clonus.

The plantar reflex is normally extensor in the newborn.

Abnormal findings

Hypotonic infants may have a 'frog-like' posture with abducted hips and extended elbows. Causes include Down's syndrome, meningitis and sepsis.

Increased tone may cause back and neck arching and limb extension; the baby feels stiff when picked up. Causes include meningitis, asphyxia and intracranial haemorrhage.

Brachial plexus injuries include Erb's palsy, which affects brachial plexus roots C5 and C6, producing reduced movement of the arm at the shoulder and elbow, medial rotation of the forearm and failure to extend the wrist (Fig. 15.12). Klumpke's palsy may be seen after breech delivery due to damage to roots C8 and T1, with weakness of the forearm and hand. These injuries can be associated with ipsilateral Horner's syndrome and/or diaphragmatic weakness in severe cases. Most perinatal brachial plexus injuries recover over subsequent weeks.

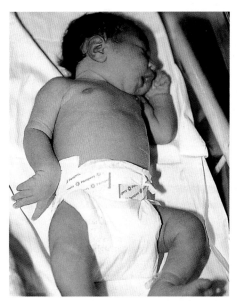

Fig. 15.12 Erb's palsy. The right arm is medially rotated and the wrist is flexed. *From Lissauer T, Clayden G. Illustrated Textbook of Paediatrics. 2nd edn. Edinburgh: Mosby; 2001.*

Facial nerve palsy causes reduced movement of the cheek muscles, and the side of the mouth does not turn down when the baby cries. Most cases are transient.

Primitive reflexes in newborn and young infants

The primitive reflexes are lower motor neurone responses that are present at birth but that become suppressed by higher centres by 4–6 months. They may be absent in infants with neurological depression or asymmetrical in infants with nerve injuries. Persistence into later infancy may indicate neurodevelopmental abnormality (p. 141). There are many examples and there is no need to elicit them all because their individual value is limited.

Examination sequence

Grasp responses

- Gently stimulate the palm or sole with your finger to produce a palmar or plantar grasp.

Ventral suspension/pelvic response to back stimulation

- Hold the baby prone and look for neck extension. Stroke the skin over the vertebral column to produce an extensor response with pelvic elevation.

Place-and-step reflexes

- Hold the baby upright and touch the dorsum of their foot against the edge of a table. The baby will flex the knee and hip, placing their foot on the table (Fig. 15.13A).
- Lower the upright baby towards the table surface. When the feet touch the surface, a walking movement occurs.

Moro reflex

- Support the supine baby's trunk and head in a semi-upright position. Let their head fall backwards slightly. The baby will quickly throw out both arms and spread their fingers (Fig. 15.13B).

Root-and-suck responses

- Gently stroke the baby's cheek. The baby turns to that side and their mouth opens, as though looking for a nipple. This is 'rooting'. If you place your finger in a healthy infant's mouth, they will suck it vigorously.

Asymmetric tonic neck reflex

- Turn the supine infant's head to the side. The arm and leg on the same side will extend and the arm and leg on the opposite side will flex. This reflex is present at term and maximal at 1 month (Fig. 15.13C).

Limbs

Examination sequence

- Inspect the limbs and count the digits.
- If the foot is abnormally positioned, gently try to place it in a normal position. If the abnormal position is at all fixed, refer to a specialist.
- Examine the hips to check for developmental dysplasia of the hip (DDH):
  - Lay the baby supine on a firm surface.
  - Inspect the skin creases of the thighs for symmetry.

15

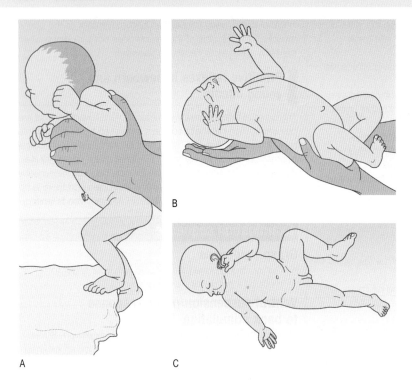

A   C

Fig. 15.13 Primitive reflexes. A Placing reflex. B The Moro reflex. C Tonic neck reflex.

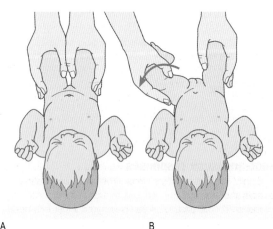

A   B

Fig. 15.14 Examination for developmental dysplasia of the hip.
A The hip is dislocated posteriorly out of the acetabulum (Barlow manœuvre). B The dislocated hip is relocated back into the acetabulum (Ortolani manœuvre).

- Examine each hip separately. Hold the thigh with the knee and hip flexed and your thumb on the medial aspect of the thigh.
- Move the proximal end of the thigh laterally and then push down towards the examining table (Barlow manœuvre, Fig. 15.14A); a clunk indicates that the hip is dislocatable.
- Now abduct the thigh; if you feel a clunk, this is the head of the femur returning into the acetabulum (Ortolani manœuvre, Fig. 15.14B). If the femoral head feels lax and you feel a clunk with an Ortolani manœuvre without first performing the Barlow manœuvre, then the hip was already dislocated.

Normal findings

A small percentage of normal babies have single palmar creases but this is also associated with Down's syndrome (see Fig. 3.31B) and other chromosomal abnormalities. Tibial bowing is common in the newborn.

It is common to hear or feel minor ligamentous clicks during hip examination. These are of no consequence and feel quite different to the dislocation and relocation of DDH. If in any doubt, obtain an expert opinion. Never use the term 'clicky hips'.

Abnormal findings

Oligodactyly (too few digits), polydactyly (too many) or syndactyly (joined digits) may occur. In talipes equinovarus the foot is plantar-flexed and rotated, with the sole facing medially. In talipes calcaneovalgus the foot is dorsiflexed so that the heel is prominent and the sole faces laterally.

Many cases of DDH have associated risk factors, including a family history, breech delivery, positional talipes (especially calcaneovalgus) or oligohydramnios.

Some centres offer hip ultrasound screening.

Weighing and measuring

Examination sequence

- Weigh the infant fully undressed using electronic scales accurate to 5 g.
- Use a paper tape to measure the maximal occipitofrontal circumference round the forehead and occiput (Fig. 15.15). Repeat the measurement three times, noting the largest measurement to the nearest millimetre.
- Measure the crown–heel length using a neonatal stadiometer (Fig. 15.16). Ask a parent or assistant to hold the baby's head still and stretch out the legs until the baby

15.5 Developmental attainment of preschool children at different ages*

Skills	4 months	6 months	10 months	1–2 years	2–3 years	3–5 years
Gross motor	Has good head control on pull to sit Keeps back straight when held in sitting position	Supports weight on hands when laid prone Rolls front to back	Sits unsupported Pulls to stand	Walks without support	Runs Bounces on trampoline	Pedals a tricycle
Fine motor	Opens hands Holds objects placed in hand	Transfers objects from hand to hand and to mouth	Uses pincer grip bilaterally without hand preference	Holds a crayon and scribbles	Can draw a circle	Can draw a cross, square, face/person
Personal social	Shows interest in toys Laughs, vocalises	Has a variety of speech noises Plays peep-bo	Starts to understand some words Claps hands	Has 10–20 recognisable words	Can communicate verbally	Has 500–1500 words Is dry by day

*Development is extremely variable and failure to attain only one milestone is of little significance whereas failure to attain several milestones is cause for concern.

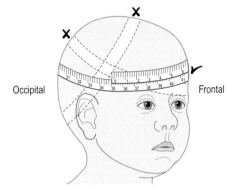

Occipital Frontal

Fig. 15.15 Measurement of head circumference.

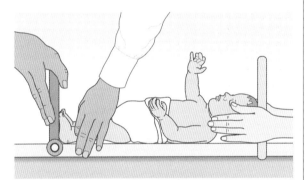

Fig. 15.16 Measuring length accurately in infants.

is fully extended (the least reproducible of the three measurements).

- Record the results on a centile chart appropriate to the infant's ethnic background.

Final inspection

Perform a final top-to-toe inspection to avoid missing anything and to allow the parents a further opportunity to ask questions.

The physical examination of infants beyond the newborn period

Examination of young infants beyond the newborn period is similar to the newborn examination. Transient neonatal findings will no longer be present. Older infants are usually happier when examined on their parent's lap than on an examination table. The examination of the ears should include otoscopy (p. 314). You should check the hips whenever you examine an infant until they are walking normally. After the first few months the Ortolani and Barlow manœuvres cannot be performed and the most important signs are limitation of abduction in the hip, and thigh skin crease asymmetry. Neurological history and examination should take account of the developmental stage of the child. The primitive reflexes disappear by 4–6 months. In later infancy, ask additional questions to obtain information about neurodevelopmental progress (Box 15.5).

OLDER CHILDREN

Individuals between 12 months and 16 years are known by non-specific terms, including toddlers, preschoolers, schoolchildren, adolescents, teenagers or young adults.

The history

Obtaining a history from children compared with adults

There are many similarities in taking a history from a child and from an adult. Introduce yourself to the child and accompanying adult, and begin to observe the child. Establish who the adult is – a parent, grandparent or foster carer, for example – and consider to what extent the child will be able to contribute to the history. Let the child become accustomed to you before asking specific questions.

Start with open-ended questions. Most often a parent will wish to explain their perspective on their child's problem and it is important to enable them to do so. Some teenagers may welcome this but most often they do not. Once the presenting symptoms have been outlined, the history should focus on questions that aim to elucidate the differential diagnosis; children are often good at helping with these more specific questions. Respect age ability to recall events and adopt a balanced perspective on whether

15

answers from parents are more likely to be accurate than those from the child. Children under 6 years often provide little history, those aged 6–11 years can do so if they are sufficiently confident, and those aged 12 years and above should be able to provide a valuable history in the correct environment and with the use of questions that are framed in appropriate terminology. As you would for adult history taking, include reflective summing up: for example, 'So what you are saying is that …'.

A paediatric history includes elements that are not part of the adult history (obstetric, developmental, immunisation histories), systematic enquiry has different components from those in adults (see later), and the differential diagnosis may include conditions seen only in children such as abdominal migraine, toddler diarrhoea, croup, viral wheeze and febrile convulsion. Most other diagnoses also occur in adults.

Common presenting symptoms

Diagnosis is built on patterns of symptoms; rarely will any one symptom or sign lead to a 'spot diagnosis'. The initial history suggests a differential diagnosis and prompts additional questions to assess the probability of particular diagnoses. As with adults, presenting symptoms should be described in terms of onset, frequency, severity, duration, aggravating and relieving factors, associated features and impact on function. Pain and the need for analgesia can be particularly difficult to assess in young children; objective scoring systems may help (Box 15.6).

The most common presenting problems in the child affect the respiratory, gastrointestinal and nervous systems (covered in Boxes 15.7–15.9), and the skin.

15.6 Pain assessment tool: FLACC scale

	0	1	2
Face	No particular expression or smile	Occasional grimace or frown, withdrawn, uninterested	Frequently or constantly quivering chin, clenched jaw
Legs	Normal position or relaxed	Uneasy, restless, tense	Kicking or legs drawn up
Activity	Lying quietly, normal position, moves easily	Squirming, shifting back and forth, tense	Arched, rigid or jerking
Cry	No cry (awake or asleep)	Moans or whimpers, occasional complaint	Crying steadily, screams or sobs, frequent complaints
Consolability	Content, relaxed	Reassured by occasional touching, hugging or being talked to, distractible	Difficult to console or comfort

Each category is scored on a 0–2 scale to give a total score of 0–10: 0 = no pain; 1–3 = mild pain; 4–7 = moderate pain; 8–10 = severe pain.

15.7 Respiratory system

Symptom[a,b]	Frequency	Diagnostic significance	Significance heightened if associated with	Differential diagnosis
Acute				
Short of breath at rest (SOBar)	***	High (indicates loss of all respiratory reserve)		LRTI, asthma, acute episodic wheeze, inhaled foreign body. Rarely, supraventricular tachycardia, congenital heart disease, heart failure or muscular weakness
Cough	***	Low	SOBar, fever	LRTI, asthma, acute episodic wheeze, foreign body
Wheeze	***	Moderate	SOBar, fever	LRTI, asthma, acute episodic wheeze, foreign body
Chest pain	*	High	Exercise Fever	Musculoskeletal pain, empyema, reflux oesophagitis, cardiac ischaemia
Stridor	***	High	URTI, high fever, choking	Croup, foreign body, epiglottitis (if not immunised)
Chronic				
Short of breath on exercise (SOBoe)	**	Low	Cough, wheeze, failure to thrive	Lack of fitness, respiratory pathology, cardiac pathology, neurological weakness
Cough	***	Low	Wheeze, SOBoe, failure to thrive	Isolated cough with sputum suggests infection, commonly bronchitis, rarely bronchiectasis, cystic fibrosis, inhaled foreign body. If also wheezy, consider asthma or viral-induced wheeze
Wheeze	***	Moderate	SOBoe, failure to thrive	Isolated, persistent 'wheeze' usually arises from the nose (stertor, e.g. adenoidal hypertrophy) or the largest airways (stridor, e.g. laryngomalacia). Episodic wheeze with cough suggests asthma or viral-induced wheeze
Chest pain	*	High	Exercise	Non-specific chest pain, musculoskeletal chest pain, very rarely cardiac ischaemia

[a]Respiratory sounds: clarify what noise the parent or child is describing. The history sometimes reveals the source, e.g. nose (stertor), throat (stridor) or chest (rattle or wheeze). A constant respiratory sound is more likely to be stertor, stridor or rattle (a sound associated with vibration of the chest). A very loud sound, such as one heard in the next room, is not genuine wheeze. [b]Coexistent failure to thrive or weight loss always increases the significance of any symptom.
LRTI/URTI, lower/upper respiratory tract infection.

15.8 Gastrointestinal system

Symptom	Frequency	Diagnostic significance	Significance heightened if associated with	Differential diagnosis
Acute				
Vomiting	***	Low: a very non-specific symptom in children	Fever, drowsiness, dehydration[a]	Acute gastritis/gastroenteritis, any infection (otitis media, pneumonia, urinary tract infection, meningitis), head injury, encephalitis
Diarrhoea	***	Moderate	Fever, dehydration[a]	Acute gastroenteritis/colitis, appendicitis
Abdominal pain[b]	**	Moderate	Fever, bloody stools	Acute gastroenteritis/colitis, acute surgical causes, e.g. appendicitis, intussusception
Chronic				
Vomiting	***	Moderate	Failure to thrive[c] Headache	Gastro-oesophageal reflux (rare in older children compared with infants), raised intracranial pressure, food allergy
Diarrhoea	***	Moderate	Failure to thrive[c]	Commonly toddler's diarrhoea, also lactose intolerance. If failure to thrive, consider coeliac disease, inflammatory bowel disease
Abdominal pain[b]	***	Low	Pain that is not periumbilical Headaches Diarrhoea and vomiting Failure to thrive[c]	If isolated and periumbilical, non-specific abdominal pain is common and other diagnoses include abdominal migraine, renal colic. If associated with other symptoms and/or failure to thrive, consider coeliac disease, inflammatory bowel disease, constipation

[a]Symptoms of dehydration include dry mouth, foul-smelling breath, anuria and lethargy. [b]Abdominal pain can be difficult to identify in young children who are not able to express themselves. [c]Coexisting failure to thrive or weight loss always increases the significance of any symptom.

15.9 Nervous system

15

Symptom	Frequency	Diagnostic significance	Significance heightened if associated with	Differential diagnosis
Acute				
Headache	**	Low		Acute (simple) headache, migraine, meningitis/encephalitis
Unsteady gait	*	High	Vomiting, fever, neck stiffness, photophobia	Varicella encephalomeningitis, vestibular neuronitis
Seizure[a]	*	High		Febrile seizure, meningitis/encephalitis Epilepsy, metabolic disorder
Disturbed level of consciousness	*	High		Encephalitis, intoxication/drug ingestion (accidental/ deliberate)
Chronic				
Headache[b]	**	Low	Vomiting Abdominal pain	Brain tumour, migraine, chronic non-specific headache
Failure to pass developmental milestones	*	Moderate	Widening gap between age and age when 'normal' milestone should have been passed	Cerebral palsy, neglect
Developmental regression	*	High		Muscular dystrophy, inborn error of metabolism, neurodegenerative conditions
Seizure	*	High		Epilepsy; rarely, long QT syndrome or inborn error of metabolism

[a]An acute seizure can be confused with a rigor in a febrile child. A seizure involves slow (1 beat per second), coarse, jerking that cannot be stopped, loss of consciousness and postictal drowsiness. A rigor is characterised by rapid (5 beats per second), fine jerking that can be stopped by a cuddle with no loss of consciousness. [b]Chronic headache can also arise from the mouth (e.g. dental abscess) or face.

Skin symptoms can be acute or chronic. Acute-onset rash is common in children and can be described using the same terminology as for adults (p. 286). Most rashes are viral and resolve spontaneously.

Rash with blisters is often itchy. It may be urticaria (with an environmental, viral, food or medicine trigger) or an insect bite. Blisters with associated yellow crusting may be infected bullous impetigo (most commonly caused by *Staphylococcus aureus*).

Red, circular lesions with a pink centre are most often erythema multiforme (target lesions). Petechial or purpuric rashes that do not blanch with pressure are of most concern. These may be viral in origin but importantly can be an early sign of meningococcal disease (particularly if the child is febrile). A differential diagnosis of a purpuric rash is idiopathic thrombocytopenic purpura.

Chronic skin excoriation, most commonly in the flexures, suggests eczema, while plaques on the elbows/knees may indicate psoriasis.

Hair loss is distressing to a child. If associated with itch, it is often due to tinea capitis; with a history of preceding illness, alopecia is a likely cause.

Past medical history

Has the child regularly seen a healthcare professional (current or past) or are they currently taking any regular medication? Have they been in hospital before, and if so, why?

Birth history

The impact of preterm birth goes beyond early childhood and so it is helpful to ask:

- Was the child born at term or preterm (if so, at what gestation)?
- Was the neonatal period normal? For example, did the child need to go to a special care baby unit?
- If the child is under 3 years of age: what was the birthweight and were there any complications during pregnancy?

Vaccination history

Are the child's immunisations up to date according to country-specific schedules? If not, explore why and consider how best to encourage catch-up.

Developmental history

This is particularly important for children under 3 years of age or those with possible neurodevelopmental delay (see p. 307 and Box 15.5).

Drug history

Prescribing errors often arise from poor reconciliation of medication lists between different healthcare professionals. It is a doctor's duty to ensure that medicines are accurately reconciled within documentation. Transcribe the medication, dose and frequency direct from the medication package or referral letter if possible. Enquire about any difficulties in taking medication to establish adherence. Clarify any adverse or allergic reactions to medications.

Family and social history

Ask:

- Who lives in the family home and who cares for the child?
- Does anyone smoke at home?
- Are there any pets? Are any symptoms associated with pet contact?
- Are there any similar symptoms in the child's first- or second-degree relatives?

Sketch a family tree, noting any step-parents, step-siblings or shared care arrangements Consider parental consanguinity, which is not uncommon in some ethnic groups. Children at risk of neglect may have complex domestic arrangements such as several caregivers.

Occasionally, chronic symptoms are associated with anxiety or potential 'secondary' gain for the child; these include chronic cough, abdominal pain and headache in a well-looking 8–12-year-old in whom examination is normal. Look carefully at the child's facial expression, eye contact and body language when asking questions. Ask specifically about school (avoidance and bullying), social interactions (does the child have many friends?) and out-of-school activities. School avoidance should be addressed if it is related to anxiety or if the pretext of medical symptoms is used.

Systematic enquiry

This screens for illnesses or symptoms that may be not recognised as important or relevant by the child or parents. For children aged over 12 years, the questions used for adults are appropriate. In younger children, ask age-related questions. Specific areas include:

- Ear, nose and throat: ask the parents about their perception of a child's hearing ability (reduced in chronic otitis media) or the presence of regular snoring with periods of struggling to breathe (symptomatic obstructive sleep apnoea).
- Gastrointestinal system: ask whether growth is as expected and whether there is pain or difficulty in opening the bowels (constipation).
- Respiratory system: ask whether the child has regularly coughed when otherwise well or had wheeze on a recurrent basis (consider asthma).
- Urinary system: 15% of children at 5 years of age will continue to have primary nocturnal enuresis.

The physical examination

Normal growth and development

An understanding of child development is vital to identifying whether symptoms and signs are consistent with age.

Infants born prematurely should have their age adjusted to their expected date of delivery instead of their date of birth for the first 2 years of life when growth and development are assessed. Failure to make this correction would otherwise create a false impression of poor growth and developmental delay. Prematurely born infants are at increased risk of impaired growth and development, and merit increased surveillance; most develop normally, however.

Growth

Growth after infancy is extremely variable. Use gender- and ethnic-specific growth charts (such as those shown in Fig. 15.17). These compare the individual with the general population and with their own previous measurements. Each child should grow along a centile line for height and weight throughout childhood. Failure to thrive is failure to attain the expected growth trajectory. A child on the 0.4th centile for height may be thriving if this has always been their growth trajectory, while a child on the 50th centile for height may be failing to thrive if previously they were on the 99.6th centile.

A child's height is related to the average of their parents' height centile ± 2 standard deviations. Parents whose average height lies on the 50th centile will have children whose height will normally lie between the 2nd and 98th centiles (approximately 10 cm above and below the 50th centile).

Neurological development

Normal development is heterogeneous within the population, which makes identifying abnormalities difficult. Important determinants are the child's environment and genetic potential. Developmental

Weight-for-age BOYS
Birth to 2 years (z-scores)

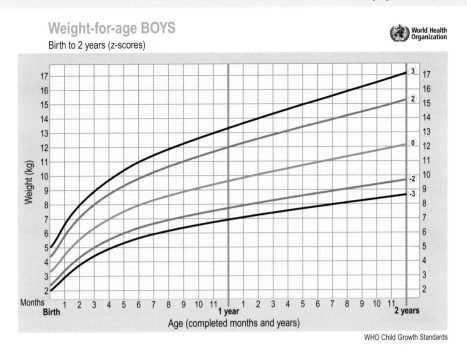

WHO Child Growth Standards

Weight-for-age GIRLS
Birth to 2 years (z-scores)

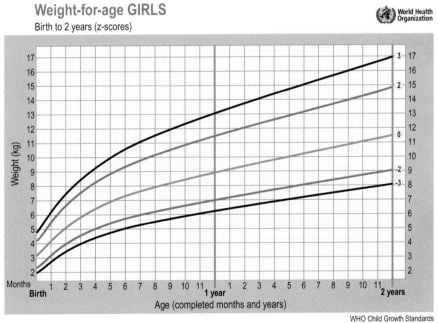

WHO Child Growth Standards

Fig. 15.17 Growth charts. World Health Organization standard centile charts for girls and boys. *From WHO Child Growth Standards. http://www.who.int/childgrowth/standards/weight_for_age/en/ © World Health Organization 2017. All rights reserved.*

assessment requires patience, familiarity with children and an understanding of the range of normality for a given age.

The preschool child (1–5 years)

At the younger end of this range, questions relating to gross motor skills are most sensitive; as the child becomes older, questions relating to fine motor and personal social skills are more meaningful. Delayed speech with normal attainment of motor milestones is not uncommon, particularly in boys, but should prompt hearing assessment (see Box 15.5).

The school-age child (5+ years)

By this age, developmental problems are usually known to parents and relevant agencies, such as educational ones, may already be engaged. However, more subtle developmental problems such as dyslexia (learning disability affecting fluency and comprehension in reading) may be unrecognised and can be a major handicap. Ask general questions such as, 'How is your child getting on at school?' and follow up by enquiring specifically about academic and social activity.

Puberty

This stage of adolescence, when an individual becomes physiologically capable of sexual reproduction, is a time of rapid physical and emotional development. The age at the onset and end of puberty varies greatly but is generally 10–14 years for girls and 12–16 years for boys (Fig. 15.18). The average child grows 30 cm during puberty and gains 40–50% in weight.

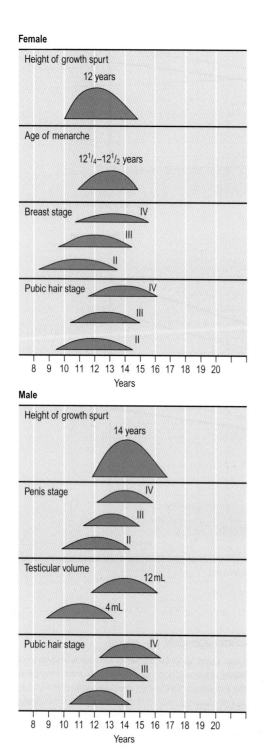

Fig. 15.18 Timing of puberty in males and females.

If required, use a chart to stage puberty (Fig. 15.19). Pubertal staging has a wide normal range, with abnormalities apparent only on follow-up. Delayed or precocious puberty is not uncommon.

Physical examination techniques in children

Children usually present with a symptom. Children with acute symptoms often have physical signs such as wheeze, but examination is normal in the majority of children with chronic symptoms. Routine screening examination after infancy is unhelpful, as many paediatric diseases only produce signs late in the illness.

Similarities in examination between children and adults

The techniques used when examining children are the same as those in adults, with some exceptions. Examining a child is a skill that takes time to learn. The key skills involve being:

- Observant of the child during discussion or play, to identify elements of the examination that are naturally displayed and so can be partitioned from the formal examination process, reducing the duration of what is often a stressful encounter for the child.
- Opportunistic, to examine systems as the child presents them. Chest and cardiac auscultation may be better earlier in the examination in younger children before they become restless or upset.
- Adaptive to a child's mood and playfulness. A skilled practitioner can glean most examination findings from even the most uncooperative child. Usually the history suggests the diagnosis; the examination confirms it.

Differences in examination between children and adults

The appropriate approach varies with the child's age.

1–3 years

All children at this age can be reluctant to be approached by strangers, and particularly dislike being examined. Early on, let children gradually become used to your presence and see that your encounter with their parents is friendly. Carefully observe the child's general condition, colour, respiratory rate and effort, and state of hydration while taking the history: that is, when the child is not focused on your close attention. For the formal examination, ask the parent to sit the child on their knees. Examine the cardiorespiratory system and the abdomen with the young child sitting upright on the parent's knee. With patience, abdominal examination can be done with the child lying supine on the bed next to a parent or on the parent's lap. Taking your stethoscope from around your neck to use it can upset the child, so make slow, non-threatening moves. If the child starts crying, chest auscultation and abdominal palpation become very difficult; take a pause. Ear, nose and throat examination often causes upset and is best left till last; suggesting that ear examination will tickle can help with older children.

3–5 years

Some children in this age range have the confidence and maturity to comply with some aspects of adult examination. They may cooperate by holding up their T-shirts for chest examination

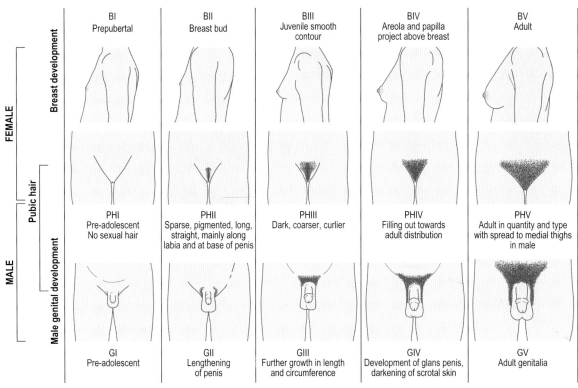

Fig. 15.19 Stages of puberty in males and females. Pubertal changes according to the Tanner stages of puberty.

15

15.10 Serious signs requiring urgent attention

- Poor perfusion with reduced capillary refill and cool peripheries (indicating shock)
- Listless, poorly responsive, whimpering child (suggesting sepsis)
- Petechial rash over the trunk (suggesting meningococcal sepsis)
- Headache with photophobia or neck stiffness (suggesting meningitis)
- Respiratory distress at rest (rapid rate and increased respiratory effort, indicating loss of respiratory reserve due to pneumonia or asthma)

and turning round; if so, comment warmly on this cooperation and provide positive feedback on helpful behaviour. Children's social skills regress when they are unwell and some are very apprehensive of strangers.

5+ years

The child may comply with a full adult-style examination. Although children under 11 years are often not able to express themselves well, those over 5 years are able to understand and comply with requests such as finger-to-nose pointing, heel-to-toe walking, and being asked to 'sit forward' and 'take a deep breath in and hold it'.

The acutely unwell child

There are many non-specific signs that are common to a range of conditions from a simple cold to meningitis. These include a runny nose, fever, lethargy, vomiting, blanching rash and irritability. However, some signs are serious, requiring immediate investigation and management (Box 15.10).

Children become ill quickly. If a child has been unwell for less than 24 hours and initial examination reveals only non-specific

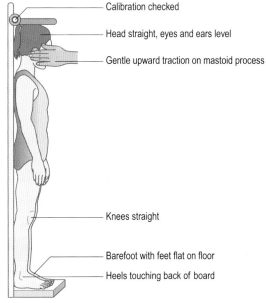

Fig. 15.20 Stadiometer for measuring height accurately in children.

signs, they should ideally be reassessed in 1–2 hours if there is a high level of parental or clinical anxiety that the signs are out of keeping with a simple viral illness in a child of that age.

General examination

Height

Use a stadiometer (Fig. 15.20).

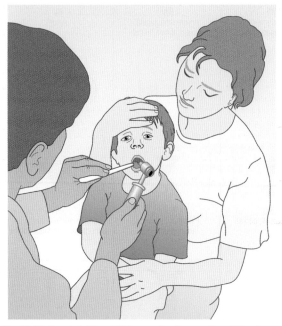

Fig. 15.21 How to hold a child to examine the mouth and throat.

15.11 Physiological measurements in children of different ages			
Age (years)	Pulse (bpm)	Respiratory rate (breaths per minute)	Systolic blood pressure (mmHg)
0–1	110–160	30–60	70–90
2–5	60–140	25–40	80–100
6–12	60–120	20–25	90–110
13–18	60–100	15–20	100–120

Vital signs

Normal ranges for vital signs vary according to age (Box 15.11).

Ears, nose and throat

The preschool child

Throat

Examination sequence

- Ask the parent to:
  - Sit the child on their knees, both facing you.
  - Give an older child the opportunity to open their mouth spontaneously ('Roar like a lion!'). If this is not successful, proceed as described here.
  - Place one arm over the child's upper arms and chest (to stop the child pushing you away, Fig. 15.21).
  - Hold the child's forehead with their other hand (to stop the child pulling their chin down to their chest).
- Hold the torch in your non-dominant hand to illuminate the child's throat.
- Slide a tongue depressor inside the child's cheek with your dominant hand. The child should open their clenched teeth (perhaps with a shout), showing their tonsils and pharynx.

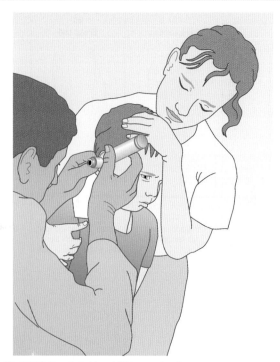

Fig. 15.22 How to hold a child to examine the ear.

Abnormal findings

Healthy tonsils and pharynx look pink; when inflamed, they are crimson–red.

Inspecting the throat reveals the presence, but not the cause, of the infection; pus on the tonsils and pharynx does not differentiate a bacterial from a viral infection (p. 185).

Ears

Examination sequence

- Ask the parent to:
  - Sit the child across their knees with the child's ear facing you.
  - Place one arm around the child's shoulder and upper arm that are facing you (to stop them pushing you away, Fig. 15.22).
  - Place their other hand over the parietal area above the child's ear that is facing you (to keep the child's head still).
- Use an otoscope with the largest speculum that will comfortably fit the child's external auditory meatus.
- To straighten the ear canal and visualise the canal and tympanic membrane, hold the pinna gently and pull it out and down in a baby or toddler with no mastoid development, or up and back in a child whose mastoid process has formed.

Lymphadenopathy

Normal findings

Palpable neck and groin nodes are extremely common in children under 5 years old. They are typically bilateral, less than 1 cm in diameter, hard and mobile with no overlying redness, and can persist for many weeks. In the absence of systemic symptoms such as weight loss, fevers or night sweats, these are typically a normal, healthy immune response to infection. Only rarely are they due to malignancy (Box 15.12).

15

15.12 Causes of lymph node enlargement

Cervical lymphadenopathy

- Tonsillitis, pharyngitis, sinusitis
- 'Glandular fever' (infectious mononucleosis/cytomegalovirus)
- Tuberculosis (uncommon in developed countries)

Generalised lymphadenopathy

- Febrile illness with a generalised rash
- 'Glandular fever'
- Systemic juvenile chronic arthritis (Still's disease)
- Acute lymphatic leukaemia
- Drug reaction
- Mucocutaneous lymph node syndrome (Kawasaki disease)

15.13 Clinical signs associated with severe illness in children

- Fever >38°C
- Drowsiness
- Cold hands and feet
- Petechial rash
- Neck stiffness
- Shortness of breath at rest
- Tachycardia
- Hypotension (a late sign in shocked children where blood pressure is initially maintained by tachycardia and increased peripheral vascular resistance)

Cardiovascular examination

Feel the brachial pulse in the antecubital fossa in children below 2–3 years. Do not palpate the carotid or radial pulses in young children. Measure blood pressure using a cuff sized two-thirds the distance from elbow to shoulder tip. Repeat with a larger cuff if the reading is elevated. If in doubt, use a larger cuff, as smaller cuffs yield falsely high values.

Respiratory examination

Abnormal findings

The child under 3 years has a soft chest wall and relatively small, stiff lungs. When the lungs are made stiffer (by infection or fluid), the diaphragm must contract vigorously to draw air into the lungs. This produces recession (ribs 'sucking in' – tracheal, intercostal and subcostal) and paradoxical outward movement of the abdomen (wrongly called 'abdominal breathing'). These important signs of increased work of breathing are often noticed by parents. Older children may be able to articulate the accompanying symptom of dyspnoea.

Children's small, thin chests transmit noises readily, and their smaller airways are more prone to turbulence and added sounds. Auscultation may reveal a variety of sounds, including expiratory polyphonic wheeze (occasionally inspiratory too), fine end-expiratory crackles, coarse louder crackles transmitted from the larger airways, and other sounds described as pops and squeaks (typically in the chest of recovering patients with asthma).

Abdominal examination

In children aged 6 months to 3 years, examine the abdomen with the child sitting upright on their parent's knee. In the young child, splenic enlargement extends towards the left iliac fossa. In older children the enlarged spleen edge moves towards the right iliac fossa. Faecal loading of the left iliac fossa is common in constipation. Rectal examination is rarely indicated in children.

Neurological examination

Test power initially by watching the child demonstrate their strength against gravity. Ask them to lift their arms above their head, raise their leg from the bed while they are lying down, and stand from a squatting position. If appropriate, test power against your strength.

Neck stiffness in a child is usually apparent when you are talking to them or their parents. A child with meningitis will not

---

15.14 Signs that may suggest child neglect or abuse

Behavioural signs

- 'Frozen watchfulness'
- Passivity
- Over-friendliness
- Sexualised behaviour
- Inappropriate dress
- Hunger, stealing food

Physical signs

- Identifiable bruises, e.g. fingertips, handprints, belt buckle, bites
- Circular (cigarette) burns or submersion burns with no splash marks
- Injuries of differing ages
- Eye or mouth injuries
- Long-bone fractures or bruises in non-mobile infants
- Posterior rib fracture
- Subconjunctival or retinal haemorrhage
- Dirty, smelly, unkempt child
- Bad nappy rash

---

want to move, and if they are forced to do so, the neck remains aligned with the trunk. With a young child, move a toy to catch their attention and see if they move their head.

Spotting the sick child

It can be difficult to identify a child with severe illness. With experience you will learn to identify whether a child is just miserable or really ill. Early-warning scores (such as PEWS or COAST, Fig. 15.23) can help. Certain features correlate with severe illness (Box 15.13).

Child protection

Children who experience neglect or physical and/or emotional abuse are at increased risk of health problems. At-risk children are often already known to other agencies but this information may not be available to you in the acute setting. Injuries from physical abuse can be detected visually. Consider non-accidental injury if the history is not consistent with the injury, or the injury is present in unusual places such as over the back. It may be difficult to detect neglect during a brief encounter but consider it if the child appears dirty or is wearing dirty or torn clothes that are too small or large. The parent–child relationship gives insight into neglect; the child is apparently scared of the parent ('frozen watchfulness') or the parent is apparently oblivious to the child's attention (Box 15.14).

PRESCHOOL (1–4 years)

COAST: CHILDREN'S UNIT

CHILDREN'S OBSERVATION AND SEVERITY TOOL

Patient details
Name
DOB
Hosp No

CHILDREN'S
UNIT

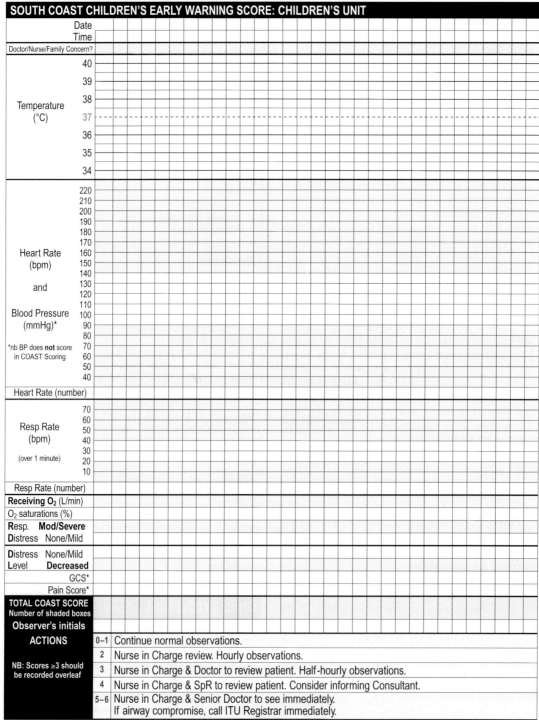

SOUTH COAST CHILDREN'S EARLY WARNING SCORE: CHILDREN'S UNIT

Date		
Time		
Doctor/Nurse/Family Concern?		

Temperature (°C)
40 / 39 / 38 / 37 / 36 / 35 / 34

Heart Rate (bpm) and Blood Pressure (mmHg)*
220 / 210 / 200 / 190 / 180 / 170 / 160 / 150 / 140 / 130 / 120 / 110 / 100 / 90 / 80 / 70 / 60 / 50 / 40

*nb BP does **not** score in COAST Scoring

Heart Rate (number)

Resp Rate (bpm) (over 1 minute)
70 / 60 / 50 / 40 / 30 / 20 / 10

Resp Rate (number)

Receiving O₂ (L/min)

O₂ saturations (%)

Resp. **Mod/Severe**
Distress None/Mild

Distress None/Mild
Level **Decreased**

GCS*

Pain Score*

TOTAL COAST SCORE
Number of shaded boxes

Observer's initials

ACTIONS		
	0–1	Continue normal observations.
	2	Nurse in Charge review. Hourly observations.
NB: Scores ≥3 should be recorded overleaf	3	Nurse in Charge & Doctor to review patient. Half-hourly observations.
	4	Nurse in Charge & SpR to review patient. Consider informing Consultant.
	5–6	Nurse in Charge & Senior Doctor to see immediately. If airway compromise, call ITU Registrar immediately.

*nb: BP, GCS and Pain Score values do not contribute to the overall COAST score.

Fig. 15.23 Rapid cardiopulmonary evaluation. *BP,* blood pressure; *bpm,* beats/breaths per minute; *GCS,* Glasgow coma scale score; *ITU,* intensive treatment unit; *SpR,* specialist registrar. *Courtesy Dr Sandell.*

OSCE example case 1: Cyanotic episodes

Charlie, 4 months old, is brought in to see you by his mother Helen. She is anxious, as he has 'turned blue' on three occasions since discharge from hospital. Two of the episodes have been during breastfeeding, when he has become agitated and breathless.

Please perform a newborn examination, focusing on the cardiovascular system

- Introduce yourself to the parent and clean your hands
- Carry out a general inspection: are there any signs of congenital heart disease?
  - Look for signs of respiratory distress (tachypnoea, indrawing, accessory muscle use).
  - Check for scars on the chest.
  - Look at the colour and perfusion of the patient (cyanosis, pallor, sweatiness).
  - Look for signs of dysmorphic features that might indicate an associated chromosomal abnormality.
  - Look for signs of poor weight gain.
- Palpate: is the infant warm and well perfused? Are there any palpable cardiac abnormalities?
  - Check central capillary refill. Feel the temperature.
  - Palpate peripheral pulses (brachial, femoral).
  - Palpate the precordium for palpable murmurs (thrills), ventricular heave or abnormal position of the apex.
  - Assess whether there is palpable hepatomegaly or finger clubbing.
- Auscultate: is there a murmur?
  - Auscultate the heart in a systematic fashion.
  - Describe any murmur by documenting timing, grade (1–6), character, location, radiation, and variation with position and respiration.
  - Auscultate the back to check whether the murmur radiates.
- Clean your hands and thank the parent.

Suggest a diagnosis

Congenital heart disease is possible with this presentation. There are many possible types and further investigation is needed for diagnosis. Tetralogy of Fallot consists of four features: ventricular septal defect, right ventricular outflow obstruction, right ventricular hypertrophy and an overriding aorta. It requires surgical correction. Children with tetralogy of Fallot are more likely to have chromosome disorders (Down's syndrome or Di George syndrome). Finger clubbing is not usually present in young infants.

Suggest investigations

Pulse oximetry, echocardiogram, electrocardiogram, chest X-ray.

15

OSCE example 2: Asthma

John, 8 years old, who has been diagnosed with asthma, is brought to see you by his parent. He has had more frequent episodes of wheeze and night-time cough over the last 3 months, each lasting longer and responding less well to regular doses of bronchodilator.

Please perform a chest examination, focusing on the respiratory system

- Introduce yourself to the parent and patient, and clean your hands.
- Carry out a general inspection: are there any signs of acute or chronic respiratory distress?
  - Look for chest wall deformity (pectus excavatum, Harrison's sulcus).
  - Look for signs of respiratory distress (tachypnoea, indrawing, accessory muscle use).
  - Count the respiratory rate over 1 minute.
  - Look at the colour and perfusion of the patient (cyanosis, pallor, sweatiness).
  - Look for finger clubbing and poor weight gain.
- Palpate: consider palpation if there are chest-wall abnormalities or differential chest expansion on inspection, to look for differential chest-wall movement.
- Auscultate: warm the stethoscope.
  - Auscultate the respiratory system in all lung regions, anteriorly and posteriorly, with the chest fully exposed.
  - Wheeze is auscultated in all lung regions. No crepitations are heard. Air entry is reduced to all lung regions. The respiratory rate is raised at 40 breaths per minute.
  - Heart sounds are normal with no murmur.
- Clean your hands and thank the parent and patient.

Summarise your findings

This child has tachypnoea and a widespread, loud, polyphonic wheeze on expiration.

Suggest a diagnosis

Acute asthma attack on the background of unstable asthma is the likely diagnosis with these symptoms and signs. This requires treatment of the acute episode with bronchodilator and oral glucocorticoids, and consideration of how to improve background control. Stabilising background control includes an assessment of adherence and technique for current therapies, consideration of new triggers and how exposure may be reduced (by history and/or skin-prick testing) and, if required, a trial of a stepwise increase in baseline asthma therapy.

Suggest initial investigations

Peak expiratory flow or spirometry, and oxygen saturation.

Integrated examination sequence for the newborn child

- Perform a general examination:
  - Looks well and is well grown? Dysmorphic features? Posture and behaviour? Does the cry sound normal?
  - Skin: note cuts, bruising, naevi (haemangiomas or melanocytic), blisters or bullae.
  - Head: check shape, swellings, anterior fontanelle, cranial sutures.
  - Eyes: check for jaundice, ocular movements and vestibular function; perform ophthalmoscopy.
  - Nose: check patency.
  - Mouth: check mucosa, tongue, palate, jaw and any teeth.
  - Ears: note size, shape and position; check the external auditory meatus.
  - Neck: inspect and palpate for asymmetry, sinuses and swellings.
- Examine the cardiovascular system:
  - Inspect: pallor, cyanosis and sweating.
  - Palpate: apex, check for heave or thrill, count heart rate, femoral pulses, feel for hepatomegaly.
  - Auscultate: heart sounds I and II, any additional heart sounds or murmurs.
- Examine the respiratory system:
  - Inspect: chest shape, symmetry of movement, respiratory rate, respiratory distress: tachypnoea, suprasternal, intercostal and subcostal recession, flaring of nostrils.
  - Auscultate anteriorly, laterally and posteriorly, comparing sides.
- Examine the abdomen:
  - Inspect: abdomen, umbilicus, anus and groins, noting any swellings.
  - Palpate: superficial, then deeper structures. Spleen, then liver.
- Examine the perineum:
  - Both sexes: check normal anatomy.
  - Male: assess the penis, noting shape; check the urethral meatus is at the tip. Do not retract the foreskin. Palpate the testes, and the inguinal canal if the testes are not in the scrotum. Transilluminate scrotal swellings.
- Examine the spine and sacrum:
  - With the infant in the prone position, inspect and palpate the entire spine for neural tube defects.
- Examine the neurological system:
  - Inspect: asymmetry in posture and movement, any muscle wasting.
  - Pick the baby up to note any stiff or floppy tone.
  - Sensation: does the baby withdraw from gentle stimuli?
  - In dim light, the eyes should open; in bright light, babies screw up their eyes.
- Check the primitive reflexes:
  - Check grasp responses, ventral suspension/pelvic response to back stimulation, place-and-step reflexes, Moro reflex, root-and-suck responses.
- Inspect the limbs:
  - Inspect: limbs, counting digits and checking feet are, or can be, normally positioned.
  - Check hips for developmental dysplasia/dislocation.
- Weigh and measure:
  - Weigh the infant to the nearest 5 g.
  - Measure: occipitofrontal circumference, crown–heel length (neonatal stadiometer).
  - Record on a centile chart.

Stephen Potts

16

The patient with mental disorder

Mental disorders are very common, frequently coexist with physical disorders and cause much mortality and morbidity. Psychiatric assessment is therefore a required skill for all clinicians. It consists of four elements: the history, mental state examination, selective physical examination and collateral information. Each element can be expanded considerably, so the assessment must be adapted to its purpose. Is it a quick screening of a patient presenting with other problems, a confirmation of a suspected diagnosis or a comprehensive review for a second opinion?

The history

General approach

The distinction between symptoms and signs is less clear in psychiatry than in the rest of medicine. The psychiatric interview, which covers both, has several purposes: to obtain a history of symptoms, to assess the present mental state for signs, and to establish rapport that will facilitate further management.

A comprehensive history covers a range of areas (Box 16.1), but the nature of the presenting problem and/or the referral question, and the setting in which the history is being taken, will determine the degree of detail needed for each. When seeing someone in the accident and emergency department with a first episode of psychosis, the focus is on symptoms, recent changes of function, family history and drug use; when interviewing someone in an outpatient clinic with a possible personality disorder, assessment concentrates instead on their personal history, which is essentially a systematised biography (Box 16.2).

Sensitive topics

Some subjects require particular skill. The common theme is reluctance to disclose, which can arise because the information is private, and disclosure is potentially embarrassing (such as sexual dysfunction, gender identity), distressing (major traumatic experiences, such as rape, childhood sexual abuse, witnessing a

death) or incriminating (illicit drug misuse, other crime, homicidal ideas). For interviews undertaken in non-clinical settings such as police stations or prisons, or for the provision of court reports, the latter is obviously especially pertinent, and it is important to be clear with the patients about any limits to confidentiality in your interview.

Try to develop rapport early in the interview, if possible, and to consolidate it before raising a sensitive topic, although sometimes you must cover such material without delay. It is particularly important to ask about suicidal thoughts.

The uncooperative patient

Adapt your approach to a patient who is mute, agitated, hostile or otherwise uncooperative during the interview, by relying more on observation and collateral information. The safety of the patient, other patients and staff is paramount, so your initial assessment of an agitated or hostile patient may be only partial.

The mental state examination

The mental state examination (MSE) is a systematic evaluation of the patient's mental condition at the time of interview. The aim is to establish signs of mental disorder that, taken with the history, enable you to make, suggest or exclude a diagnosis. While making your specific enquiries, you need to observe, evaluate and draw inferences in the light of the history. This is daunting, but with good teaching, practice and experience you will learn the skills.

The MSE incorporates elements of the history, observation of the patient, specific questions exploring various mental phenomena and short tests of cognitive function. Like the history, its focus is determined by the potential diagnoses. For example, detailed cognitive assessment in an elderly patient presenting with confusion is crucial; similarly, you should carefully evaluate mood and suicidal thoughts when the presenting problem is depression.

Appearance

Think of this as a written account of a still photograph, prepared for someone who cannot see it. Observe:

- general elements such as attire and signs of self-neglect
- facial expression
- tattoos and scars (especially any that suggest recent or previous self-harm)
- evidence of substance misuse (such as injection tracks from intravenous drug use; spider naevi and jaundice from alcoholic liver disease)
- possibly relevant physical disease (such as exophthalmos from thyrotoxicosis).

Behaviour

Think of this as a written account of a video, observing such features as:

- cooperation, rapport, eye contact
- social behaviour (such as aggression, disinhibition, fearful withdrawal)
- apparent responses to possible hallucinations or unobserved stimuli

---

16.1 Content of a psychiatric history

- Referral source
- Reason for referral
- History of presenting symptom(s)
- Systematic enquiry into other relevant problems and symptoms
- Past medical/psychiatric history
- Prescribed and non-prescribed medication
- Substance use: illegal drugs, alcohol, tobacco, caffeine
- Family history (including psychiatric disorders)
- Personal history

16.2 Personal history

- Childhood development
- Losses and experiences
- Education
- Occupation(s)
- Financial circumstances
- Relationships
- Partner(s) and children
- Housing
- Leisure activities
- Hobbies and interests
- Forensic history

16.3 Behaviour: definitions

Term	Definition
Agitation	A combination of psychic anxiety and excessive, purposeless motor activity
Compulsion	A stereotyped action that the patient cannot resist performing repeatedly
Disinhibition	Loss of control over normal social behaviour
Motor retardation	Decreased motor activity, usually a combination of fewer and slower movements
Posturing	The maintenance of bizarre gait or limb positions for no valid reason

16.4 Speech: definitions

Term	Definition
Clang associations	Thoughts connected by their similar sound rather than by meaning
Echolalia	Senseless repetition of the interviewer's words
Mutism	Absence of speech without impaired consciousness
Neologism	An invented word, or a new meaning for an established word
Pressure of speech	Rapid, excessive, continuous speech (due to pressure of thought)
Word salad	A meaningless string of words, often with loss of grammatical construction

16.5 Mood: definitions

Term	Definition
Blunting	Loss of normal emotional sensitivity to experiences
Catastrophic reaction	An extreme emotional and behavioural over-reaction to a trivial stimulus
Flattening	Loss of the range of normal emotional responses
Incongruity	A mismatch between the emotional expression and the associated thought
Lability	Superficial, rapidly changing and poorly controlled emotions

16.6 Thought form: definitions

Term	Definition
Circumstantiality	Trivia and digressions impairing the flow but not direction of thought
Concrete thinking	Inability to think abstractly
Flights of ideas	Rapid shifts from one idea to another, retaining sequencing
Loosening of associations	Logical sequence of ideas impaired. Subtypes include knight's-move thinking, derailment, thought blocking and, in its extreme form, word salad
Perseveration	Inability to shift from one idea to the next
Pressure of thought	Increased rate and quantity of thoughts

16

- over-activity (agitation, pacing, compulsive hand washing)
- under-activity (stupor, motor retardation)
- abnormal activity (posturing, involuntary movements, Box 16.3).

Speech

This is not a description of what the patient says (that is, content), but of how they say it (form). Assess:
- articulation (such as stammering, dysarthria)
- quantity (mutism, garrulousness)
- rate (pressured, slowed)
- volume (whispering, shouting)
- tone and quality (accent, emotionality)
- fluency (staccato, monotonous)
- abnormal language (neologisms, dysphasia, clanging, Box 16.4).

Mood

Mood is the patient's pervasive emotional state, while affect is the observable expression of their emotions, which is more variable over time. Think of mood as the emotional climate and affect as the weather. Both have elements of subjective experience (that is, how the patient feels, according to their own report and your specific questions) and how the patient appears to feel, according to your own objective observation. So a depressed patient might describe feeling sad, hopeless and unable to enjoy any aspect of life, and at interview appear downcast, withdrawn and tearful, with little brightening even when talking about their much-loved children.

Pervasive disturbance of mood is the most important feature of depression, mania and anxiety, but mood changes commonly occur in other mental disorders such as schizophrenia and dementia. You might ask patients 'How has your mood been lately?', 'Have you noticed any change in your emotions recently?' and 'Do you still enjoy things that normally give you pleasure?' Abnormalities of mood include a problematic pervasive mood, an abnormal range of affect, abnormal reactivity and inappropriateness or incongruity. Some terms relating to mood are defined in Box 16.5.

Some patients prompt affective responses in the interviewer, via the process of countertransference. The elated gaiety of some hypomanic patients can be infectious, as can the hopeless gloom of some people with depression. Recognising these responses in yourself can be helpful in understanding how the patient relates to others and vice versa.

Thought form

As with speech, this is a not an assessment of what the patient is thinking about, but how they think about it. Assess it by observing how thoughts appear to be linked together, and the speed and directness with which the train of thought moves, considering rate, flow, sequencing and abstraction. Some terms relating to thought form are defined in Box 16.6.

Thinking may appear speeded up, as in hypomania, or slowed down, as in profound depression. The flow of subjects may be understandable but unusually rapid, as in the *flight of ideas* that characterises hypomania, or unduly 'single track' and perseverative, as in some cases of dementia. Sometimes thinking appears to be very circumstantial, and the patient hard to pin down, even when asked simple questions.

More severe disruption of the train of thought is termed loosening of associations or formal thought disorder, in which the patient moves from subject to subject via abrupt changes of direction that the interviewer cannot follow. This is a core feature of schizophrenia. Concrete thinking, in the sense of difficulty handling abstract concepts, is a common feature of dementia, and can be assessed by asking the patients to explain the meaning of common proverbs.

It may help to illustrate your assessment with verbatim examples from the interview, chosen to illustrate the patient's manner of thinking and speaking.

Thought content

Thought content refers to the main themes and subjects occupying the patient's mind. It will become apparent when taking the history but may need to be explored further via specific enquiries. It may broadly be divided into preoccupations, ruminations and abnormal beliefs. These are defined in Boxes 16.7 and 16.8.

Preoccupations

Preoccupations occur in both normal and abnormal mood states. Sadly dwelling on the loss of a loved one is entirely normal in bereavement; persisting disproportionate guilty gloom about the state of the world may be a symptom of depression.

Ruminations

These are preoccupations that are in themselves abnormal – and therefore symptoms of mental disorder – by reason of repetition (as in obsessional disorders) or groundlessness (as in hypochondriasis).

Abnormal beliefs

These beliefs fall into two categories: those that are not diagnostic of mental illness (such as overvalued ideas, superstitions and magical thinking) and those that invariably signify mental illness (that is, delusions).

The main difference between them is that delusions either lack a cultural basis for the belief or have been derived from abnormal psychological processes.

Overvalued ideas

These are usually beliefs of great personal significance. They fall short of being full delusions but are abnormal because of their effects on a person's behaviour or wellbeing. For example, in anorexia nervosa, people may still believe they are fat when they are seriously underweight – and then respond to their belief rather than their weight, by further starving themselves.

Delusional beliefs

These beliefs also matter greatly to the person, resulting in powerful emotions and important behavioural consequences; they are always of clinical significance. They are classified by their content, such as:

- paranoid
- religious
- grandiose
- hypochondriacal
- of guilt
- of love
- of jealousy
- of infestation
- of thought interference (broadcasting, insertion and withdrawal)
- of control.

Bizarre delusions are easy to recognise, but not all delusions are weird ideas: a man convinced that his partner is unfaithful may or may not be deluded. Even if a partner were unfaithful, it would still amount to a delusional jealousy if the belief were held without evidence or for some unaccountable reason, such as finding a dead bird in the garden.

16.7 Thought content: definitions	
Term	**Definition**
Hypochondriasis	Unjustified belief in suffering from a particular disease in spite of appropriate examination and reassurance
Morbid thinking	Depressive ideas, e.g. themes of guilt, burden, unworthiness, failure, blame, death, suicide
Phobia	A senseless avoidance of a situation, object or activity stemming from a belief that has caused an irrational fear
Preoccupation	Beliefs that are not inherently abnormal but which have come to dominate the patient's thinking
Ruminations	Repetitive, intrusive, senseless thoughts or preoccupations
Obsessions	Ruminations that persist despite resistance

16.8 Abnormal beliefs: definitions	
Term	**Definition**
Delusion	An abnormal belief, held with total conviction, which is maintained in spite of proof or logical argument to the contrary and is not shared by others from the same culture
Delusional perception	A delusion that arises fully formed from the false interpretation of a real perception, e.g. a traffic light turning green confirms that aliens have landed on the rooftop
Magical thinking	An irrational belief that certain actions and outcomes are linked, often culturally determined by folklore or custom, e.g. fingers crossed for good luck
Overvalued ideas	Beliefs that are held, valued, expressed and acted on beyond the norm for the culture to which the person belongs
Thought broadcasting	The belief that the patient's thoughts are heard by others
Thought insertion	The belief that thoughts are being placed in the patient's head from outside
Thought withdrawal	The belief that thoughts are being removed from the patient's head

Delusions can sometimes be understood as the patient's way of trying to make sense of their experience, while the content of the delusions often gives a clue that may help type the underlying illness: for example, delusions of guilt suggest severe depression, whereas grandiose delusions typify mania.

Some delusions are characteristic of schizophrenia. They include a delusional perception (or primary delusion) and 'passivity phenomena': namely, the belief that thoughts, feelings or acts are no longer controlled by a person's own free will.

Perceptions

People normally distinguish between their inner and outer worlds with ease: we know what is real, what reality feels like, and what resides in our 'mind's eye' or 'mind's ear'. In mental illness this distinction can become disrupted, so that normal perceptions become unfamiliar, while abnormal perceptions seem real.

Abnormal perceptions are assessed via the history and specific enquiries, backed up by observation. They fall into several categories, defined in Box 16.9.

Perceptions may be altered (as in sensory distortions or illusions) or false (as in hallucinations and pseudohallucinations). In a third category, what is altered is not a perception in a specific sensory modality but a general sense of disconnection and unreality in oneself (depersonalisation), the world (derealisation) or both.

People find depersonalisation and derealisation intensely unpleasant but hard to describe. They may occur in association with severe tiredness or intense anxiety but can also arise in most types of mental illness. Ask, for example, 'Have you ever felt that you were not real or that the world around you wasn't real?'

With altered perceptions there is a real external object but its subjective perception has been distorted. Sensory distortions, such as unpleasant amplification of light (photophobia) or sound (hyperacusis), can occur in physical diseases, but are also common in anxiety states and drug intoxication or withdrawal. Diminution of perceptions, including pain, can occur in depression and schizophrenia.

Illusions, in which, for example, a bedside locker is misperceived as a threatening animal, commonly occur among people with established impairment of vision or hearing. They are also found in predisposed patients who are subjected to sensory deprivation, notably after dark in a patient with clouding of consciousness. They are suggestive of an organic illness such as delirium, dementia or alcohol withdrawal.

True hallucinations arise without external stimuli. They usually indicate severe mental illness, although they can occur naturally when going to sleep (hypnagogic) or waking up (hypnopompic). Hallucinations are categorised according to their sensory modality as auditory, visual, olfactory, gustatory or tactile.

Any form of hallucination can occur in any severe mental disorder. The most common are auditory and visual hallucinations, the former associated with schizophrenia and the latter with delirium. Some auditory hallucinations are characteristic of schizophrenia, such as voices discussing the patient in the third person or giving a running commentary on the person's activities ('Now he's opening the kitchen cupboard'). Ask, for example, 'Do you ever hear voices when nobody is talking?' and 'What do they say?'

Pseudohallucinations are common. The key distinction from a true hallucination is that they occur within the patient, rather than arising externally. They have an 'as if' quality and lack the vividness and reality of true hallucinations. Consequently, the affected person is not usually distressed by them, and does not normally feel the need to respond, as often happens with true hallucinations.

Cognition

If the history and observation suggest a cognitive deficit, it must be evaluated by standard tests. History, observation, MSE and rating scales (see later) are then used together to diagnose and distinguish between the '3Ds' (dementia, delirium and depression), which are common in the elderly and in hospital inpatients.

Core cognitive functions include:
- level of consciousness
- orientation
- memory
- attention and concentration
- intelligence.

Level of consciousness

Mental disorders are rarely associated with a reduced (or clouded) level of consciousness, such as drowsiness, stupor or coma. The exception is delirium (which is both a physical and a mental disorder), where it is common.

Orientation

This is a key aspect of cognitive function, being particularly sensitive to impairment. Disorientation is the hallmark of the 'organic mental state' found in delirium and dementia. Abnormalities may be evident during the interview but some patients are adept at hiding them in social interactions. Check the patient's orientation to time, place and person by evaluating their knowledge of the current time and date, recognition of where they are, and identification of familiar people.

Memory

Memory function is divided into three elements:
- Registration is tested by asking the patient to repeat after you the names of three unrelated objects (apple, table, penny); any mistake is significant. Alternatively, in the digit span test, ask the patient to repeat after you a sequence of random single digit numbers. Make sure you speak slowly and clearly. A person with normal function can produce at least five digits.
- Short-term memory (where short-term is defined as a matter of minutes) is tested by giving the patient some

16

16.9 Perceptions: definitions	
Term	**Definition**
Depersonalisation	A subjective experience of feeling unreal
Derealisation	A subjective experience that the surrounding environment is unreal
Hallucination	A false perception arising without a valid stimulus from the external world
Illusion	A false perception that is an understandable misinterpretation of a real stimulus in the external world
Pseudohallucination	A false perception that is perceived as part of one's internal experience

new information; once this has registered, check retention after 5 minutes, with a distracting task in between. Do the same with the names of three objects; any error is significant. Alternatively, use a six-item name and address (in the format: Mr David Green, 25 Sharp Street, Durham). More than one error indicates impairment.

- Long-term memory is assessed mainly from the personal history. Gaps and mistakes are often obvious but some patients may confabulate (that is, fill in the gaps with plausible but unconsciously fabricated facts), so check the account with a family member or other informant if possible. Confabulation is a core feature of Korsakoff's syndrome, a complication of chronic alcoholism. Failing long-term memory is characteristic of dementia, although this store of knowledge can be remarkably intact in the presence of severe impairment of other cognitive functions.

Impaired attention and concentration

These occur in many mental disorders and are not diagnostic. Impaired attention is observed as increased distractibility, with the patient responding inappropriately to intrusive internal events (memories, obsessions, anxious ruminations) or to extraneous stimuli, which may be either real (a noise outside the room) or unreal (auditory hallucinations).

Concentration is the patient's ability to persist with a mental task. It is tested by using simple, repetitive sequences, such as asking the patient to repeat the months of the year or days of the week in reverse, or to do the 'serial 7s' test, in which 7 is subtracted from 100, then from 93, then 86 and so on. Note the finishing point, the number of errors and the time taken.

Intelligence

This is estimated clinically from a combination of the history of educational attainment and occupations, and the evidence provided at interview of vocabulary, general knowledge, abstract thought, foresight and understanding. If in doubt as to whether the patient has a learning disability, or if there is a discrepancy between the history and presentation, a psychologist should formally test IQ.

Insight

Insight is the degree to which a patient agrees that they are ill. It can be broken down into the recognition that abnormal mental experiences are in fact abnormal, agreement that these abnormalities amount to a mental illness, and acceptance of the need for treatment. Insight matters, since a lack of it often leads to non-adherence, and sometimes to the need for compulsory detention. You might ask 'Do you think anything is wrong with you' or 'If you are ill, what do you think needs to happen to make you better?'

Risk assessment

Risk assessment is a crucial part of every psychiatric assessment. Consider:

- Who is at risk?
- What is the nature of the risk?
- What is the likelihood of the risk?

The person usually at risk, if anyone, is the patient themselves. The risk posed to others by people with mental disorder must be neither overstated nor ignored. Any others at risk are most likely to be family or, less commonly, specific individuals (such as celebrities in cases of stalking) or members of specific groups (defined by age, ethnicity, occupation and so on). Sometimes the risk applies non-specifically to strangers, or to anyone preventing the patient from achieving their goals.

There may be direct risk to life and limb (as in suicide, self-harm or violence to others), or it may be an indirect risk, either to health (through refusal of treatment for physical or mental illness) or welfare (through inability to provide basic care – food, warmth, shelter, hygiene – for oneself or one's dependents). The risk may be imminent, as in a patient actively attempting self-harm, or remote, as in a patient refusing prophylactic medical treatment. Direct risks tend to be imminent and indirect risks remote, although this is not always so. A patient declining renal dialysis because their depression makes them feel unworthy is at imminent but indirect risk of death. Finally, the likelihood of the risk may range from near certainty to hypothetical possibility.

A risk assessment should readily distinguish between cases where there is an imminent, direct and near-certain risk to the patient's life (such as a man actively trying to throw himself from the window to escape delusional persecutors), and those where any risks apply to the welfare of other people, at some point in the future, and amount to possibilities (such as a depressed woman who may be neglecting her frail elderly father). The former case calls for urgent intervention, probably via mental health legislation; the latter requires engagement over time, preferably in a voluntary way.

While all psychiatric evaluations require some assessment of risk, it should be considered in depth whenever the presentation includes acts or threats of self-harm or reports of command hallucinations, the past history includes self-harm or violent behaviour, the social circumstances show a recent, significant loss, or the mental disorder is strongly associated with risk (as in severe depression).

Assessing suicidality is the element of risk assessment that is most often needed. If a patient presents after an act of self-harm or overdose, the questions arise naturally ('What did you want to happen when you took the tablets? Did you expect to die? Is that what you wanted? How do you feel about that now? Do you still feel you'd be better off dead? Have you had thoughts about doing anything else to harm yourself?').

In other circumstances the subject will need to be introduced, but do not fear that you may be putting ideas in the patient's mind ('You've told me how bad you have been feeling. Have you ever felt life is not worth living? Have you had any thoughts about ending your life? How close have you come? What has stopped you acting on those thoughts so far?').

Capacity

Assessing capacity is a skill required of all doctors and should not be delegated to psychiatrists. The legal elements vary between jurisdictions but there are key clinical principles in common. The first is the presumption of capacity: clinicians should treat patients as retaining capacity until it is proven that they have lost it. Secondly, capacity is decision-specific: patients may not be able to understand the risks and benefits of complex medical treatment options, while retaining the ability to decide whether or not to enter a nursing home. Thirdly, residual capacity should be maximised: if a patient's ability to understand is impaired by sensory deficits or language barriers, these should be corrected as far as possible by visual corrections, hearing aids and interpreters.

The central matters to be assessed are essentially cognitive: can the patient make, understand, remember and communicate decisions about medical treatment or other options before them?

Determining that a patient lacks capacity for a particular decision leads to the next stage: making that decision on their behalf. The key principles here are to ensure that any treatment proposed must benefit the patient and be the least restrictive option available; it should take account of any wishes the patient has previously expressed, as well as the views of family members and any other relevant others (such as nursing home staff).

The physical examination

Physical and mental disorders are associated, so always consider the physical dimension in any patient presenting with a psychiatric disorder, and vice versa. The setting and the patient's age, health and mode of presentation will determine the extent of physical assessment required.

In psychiatric settings, general physical observation, coupled with basic cardiovascular and neurological examination, will usually suffice. Bear in mind that some physical disorders can present with psychiatric symptoms (such as thyrotoxicosis manifesting as anxiety – look for exophthalmos, lid lag, goitre, tachycardia and so on). For older patients with multiple medical problems, or those with alcohol dependence and associated physical harm, a more detailed examination is clearly needed.

In primary care and acute hospital settings, patients will usually undergo physical examination tailored to the presenting problem, but it is important to be aware that some psychiatric disorders can present with physical symptoms, such as chest pain and transient neurological symptoms as manifestations of panic attacks.

Collateral history

Collateral history is important whenever assessment is limited by:
- physical illness, acute confusional state or dementia
- severe learning disability or other mental disorder impairing communication
- disturbed, aggressive or otherwise uncooperative behaviour.

Sources of third-party information will usually include family and other carers, as well as past and present general practitioners and other health professionals. Previous psychiatric assessments are particularly valuable when a diagnosis of personality disorder is being considered, as this depends more on information about behaviour patterns over time than the details of the current presentation (Box 16.10).

16.10 Personality disorder: definition

Patterns of experience and behaviour that are:
- pathological (i.e. outside social norms)
- problematic (for the patient and/or others)
- pervasive (affecting most or all areas of a patient's life)
- persistent (adolescent onset, enduring throughout adult life and resistant to treatment)

Psychiatric rating scales

The use of psychiatric rating scales as clinical tools in psychiatric assessment is increasing. Most were developed in research studies to make a confident diagnosis or to measure change in severity of illness. Some require special training; all must be used sensibly. In general, scales are too inflexible and limited in scope to replace a well-conducted standard psychiatric interview but they can be useful adjuncts for screening, measuring response to treatment or focusing on particular areas.

In routine practice, scales are most widely used to assess cognitive function when an organic brain disorder is suspected. They include:
- Abbreviated Mental Test (AMT): takes less than 5 minutes (Box 16.11)
- Mini-Mental State Examination (MMSE) or Montreal Cognitive Assessment (MoCA): takes 5–15 minutes.

Well-known instruments assessing areas other than cognition include:
- general morbidity:
  - General Health Questionnaire (GHQ)
- mood disorder:
  - Hospital Anxiety and Depression Scale (HADS)
  - Beck Depression Inventory (BDI)
- alcohol:
  - CAGE questionnaire (Box 16.12)
  - FAST questionnaire (Box 16.13).

Putting it all together: clinical vignettes

Examples in practice are provided in Boxes 16.14–16.17.

16.11 The Abbreviated Mental Test

- Age
- Date of birth
- Time (to the nearest hour)
- Year
- Hospital name
- Recognition of two people, e.g. doctor, nurse
- Recall address
- Dates of First World War (or other significant event)
- Name of the monarch (or prime minister/president as appropriate)
- Count backwards 20–1
  Each question scores 1 mark; a score of 8/10 or less indicates confusion.

From Hodkinson HM. Evaluation of a mental test score for assessment of mental impairment in the elderly. Age and Ageing 1972; 1(4):233–238, by permission of Oxford University Press.

16.12 The CAGE questionnaire

- <u>C</u>ut down: Have you ever felt you should cut down on your drinking?
- <u>A</u>nnoyed: Have people annoyed you by criticising your drinking?
- <u>G</u>uilty: Have you ever felt bad or guilty about your drinking?
- <u>E</u>ver: Do you ever have a drink first thing in the morning to steady you or help a hangover (an 'eye opener')?
  Positive answers to two or more questions suggest problem drinking; confirm this by asking about the maximum taken.

16

16.13 The fast alcohol screening test (FAST) questionnaire

For the following questions please circle the answer that best applies

1 drink = $\frac{1}{2}$ pint of beer or 1 glass of wine or 1 single measure of spirits

1. Men: How often do you have eight or more drinks on one occasion?
   Women: How often do you have six or more drinks on one occasion?
   - Never (0)
   - Less than monthly (1)
   - Monthly (2)
   - Weekly (3)
   - Daily or almost daily (4)
2. How often during the last year have you been unable to remember what happened the night before because you had been drinking?
   - Never (0)
   - Less than monthly (1)
   - Monthly (2)
   - Weekly (3)
   - Daily or almost daily (4)
3. How often during the last year have you failed to do what was normally expected of you because of drinking?
   - Never (0)
   - Less than monthly (1)
   - Monthly (2)
   - Weekly (3)
   - Daily or almost daily (4)
4. In the last year, has a relative or friend, or a doctor or other health worker, been concerned about your drinking or suggested you cut down?
   - Never (0)
   - Yes, on one occasion (2)
   - Yes, on more than one occasion (4)

Scoring FAST

First stage
- If the answer to question 1 is 'Never', then the patient is probably not misusing alcohol
- If the answer is 'Weekly' or 'Daily or almost daily', then the patient is a hazardous, harmful or dependent drinker
- 50% of people are classified using this one question

Second stage
- Only use questions 2–4 if the answer to question 1 is 'Less than monthly' or 'Monthly':
- Score questions 1–3: 0, 1, 2, 3, 4
- Score question 4: 0, 2, 4
- Minimum score is 0
- Maximum score is 16
- Score for hazardous drinking is 3 or more

16.14 Clinical vignette: overdose

A 19-year-old woman attends the accident and emergency department, having taken a medically minor overdose. She has presented in this way three times in the last 2 years. She needs no specific medical treatment.

Your assessment should concentrate first on the circumstances of the overdose and her intentions at the time. Collateral information should include assessments after previous presentations and any continuing psychiatric follow-up. Mental state examination should screen for any new signs of mental disorder emerging since her last assessment, and in particular any mood problems or new psychotic symptoms. She will clearly have undergone a detailed physical assessment, but even if the overdose appears medically trivial, you need to undertake a risk assessment to judge the chances of further self-harm or completed suicide in the near future. She probably does not need a detailed cognitive assessment or psychiatric rating scales.

16.15 Clinical vignette: confusion, agitation and hostility

An 85-year-old man in a medical ward, where he is undergoing intravenous antibiotic treatment for a chest infection, now appears confused, agitated and hostile, in a way not previously evident to his family.

You need to approach him carefully to establish rapport and to interview him as much as he will allow, while anticipating that you may have to rely heavily on collateral information, and a mental state examination limited to observation of appearance and behaviour. It will be crucial to talk to his family to establish his normal level of cognition and independence, and to the nursing staff to establish the diurnal pattern of his problems. If there is any history of previous episodes, acquire the results of previous assessments. He will need a neurological examination and assessment of his cognition via a standard scale. Risk assessment should focus on the indirect risks to his health if he tries to leave hospital against advice, generating a view about his detainability under mental health legislation. A capacity assessment of his ability to consent to continuing antibiotic treatment is required, and may result in the issue of an incapacity certificate.

16.16 Clinical vignette: fatigue

A 35-year-old woman attends her general practitioner, presenting with fatigue.

Assessment of possible physical causes is required, via history, examination and appropriate blood tests, but as these proceed, the interview should also cover possible symptoms of depression, previous episodes, family history and recent stressors. Mental state examination should concentrate on objective evidence of lowered mood. Formal assessment of cognition is probably not necessary, but a standard rating scale for mood disorder may help establish a diagnosis and a baseline against which to measure change. Risk assessment is not a prominent requirement, unless a depressive illness is suspected and she reports thoughts of self-harm, or is responsible for young children, in which case the chance of direct or indirect harm to them needs to be considered.

16.17 Clinical vignette: paranoid thoughts

A 42-year-old man attends a psychiatric outpatient clinic for the first time, having been referred by his general practitioner for longstanding paranoid thoughts.

It will be particularly important to establish rapport with a patient who is likely to be very wary. The interview needs to cover the psychiatric history in some detail, considering substance misuse, family history of mental illness and a full personal history in particular. Mental state examination should explore the paranoid thoughts in detail, to establish whether they are preoccupations or overvalued ideas (suggesting a personality disorder), or delusions (suggesting a psychotic illness). Risk assessment should concentrate on the risk to others about whom the patient has paranoid fears. Neither detailed cognitive assessment nor a specific rating scale is likely to add much to the initial assessment.

OSCE example 1: Assessing suicidal risk

Miss Gardiner, 27 years old, presented to the accident and emergency department the previous day after taking an overdose of paracetamol while intoxicated with alcohol. She has undergone treatment with acetylcysteine overnight and is now medically fit for discharge.

Please assess her risk of self-harm and suicide

- Introduce yourself and clean your hands.
- Explain the purpose of your assessment; try to gain rapport.
- Enquire how she is feeling physically (specifically asking about nausea, vomiting and abdominal pain).
- Tactfully introduce the subject of the overdose.
- Establish the number and type of tablets taken.
- Establish how much alcohol she drank, whether this was with the tablets (to 'wash them down') or whether she was already intoxicated at the time of the overdose.
- Clarify the circumstances. Who else was present or expected? Did she write a note or otherwise communicate what she had done or was planning to do?
- Clarify how she was found and either came or was brought to hospital.
- Explore recent or chronic stressors.
- Establish her intent at the time of the overdose. Did she expect to die? Is that what she wanted?
- Confirm her view now. Does she still wish to die? Does she have any thoughts about another overdose or other form of self-harm?
- Establish relevant past history. Are there any previous overdoses? Any previous or continuing psychiatric follow-up?
- Confirm whether she has parental or caring responsibilities for young children. Tactfully enquire about any thoughts of harming them.
- Establish who will be with her when she leaves hospital.
- Thank the patient and clean your hands.

Summarise your findings

The risk assessment should concentrate most on the short-term risk of suicide.

Advanced level comments

More advanced students would be expected to tabulate short- and long-term risk of both suicide and further self-harm, and to quote the risk of completed suicide in the first year after an act of self-harm (1–2%).

16

OSCE example 2: Assessing delirium

Mr Duncan, 82 years old, is admitted to an orthopaedic ward after falling and breaking his hip. Forty-eight hours after surgery he became restless and agitated overnight, pulling out his intravenous line. He is now settled and cooperative.

Please assess the likely cause of this episode

- Introduce yourself and clean your hands.
- Explain the purpose of your assessment; try to establish rapport.
- Enquire how he is feeling physically (specifically asking about pain, fever, constipation, and urinary and respiratory symptoms).
- Establish his awareness of where he is, why he is there and how long he has been in hospital.
- Ask how much he remembers of the night's events and enquire specifically about any recollection of hallucinations or persecutory fears.
- Enquire about any continuing hallucinations or fears.
- Ask about any previous similar episodes.
- Clarify how active he was before his fall, and whether there is any awareness of memory impairment leading up to it.
- Ask about alcohol intake.
- Administer simple tests of cognitive function, especially of attention and memory (advanced performers should know the Abbreviated Mental Test questions).
- Undertake a basic physical examination, assessing for tremor, ophthalmoplegia and nystagmus.
- Gain the patient's permission to speak to his next of kin, general practitioner and others.
- Thank the patient and clean your hands.

Summarise your findings

The diagnosis is delirium, with further enquiries needed to establish the likely cause (which may be alcohol withdrawal, given the timing), as well as the possibility of pre-existing cognitive impairment as a vulnerability factor.

Integrated examination sequence for the psychiatric assessment

- Review the relevant information to clarify the reason for referral or mode of self-presentation.
- Establish rapport to reduce distress and assist assessment.
- Cover the key headings for the history (presenting symptoms, systematic review, past medical and psychiatric history, current medication, substance misuse, family history, personal history).
- Cover the headings for the personal history (childhood development, losses and experiences, education, occupation, financial circumstances, relationships, partner(s) and children, housing, leisure activities, hobbies and interests, forensic history).
- Make the extent, order and content of the assessment appropriate to the presentation and setting.
- Observe closely to gain objective evidence of mental state, especially non-verbal information.
- Cover the headings for the mental state examination systematically (appearance and behaviour, speech, mood, thought form and content, perceptions, cognition and insight).
- Use brief formal tests to assess cognitive function (Abbreviated Mental Test, Mini-Mental State Examination, Montreal Cognitive Assessment).
- Consider your own emotional response to your patient.
- Consider standardised rating scales as a screening tool (and sometimes to monitor progress).
- Undertake physical examination as appropriate to the setting and the presentation.
- Gather further background information from other sources to the degree necessary (with permission).
- As well as a diagnosis and management plan, be sure to consider:
  - assessment of risk to self or others
  - capacity to take decisions
  - need to use mental health or incapacity legislation.

The frail elderly patient

Assessment of the frail elderly patient

Comprehensive geriatric assessment is an evidence-based process that improves outcomes. It involves taking the history from the patient and, with the patient's consent, from a carer or relative, followed by a systematic assessment of:

- cognitive function and mood
- nutrition and hydration
- skin
- pain
- continence
- hearing and vision
- functional status.

The extent and focus of the assessment depend on the clinical presentation. In non-acute settings such as the general practice or outpatient clinic or day hospital, focus on establishing what diseases are present, and also which functional impairments and problems most affect the patient's life.

In acute settings such as following acute hospital referral, focus on what has changed or is new. Seek any new symptoms or signs of illness and any changes from baseline physical or cognitive function.

The complexity of the problems presented, and the need for comprehensive and systematic analysis, mean that assessment is divided into components undertaken at different times, by different members of the multiprofessional team (Box 17.1).

There is no specific age at which a patient becomes 'elderly'; although age over 65 years is commonly used as the definition, this has no biological basis, and many patients who are chronologically 'elderly' appear biologically and functionally younger, and vice versa.

Frailty becomes more common with advancing age and is likely to be a response to chronic disease and ageing itself. A frail elderly person typically suffers multimorbidity (multiple illnesses) and has associated polypharmacy (multiple medications). They often have cognitive impairment, visual and hearing loss, low bodyweight and poor mobility due to muscular weakness, unstable balance and poor exercise tolerance. Their general functional reserve and the capacity of individual organs and physiological systems are impaired, making the individual vulnerable to the effects of minor illness.

Factors influencing presentation and history

Classical patterns of symptoms and signs still occur in the frail elderly, but modified or non-specific presentations are common due to comorbidity, drug treatment and ageing itself. As the combination of these factors is unique for each individual, their presentations will be different. The first sign of new illness may be a change in functional status: typically, reduced mobility, altered cognition or impairment of balance leading to falls. Common precipitants are infections, changes in medication and metabolic derangements but almost any acute medical insult can produce these non-specific presentations (Fig. 17.1). Each of these presentations should be explored through careful history taking, physical examination and functional assessment.

Disorders of cognition, communication and mood are so common that they should always be considered at the start of the assessment of a frail older adult.

Communication difficulties, cognition and mood

Communication can be challenging (Box 17.2). The history can be incomplete, difficult to interpret or misleading, and the whole assessment, including physical examination, may be time-consuming.

Whenever possible, assess the patient somewhere quiet with few distractions. Make your patient comfortable and ensure they understand the purpose of your contact. Provide any glasses, hearing aids or dentures that they need and help them to switch

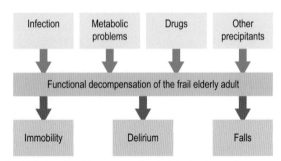

Fig. 17.1 Functional decompensation in frail elderly people.

17.1 The multiprofessional team	
Professional	**Key roles in assessment of**
Physician	Physical state, including diagnosis and therapeutic intervention
Psychiatrist	Cognition, mood and capacity
Physiotherapist	Mobility, balance, gait and falls risk
Occupational therapist	Practical functional activities (self-care and domestic)
Nurse	Skin health, nutrition and continence
Dietician	Nutrition
Speech and language therapist	Speech and swallowing
Social worker	Social care needs

17.2 Communication difficulties: the seven Ds	
Problem	**Comment/causes**
Deafness	Nerve or conductive
Dysphasia	Most commonly due to stroke disease but sometimes a feature of dementia
Dysarthria	Cerebrovascular disease, motor neurone disease, Parkinson's disease
Dysphonia	Parkinson's disease
Dementia	Global impairment of cognitive function
Delirium	Impaired attention, disturbance of arousal and perceptual disturbances
Depression	May mimic dementia or delirium

on and adjust their hearing aid if necessary. If they still cannot hear you clearly, use an electronic communicator, or if they can read easily, write down simple questions and instructions.

Cognitive function includes the processes of perception, attention, memory, reasoning, decision making and problem solving (p. 323). Cognitive impairment increases with age and has implications for assessment, treatment, consent and prognosis. Consider cognitive impairment if a patient has limited ability to cooperate with you, cannot recall their medical history or seems to deny all symptoms, even when they are clearly unwell. Other problems, including impaired hearing, low mood or dysphasia, can mimic cognitive impairment. Some patients present with apparently good social skills or 'façade' and cover their impaired memory by diverting the conversation to another topic. Do not ascribe changes in cognition to age alone without excluding dementia or delirium (p. 323).

Depression is common in frail elderly people and may be difficult to diagnose. Consider this if your patient struggles to concentrate, or is withdrawn or reluctant to interact. A formal psychiatric assessment and corroborating history from a carer or friend may be valuable. Standardised rating scales are available such as the Geriatric Depression Scale.

Patients are often fearful that they will be admitted to hospital or not return home after admission, and may play down their symptoms or functional limitations. Always try to corroborate the history from a carer, relative or friend, with the patient's consent.

The history

The presenting symptoms

Frail elderly patients often have multiple symptoms. Take time to detail each symptom, and separate those arising from new acute illness from those due to background disabilities.

Ask:

- How long have you had a particular symptom?
- Has it changed recently?
- When were you last totally free of the symptom?

Try to establish what the patient's symptoms, functional abilities and mental status were before the new presenting problem. This helps set realistic goals for treatment and rehabilitation.

The patient's perspective may vary from yours, particularly in acute settings. For example, a patient referred following sudden loss of consciousness may be unconcerned by this but anxious about longstanding back pain. These symptoms are not coincidental; if it is important to your patient, it should be important to you.

Common presenting symptoms

Decreased mobility

Ask about:

- the patient's usual mobility, when it changed and if the change was abrupt
- any falls
- use of walking aids
- history of recent head injury, fevers or rigors, dizziness or poor balance
- lower limb weakness, numbness or paraesthesia
- joint pain, especially in the back, neck or lower limbs

- any bladder or bowel symptoms
- current drug treatment and whether this has changed recently
- how the change in mobility is affecting their daily life.

Confusion

Check that the patient can hear you clearly and ask if they would like a friend or relative to be with them. Although a confused patient may struggle to give an accurate history or clear description of symptoms, never ignore what they tell you, as their perspective remains important to your care. Take a collateral history.

Establish:

- the person's normal cognitive state and whether the change has been abrupt or gradual
- any symptoms of common infections, such as urinary frequency, productive cough, fever or rigors
- whether the person has any pain, and if so, where
- current drug treatment and adherence, with any recent changes.

Falls

A collateral history is helpful if a fall has been witnessed.

Establish:

- the patient's usual mobility
- how many falls they have had, over what timescale and whether injuries, including head injury, have been sustained
- the presence of dizziness or lightheadedness, and whether the problem is true vertigo or worse on standing (p. 123)
- the presence of palpitations, limb weakness, paraesthesia or any joint pain, especially in the back, neck or lower limbs
- quality of vision
- any problems with the feet
- any recent symptoms of infection (see earlier)
- current drug treatment and any recent changes.

Past medical history

Detail the past history and known comorbidities from all available sources, including any previous records. Comorbidities may not be directly relevant to the current problem but may influence prognosis and the feasibility and appropriateness of potential investigations and treatments (Box 17.3).

Drug history

Polypharmacy is associated with drug interactions, adverse events and difficulties with adherence. Take a detailed drug history, supplemented by the following:

- Identify all medications, including over-the-counter preparations.
- Ask whether any drugs have been started or stopped recently, or doses of regular medications altered.
- Explore the patient's ability to self-administer drugs; ask if they use a dosette box or if a carer helps with administration.
- Explore the ability to read labels, open bottles or use inhalers correctly.

17

17.3 How comorbidities or drugs can influence symptoms

Comorbidity/drug	Effect of comorbidity or drug	Effect on presentation of new disease
Osteoarthritis of weight-bearing joint	Limited mobility	Patient does not experience exertional dyspnoea, resulting in late presentation of heart disease
Cognitive impairment	Poor recall or no recognition of symptoms	Patient does not describe symptoms of disease and diagnosis is not recognised
Anticholinergics Diuretics Some calcium antagonists	Dry mouth Urinary frequency Ankle swelling	A symptom is caused by drug treatment rather than disease
Vasodilators, diuretics Beta-blockers L-dopa (usually long-term)	Postural hypotension Bradycardia Dyskinetic limb movements	A sign is caused by drug treatment rather than disease
Beta-blockers	No tachycardia in gastrointestinal bleeding	An expected sign does not occur because of drug treatment

- If patients have their drugs with them, go through them together. Ask patients what they believe each one is for, how it affects them and how often they take it.
- Ask if there are any drugs that they sometimes omit, such as diuretics on days when they are going out.
- Ask carers if there are partially used supplies of drugs in the house.
- Clarify any 'allergies' or previous adverse events. Explore what symptoms the patient believes to be caused by their drugs, as some may be unrelated. If in doubt, regard the allergy as significant.
- Contact the prescriber, if necessary, to confirm details of the drug history.

Family history

A first presentation of disease with a strong genetic basis is unlikely, but family history is still important to patients who have lost siblings or children to specific conditions and who may believe that their own symptoms are related.

Social and functional history

Complement a comprehensive social history with information about the patient's functional ability, as this affects their capacity to cope at home, and what assistance they need to support their function there.

Ask about:

- Their normal mobility and whether they transfer from chair to bed or toilet, and walk alone.
- Use of a walking aid and whether they can manage stairs
- Their current level of function, what it was before, and the time course of any functional deterioration.
- How they manage day-to-day activities:
  - Can they wash and dress?
  - Do they do their own shopping and prepare their own meals?

Abrupt functional decline suggests a more acute underlying precipitant or disease. Insidious decline suggests alternate pathologies or progression of underlying chronic disease. Seek corroboration from a friend, relative or carer, but interpret all information obtained in association with objective functional assessment by yourself and other members of the multiprofessional team (see Box 17.1).

The elderly patient's home environment is important:

- Does anyone else live with the patient? Patients who live alone often require more support.
- Have they lived in their current home for long?
- What is access like to the house/bedroom/toilets? Do they use stairs, inside or outside?
- What carer support does the patient have (home help, family or friends)? How often does any carer visit and what does each person do for the patient?
- If in sheltered accommodation:
  - Are meals provided?
  - Is there an on-site warden or personal safety alarms?
  - How does the patient feel about living there and do they wish to return?
- Do they still have a job, and if so, what is it?
- If they are retired, find out what they did, as it may be relevant to their condition and gives insight into their past life. Retirement can lead to social isolation, which contributes to mood disorders.
- Can the patient still get out by themselves or accompanied, or are they house-bound? How many visitors do they have?

Consider that patients may still be driving and there will be safety issues in the presence of visual or cognitive defects. Establish lifestyle information. Alcohol overuse is not infrequent and there may be many pack-years of cigarette use.

Systematic enquiry

Many diseases in frailer people present with non-specific functional deterioration such as immobility. The systematic enquiry is important, as it may provide clues to specific underlying precipitants. Supplement the standard systematic enquiry with questions in the following areas:

- Cognition and mood: has the patient noticed any memory problems or has anyone else commented on their memory? Does anyone help them with letters and bills? Ask about how they sleep at night. How would they describe their mood and appetite? Are they still interested in previous pursuits, such as reading or following favourite television programmes?
- Nutrition: has their weight been steady over the past few months? Have they noticed their clothes getting loose? How many meals do they have in the day and do they eat

17.4 Modified signs in acutely unwell frail elderly patients

Feature	Clinical context	Modification
Temperature	Possible sepsis	Systemic inflammatory response obtunded, may not mount pyrexia (or may become hypothermic) Core temperature normally lower and diurnal variation lost: ↑ temperature may occur but not >37°C
Pulse rate	Volume status, response to sepsis or pain	Altered baroreceptor function may attenuate the rise in heart rate typically associated with these stressors
Blood pressure	Volume status, response to sepsis or pain	Altered baroreceptor function may modify blood pressure response to acute illness
Postural hypotension	Volume status	May be found in volume-replete patients due to primary autonomic dysfunction. Less reliable indicator of volume depletion
Skin turgor	Hydration	↓ but less specific because of reduction in subcutaneous fat

meat, fish, vegetables and fruit? Who prepares their meals? Do they have any problems with their teeth or gums? If they wear dentures, do they fit well? Is their mouth dry?

- Pain: always ask specifically about pain, as this may affect mobility and sleep.
- Continence: ask whether they ever notice incontinence or leakage from their bladder or bowels. Are they aware when they are about to pass urine or a stool? Do they ever find it hard to get to the toilet in time? Ask men about prostatic symptoms (p. 235) in particular. Do these problems stop them doing activities?
- Sensory impairment: ask about any problems with vision and whether they wear glasses. Can they can see the television and read a newspaper? If they wear a hearing aid, find out if it is working and whether they are wearing it.
- Balance and falls: do they ever feel unsteady on their feet? Ask specifically about any falls in the past year and obtain a careful description of these (p. 331). Find out how they would call for help if they fell and could not get up.

The physical examination

It takes time and patience to perform a detailed assessment of a frail elderly patient. Physical examination is easiest when your patient can comply with your instructions. All patients benefit from clear, careful instruction and this is particularly important for the frail elderly, who may have communication problems or find the examination routine demanding. Many have low levels of stamina and movement may be limited. Integrate your physical examination to minimise movement for patients and maximise their understanding and cooperation. Help them to move around the room and to get on and off the examination couch. Remember that they will take longer to undress and dress. Some patients feel more comfortable if a family member, carer or friend is present, but always check if this is what they wish.

Use the physical examination to find evidence of established comorbidities, and explanations for functional problems, current symptoms, or concerns voiced by a carer. Some elderly people have difficulty maintaining personal hygiene, grooming or appearance. Their hair and clothes may be unclean, nails unkempt and facial hair longer than in younger life. These findings may reflect underlying functional or cognitive impairment, social isolation or low mood, and are relevant to the patient's overall functional status, condition and outlook, or need for social support.

17.5 Assessment of dehydration

Classical feature of dehydration	Interpretation in frail elderly
Postural hypotension	Less specific than in younger patients; may be caused by drugs, disease or age-related abnormal autonomic responses to postural change
Decreased skin turgor	Decreased collagen elasticity and reduced subcutaneous fat can mimic reduced turgor. Best assessed at the sternum
Impaired capillary refill time	Less reliable in the frail elderly because less specific
Dry mouth	A non-specific finding caused by other problems such as anticholinergic drugs or mouth breathing
Tachycardia in hypovolaemia	Less sensitive due to drug- or age-related abnormal autonomic responses

Be aware of the common clinical signs found in frail elderly patients. Just as the history uncovers multiple diverse and unexpected symptoms, a careful examination will often reveal many clinical signs in different clinical systems. In acute presentations, be alert to typical signs of acute illness that may misleadingly be absent in older patients (Box 17.4).

Document all examination findings, as this will help doctors who assess the patient in the future. Assume that the physical signs you find are due to disease, which may be treatable, rather than ageing, which is not.

General examination

Hydration and nutrition

Disorders of hydration are common in frail elderly patients but accurate clinical assessment is difficult and classical signs less reliable (Box 17.5).

Undernutrition and low bodyweight are common features of frailty that may develop rapidly in hospitalised patients. Screening tools are used to assess the risk of malnutrition (Fig. 17.2). Seek reversible causes. Consider chronic disease such as chronic obstructive pulmonary disease, new serious disease such as cancer, poor social support or isolation and depression, as these may present with low bodyweight. Other factors that may contribute include poor oral health, poor function (being unable to

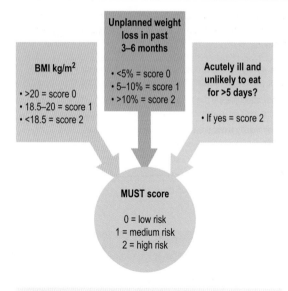

Fig. 17.2 The Malnutrition Universal Screening Tool (MUST) score for assessment of risk of malnutrition. *BMI, body mass index. The 'Malnutrition Universal Screening Tool' ('MUST') is reproduced here with the kind permission of BAPEN (British Association for Parenteral and Enteral Nutrition). For further information on 'MUST' see www.bapen.org. uk. Copyright © BAPEN 2012.*

17.6 Signs and behaviour associated with pain

Type	Description
Autonomic changes	Pallor, sweating, tachypnoea, altered breathing patterns, tachycardia, hypertension
Facial expressions	Grimacing, wincing, frowning, rapid blinking, brow raising, brow lowering, cheek raising, eyelid tightening, nose wrinkling, lip corner pulling, chin raising, lip puckering
Body movements	Altered gait, pacing, rocking, hand wringing, repetitive movements, increased tone, guarding,[a] bracing[b]
Verbalisation/vocalisation	Sighing, grunting, groaning, moaning, screaming, calling out, aggressive/offensive speech
Interpersonal interactions	Aggression, withdrawal, resistance
Changes in activity patterns	Wandering, altered sleep, altered rest patterns
Mental status changes	Confusion, crying, distress, irritability

[a]Guarding = abnormal stiff, rigid or interrupted movement while changing position. [b]Bracing = a stationary position in which a fully extended limb maintains and supports an abnormal weight distribution for at least 3 seconds.

obtain or prepare food) and cognitive impairment (being unable to prepare food or remember to eat it).

The skin

Bruising may suggest glucocorticoid use but is often simply age-related and caused by the reduction in subcutaneous supporting tissue. Rarely, it is due to scurvy (p. 28). Soft-tissue infections often cause functional decompensation and confusion, immobility and falls (see Fig. 17.1). Leg ulcers are common and frequently have multifactorial causes (p. 72). Pain from ulcers may reduce mobility. On admission to hospital, many frail elderly patients have skin wounds that have been dressed in the community. Always remove these dressings, with the help of a nurse, and assess the underlying lesion.

Frail elderly patients with limited mobility are vulnerable to the rapid development of pressure sores, particularly when acutely ill. Standardised assessment scores such as the Waterlow score help identify patients at risk of skin breakdown.

Pain behaviour

In patients with impairment of communication or cognition, always look for pain-related behaviour, as the patient may not volunteer or admit to pain or discomfort (Box 17.6).

Vision and hearing

Hearing loss and visual symptoms, including impairment of visual acuity, are common (Box 17.7) but often overlooked, and this can adversely affect communication, interaction and function.

17.7 Sensory problems

Sensory modality	Underlying disease process
Visual	
Loss of near vision (presbyopia)	Common in elderly because lens is less pliable
Loss of central vision	Macular degeneration
Loss of peripheral vision	Glaucoma Stroke disease (homonymous hemianopia)
Glare from lights at night	Cataracts
Eye pain	Glaucoma
Auditory	
High-frequency loss	Presbyacusis Conductive deafness more common due to otosclerosis
Generalised loss	Conductive – otosclerosis, wax Nerve – Paget's disease, drug-induced ototoxicity, acoustic neuroma

Use a Snellen chart or ask the patient to read from a newspaper to assess their vision. Hearing loss may be misinterpreted as cognitive impairment and vice versa. Make sure the external auditory meatus is not blocked with wax. Ensure patients wear their hearing aids with a functioning battery. Assess hearing using the whispered voice test if they do not have hearing aids (p. 177).

Systems examination

Fully examine each system, and be aware of differences found in the frail elderly compared to younger patients.

Cardiovascular examination

Corneal arcus (see Fig. 4.6C) increases in prevalence in the elderly but is an unreliable sign of dyslipidaemia. A widened pulse pressure occurs because there is decreased arterial compliance. Isolated systolic hypertension and postural hypotension occur more frequently. The latter may result from age-related baroreceptor reflex change, disease or drugs. It may not be symptomatic but increases the risk of a fall.

Medial sclerosis and arterial calcification can make it difficult to feel peripheral pulses but do not cause impaired perfusion and circulation in isolation. The carotid artery may become more tortuous and its pulsations more easily visible. This can create a false impression of arterial dilatation.

Atrial contribution to left ventricular filling increases with age, partly due to diastolic dysfunction of the heart, and a fourth heart sound (S_4) is more commonly heard.

Respiratory examination

Localised crackles are common, and although they may not represent acute disease, you should never disregard new respiratory pathology as a possible cause.

Gastrointestinal examination

Dry mouth and tongue are common side effects of drugs and may affect taste and swallowing. Abnormal dentition, oral thrush or mouth ulcers may reduce oral intake and nutrition.

Neurological examination

Cognitive impairment may reduce the accuracy of the history and affect consent for investigation and treatment. Impaired vibration and position sense occur in old age and may impair balance and increase the risk of falls. Always exclude correctable causes such as vitamin B_{12} deficiency. Bilateral absent ankle reflexes may be normal but unilateral loss is likely to indicate pathology.

Musculoskeletal examination

Low muscle mass is a frailty indicator and a risk factor for falls. Osteoarthritic changes in the hands and weight-bearing joints may predispose to falls or unsteadiness, even if relatively asymptomatic or painless. Gouty tophi may be asymptomatic and reflect underlying renal dysfunction and influence the choice of

drug therapy. Kyphosis often occurs from painless osteoporotic vertebral collapse and may affect postural stability and respiratory function.

Always examine the feet. Bunions, onychomycosis with or without nail overgrowth, and foot ulcers are common. All can compromise mobility and stability, be a source of sepsis or pain, and affect gait. Observe your patient walking. A wide variety of pathologies can produce distinctive abnormalities of gait, including Parkinson's disease (see Fig. 7.17). Gait abnormalities are a risk factor for falls and can exacerbate joint problems.

Functional assessment

Functional assessment is divided into an analysis of:
- mobility
- ability to undertake activities of daily living (ADLs):
  - personal ADLs: washing, dressing, feeding and toileting
  - domestic ADLs: preparing food, laundering clothes and cleaning the house.

Mobility is a key determinant of physical function. Many different pathologies can impair mobility, including neurological, muscular or joint disease. Frailty itself causes generally impaired muscle strength, function and poor mobility without specific clinical findings on examination of muscles, nerves, joints or gait.

Standardised rating scales are used to assess components of function and include the modified Barthel Index for ADLs and the Elderly Mobility Score. The Timed Get Up and Go Test is easy to perform and assesses both mobility and falls risk (Fig. 17.3). Use these scales to describe the patient's abilities succinctly and, using sequential recording over time, objectively assess improvement or deterioration.

Examination sequence
The frail elderly person with decreased mobility
- General examination: look particularly for signs of acute illness (see Box 17.4). If patient is able to walk, assess the

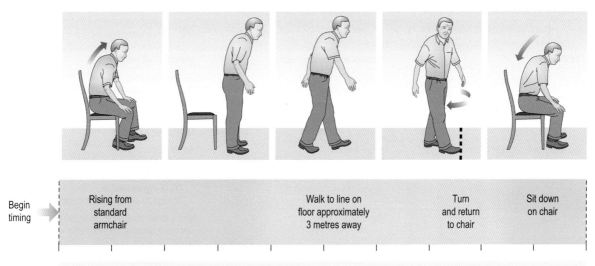

| Begin timing | Rising from standard armchair | Walk to line on floor approximately 3 metres away | Turn and return to chair | Sit down on chair |

The normal time to finish the test is between 7 and 10 seconds.
Patients who cannot complete the task in that time probably have some mobility problems, especially if they take more than 20 seconds.

Fig. 17.3 The Timed Get Up and Go Test.

posture and gait and any inappropriate footwear. Are they visually impaired (see Box 17.7)? Are there signs of sepsis or a distended bladder?

- Cardiovascular system: check for postural hypotension.
- Nervous system: note any neurological signs, particularly in the lower limbs, and look for evidence of Parkinson's disease (Ch. 7).
- Musculoskeletal system: look for muscle wasting or fasciculation, joint abnormality and foot deformity.
- Consider specific investigations (Box 17.8).

The acutely confused frail elderly person

- If patients have problems with vision or hearing, ensure they wear their glasses or a working hearing aid.

- Look for signs of acute illness (see Box 17.4) and pain (see Box 17.6).
- Examine the skin, large joints, lungs, heart valves, prostheses and abdomen for signs of sepsis.
- Examine for any new neurological features.
- Perform pulse oximetry (SpO_2).
- Feel for a distended bladder.
- Consider a rectal examination (p. 111) to check for faecal impaction.
- Consider specific investigations (see Box 17.8).

The frail elderly person with falls

- Look for signs of bony or soft-tissue injury and acute illness such as sepsis (see Box 17.4).
- Cardiovascular system: check for postural hypotension, arrhythmias and aortic stenosis.
- Nervous system: are there neurological signs in lower limbs or evidence of Parkinson's disease (Ch. 7)? Is there visual impairment?
- Musculoskeletal system: look for joint or muscle abnormality and foot deformity. Is footwear appropriate? Note any posture or gait abnormality (see Fig. 7.17).
- Consider specific investigations (see Box 17.8).

The frail elderly person with incontinence

- Observe whether the patient can mobilise or transfer to the toilet.
- Are they cognitively impaired? Is there any evidence of neurological disease?
- Abdomen: palpate for any abnormal abdominal masses. Is the bladder palpable?
- Examine the perineal skin and see if it is intact. Perform a rectal examination for anal fissures, haemorrhoids or other local disease. Note if the rectum is empty or impacted with faeces; assess anal tone and sensation. In a man, assess prostate enlargement; in a woman, look for vaginal prolapse or atrophy.
- Consider specific investigations (see Box 17.8).

17.8 Specific investigations in the frail elderly	
Presentation	**Investigations**
Immobility and/or falls	Septic screen – include urinalysis and WCC Electrolytes and renal function Mental state assessment (p. 325) CT head[a] MRI spine[b]
Confusion	Septic screen – include urinalysis and WCC Electrolytes and renal function Mental state assessment (p. 325) CT head[a]
Urinary incontinence	Urinalysis, urine culture Voiding chart (frequency and volume) Bladder ultrasound (postresidual volume) Consider prostate-specific antigen in men
Faecal incontinence	Stool culture if diarrhoea Abdominal X-ray if high impaction is suspected

[a]If new neurological signs or head injury are suspected. [b]If cord pathology is suspected.
CT, computed tomography; MRI, magnetic resonance imaging; WCC, white cell count.

17.9 A problem-based approach in a frail elderly patient with immobility and confusion		
Problem	**Potential contributory factors**	**Management plan**
Urinary incontinence	Urinary tract infection Faecal impaction	Perform urinalysis Send a midstream specimen of urine to confirm Carry out a rectal examination
Hyponatraemia	Bendroflumethiazide	Withhold bendroflumethiazide Monitor serum sodium

Confusion with features of delirium	Urinary infection
	Hyponatraemia
	Underlying dementia
		As above plus:
		  Check Mini Mental State Examination
		  Obtain a collateral history from a carer
		  Check thyroid function
		  Arrange an occupational therapy review

Foot ulcer	Absent pedal pulses	Check ankle:brachial pressure index Discuss a dressing with the nurse

Poor mobility	Urinary infection
	Hyponatraemia
	Pain from foot ulcer
	Underlying cerebrovascular disease
		As above plus:
		  Prescribe simple analgesia
		  Carry out a full neurological/gait examination
		  Assess vascular risk factors
		  Arrange a physiotherapy review

Interpretation of the findings

Comprehensive geriatric assessment requires excellent communication between members of the multiprofessional team. A problem-based approach helps assimilate all the information and facilitate a clear and individualised management plan.

Start by creating a list to summarise all identified problems. Generate a provisional list after speaking with the patient and refine it after interviewing carers, undertaking the physical examination and hearing the outcome of functional assessments. Do not confine the list to medical diagnoses but include symptoms, laboratory results and presenting features (Box 17.9).

The problem list builds a complete picture of the patient and alerts you to how the different problems may interact. If a problem has several contributing factors, list them all. Use the list to develop a management plan addressing each problem and contributing factor. Include actions such as diagnostic investigations, treatment of identified disease, alteration of drug therapy and rehabilitation. Tailor your management plan specifically to the individual, considering the outcome goals you have agreed with the patient. Explain the proposed management plan to your patient and ensure that they understand and agree.

OSCE example 1: History in a frail elderly patient with falls

Mr Smith, 88 years old, presents with recent falls.

Please take a history

- Introduce yourself and clean your hands.
- Explain the purpose of the encounter.
- Make sure the patient is comfortable and can hear you clearly.
- Ask him to describe his falls:
  - number of falls and where they happen
  - what he is doing before the falls and whether he is aware he is about to fall
  - any injuries, including head injury
  - whether he can get up after falling
  - whether anyone has witnessed his falls
  - his normal mobility and any walking aid.
- Ask focused questions about associated symptoms:
  - loss of consciousness
  - dizziness or vertigo
  - palpitations
  - limb weakness
  - incontinence or tongue biting.
- Ask whether there are any problems with vision, joints or feet.
- Establish whether there is a previous history of diabetes mellitus, heart or stroke disease, or joint disorders.
- Take a drug history, including:
  - new drugs
  - recent changes in drug dosages.
- Assess his social situation, including:
  - Does he live alone?
  - Are there any stairs?
  - Does he have any family or carer support?
- Ask why he thinks he is falling. What is concerning him most?
- Enquire whether there is anything else he can add.
- Thank the patient and clean your hands.

Summarise your findings

Mr Smith is an 88-year-old man who lives alone in a ground-floor flat, supported by a twice-weekly home help. He is normally able to walk unaided within the house and a quarter of a mile to the local shop with a walking stick. He is generally healthy but takes blood pressure tablets from his doctor. In the past 3 months he has had two significant falls. On each occasion he felt drained and dizzy immediately on rising from his chair and has collapsed to the floor, sustaining minor bruising. He did not lose consciousness and felt better spontaneously within a couple of minutes. There is no history of incontinence, chest pain, breathlessness, focal weakness or palpitations associated with the falls.

Suggest a differential diagnosis

Postural hypotension secondary to excessive antihypertensive medication is the likely diagnosis. Paroxysmal arrhythmia, transient ischaemic attacks and episodes of pulmonary embolism are less likely alternatives.

OSCE example 2: Examination of an acutely confused frail elderly patient

Mrs Collins, 87 years old, has suddenly become confused.

Please examine the patient

- Introduce yourself and clean your hands.
- Find a quiet place and ask a nurse or family member to be present.
- Ensure that the patient is wearing any glasses and hearing aids.
- Observe the patient's general appearance and behaviour:
  - Is she restless or agitated? Or quiet and withdrawn?
  - Are there any non-verbal signs of pain (see Box 17.6)?
- Look for signs of acute illness:
  - temperature
  - oxygen saturation.
- Check drugs:
  - New drugs?
  - Sudden drug withdrawal?
- Check orientation with simple questions:
  - Where are you?
  - What is today's date?
  - What is your date of birth?
  - What is your age?
- Examine gently, looking for signs of sepsis or sources of pain:
  - chest: crepitations or wheeze
  - abdomen: tenderness or masses; distended bladder
  - skin: rashes, inflammation or sores
  - joints: injuries, pain or inflammation.
- Examine for new neurological features. Observation is helpful if the patient cannot cooperate with formal examination:
  - Is the speech clear?
  - Is the patient moving all limbs equally and purposefully?
  - Can she walk?
- Consider a rectal examination to look for faecal impaction.
- After the examination, help the patient to dress, reassure her and clean your hands.

Summarise your findings

Mrs Collins is an 87-year-old woman who suddenly became confused this evening. She is disorientated with regard to day, month and place, which is new for her. She appears anxious and did not fully cooperate with examination, but was moving all four limbs purposefully and could speak clearly. Her chart reveals a temperature of 39°C, which is new. She has not been given any drugs that are likely to cause confusion. There are no focal signs in the chest or abdomen.

Suggest a differential diagnosis

Acute urinary tract infection is the most likely diagnosis, but developing pneumonia is also possible as chest symptoms and signs may take time to appear.

17

Integrated clinical examination for the frail elderly patient

- Follow a standard systematic approach, including aspects that are important in frail patients. Remember that examination is tiring for frail patients and may have to be done in stages, and that they benefit from assessment by the full multiprofessional team (see Box 17.1).
- Introduce yourself and clean your hands.
- Ensure that the patient is comfortable and wearing any glasses and hearing aids. Ask if they want someone to be with them.
- Throughout the examination, observe for signs of pain (see Box 17.6) or distress.
- Assess the general appearance: ill kempt, restless or anxious, withdrawn.
- Test vision and hearing: check with the patient wearing any glasses or hearing aids.
- Assess cognition: screen for cognitive deficit (p. 323), low mood or anxiety.
- Establish nutritional status: body mass index, weight loss or dehydration (see Box 17.5).
- Check skin health: inflammation, ulcers, breaks in pressures areas.
- Look at mobility: decreased balance or gait abnormality.
- Perform a systems examination, noting particularly:
  - Chest: symmetrical air entry, added sounds.
  - Cardiovascular system: cardiac rhythm, heart murmurs, postural blood pressure.
  - Abdomen: distended bladder. Consider rectal examination.
  - Locomotor system: joints – swelling, deformity, pain or inflammation. Feet – overgrown nails, deformities or ulcers.
  - Neurology: abnormal speech, asymmetry of neurology, signs of Parkinson's disease.
- After the examination help your patient to dress.
- Thank the patient and clean your hands.

Ross Paterson
Anna R Dover

18

The deteriorating patient

A deteriorating patient is one who becomes acutely unwell in the hospital setting. This can occur at any stage of a patient's illness but is more common if the patient has been admitted as an emergency, undergone surgery or spent time in a high-dependency or intensive care setting. Common causes for deterioration include sepsis, bleeding, myocardial infarction, hypoglycaemia and pulmonary embolism.

Early assessment and intervention is required, as these patients are at high risk of cardiac arrest; once this occurs, fewer than 20% of patients survive to hospital discharge.

Vital signs

Physiological observations are monitored routinely in patients who are admitted to hospital. The vital signs that are measured include heart rate, blood pressure, respiratory rate, oxygen saturations, temperature and level of consciousness. Additional monitoring may include urine output, pain assessment and blood glucose testing.

Early warning scores

Vital signs are recorded using track-and-trigger systems in the form of early warning scores designed to assess illness severity. Measurements are made of the patient's respiratory rate, the use of oxygen therapy, oxygen saturation, temperature, heart rate, blood pressure and level of consciousness, and points are assigned for physiological derangement in each organ system. Increased frequency of observations is recommended for patients with abnormal signs, and a rising score triggers a graded response.

In the UK there is a validated track-and-trigger system, the National Early Warning Score (NEWS; Fig. 18.1). This system will trigger a graded response, due to either an aggregated high score or a single severe physiological derangement, with the urgency and seniority of the team being summoned escalating as the score rises (Box 18.1). For example, a NEWS score of between 1 and 4 is escalated to the nurse in charge of the ward, a score of 5 or 6 (or a single observation scoring 3) is escalated to the doctor covering the ward, and a score of 7 should be escalated to a senior doctor and discussed with the supervising consultant, with consideration of referral to a critical care team.

The early warning score is designed to complement clinical judgement. If you or another member of your team is concerned about a patient, do not dismiss this instinct purely because the early warning score is low. A patient may just look unwell or feel cold to the touch and, although these features are not captured by the early warning scoring systems, they may signify early deterioration, particularly in young patients with greater physiological reserve.

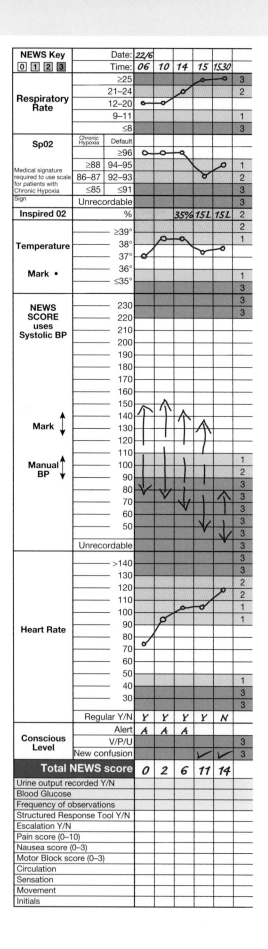

Fig. 18.1 An example of a National Early Warning Score (NEWS) chart. The scoring of physiological variables is shown. *BP,* blood pressure; *V/P/U,* responding to voice/pain/unresponsive.

18.1 Example of graded response to early warning score

Early warning score	Response
Normal	Carry out minimum 12-hourly observations
Low	Increase frequency of observations Alert nurse in charge of ward
Medium	Respond within 30 minutes Urgently call a member of the medical team responsible for the patient Initiate appropriate interventions, assess response, document ongoing management plan including level of care
High	Respond immediately Make an emergency call to a senior clinician or member of the critical care team Initiate appropriate interventions, assess response, document ongoing management plan including level of care

Initial assessment

When you are reviewing a deteriorating patient, a rapid assessment should replace the usual systematic history taking and physical examination in order to identify abnormal physiology quickly and to administer immediate life-saving interventions to prevent further deterioration and death.

The approach to the acutely deteriorating patient is time-critical and attending to this patient should be prioritised; do not wait to finish other tasks or ward rounds. Make every effort to go and see the patient for yourself, as your immediate first impressions can provide much more information than can be obtained by several minutes of discussion by telephone; if patients look sick, they probably are.

Examination sequence

- Always ensure your own safety and use the appropriate personal protective equipment.
- Approach the patient and assess their response by asking 'Are you alright?' Gently shake the patient by the shoulders and shout loudly into both ears if unresponsive. A normal response confirms that the airway is clear and there is perfusion of the brain.
- If the patient is unresponsive, check for a pulse and assess whether the patient is breathing. If in cardiac or respiratory arrest, ask a colleague to summon the cardiac arrest team and begin cardiopulmonary resuscitation in accordance with guidelines.
- Monitor the vital signs; attach an electrocardiogram (ECG) monitor, a non-invasive blood pressure monitor and a pulse oximeter as soon as possible. Ensure the patient has an intravenous cannula inserted.
- If the patient does not respond or looks unwell, seek senior help immediately.

The ABCDE approach

The ABCDE approach provides a standardised framework for simultaneously assessing and treating life-threatening problems in critically ill patients. This systematic approach will help you to break down complex and stressful clinical situations into more manageable components.

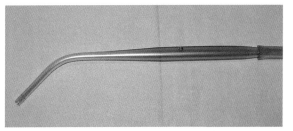

Fig. 18.2 Yankauer suction catheter. This may have a small hole to control airflow. If this is present, occlude it with your thumb to generate suction.

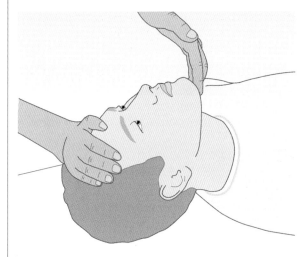

Fig. 18.3 Chin lift for opening the airway.

18

A: Airway

If a patient is able to speak normally, you can be confident that the airway is patent. If there is no response or if the patient appears to have difficulty in breathing, perform a more detailed assessment. Airway obstruction is a medical emergency; call for expert help immediately.

Examination sequence

- Look for signs of airway obstruction. There may be use of the accessory muscles of respiration, supraclavicular or subcostal indrawing, or paradoxical movements where the abdomen moves out as the chest moves in ('seesaw' breathing). Cyanosis is a late sign.
- Look in the mouth for foreign objects, blood, vomit or secretions. These can be removed by gentle suction with a Yankauer suction catheter (Fig. 18.2).
- Listen for abnormal airway noises (Box 18.2).
- Open the airway with a chin-lift or jaw-thrust manœuvre (Figs 18.3 and 18.4).
- In patients with altered consciousness it may be necessary to maintain the airway by insertion of an oropharyngeal (Guedel) or nasopharyngeal airway adjunct (Fig. 18.5), or by tracheal intubation, which must be performed by an experienced clinician.
- Administer high-concentration oxygen via a non-rebreather mask at a flow rate of 15 L/minute (Fig. 18.6).

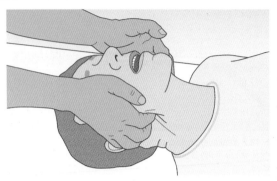

Fig. 18.4 Jaw thrust for opening the airway. Place your fingers behind the angle of the patient's jaw, and then lift it to open the airway.

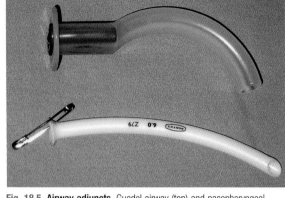

Fig. 18.5 Airway adjuncts. Guedel airway (top) and nasopharyngeal airway (bottom). Note the 'safety pin', which prevents migration of the proximal end of the airway beyond the nasal orifice.

18.2 Airway noises

No noise (the 'silent airway')

- Implies complete airway obstruction and/or absence of, or minimal, respiratory effort

Stridor

- A harsh noise, usually loudest in inspiration, caused by partial obstruction around the larynx
- In febrile patients, consider supraglottitis
- Other causes are foreign bodies, laryngeal trauma, burns or tumours

Snoring/stertor

- Caused by partial upper airway obstruction from soft tissues of the mouth and oropharynx

Gurgling

- Caused by fluids (secretions, blood or vomit) in the oropharynx

Grunting

- A grunt during expiration is a sign of respiratory muscle fatigue. It may be present after chest-wall trauma with a flail segment. Grunting improves gas exchange by slowing expiration and preventing alveolar collapse by creating positive end-expiratory pressure.

Wheeze

- A 'musical' noise, best heard on auscultation
- When loudest in expiration, relates to intrathoracic obstruction of the small bronchi and bronchioles; most often occurs in asthma and chronic obstructive pulmonary disease

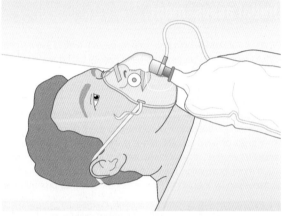

Fig. 18.6 Administering high-concentration oxygen using a non-rebreather mask with a reservoir bag. Oxygen should be delivered at a rate of 15 L/minute.

Aim for an oxygen saturation of 94–98% except in patients at risk of type 2 (hypercapnic) respiratory failure such as chronic obstructive pulmonary disease; in this case use a lower target of 88–92%.

B: Breathing

It is vital to identify and treat hypoxia, as it can lead rapidly to cardiac arrest and death. Perform a thorough assessment, looking for life-threatening respiratory compromise due to conditions such as acute severe asthma, pulmonary oedema or tension pneumothorax.

Examination sequence

- Attach a pulse oximeter to assess peripheral oxygenation. Be alert to circumstances in which this measurement may be unreliable (Box 18.3).
- Look for signs of respiratory distress: sweating, use of the accessory muscles or abdominal 'seesaw' breathing. Cyanosis is a late finding, and may be absent in severe anaemia or massive blood loss.
- Count the respiratory rate. The normal rate is 12–20 breaths per minute. A rising respiratory rate is an early and sensitive sign of deterioration. A respiratory rate of more than 30 breaths per minute is a sign of critical illness and should prompt escalation. Inadequate breathing, which is either a respiratory rate of less than 10 breaths per minute or shallow breathing, requires supported ventilation with a bag-valve mask and should prompt a call for the cardiac arrest team. Look for reversible causes. Has the patient received or taken opiates or other sedatives recently?
- Look for chest wall deformity or injury; observe the depth of inspiration and assess for symmetrical chest-wall expansion. Other breathing patterns may provide a clue to the underlying diagnosis (Box 18.4).

18.3 Situations in which pulse oximetry may give misleading values

Inadequate waveform

- Hypoperfusion – ear-lobe sensor may be better than finger probe if poor hand perfusion
- Hypothermia
- Movement artefact
- Rapid irregular pulse – e.g. atrial fibrillation

Falsely normal or high reading

- Abnormal haemoglobins:
  - Carboxyhaemoglobin (e.g. carbon monoxide poisoning)
  - Methaemoglobin[a]
  - Sulphaemoglobin[a]
- High levels of HbA_{1c}

Falsely low reading

- Abnormal haemoglobins:
  - Methaemoglobin[a]
  - Sulphaemoglobin[a]
- Severe anaemia
- Nail varnish, false fingernails
- Skin pigmentation
- Excessively dirty fingers

[a]Depending on the levels of methaemoglobin or sulphaemoglobin, pulse oximetry may underestimate or overestimate the true arterial oxygen saturation (usually low).
HbA_{1c}, haemoglobin A_{1c}, glycated haemoglobin.

18.4 Respiratory patterns: common causes

Tachypnoea

- Anxiety
- Pain
- Asthma
- Metabolic acidosis
- Chest injury
- Pneumothorax
- Pulmonary embolus
- Brainstem stroke

Bradypnoea/apnoea

- Cardiac arrest
- Opioids/other sedative overdose
- Central neurological causes (stroke, head injury)

Cheyne–Stokes respiration

- Left ventricular failure
- Central neurological causes (stroke, head injury)
- Overdose (barbiturates, gamma-hydroxybutyrate, opioids)

Kussmaul respiration

- Metabolic acidosis, e.g. diabetic ketoacidosis
- Uraemia
- Hepatic failure
- Shock (lactic acidosis)
- Overdose (methanol, ethylene glycol, salicylate)

Paradoxical respiration

- Airway obstruction
- Respiratory failure
- Flail segment
- High spinal cord lesions
- Guillain–Barré syndrome

- Palpate the trachea in the suprasternal notch. It should be central; if it is not, it suggests mediastinal displacement by pneumothorax or collapse. Gently palpate any areas of injury to assess for a flail segment, where multiple rib fractures in more than one place allow a part of the rib cage to move independently. Feel for subcutaneous emphysema due to pneumothorax or trauma.
- Percuss and auscultate the chest to identify pneumothorax, effusions, consolidation or oedema. A silent chest can occur when airflow is poor, such as in life-threatening asthma.

Consider further evaluation of gas exchange with an arterial blood gas (ABG) measurement; it will give valuable information on arterial oxygen, carbon dioxide and acid–base status but requires skill and competence to obtain. Prolonged attempts at taking an ABG sample should not detract from other aspects of the resuscitation. It is usually appropriate to obtain a portable chest X-ray in a breathless or hypoxic patient.

C: Circulation

Consider hypovolaemia as the most probable cause of shock in any acutely unwell patient.

Examination sequence

- Look at and feel the skin; a shocked patient will be cold with pale, white or mottled skin.
- Check capillary refill by pressing on a fingertip (held at the level of the heart) for 5 seconds. This will cause it to blanch. When the pressure is released the colour should return to the fingertip in less than 2 seconds. This is roughly the same time as it takes you to say 'capillary refill time'. If the capillary refill time is delayed, this indicates poor peripheral perfusion or shock.
- Assess the pulse rate and rhythm (p. 47). A heart rate of less than 50 beats per minute (bpm) or more than 90 bpm requires further investigation. A heart rate of more than 130 bpm requires immediate attention.
- Palpate peripheral and central pulses, assessing the volume and character (p. 48); poorly felt peripheral pulses may indicate hypovolaemia or poor cardiac output, whereas a bounding pulse may indicate sepsis. As blood pressure falls, peripheral pulses diminish, with loss of the radial, then femoral and finally carotid pulsation. As a rule of thumb, if the radial pulse is present, the systolic blood pressure is likely to be greater than 90 mmHg but once the femoral pulse becomes impalpable, the systolic blood pressure is likely to be less than 60 mmHg.
- Attach an ECG monitor to the patient to assess heart rate and rhythm. A 12-lead ECG should also be recorded in patients with suspected acute coronary syndrome or arrhythmia.
- Check the blood pressure (p. 49). Use a manual sphygmomanometer, as automated blood pressure devices may be inaccurate in the acutely unwell patient. Hypotension is a late and serious sign, particularly in young patients who may be able to maintain blood pressure by peripheral vasoconstriction.
- Examine the jugular venous pressure (p. 52).
- Auscultate the heart to identify added sounds or murmurs (p. 55).
- Insert one or more wide-bore (14- or 16-gauge) intravenous cannulae, and take blood for routine haematological, biochemical and coagulation tests and for cross-matching. If the patient is hypotensive, give a bolus of 250–500 mL warmed crystalloid solution.

18

- Look for other signs of inadequate organ perfusion such as reduced consciousness (see later) and oliguria (<0.5 mL/kg/hour). A fluid balance chart should be commenced. Consider urinary catheterisation. Urinary catheters have their own associated morbidity, in particular catheter-associated urinary tract infection. However, if the patient is obtunded or unable to pass urine, a catheter should be inserted.

D: Disability

Any change in a patient's conscious level should raise concern. Causes of unconsciousness can include hypoxia, hypercapnia, cerebral hypoperfusion, hypoglycaemia or the use of sedative medications such as opiates.

Conscious level is often recorded using the AVPU scale, which categorises the patient as:

- **a**lert
- responding to **v**oice
- responding to **p**ain
- **u**nresponsive.

This measure is incorporated into many early warning scores and has the advantage of being a fast and easily understood verbal description of the patient's conscious level. It is not designed as a measure to track small changes in a patient's neurological condition.

The Glasgow Coma Scale (GCS) is more sensitive to changes in a patient's conscious level but is more complex. It measures eye opening, vocal and motor responses (Box 18.5). The GCS was initially validated as a measure of conscious level in patients with traumatic brain injury. Its use has been extrapolated to many situations of altered consciousness and it may not always perform as intended.

The GCS should always be reported in its component parts – for example, E4 V5 M6 – and it can be useful to describe each component ('E4 eyes open spontaneously; V2 sounds only; M6 obeying commands') when communicating by telephone to remove ambiguity.

Testing for response to a painful stimulus should be done only if the patient is not responding to speech. The stimulus should be administered centrally by applying firm supraorbital pressure or a trapezius pinch; sternal rub should be avoided, as it can cause distressing bruising to the patient's chest. Peripheral painful stimuli should be avoided, as they can elicit misleading spinal reflexes.

Examination sequence

- Assess the patient's conscious level using either the AVPU scale or GCS.
- Examine the pupils for size, symmetry and light reflex. Pupil size will vary with ambient lighting but should be symmetrical and constrict to light. Symmetrical change in pupil size suggests a drug or metabolic cause. Constricted pupils (miosis) can be a sign of opiate overdose or organophosphate poisoning, whereas pupillary dilatation (mydriasis) may indicate toxicity from anticholinergics (such as atropine or tricyclic antidepressants) or sympathomimetics (such as cocaine). Asymmetrical pupils suggest a structural lesion. A unilateral dilated pupil in a patient with altered conscious level is a medical emergency and should prompt further investigation with emergency computed tomography of the head.
- Check the drug chart for reversible causes of reduced consciousness.
- Check the capillary blood glucose using a bedside glucose meter (Fig. 18.7 and Box 18.6). The acronym after ABC of 'DEFG' ('Don't ever forget glucose') is a good reminder. If the blood glucose is less than 4 mmol/L (72 mg/dL) and the patient is unconsciousness, administer 75–100 mL of 20% glucose intravenously over 15 minutes; thereafter, follow national guidelines for the management of hypoglycaemia.

Delirium is a common complication affecting 10–20% of hospital patients; the incidence is greatest in the elderly. It should not be overlooked or dismissed, as it may be a sign of an underlying deterioration and should prompt a search for an underlying cause such as infection, metabolic derangement, hypoxia or cerebral hypoperfusion.

18.5 Glasgow Coma Scale (GCS)	
Eye opening (E)	
4	Spontaneously
3	To speech
2	To pain
1	No response
Best verbal response (V)	
5	Orientated
4	Confused
3	Inappropriate words
2	Incomprehensible sounds
1	No verbal response
Best motor response (M)	
6	Obeys commands
5	Localises painful stimulus
4	Normal flexion
3	Abnormal flexion
2	Extends to painful stimulus
1	No response

Reproduced from Teasdale G, Jennett B. Assessment of coma and impaired consciousness: a practical scale. The Lancet 1974; 304(7872):81–84, with permission from Elsevier Ltd.

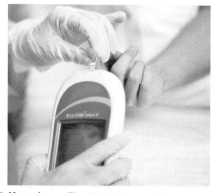

Fig. 18.7 Measuring capillary blood glucose with a glucometer.

18.6 Performing a capillary blood glucose measurement

- Prepare equipment for the procedure:
  - Gloves
  - Glucose meter
  - Test strips
  - Single-use lancet
  - Cotton swab
- Introduce yourself, explain the procedure and obtain consent
- Clean your hands and put on gloves
- Clean the patient's fingertip and allow it to dry. Note that any glucose on the patient's finger will give a falsely high reading
- Inset the test strip into the glucose meter after checking it is in date
- Prick the side of the patient's finger with the lancet (no lower than the nail bed) and gently massage (or milk) the finger to promote bleeding. Apply this drop of blood to the test strip until the meter confirms an adequate sample has been received
- Give the patient the swab to stop the bleeding and safely dispose of gloves, lancet and test strip
- Clean your hands and thank the patient for their cooperation

---

18.7 Identifying sepsis

If there is clinical suspicion of infection and 2 or more of the criteria below, think 'Could this be sepsis?'

Systemic inflammatory response syndrome (SIRS) criteria

- Temperature: $<36°C$ or $>38°C$
- Pulse: >90 beats per minute
- White cell count: $<4\times10^9$/L or $>12\times10^9$/L
- Respiratory rate: >20 breaths per minute
- Mental state: new confusion
- Blood glucose: >7.7 mmol/L (138 mg/dL) in a patient without diabetes

qSOFA score

Respiratory rate ≥22 breaths per minute
Systolic blood pressure ≤100 mmHg
Glasgow coma scale <15

E: Exposure

Examine the patient thoroughly while respecting their dignity and minimising heat loss.

Examination sequence

- Look for evidence of trauma, blood loss and rashes, in particular the non-blanching petechial rash of meningococcal bacteraemia.
- Check the temperature using an infrared tympanic thermometer. Normal mean body temperature is 36.5°C but varies diurnally (highest in the early evening) and according to the site where it is measured. A temperature below 35°C indicates hypothermia and should be confirmed by measuring a core (rectal) temperature, and treated by external rewarming using a warming system such as a Bair Hugger. Other forms of active rewarming include use of warmed intravenous fluids and heated humidified oxygen therapy. A temperature above 37.8°C indicates fever and, if acute, should prompt a search for infection and/or sepsis.

Sepsis

Sepsis is a condition that occurs as a result of the host response to infection (such as pneumonia, urinary tract infection or intra-abdominal infection). It is the reason for deterioration in approximately 40% of patients who become acutely unwell in medical wards, and carries a high mortality risk. Those at greatest risk include elderly or frail patients, those who are immunocompromised or have undergone recent surgery, and those with indwelling lines or catheters. As sepsis progresses, it can lead to shock and ultimately multiple organ failure; if it is not identified early, the chance of a good outcome falls rapidly. In a patient with signs or symptoms of infection, always think, 'Could this be sepsis?'

The most widely adopted criteria for sepsis are based on the systemic inflammatory response syndrome (SIRS) criteria, although

---

18.8 'Sepsis Six' therapeutic bundle

Resuscitate = 'Sepsis Six' within 1 hour

- Give O_2 to target saturation $>94\%$ (N.B. Aim for 88–92% in chronic obstructive pulmonary disease)
- Administer intravenous fluids, up to 20 mL/kg
- Give intravenous antibiotics
- Take blood cultures
- Measure lactate and white cell count
- Monitor urine output; commence fluid balance chart

Reassess and escalate

- Reassess for severe sepsis
- Repeat observations
- Escalate to the consultant and/or critical care if there are signs of organ dysfunction

---

18

other scoring systems (such as qSOFA) are also used (Box 18.7). These describe a physiological response to a non-specific insult. In the presence of clinical suspicion of infection, a patient who fulfils the SIRS criteria should be assumed to have sepsis.

The assessment and initial management of sepsis are described by the 'Sepsis Six' therapeutic bundle, which aims to deliver three diagnostic and three therapeutic steps within 1 hour of the recognition of sepsis (Box 18.8). In addition to the routine vital signs, the measurement of urine output and lactate is recommended as a guide to illness severity. Lactate is the product of anaerobic metabolism and is a marker of tissue perfusion. A lactate of more than 2 mmol/L (18 mg/dL) is abnormal and a level of more than 4 mmol/L (36 mg/dL) is associated with 30% mortality. A careful search must be undertaken to identify the underlying infection in order to aid diagnosis and guide appropriate choice of antibiotics.

Initial investigations should include ABGs, glucose and lactate measurement, blood cultures, full blood count, C-reactive protein, urea and electrolytes, and a clotting screen.

Treatment of sepsis with early and appropriate antibiotics, oxygen and intravenous fluids reduces mortality. Patients who fail to respond to initial treatment may require a higher level of care and should be discussed with a senior clinician.

Ongoing management

The management of a deteriorating patient must include not simply the initiation of appropriate interventions but also frequent review of response to therapy. Once you have completed the ABCDE approach, return to the beginning to reassess, if the patient is not improving.

Clear goals of interventions should be communicated to the team (for example, 'The goal of this fluid bolus is to achieve a systolic blood pressure of over 100 mmHg; if this is not achieved, please let me know and we will give a further fluid bolus'). A written management plan should be documented, which should also include a stipulation of the frequency of observations (such as every 15 minutes until stabilised).

It is particularly important to work as a team when a patient is deteriorating rapidly. A structured approach to communication will help you organise your thoughts and is an effective way to communicate the urgency of the situation to the person you are escalating to. The SBAR tool is particularly useful in this setting (p. 365).

Finally, consideration should be given to patients with limited reversibility in whom intensive treatment may not be appropriate. It is important to acknowledge the uncertainty of outcomes in these cases (p. 349) and to ensure early discussion of resuscitation status and agreed ceilings of care.

OSCE example: The unwell patient

Mr Green, 50 years old, had a laparotomy and small-bowel resection 5 days ago. He has an elevated temperature of 38.6°C and is tachycardic with a heart rate of 98 beats per minute.

Please assess this unwell patient

- Prioritise seeing this patient.
- Introduce yourself and clean your hands.
- Is the patient responsive? If unconscious, are they in cardiac arrest?
- Assess the airway. Is the patient speaking to you? Look for airway obstruction, supraclavicular or subcostal indrawing, or paradoxical movements of the chest and abdomen.
- Assess breathing for rate and depth. Attach pulse oximeter. Look for chest asymmetry. Palpate the trachea in the suprasternal notch. Percuss and auscultate, looking for pneumothorax, consolidation or effusion.
- Assess the circulation. Examine for skin pallor, clamminess and capillary refill time. Assess the pulse for tachycardia. Measure the blood pressure with a manual sphygmomanometer.
- Assess conscious level. Is the patient confused?
- Measure blood glucose.
- Comment on the presence of systemic inflammatory response syndrome (SIRS) criteria and signs of systemic infection.
- Examine the abdomen for signs of infection or bleeding.
- Call for senior help and document the management plan.

Summarise your findings

Mr Green is a 50-year-old man who had a small-bowel resection 5 days ago, and has now become drowsy and febrile. He is hypotensive at 95/60 mmHg, with a tachycardia of 98 beats per minute, and an elevated respiratory rate at 28 breaths per minute. He is rousable and responds appropriately to questions but looks unwell. Abdominal examination reveals a recent laparotomy scar and generalised tenderness with rebound.

Suggest a differential diagnosis

The likely problem is sepsis from an intra-abdominal infection. This is an emergency situation requiring urgent resuscitation.

Suggested investigations

Lactate, full blood count, blood cultures.

Advanced level comments

Immediate resuscitation is appropriate as per the 'Sepsis Six' bundle: oxygen, fluids and antibiotics. Review the effects of resuscitation on blood pressure and urine output, and repeat the measurement of lactate concentration. Escalation to critical care should be considered, and exploratory surgery may be required for source infection control.

Integrated examination sequence for the deteriorating patient

- General appearance:
  - If the patient is unconscious, are they in cardiac arrest?
  - If they look unwell, call for help.
- Airway:
  - Is the airway clear?
  - Is patient able to speak?
  - Look for signs of airway obstruction: supraclavicular, subcostal indrawing or paradoxical movements, or 'seesaw' breathing.
  - Listen for abnormal airway noises.
  - Open the airway with airway manœuvres if required.
  - Administer high-flow oxygen.
- Breathing:
  - Measure the respiratory rate and assess peripheral oxygenation using pulse oximetry.
  - Look for signs of respiratory distress: use of accessory muscles, abdominal 'seesaw' breathing, chest deformity or trauma, asymmetrical movement.
  - Palpate the trachea in the suprasternal notch and palpate any areas of injury.
  - Percuss and auscultate the chest.
- Circulation:
  - Examine the skin: is it cold, pale or mottled? Check capillary refill time.
  - Assess the rate and volume of the pulse; palpate peripheral pulses.
  - Check the blood pressure.
  - Examine the jugular venous pressure and auscultate the heart.
  - Measure the urine output and assess cerebral perfusion.
  - Obtain intravenous access and perform a 12-lead electrocardiogram.
- Disability:
  - Assess conscious level using the AVPU or Glasgow Coma Scale scores.
  - Examine pupils for symmetry, size and reaction to light.
  - Measure capillary blood glucose.
  - Check the drug chart for reversible causes of reduced consciousness.
- Exposure:
  - Check the temperature.
  - Look for trauma, bleeding and rashes.

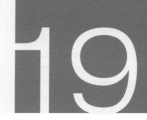

Anthony Bateman
Kirsty Boyd

The dying patient

Around 1% of the population in economically developed countries die each year. Some deaths are unexpected but the majority are the result of one or more advanced progressive illnesses. It is important to identify whether an acute deterioration in the context of chronic disease is reversible, or represents an inevitable decline and that the person will die soon. Recognising where a person is on their current illness trajectory allows pragmatic decisions to be made about what further investigations and treatments are appropriate and informs discussions with the patient and their relatives.

Assessing the dying patient

Physiology

There are three broad illness trajectories (Fig. 19.1):

- predictable progression of a life-limiting condition with a clear terminal phase: for example, progressive cancer
- fluctuating decline with intermittent, potentially life-threatening, acute exacerbations that may result in a seemingly unexpected death: for example, advanced respiratory disease or heart failure
- prolonged, gradual decline, sometimes with a more acute terminal event: for example, dementia or general frailty, and some advanced neurological conditions.

Many physiological changes occur towards the end of life. General indicators of decline include:

- deteriorating performance status, with the person in bed or in a chair for more than 50% of the day
- unplanned, emergency hospital admissions
- persistent symptoms despite optimal treatment of underlying illnesses
- significant weight loss.

Some patients are close to death when they first present, or fail to improve with treatment so that it becomes clear that they will die soon. What matters is that we recognise when this person is so unwell that they could die.

The history

To understand the patient's situation fully and to plan appropriately, the approach to the history needs to be adapted to include background and context.

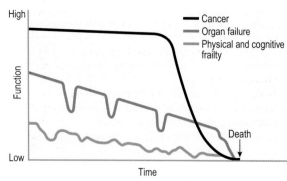

Fig. 19.1 Illness trajectories towards the end of life. *Adapted from Lynn J, Adamson DM. Living well at the end of life. Adapting health care to serious chronic illness in old age. Washington: Rand Health, 2003. With permission from RAND Corporation, Santa Monica, California, USA. https://www.rand.org/pubs/white_papers/WP137.html.*

Background information

Use all available sources to determine the patient's previous health status in addition to their presenting problems. Review referral letters, hospital records and previous discharge summaries. Check for advance directives or anticipatory care plans. Look for any record of previous discussions or decisions about cardiopulmonary resuscitation (CPR). Find out if the person has a pacemaker or any other device that will need to be removed after death, and record this clearly.

Establishing the broader context

Build up a picture of the patient's overall health status, not just the presenting symptoms. If a family member or friend is present, they can provide valuable additional information and also support the patient. If the patient cannot provide information, contact someone who knows them such as their general practitioner. Find out what the person and their family know about their condition and what their hopes, fears and expectations of treatment are. The key questions to ask are shown in Box 19.1.

It is also helpful to ask yourself the 'surprise question': 'Would you be surprised if this person died in the next few months, weeks or days?' If the answer is no, then it is time to find out what things matter most to the patient and how they and their family can best be supported during this time.

The physical examination

People may retain some awareness, even when close to death. Speak to the patient by name and to others in the room as you would when your patient is awake. Always introduce yourself and explain your role in the team. Your assessment begins with observing whether the person looks comfortable, and checking with other staff and the family. Non-verbal ways of showing concern for the person have a big impact (tone, gentle touch, gestures of kindness), for both the person and their family.

It can be difficult to decide when a person has entered the last days of life but there are signs that suggest a patient will die soon (Fig. 19.2). Even when this is the situation, a focused examination looking for reversible causes of deterioration is always indicated (see the integrated examination sequence at the end of the chapter). Common potentially reversible causes of deterioration in advanced illness are shown in Box 19.2.

Some patients will benefit from carefully selected tests to allow us to see if their condition is partly reversible, to guide specific palliative treatment or to clarify the prognosis.

19.1 Key questions towards the end of life

- How have you been doing recently?
- What has changed?
- How were you a month ago?
- What do you know about your health problems?
- What are you expecting to happen now/in the future?
- What things are important to you that we should know about?
- We hope the treatment will work but I am worried you might get more unwell. Can we talk about that?
- Is there anything or anyone you are worried about?
- Do you have a family member or a close friend who helps you when you are less well?
- Is there someone we should speak to about your treatment and care?

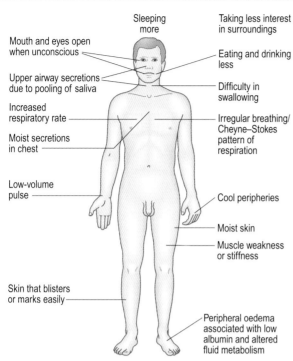

Sleeping more

Taking less interest in surroundings

Mouth and eyes open when unconscious

Eating and drinking less

Upper airway secretions due to pooling of saliva

Difficulty in swallowing

Increased respiratory rate

Irregular breathing/ Cheyne–Stokes pattern of respiration

Moist secretions in chest

Low-volume pulse

Cool peripheries

Moist skin

Muscle weakness or stiffness

Skin that blisters or marks easily

Peripheral oedema associated with low albumin and altered fluid metabolism

Fig. 19.2 Signs that suggest a patient will die soon.

19.2 Common potentially reversible causes of deterioration in advanced illness

- Dehydration
- Infection
- Opioid toxicity or other drug toxicity or poisoning
- Glucocorticoid withdrawal or a new diagnosis of adrenal insufficiency
- Acute kidney injury
- Delirium
- Hypercalcaemia
- Hypoglycaemia or hyperglycaemia
- Hyponatraemia

Care in the last days of life

If the patient is likely to die soon, their care needs to be planned to anticipate problems. It is important to review a patient who is dying at least daily, and more often if they are unsettled or have complex clinical problems. If a patient deteriorates rapidly or their symptoms change, urgent assessment is required. Find out if the other people who are caring for the dying patient have any concerns and work with them to maintain the person's comfort and dignity. Involve and support family members and close friends.

Cultural, religious and spiritual care is very important when a person is dying, at the time of death and afterwards. Always ask the person and those close to them about their wishes and what you and other staff members can do to help support them. This may include wishes about how the person is touched or cared for after death.

Communication with patients and families

Find out what the patient and their family know and what they expect. Explain what happens when a person is dying. Talk about the changes that will be seen and what they mean. Explain

why the focus of treatment, monitoring and care will change to making sure the person is comfortable. Explain what to expect when the person dies and what to do if the person is at home. Most people stop breathing gradually but may take a final breath after a long pause. A brief muscle spasm may be observed at that time, so warn relatives about this.

Confirming and certifying death

The confirmation and certification of death are important to allow the legal requirements and cultural and religious traditions that happen after a person has died to be fulfilled. Some people will have decided to be organ donors. Notification of the relevant team in advance and the prompt diagnosis of death can make this possible for many of them.

In the UK death is defined as 'the irreversible loss of the essential characteristics necessary to the existence of a living person – to be able to sense and interact with the environment and to maintain the fundamental bodily functions of respiration and circulation'.

Consciousness and respiratory and circulatory function are controlled within the brainstem. Irreversible damage to the brainstem, either after cardiorespiratory arrest or due to direct damage to the brainstem itself, always results in death.

The history

A decision will usually have been made and documented in advance, stating that CPR will not be given because it would not work or would have a very poor outcome for this person. Occasionally, a person with one or more advanced illnesses deteriorates more rapidly than expected or a decision that CPR will not be given has not been made in advance. In those situations the professionals who are present decide if CPR should not start or should be stopped.

If you are not familiar with the patient and their recent medical history, read their records before going to see them or speaking to their family. Being aware of whether the death was sudden or expected and how the person has been during their final illness helps you to prepare for speaking with the family.

The physical examination

After the person has died, it is important for the clinical team to continue to care for them as they would any other patient. This includes speaking about the person by name to family members who are present at the time of death or while you are carrying out the examination to confirm death. Some relatives choose to remain in the room and you need to explain each part of the examination in simple terms and conduct it in a respectful and professional manner.

The person who has died should be observed for a minimum of 5 minutes to establish that irreversible cardiorespiratory arrest has occurred. This provides an opportunity for you to spend time supporting and listening to any family members who are present. After death the body cools gradually and stiffens; bowel sounds may persist for a time until the sphincters relax and the bowels and bladder empty.

Brainstem death

The diagnosis of brainstem death must be made by at least two doctors who have been fully registered for at least 5 years. They

19

should have experience in the assessment of brainstem function. One of the doctors must be a consultant or equivalent senior physician. The tests are performed on two occasions. The first set of tests is to diagnose brainstem death. The second set is to confirm the diagnosis. There is no minimum time required between tests; they can occur concurrently. If the tests demonstrate that brain death has occurred, then the time of death is recorded as the time of diagnosis: that is, the time at which the first set of tests was completed.

Communication with families

Communicating with family members to tell them that someone has died should be done as soon as possible. Speak to relatives in a quiet, private room and try to avoid interruptions. If the death is sudden and unexpected, this will be breaking bad news so it needs to be done clearly and sensitively. If contacting a family member by telephone to inform them of a patient's death, it is important to decide if it is safe to do so or whether it would be better instead to contact someone such as the police and ask them to go and inform the family member in person about a sudden death. Explain what has happened and what will happen next. Offer the family time with the person who has died if they wish.

Documentation

Document the place, time and date of death in the patient's medical record. In some countries the time of death is when the person was observed to have died by those present or the person was found to have died. In other countries the time of death is when death is confirmed by a doctor, so make sure you know which time to record. Include details of who was present when the person died and what the primary and main secondary causes of death were. The cause of death should always be discussed and confirmed with a senior colleague. Some medical certificates of death require additional information such as the duration of the final illness, so make sure you are familiar with these requirements. You should also know or seek advice about when a medical certificate of death should not be issued because the death has to be reported (Box 19.3).

Looking after yourself and others

Caring for a patient who is dying and their family is very rewarding but can also be stressful and emotionally demanding. It is important to recognise this and look for help and support when you need it. You may need advice on how to manage a patient's symptoms, decide on a care plan or communicate sensitively and effectively with people who are experiencing loss and bereavement. Talk to colleagues and support them too.

19.3 Deaths that may require further investigation

- The cause of death is unknown
- Death was violent or unnatural
- Death was sudden and unexplained
- The person who died was not visited by a medical practitioner during their final illness
- A medical certificate is not available
- Death occurred during an operation or before the person came round from the anaesthetic
- The medical certificate suggests that the death may have been caused by an industrial disease or industrial poisoning
- Death occurred in legal custody
- A complaint has been received over the medical treatment or standards of care received by the deceased
- Death was due to a notifiable disease

OSCE example 1: Informing relatives that a patient is nearing death

Mr Jenkins, 80 years old, has severe chronic obstructive pulmonary disease. He is on domiciliary oxygen therapy. He was admitted to the ward 3 days ago with severe pneumonia. After initially responding to treatment, his condition has deteriorated. He is becoming breathless, confused and distressed. He has been seen by the intensive care consultant, who has stated, 'The patient would not benefit from ICU care.' She has suggested that Mr Jenkins should be treated with a focus on good symptom control and care appropriate for the last days of life. The nurses ask you to speak to Mr Jenkins's son about what has happened and what the next steps should be in terms of treatment. You should talk about cardiopulmonary resuscitation and explain why this would not be the right treatment when his father dies.

- To prepare:
  - Ask for a private room.
  - Ask if you can leave your bleep and /or telephone with the nursing staff.
  - Ask for a nurse to accompany you.
  - Introduce yourself to the son and clarify his relationship to the dying person:
    - 'Hello. My name's Dr Smith. Are you Mr Jenkins's son, John? Thank you for seeing me, Mr Jenkins. I'm sorry to tell you that your father has become much more unwell today. Is there anyone else you'd like to be with you at this time?'
- Establish the son's perceptions:
  - 'What do you understand about your father's illness and what's happened so far?'
- Explain the medical facts in lay terms:
  - 'He's been unwell for a while, not really getting out of the house for a long time. He's been in and out of hospital a lot lately and never really seemed to get better.'
  - Inform the son of the severity of his father's illness and what the frequent hospital admissions reflect about its progression.
  - Explain that, because his father has advanced lung disease and is not responding to antibiotics, he is likely to deteriorate further.
  - Pause.
  - Explain that this means Mr Jenkins is likely to die.
- Allow time for silence.
- Express your condolences.
- Gently rebuff any false hopes.

OSCE example 1: Informing relatives that a patient is nearing death – *cont'd*

- Sensitively cover the following additional points:
  - Say that you are not sure how quickly he will die, but it could be in the next few days or even sooner.
  - Explain that some people can improve for a short while and then become less well again, and that occasionally unexpected recovery occurs but this is now unlikely.
  - State that the most important thing now is to make sure his father has the right nursing care and medicines to make sure he is as comfortable and as free of symptoms as possible.
  - Outline what palliative treatments he might receive, and say that you would like to start those treatments as soon as possible.
  - Explain that when a person is dying, their heart and breathing stop. Giving treatment to restart the heart does not work and is not the best way to care for them, so that decision is made in advance and recorded so that everyone knows about it.
  - Ask about any religious or cultural practices.
  - Ask if he would like you to talk to anyone else.
  - Ask if there are any questions.
  - State that if he has any questions later, someone will be available to try to answer them.

OSCE example 2: Confirming death

The nurse-in-charge calls you to tell you that Mr Williams, an 83-year-old inpatient, has died.

Please describe the process for establishing and certifying death, and how you would communicate with staff and family

- Introduce yourself to the nursing team on the ward:
  - 'Hello, my name's Dr Smith. I'm here to see Mr Williams.'
- Ask if the death was expected.
- Confirm that the patient was not for resuscitation.
- Ask if the team know why Mr Williams was in hospital and what the likely cause of death might be.
- Ask for the patient's notes and check you have the correct name, hospital number and date of birth.
- On entering the patient's bed space:
  - Clean your hands and introduce yourself to any relatives or staff present.
  - Express your condolences and explain why you need to examine the patient:
    - 'I'm sorry to intrude at a sad time. I'm here to examine Mr Williams to confirm that he's died. If you have any questions about what I'm doing or what happens next, please ask me and I'll do my best to answer.'
  - Check the patient's identity on their wristband.
  - From the end of the bed, respectfully inspect the patient. If necessary, make sure the patient looks dignified before continuing with examination: for example, position their head, clean any obvious secretions, and lift their limbs into appropriate and peaceful positions.
  - Gently stimulate the patient and say their name:
    - 'Mr Williams, Mr Williams, can you hear me?'
  - Inspect for any respiratory effort, carotid pulsation or limb movement.
  - Note the colour and temperature of the skin.
  - Say:
    - 'I'm just going to look into your eyes.'
  - Respectfully retract the eyelids and inspect the eyes. The pupils should be dilated and unresponsive.
  - Shine a torch into each eye, looking for both a direct response and a consensual response.
  - Test for corneal reflexes by stimulating the cornea with cotton wool and look for a motor response. To ensure that the cornea is stimulated, the cotton wool must touch the area over the iris. Close the eyelids after examination.
  - Apply supraorbital pressure and check for a response.
  - Respectfully expose the upper anterior chest wall and palpate for a pacemaker on both sides. This is felt as a firm, subcutaneous object with a clear geometrical shape and an associated linear operation scar.
  - Palpate for carotid pulsation for 1 minute.
  - Listen for heart sounds for 1 minute.
  - Listen for breath sounds for 1 minute.
  - Cover the patient in a dignified manner.
  - Clean your hands.
- Document the examination and confirmation of death in the notes:
  - Date and time of death:
    - Mr Williams died at 01:00h on 1 January 2016.
    - No response to stimulation.
    - Pupils unreactive to light and dilated.
    - No corneal reflex.
    - No central pulse palpated for 1 minute.
    - No heart sounds auscultated for 1 minute.
    - No breath sounds auscultated for 1 minute.
  - Write your full name, qualifications, contact number and formal signature.
  - If appropriate, write the cause of death in the notes, indicating that this will need to be discussed with a senior member of the team before a death certificate can be issued.
- If appropriate, make arrangements for the patient's relatives to be informed.
- Thank the nursing staff on the ward.

19

Integrated examination sequence for the patient nearing the end of life

- Look at how the patient is breathing. Does their chest sound moist? You do not need to auscultate the chest to identify chest secretions.
- Is the respiratory rate raised (sepsis, metabolic disorders, persistent hypoxia or brain injuries)?
- Is the breathing pattern changing? Irregular breathing, with phases of rapid or deeper breathing followed by periods of apnoea, is Cheyne–Stokes breathing.
- If secretions are present and clinically assisted hydration or nutrition is being given, explain why this will be stopped to avoid worsening symptoms due to fluid overload and reduced excretion.
- Review monitoring charts and decide when pulse, temperature and blood pressure monitoring can stop. For many people with diabetes, blood glucose monitoring can be stopped along with medications. A once-daily test in insulin-dependent patients with diabetes may be needed, along with a small dose of maintenance insulin.
- Skin care: patients are moved for comfort and a special mattress may be used.
- Bladder care: you may need to check for signs of urinary retention (lower abdominal discomfort and bladder dullness on suprapubic percussion).
- Bowel care: the bowels may still open even after a person stops eating, so consider a gentle rectal examination and a suppository if this could be causing discomfort or restlessness.
- Mouth care: check the lips and mouth are clean and being moistened regularly.
- Check for reduced blinking and drying of the eyes.
- Ensure that medication for symptom control is prescribed and review it in line with 'as-needed' use.
- If the patient has a subcutaneous infusion of palliative medication, check this is running correctly and that the site is not red or swollen. The infusion may need to be resited.

Integrated examination sequence for confirming death

- Review the clinical notes and check there is a 'Do not attempt cardiopulmonary resuscitation' (DNACPR) form or appropriate documentation.
- Confirm the patient's name on their wristband.
- Look for any obvious signs of life: spontaneous movement, respiratory effort.
- Look for any obvious signs of death: rigor mortis, pallor mortis – dependent pooling of blood causing distinct paleness, decomposition.
- Approach the person and say their name.
- Gently stimulate the person, such as by gently shaking their shoulder and repeating their name.
- Press firmly over the supraorbital ridge and look for a motor response to stimulation.
- Gently retract the eyelid and shine a bright light into each eye, looking for both direct (constriction of the pupil that the light is being shone into) and indirect pupillary responses (constriction of the opposite pupil to that which the light is being shone into).
- Test for corneal reflexes by stimulating the cornea with cotton wool and look for a motor response. To ensure that the cornea is stimulated, the cotton wool must touch the area over the iris.
- Listen for heart sounds for 1 minute.
- Feel for a central pulse (carotid or femoral) for 1 minute.
- Listen for breath sounds for 1 minute.
- Make sure the person is lying in a dignified position with a cover over their body.
- Document the confirmation of death in the notes: the person's name, the date and time of death, persons present at the time of death and, if appropriate, primary and secondary causes of death.

Section 4

Putting history and examination skills to use

Anna R Dover
Janet Skinner

20

Preparing for assessment

General principles

Clinical assessments are integral to undergraduate and postgraduate medical education and training, and are designed to verify that those involved in the care of patients meet safe clinical standards. Assessments can be formative and/or summative. Formative assessments (such as workplace-based assessments) allow you to receive feedback on and monitor your own performance. Assessments such as these can be highly effective adjuncts to learning if they promote reflection on your own performance and recognition of areas for improvement and further development. Summative assessments, on the other hand, are used to evaluate whether you have achieved a required competence or standard in terms of knowledge, skills or performance, which may be set by licensing bodies such as the General Medical Council in the UK or postgraduate colleges. Assessment can also be used to provide evidence of safe practice: for example, simulation assessments for doctors in difficulty, or for recruitment and selection into specialty training.

This chapter provides an overview of the spectrum of clinical assessment methods, with a particular emphasis on objective structured clinical examinations (OSCEs) and clinical simulation scenarios. Guidance is offered on how to prepare for formal assessment, including the role of deliberate rehearsal, along with hints for optimising your performance in clinical and communication skills assessment.

Methods of assessment

The most widely used clinical assessment methods include OSCEs, short cases, long cases and clinical simulation scenarios (Box 20.1), during which you may be observed performing an integrated sequence of clinical, practical and/or communication skills.

Different assessment formats test different aspects of your professional competence or expertise. Short cases, for example,

will usually focus on testing either your clinical examination skills or your ability to take a history from a patient. Modern assessment methods such as OSCEs and clinical simulation allow assessment of knowledge, skills and attitudes in an integrated manner and can permit candidates to demonstrate a higher level of performance through 'showing how' and 'doing' (Fig. 20.1).

Assessments are linked to the learning outcomes of a course or curriculum, and 'blueprinting' is used to ensure there is appropriate coverage of the required knowledge, skills and behaviours across the examination. In order to perform well in clinical assessments, it is therefore crucial that you familiarise yourself with both the curriculum and the domains or skills on which you are being assessed. Not all skills will be assessed at each examination (Box 20.2).

Once you have achieved a level of competence in a clinical skill or domain, you may be considered to be 'entrustable' in this professional activity. For example, a final-year medical student may be 'entrusted' to perform peripheral cannulation on a patient if they have demonstrated competence in the specified domains (such as obtaining consent from a patient for the procedure and technical competence in the procedure itself).

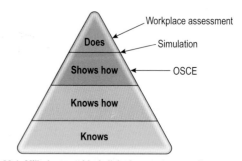

Fig. 20.1 Miller's pyramid of clinical competence and assessment methods. *Adapted from Miller G. The assessment of clinical skills/competence/performance. Academic Medicine 1990; 65(suppl):S63–S67.*

20.1 Clinical assessment formats			
Assessment format	**Patient/mannequin**	**Marking structure**	**Example**
Objective structured clinical examination	Either, in multiple stations testing different domains	Checklist or global judgement	8-minute OSCE station where the candidate is required to obtain consent from a simulated patient for venepuncture and then perform this procedure on a part-task trainer (often 6–12 stations per OSCE)
Short case	Patient	Global judgement (usually two examiners independently mark the student on several cases)	20-minute station where the candidate is required to examine three patients with evident physical signs (systolic murmur, abdominal mass and abnormal gait) and present the findings
Long case	Patient	Global judgement	60-minute station where the candidate is required to take a full history and examine a patient with chronic liver disease. The candidate is expected to formulate a differential diagnosis and plans for investigation and management (not normally during the case but the candidate presents to the examiner afterwards)
Clinical simulation scenario	Mannequin	Often global judgements of domains, e.g. behavioural marker system with areas such as communication, leadership, situation awareness, task management	20-minute station in which the candidate is required to assess and treat a simulated mannequin patient who is having an anaphylactic reaction

20.2 Example OSCE blueprint

OSCE station	Gastroenterology curriculum	Respiratory curriculum	Cardiology curriculum	Procedural skills	Resuscitation skills	Communication skills
1. Venepuncture				✓		✓
2. Cardiovascular examination			✓			
3. History taking		✓				✓
4. Abdominal examination	✓					
5. Advanced life support			✓		✓	
6. Explanation and advice		✓				✓

Clinical simulation

Clinical simulation, using either high-fidelity patient mannequins or simulated patients, is increasingly employed for teaching and learning in healthcare, as it supports deliberate rehearsal of clinical skills in a realistic setting without compromising patient safety. Experiential learning such as this ('learning by doing') also supports the transition from theory to practice. Clinical simulation is commonly included in both undergraduate and postgraduate assessments to evaluate a candidate's ability to integrate a number of complex skills or domains, which may include clinical examination, practical skills and drug or fluid prescribing. Often the scenario will involve an acutely unwell patient who is experiencing a medical emergency such as life-threatening asthma, where the use of a real patient is not feasible (Box 20.3). The patient mannequin is set up in a realistic clinical environment (such as a simulated ward), with real props and equipment (such as a nebuliser mask), and there is often an additional member of staff in the room (playing the role of the nurse, for example) who can perform tasks and provide results of investigations if requested by the candidate. Sometimes a facilitator may also be the 'voice' of the patient, giving important prompts ('I can't breathe' or simulating audible wheeze). The examination brief will clarify what is expected of you during the station but it is likely that you will be assessed on your competence in physical assessment, communication skills and the initial management of the patient.

OSCEs

These are widely used in undergraduate and postgraduate assessments, and are commonly designed to assess communication/consultation skills, practical skills, examination skills or an integrated combination of all of these. OSCEs consist of multiple clinical encounters or 'stations' (generally between 6 and 12). Candidates rotate through each station, which will be assigned a fixed duration (usually 8–12 minutes).

OSCEs may use a combination of real patients with good clinical signs, simulated patients who often participate in the communication skills stations, simulation mannequins (who may be put in the role of an acutely unwell patient where using a real patient is not feasible or safe) and/or part-task trainers (lifelike models of body parts) for assessment of procedural skills such as venepuncture (Box 20.4).

Marking structures

Examiners award marks for your performance in assessments using a standardised marking structure. While this varies from

20.3 Clinical simulation station

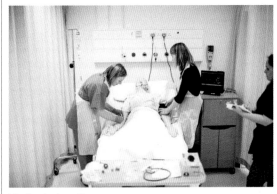

Life-threatening asthma.

You are a junior doctor on the admissions unit. The nurses ask you to see a 25-year-old male patient (the mannequin) with breathlessness whom they are concerned about. There is also a nurse present who can help you with appropriate tasks.

Typical global assessment mark sheet: life-threatening asthma simulation station

	Fail	Borderline	Good	Excellent
Structured initial assessment			✓	
Recognition of severity of illness			✓	
Initial management and resuscitation	✓			
Interpretation of results		✓		
Safe and appropriate prescribing		✓		
Escalation of care		✓		
Formulation of an ongoing management plan		✓		

Comments

Good initial A–E assessment + recognition of life-threatening asthma. Did not prescribe oxygen or nebulisers. Failed to ask for a blood gas. Called for help but quite late on. Recognised that patient needs critical care.

20

one type of examination to another, some common marking approaches are used and you should be familiar with these.

Many assessments will employ a 'checklist' format that allows the examiners to award your score objectively. These checklists are commonly used in OSCE stations, where the assessment is broken down into its individual components (for example, 'Introduces self to patient'), each component is allocated a range of marks, and your score is calculated as the sum of the component marks (Box 20.4). Often a significant number of marks will be allocated to generic aspects of the encounter (such as hand washing, obtaining consent to proceed, and demonstrating kindness and respect). There may also be some elements of the OSCE that are mandatory in order to achieve a pass (such as administering oxygen to a simulated patient with acute asthma, or addressing the patient's concerns in a communications station). By familiarising yourself with the marking structure for the examination, you can ensure that you tailor your preparation to maximise your chance of success.

Another common examination marking approach is the use of global judgement scores. Global judgements are awarded as an overall rating of performance or competence in particular domains or distinct observed behaviours (such as 'Identifying clinical signs' or 'Maintaining patient welfare', see Box 20.3). When global assessment is used, usually two or more examiners will independently mark the candidate. If the assessment has included a simulated or real patient, they may also be asked for their global judgement of your performance.

Approach to preparation

Make sure that you start to prepare well in advance and familiarise yourself with the format of the assessment: know how many stations there are, how long you have for each station and what domains or skills are being assessed. Most institutions will readily tell you what is expected from a candidate in order to pass each station, and there may be useful information available online. For example, to achieve a pass in a physical examination OSCE you may be required to perform a systematic examination, correctly identify the physical signs, create a sensible differential diagnosis and suggest an appropriate initial management plan. Remember that assessments are 'blueprinted' (that is, they will be mapped to the learning outcomes from your curriculum; Box 20.2) and you should therefore use the curriculum to guide your learning.

To some extent, the cases you are likely to be presented with in an examination can be predicted. Institutions will typically have a cohort of volunteer patients with common chronic stable diseases (such as pulmonary fibrosis or a renal transplant) or pathognomonic signs (retinitis pigmentosa or acromegaly), who have volunteered to participate. These patients may have helped in examinations before and will be well prepared to cooperate with your physical assessment. It is unusual to be asked to examine a patient who is acutely unwell, and therefore conditions such as severe asthma or pulmonary oedema will usually be tested only in simulated scenarios. Remember that there are certain rare conditions, many of which are covered in earlier sections of this book, that may be over-represented in certain examinations. Where possible, speak to other candidates who have sat the examination in the past, or refer to past papers or revision aids where they exist.

Take every opportunity you can to practise what will be expected of you on the day, informally with peers or more formally in preparatory courses if these are available to you. Many institutions

20.4 Venepuncture OSCE station

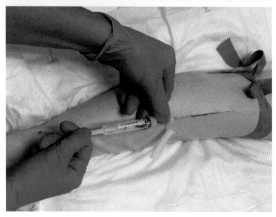

Assessment of venepuncture using a part-task trainer.

You are a junior doctor on the medical unit and have been asked to check Mrs Jones's full blood count. Please carry out the procedure on the mannequin while interacting with the actual patient.

Typical checklist mark sheet

Observed skill or behaviour	Potential score	Actual score
Cleans hands	0,1	1
Introduces self to patient	0,1,2	0
Checks patient details	0,1,2	1
Explains procedure	0,1,2,3	2
Allows patient to ask questions	0,1	1
Gains consent	0,1,2	1
Applies tourniquet to arm and chooses vein	0,1,2	2
Releases tourniquet	0,1	1
Gathers equipment and checks expiry date	0,1,2,3	2
Cleans hands and puts on appropriate PPE	0,1,2	0
Cleans skin and allows to dry	0,1	0
Reapplies tourniquet	0,1	1
Inserts needle at 15 degrees	0,1	1
Attaches blood tubes while holding needle steady	0,1,2,3,4	3
Releases tourniquet and removes blood tube	0,1,2	1
Removes needle and presses on wound with cotton swab	0,1,2	2
Immediately disposes of needle in sharps bin	0,1	1
Labels and packages bloods	0,1,2,3	3
Appropriately disposes of waste and cleans hands	0,1,2	0
Documents in patient notes	0,1	1
Simulated patient global assessment	0,1,2,3	2
TOTAL MARK (MAXIMUM 40)	40	26

PPE, *personal protective equipment*.

run revision courses or mock examinations, and these can be excellent ways to experience what the examination itself will be like. Daily clinical encounters are always opportunities for practice, as are more formal encounters with senior colleagues such as workplace-based assessments and bedside or simulation-based teaching events. Make sure you also ask colleagues for honest and critical feedback after clinical encounters so that you can reflect on which areas you can improve.

You may be offered technical and non-technical (such as team working and leadership) skills training in your local clinical skills centre, and these occasions will also allow you to practise repeatedly those techniques that you will be asked to demonstrate during assessments. Deliberate practice, repeating the skills and sequences of examination that you will be expected to execute on the day, helps to make these behaviours automatic and reduces the chances of you forgetting an aspect of history taking or physical examination under pressure.

Approach to assessment

Professionalism

Make sure you are smartly dressed, look professional and adhere to any local infection control and uniform policies (Box 20.5). Most institutions would expect you to be bare from the elbows

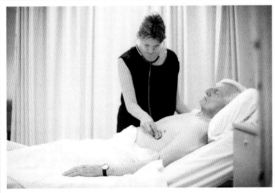

20.5 Professionalism during assessment

Observing local dress and infection control policies.

Presenting your findings: examination of the cardiovascular system

Mr Scott is a 65-year-old male. On general inspection the patient looks comfortable at rest and is not obviously breathless. Examination of the hands does not show any abnormality such as splinter haemorrhages. The pulse is regular and has a good volume with a rate of 80 per minute; there is no evidence of a collapsing pulse. The JVP is not elevated; I did not detect any central cyanosis. On inspection of the chest there is no evidence of scars, the apex beat is palpable in the fifth intercostal space and there are no thrills or heaves. On auscultation, the heart sounds are normal and there is a grade 3/6 ejection systolic murmur, loudest over the aortic area and radiating to the carotids. To conclude my examination I would like to measure the blood pressure, listen to the lung bases, check for peripheral oedema and assess peripheral pulses. The most likely diagnosis in this patient is that of aortic stenosis.

down and to have long hair tied back. Ensure that you have the appropriate clinical equipment with you (such as stethoscope, pen torch and so on) and are familiar with their use. If you are going to have physical contact with a patient during the assessment, always clean your hands with alcohol-based gel or soap and water (see Fig. 3.1) and observe basic safety principles, including the use of personal protective equipment and safe sharps disposal.

Managing time

Managing your time, both in advance of and during the assessment, can have a major impact on your performance. Make sure that you know where the examination is to be held, rehearse your journey and give yourself plenty of time to get there.

Pay particular attention to the timings within the examination and ensure that you have practised completing your assessment within the allocated time. Some assessments will be broken into different stages, and it is worth finding out as much as you can about the format; you may think you have 10 minutes to complete the OSCE station but in reality you may be allowed to spend only part of the time with the patient with the remaining time reserved for questioning from the examiners. Marks will be awarded for your answers to these questions. If you take too long assessing the patient, you may not be able to take advantage of these marks; similarly, if you finish your assessment too quickly, you risk the examiners moving on to more challenging questions to fill the remaining time. Assessments will often have short breaks between stations to allow candidates to read the instructions for the next station; once again, it is helpful to familiarise yourself with these aspects of the examination in advance.

Communication during assessment

It is vital in any assessment that you communicate with the examiners and patients in a polite and professional manner, as you would in real clinical practice. Always obtain consent from the patient to be examined, be sure not to cause any physical discomfort and thank them at the end of the station. Examiners will be assessing your communication skills and bedside manner, as well as your clinical examination technique.

Listen carefully to the instructions from the examiners, as these are often very specific ('Examine this patient's precordium'). You may also be told whether you should present your findings as you go along or at the end of your examination. When presenting your clinical findings, try to sound confident about them, avoid using language that indicates uncertainty in your own abilities ('I think I heard a systolic murmur' does not fill an examiner with confidence) and never report findings that you have not actually elicited. Use a succinct and structured format when presenting, highlighting important positive findings and describing only the relevant negative findings (see Box 20.5); listing all negatives wastes valuable time. If there is an obvious abnormality (such as a patient who is jaundiced), it is sensible to mention this early in your case presentation so that examiners see that you have noted the important finding. Do not expect any feedback from your examiners at the end of each station, as generally they are asked to avoid giving you an indication of how you have performed.

In communication stations involving simulated patients, you may be asked to take a focused history or to discuss a specific issue such as consent, or to break some difficult news. The simulated patients will have been given a standardised scenario or brief that often includes information that they will volunteer to you from the outset, and further information that they will divulge only if asked. It is therefore important to ensure that you take a structured approach to your questioning, making sure you start with open questioning and then focus on pertinent aspects, not forgetting to enquire about the patient's own concerns.

Managing unexpected difficulties

Even with thorough preparation, things may not go to plan, because of examination pressure or nerves, or through you misunderstanding the format of a station or the question you are asked. Remember that examiners generally want you to succeed and will have experienced similar assessments themselves. They will understand that you may be very nervous and will try to support you if you are finding the experience difficult. If you feel you have performed poorly in a station, try to put it behind you and focus your attention on the next one, where you may be able to recover your position. Remember that in most assessments your final mark will be a composite of all of the components of the assessment, and it is often possible to fail a station or two and still pass overall.

Putting it all together

Preparing for assessment starts long before the examination itself. Deliberate repeated practice of clinical and communication skills is key to performing well on the day. This should include timed practice within the format itself, as well as practice in presenting your findings to a surrogate examiner. A detailed understanding of the examination format and timing, as well as the marking structure, will help to ensure you are well prepared.

Take time to review the information provided in the relevant system-based chapters, as well as the more general guidance in Section 1, and watch the clinical videos for examples of comprehensive systematic examination techniques.

Good luck!

Karen Fairhurst
Gareth Clegg

21

Preparing for practice

The transition from medical student to junior doctor culminates in independent practice in a variety of clinical settings. This chapter addresses how the clinical skills described in this book are used and adapted in everyday practice.

Whatever the setting, the doctor's task is to translate patients' problems into diagnoses, therapeutic possibilities and prognoses. Undergraduate medical students first learn history taking, examination and investigation as a logical sequence, as described in preceding chapters. In reality, however, the application of these skills to a patient's clinical problem is often a less ordered, more nuanced process.

Adapting history and examination skills appropriately

History and examination skills are adapted by doctors to suit the situation. For example, elective surgical or unscheduled emergency admissions may require a systematic and comprehensive history and examination. Patients attending a specialist outpatient clinic, will already have been screened by a referring clinician, however, and a history and examination focused on the presenting condition is appropriate. If the patient is attending a review clinic, history and examination may be restricted to monitoring an existing condition. The information-gathering process may appear to be sequential: the history suggests a differential diagnosis; examination and then investigation help confirm or refute diagnostic possibilities. In reality, these elements often occur in parallel. For example, sequential history then examination may be abandoned in favour of a more opportunistic approach to avoid distressing a reluctant child. In critically ill patients a highly focused history and examination aimed at rapidly identifying the main problems while initiating resuscitation is imperative.

Integrated examination

Although in an individual it is rarely necessary to carry out a comprehensive history and examination of all systems, a rapid screening examination may be useful to direct more detailed examination if the diagnosis is unclear or when patients are being admitted to hospital. There is no single correct procedure for performing a physical examination and you will develop your own approach, but a reasonable routine is outlined in Box 21.1.

21.1 A personal system for performing a physical examination

- Handshake and introduction
- Note general appearances while talking:
  - Does the patient look well?
  - Any immediate and obvious clues, e.g. obesity, plethora, breathlessness
  - Complexion
- Hands and radial pulse
- Face
- Mouth and ears
- Neck
- Thorax:
  - Breasts
  - Heart
  - Lungs
- Abdomen
- Lower limbs:
  - Oedema
  - Circulation
  - Locomotor function and neurology
- Upper limbs:
  - Movement and neurology
- Cranial nerves, including fundoscopy
- Blood pressure
- Temperature
- Height and weight
- Urinalysis

Diagnostic strategies

Doctors recognise patterns of symptoms and signs, then apply clinical reasoning to interpret them and to formulate diagnostic possibilities or probabilities. Sometimes doctors instantly recognise a condition based on previous experience ('spot diagnoses', p. 34). Visual patterns are particularly likely to lead to such recognition: for example, a typical rash. More commonly, elements of the history and examination together trigger pattern recognition. This process relies on comparing a patient's presentation to cases encountered before and remembered as 'illness scripts'. With increasing experience, less typical presentations are encountered and recalled, and doctors are increasingly able to recognise more exceptional cases.

Pre-test probability

Where doctors are unable to recognise patterns in presentations quickly, various refinement strategies are used to arrange the possible diagnoses in order of probability. The pre-test probability of a disease in an individual depends on the context in which the symptom has appeared because the prevalence of disease varies between populations. In general practice populations the incidence of serious disease is much lower than in hospital populations; serious conditions still usually need to be excluded, however. This may involve identification of 'red flag' symptoms and signs for serious disease, or the use of clinical prediction rules such as the Wells score for deep vein thrombosis. Positive 'red flag' features or above-threshold prediction scores increase the probability of a disease in individuals and generally trigger further investigations.

Additional factors affecting the pre-test probability of disease in patients with the same presenting symptoms include age, gender, past medical history, family history and lifestyle. Few doctors use formal probabilistic reasoning in making diagnoses, but most know the relationship between these factors and the likelihood of a specific disease and use this understanding intuitively to select likely diagnoses (hypotheticodeductive reasoning, Fig. 21.1). History, examination and investigation results are used to support or refute putative diagnoses. These components are rarely independent, however, and returning to clarify the history or re-examine when signs are ambiguous allows an iterative approach to accurate diagnosis.

Rare diseases

While diagnosis by probability works in most cases, rare diseases also occur, and to the affected patients and their families they are not rare. Avoid the trap of thinking that all patients have common conditions and that symptoms that do not fit with common diagnoses are less important. Indeed, occasional patients with a credible and consistent history of unusual symptoms may actually merit more, not less, investigation. The art is to listen carefully, keep an open mind, and pick up the uncommon situation when the usual patterns of presentation really do not fit the facts of a case.

Other factors that complicate the application of clinical skills in diagnosis include:

- clinical problems involving many organ systems rather than one
- new disease occurring in the context of existing physical and psychological comorbidities

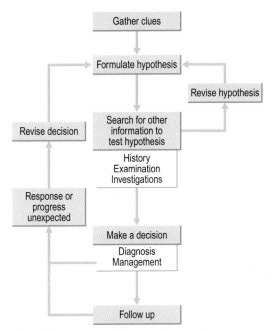

Fig. 21.1 The hypotheticodeductive method of decision-making.

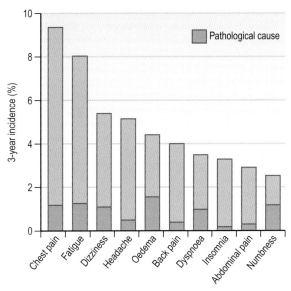

Fig. 21.2 Percentage of symptoms presenting in primary care with an underlying pathological cause.

- the presentation being embedded in the context of an individual patient's story
- symptoms arising in the absence of underlying pathology (see the next section).

Approach to the patient with medically unexplained symptoms

Much of this book deals with the association between a patient's history and examination findings and the presence of underlying disease. Symptoms are not synonymous with disease, however, but are subjective experiences with many possible sources: pathological, physiological, psychological, cultural, behavioural and external. Many patients experience symptoms that impair function but do not fit characteristic patterns of disease, and persist despite normal examination and investigations. These are called 'functional' or 'medically unexplained symptoms' (MUS, Fig. 21.2). Over 30% of patients attending their general practitioner have MUS and they are also common in secondary care, although disease prevalence is much higher there. Some symptoms are more likely to be medically unexplained than others: for example, persistent fatigue, abdominal pain and back pain. The causes of MUS are poorly understood but various predisposing and precipitating factors (Box 21.2) may contribute. Most functional symptoms are transient but some become persistent, causing similar disability to those resulting from disease and also significant emotional distress. If MUS are not recognised and managed appropriately, attempts to alleviate them can result in harm from fruitless investigations, inappropriate interventions or drugs, and increased fear of disease.

Patients with MUS commonly feel that doctors do not think their symptoms are real, leading to a breakdown in trust between patient and doctor, and frustration for both. Crucially, doctors must use an empathic and non-judgemental approach so the patient feels believed. Keep an open mind and accept all the

21.2 Aetiological factors for medically unexplained symptoms

- Precipitating: stress, depression, anxiety and sometimes disease and injury, especially if associated with fears of, or belief in, disease
- Predisposing: fear of disease from previous experience
- Perpetuating: inappropriate attempts to alleviate symptoms, e.g. excessive rest, failure to address patient's concerns

patient's symptoms at face value. Remember that patients with MUS may also have or develop disease. Even if a functional diagnosis is suspected, a comprehensive history and examination remain imperative. This helps patients to feel that they are being taken seriously; in addition, organic disease, however unlikely, is less likely to be missed.

Patients' illness beliefs matter hugely and should be explicitly acknowledged. What do they think is wrong? Why have they come to you now and what do they hope you can do for them? Inconsistencies in the history should be explored with the patient; for example, a patient with severe chest pain and normal coronary angiography may still firmly believe they have angina. Normal investigations need to be explained clearly to help demonstrate that the evidence does not support their belief.

Patients may complain about previous doctors or treatments. Allowing a patient to express dissatisfaction shows interest, and helps to avoid suggesting treatments they are likely to reject. Always remain professional and avoid being drawn into criticism of other healthcare providers.

Patients can be acutely sensitive to questions that suggest a doctor thinks there is a psychological basis for their symptoms ('all in the mind'). Frame questions carefully in terms of their symptoms: for example, 'Do your symptoms ever make you feel down or frustrated?' rather than 'Do you ever feel depressed?' Abuse is one possible precipitant of MUS but seek this history judiciously. Follow local guidelines for any abuse you discover.

The physical assessment includes observing the patient throughout the consultation. Watch for inconsistent signs, though this does not indicate whether they are consciously or subconsciously produced. Usually there are no physical signs

21

but some non-pathological signs are associated with MUS; for instance, in irritable bowel syndrome you may find evidence of bloating and some tenderness, but otherwise gastrointestinal examination will be normal. The history often suggests MUS, so focus on excluding any unexpected physical findings, as well as demonstrating to patients that you are taking them seriously. Any signs you do find may vary between examinations but overall the examination is commonly normal with MUS.

Investigations are used in MUS mainly to reassure both physician and patient. Exhaustive investigations to exclude all physical illness are costly and unhelpful, risk side effects and do not reassure patients in the longer term. Before requesting investigations, discuss with the patient the likelihood and significance of a normal result. Patients are more likely to be satisfied when your explanation makes sense to them, removes blame and helps generate ideas about how they can manage their symptoms.

Assessment of a patient with minor injury or illness

In patients with minor injury or illness, usually presenting in the accident and emergency department or general practice, a history and examination focused on the presenting symptoms are usually sufficient. It is, however, crucial to establish the reason for the patient's presentation, as well as clearly defining their clinical problem, as their concerns about their symptoms and their expectations of investigation and treatment influence the outcome.

Carefully eliciting the mechanism of injury, progression of symptoms and their impact on the patient (for example, whether they can walk and go to work/school) will help detect problems that are not as 'minor' as they might seem. Be wary of the apparently minor injury or illness that is actually the tip of a diagnostic iceberg, for example:

- a clavicular fracture caused by minimal trauma, which is in fact a pathological fracture secondary to an underlying lung malignancy
- a fall with wrist injury that was actually a syncopal episode caused by cardiac arrhythmia
- shoulder pain that initially sounds musculoskeletal but is in fact the first presentation of angina
- a pattern of soft-tissue injury in a toddler that is completely at odds with the history, suggesting possible non-accidental injury.

Focus your examination on the system or body part implicated in the history, as outlined in previous chapters. If the findings are not consistent, carry out a more comprehensive history and examination. If the system affected is unclear (such as arm pain, which may be musculoskeletal, vascular, neurological or referred cardiac pain), examine all of these systems.

As you formulate a differential diagnosis, check for other systemic features of disease in addition to examining the obvious source of symptoms. A swollen ankle may trigger a systematic enquiry and examination if the history suggests a reactive arthropathy rather than a simple sprain.

Focusing the clinical examination comes with practice, but if in doubt, be comprehensive. Start with the body part that is causing the most trouble and follow leads. Elements of the examination likely to cause discomfort should be left until last.

A careful and courteous examination can also increase trust between the patient and clinician. Even when you feel it is unlikely to yield important information, examination reassures the patient that they are being taken seriously and assessed thoroughly. Conversely, not examining a patient risks them feeling you are being dismissive of their problems.

Assessment of a critically ill patient

A critically unwell patient requires a very different approach to those with minor ailments. Examination and interventions often occur simultaneously as the clinician attempts to identify the main problems. Initially, your aim is to gain control of the situation and stabilise the patient's condition. A fuller history and clinical examination can follow after initial resuscitation.

The approach to recognising and assessing the acutely ill and deteriorating patient is covered in detail in Chapter 18.

Documenting your findings

Documenting clinical findings in a clear and concise medical record is a crucial aspect of medical practice. It should include a structured account of the history and examination – both positive and important negative findings. Some circumstances demand additional detail: for example, forensic documentation of the length and position of wounds.

The appropriate level of detail varies with the context but adopt and use a consistent format. This format quickly becomes a habit, reduces your need to think about what to record next, and lessens the likelihood of forgetting something important. A consistent format also allows others to locate specific information quickly in your documentation. An example of clear and comprehensive clinical documentation of a case is shown in Fig. 21.3.

One widely used overall structure for organising your written documentation is SOAP, an acronym for subjective, objective, assessment and plan.

Subjective

This records information you obtain directly from the patient (or someone speaking on their behalf). It constitutes the body of the history, as covered in Chapter 2. What is the patient's chief symptom? What is the patient's current condition? It is best to avoid describing the problem in medical terms at this point and more useful to record the patient's own words. What is the history of the problem? If an injury, what was the mechanism?

Past medical history, family medical history, social history (including smoking and alcohol or recreational drug use), current medications and any allergies should also be noted here.

Objective

This is information you gather about the patient. Here you record vital signs, findings from your physical examination and the results of any initial investigations. Again, it is useful to use a standard format to record physical findings, so others can find specific information quickly.

Assessment

This starts with a brief summary of the information obtained. It then lists the patient's main symptoms, together with a differential diagnosis. If the patient has several pressing issues, compile a 'problem list'. Not all of these problems may be medical but they will all influence the best plan for what to do next. For example, 'worsening soft-tissue infection of the left lower leg' is a problem with a diagnosis, but 'not taken any of the prescribed antibiotics as unable to swallow tablets' is a different kind of problem, which is nevertheless crucial to negotiating a successful plan.

The differential diagnosis list should include the following:

- What is the most likely cause of this patient's problems?
- Are there possible underlying causes that are less likely but would have serious consequences if missed?
- What other medical problem could this be? It is often worth taking a moment to reflect on whether there is another condition that may present in a similar way, particularly if an obvious diagnosis suggests itself quickly.
- Is the main problem medical? Could the main issue underlying the presentation be a social, psychological or emotional one?

Plan

This should include all relevant actions: procedures performed, medications given, explanations and advice offered, referrals and recommendations made. Additionally, record here any further investigations and information still required to refine the diagnosis and inform further management.

Sign and date your notes, including your position and contact details (pager number, for example).

Communicating with colleagues

An essential part of a doctor's work is the accurate and timely sharing of information about patients with colleagues. Communication failures are strong predictors of healthcare-related harm.

Typical situations include:

- referral of a patient from the community to hospital (Box 21.3)
- request for advice or immediate help
- discharge of a patient back to the community from hospital (Box 21.4)
- outpatient clinic letter to the general practitioner or referring consultant
- referral of a patient to another consultant
- referral of a patient to other hospital or community services (such as a social work referral or referral to a specialist service such as palliative care).

Verbal communication

Verbal communication about a patient needs to be structured and concise to be effective. Be clear about your expectations of the person you are communicating with, especially if you are requesting that they do something, such as coming to review the patient.

SBAR (situation, background, assessment, recommendation) is a simple tool to help standardise communication. It is recommended by the World Health Organization for use as a tool to increase patient safety. It allows staff to share similar expectations about what is to be communicated and how the communication is structured. SBAR can be used face to face, over the telephone or even in some written communication.

Using SBAR

- Firstly, collect the information you need to pass on, and think through what you want to achieve by the communication: for example, informing a colleague, asking for immediate help or requesting advice. Consider some brief notes under the SBAR headings.
- Attract the attention of the person you are communicating with. Introduce yourself. If face to face, make eye contact. If possible, use the person's name.
    - 'Hello, Dr Jones. My name is Dr Smith. I'm one of the junior doctors in the emergency department.'
- **Situation:** give a one- or two-sentence description covering why you are calling, what is happening and what the acute change is.
    - 'I'm concerned about a 53-year-old man who came into the emergency department this morning complaining of severe headache. His headache's getting worse and he's begun to vomit.'

21

21.3 Contents of a referral letter

- Demographic details about the patient and the referring doctor practice
- Consultant/receiving practitioner and/or clinic, ward or specialty
- The urgency of the referral
- Clinical information:
    - History of presenting symptoms/examination findings/results of any investigation
    - Reason for referral and expected outcome
    - Past medical history
    - Current and recent medication (including any complementary therapies and self-medication known to the referring doctor)
    - Clinical warnings, e.g. allergies, blood-borne viruses
    - Smoking status/alcohol history
    - Additional relevant information, e.g.:
        - Relevant social or personal circumstances
        - Patient/family's understanding of the condition and their expectations
        - Information about any advanced directives or resuscitation orders

Similar information will be required when a patient is referred internally to another hospital consultant.

21.4 Contents of a patient discharge letter following a hospital admission

- Demographic information about the patient, the consultant and the preferred GP (the GP who has been most involved, if known)
- Ward
- Date of discharge/transfer or date of death
- Reason for admission/transfer
- Mode of admission: elective, emergency or transfer
- Source of admission
- Diagnosis/problem list
- Significant operations/procedures (dates)
- Relevant investigations
- Complications/adverse reactions
- Medication (including start and stop dates, recommendations for altering dose or stopping medication after discharge, use of aids such as a dosette box)
- Discharge plans:
    - Further information about destination
    - Care package
    - Primary care support needed
- Information given to patient/carers
- Results awaited
- Hospital review plan/referral to other hospital services
- Other relevant clinical or personal information
- Contact name and telephone number of author

Date : 03.08.13
Time : 14.00

MARY BROWN aged 78
32 Tartan Cresc.
Edinburgh
DOB 12.09.35
CHI120935xxxx

Emergency admission to CCU via GP: Dr Wells, High St, Edinburgh

History from patient

PC Chest pain   2 hours
        Breathlessness   1 hour
        Dizziness   30 mins

HPC
Severe pain 'like a band around chest' while watching TV, which has now lasted 2 hours despite using GTN, aspirin and diltiazem.
Radiates to jaw and inner aspect of L arm.
Has gradually become breathless over the last hour and dizzy in last 30 minutes.

First began 6 months ago: episode of lower retrosternal chest pain after walking about $^1/2$ mile uphill:
        • no associated palpitation or SOB.
Two further episodes over the next 3 months.

3 months ago: increasing frequency of pain
        • now brought on by walking 200 m on the flat or climbing 1 flight of stairs
        • worse after heavy meals
        • other features of pain as before.

2 months ago: visited GP who diagnosed angina. Prescribed GTN, which gave effective relief.

1 week ago: three episodes of chest pain at rest, all immediately relieved by GTN.
°Blackouts, °pain in calves on exertion.

PH Tonsillectomy   1952   Hospital X
        Perforated peptic ulcer   1977   Hospital Y
        COPD   Since 1990   General practitioner

        °MI, °DM, °J, °HBP, °Stroke, °RF, °TB

DH   DOSE   FREQUENCY   DURATION
        Salbutamol inhaler   2 puffs   As necessary   3 years
        Zopiclone   7.5mg   At night   6 months
        Senokot (self-medication) 2 tabs   2–3 times per week   10 years
        GTN spray   1 puff   As required   2 months
        Aspirin   75mg   Once daily   2 months
        No allergies

FH
        Pit accident   ☐   ⊘ Heart failure
        aged 36   age 83

                    ⊘   ☐   ⊠   ●
                Breast cancer 79
                aged 50
        1 aunt died aged 57 of acute MI   ☐ ☐ ○ ☐

1

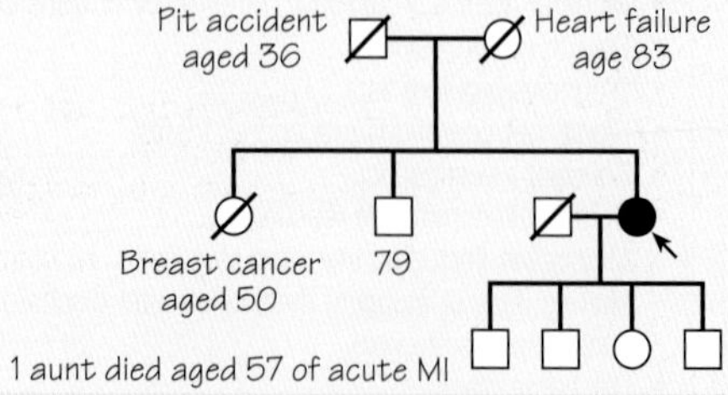

Fig. 21.3 Case notes example. *CCU,* coronary care unit; *CHI,* community health index.

Demographic details

Always record:
- The patient's name and address, date of birth (DOB) and age
- Any national health identification number, such as Community Health Index number in Scotland or National Health Service number in England and Wales
- Source of referral, e.g. from emergency department or general practitioner
- General practitioner's name and address
- Source of history, e.g. patient, relative, carer
- Date and time of examination

Presenting complaint (PC)

State the major problem in one or two of the patient's own words (or give a brief list), followed by the duration of each. Do not use medical terminology.

History of presenting complaint (HPC)

Describe the onset, nature and course of each symptom.
Paraphrase the patient's account and condense it if necessary.
Omit irrelevant details.
Put particularly telling comments in inverted commas.
Include other parts of the history if relevant, such as the smoking history in patients with cardiac or respiratory presentations, or family history in disorders with a possible genetic trait such as hypercholesterolaemia or diabetes.
Correct grammar is not necessary.

GTN – Glyceryl trinitrate

SOB – Shortness of breath

Past history (PH)

Tabulate in chronological order.
Include important negatives, e.g. in a patient with chest pain ask about previous myocardial infarction, angina, hypertension or diabetes mellitus and record whether these are present or absent.
Jaundice is important because it may pose a risk to healthcare workers if due to hepatitis B or C.

COPD – Chronic obstructive pulmonary disease
  MI – Myocardial infarction
  DM – Diabetes mellitus
   J – Jaundice
 HBP – Hypertension
  RF – Rheumatic fever
  TB – Tuberculosis

Drug history (DH)

Tabulate this and include any allergies, particularly to drugs.
Record any previous adverse drug reactions prominently on the front of the notes as well as inside.

21

Family history (FH)

Record the age and current health or the causes of or the ages at death of the patient's parents, siblings and children.
Use the symbols shown in Figure 2.1 to construct a pedigree chart.

Fig. 21.3 (Continued)

SH

Retired cleaner.
Widow for 3 years. Lives alone in sheltered housing.
Smoked 20/day from age 19.
Teetotal.
HH once a week for cleaning and shopping. Daughter nearby visits regularly.

SE

CVS: See above.

RS: Longstanding cough most days with white sputum on rising in morning only. °Haemoptysis.
Wheezy in cold weather.

GI: Weight steady.
Nil else of note.

GUS: PARA 1 + 0. °PMB, °urinary symptoms.

CNS: Nil of note.

MSS: Occasional pain and stiffness in right knee on exertion for 5 years.

ES: Nil of note.

O/E

Anxious, frail, cachectic lady.
Weight 45 kg. Height 1.25 m.
2 cm craggy mass in upper, outer quadrant L breast. Fixed to underlying tissues.
Patient unaware of this
1 cm node in apex of left axilla.
°Pallor, °cyanosis, °jaundice, °clubbing.

CVS

P90 reg, small volume, normal character.
BP 140/80 JVP + 3 cm normal character, °oedema, AB 5ICS MCL, °thrills.
HS I + II + 2/6 ESM at LLSE °radiation.
°Bruits.
PP:

	Radial	Brachial	Carotid	Femoral	Popliteal	Post. Tibial	Dorsalis pedis
R	+	+	+	+	+/-	+/-	+/-
L	+	+	+	+	+	+	+

(Normal +, Reduced +/-, Absent -)

RS

Trachea central. Reduced cricosternal distance and intercostal indrawing on inspiration.
Expansion reduced but symmetrical.
PN resonant.
Breath sounds normal, no wheeze or crackles heard.
VR normal and symmetrical.

2

Fig. 21.3 (Continued)

Social history (SH)
- Occupation
- Marital status
- Living circumstances: type of housing and with whom
- Smoking
- Alcohol
- Illicit drug use (if appropriate)
- Social support in the frail or disabled

HH – Home help

Systematic enquiry (SE)
Document positive responses that do not feature in the HPC.

CVS – Cardiovascular system
RS – Respiratory system
GI – Gastrointestinal system
GUS – Genitourinary system
PMB – Postmenopausal bleeding
CNS – Central nervous system
MSS – Musculoskeletal system
ES – Endocrine system

General / On examination (OE)
- Physical appearance, e.g. frail, drowsy, breathless
- Mental state, e.g. anxious, distressed, confused
- Under-nourished, cachectic, obese
- Abnormal smells, e.g. ketones, alcohol, uraemia, fetor hepaticus
- Height, weight and waist circumference
- Skin, e.g. cyanosis, pallor, jaundice, any specific lesions or rashes
- Breasts: normal or describe any mass
- Hands: finger clubbing, or abnormalities of skin and nails
- Lymph nodes: characteristics and site

Cardiovascular system (CVS)
- Pulse (P): rate, rhythm, character and volume
- Blood pressure (BP)
- Jugular venous pressure (JVP): height and character
- Presence or absence of ankle oedema
- Apex beat (AB): position, character, presence of thrills
- Heart sounds (HS): any added sounds, murmurs and grade
- Peripheral pulses (PP) and bruits

5ICS – 5th intercostal space
MCL – Mid-clavicular line
ESM – Ejection systolic murmur
LLSE – Lower left sternal edge

21

Respiratory system (RS)
- Any chest-wall deformity
- Trachea central or deviated
- Signs of hyperinflation
- Expansion and its symmetry
- Percussion note (PN) and site of any abnormality
- Breath sounds (BS): any added sounds and site of abnormality
- Vocal resonance (VR) and site of abnormality

Fig. 21.3 (Continued)

AS
Normal oral mucosa
Upper midline scar
Hernial orifices intact
°Tenderness or guarding
°Masses
°LKKS or ascites
BS normal
PR not done
PV not performed

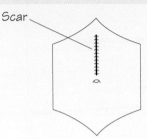

Scar

CNS
AMT 9/10
Cranial nerves II–XII: PERLA, NAD
Speech normal

	RIGHT		LEFT	
	UL	LL	UL	LL
Power	5	5	5	5
Tone	normal (n)	n	n	n
Light touch	n	n	n	n
Position	n	n	n	n
Coordination	n	n	n	n

Reflexes	K	A	B	T	S	Pl
R	++	+	++	+	+	flexor
L	++	+	++	+	+	flexor

(increased +++, normal ++, diminished +, absent -)

MSS
Heberden's nodes on index and middle fingers bilaterally.
Full ROM in all joints.
Crepitus in right knee. No other bony abnormality.

IMPRESSION △

Active problems
1 Chest pain suggestive of acute coronary syndrome
2 Left breast lump and axillary node suspicious for cancer
3 Smoker

Inactive problems
1 Stable COPD
2 Perforated duodenal ulcer 1977
3 Possible osteoarthritis of right knee

3

Fig. 21.3 (Continued)

Abdominal system (AS)
Mouth:
 • Any abnormality; own teeth or dentures
Abdomen:
 • Scars and site
 • Shape: distended or scaphoid
 • Hernial orifices
 • Tenderness and guarding; site of these
 • Masses and description of these
 • Enlargement of liver, kidneys or spleen (LKKS)
 • Ascites if present
 • Bowel sounds (BS): presence and character
 • Rectal examination (per rectum, PR): record whether or not it was
   performed and your findings; should not be done in patients
   with cardiac disease, as it may provoke an arrhythmia
 • In women: vaginal examination (per vaginam, PV) is only carried
   out if relevant
 • In men: external genitalia

Central nervous system (CNS)
In older patients, record the abbreviated mental test (AMT) score.
In impaired consciousness, head injury or possible raised
intracranial pressure, record the Glasgow Coma Scale (GCS) score.

 • Abnormal speech
 • Cranial nerves: record abnormalities only
 • Fundoscopy
 • Tabulate the remaining examination

If it is relevant, record the presence or absence of tremor, gait
abnormality, fasciculation, dyspraxia, two-point discrimination,
stereognosis or sensory neglect.

PERLA – Pupils equal and react to light and accommodation
  NAD – No abnormality detected
   UL – Upper limb
   LL – Lower limb
    K – Knee
    A – Ankle
    B – Biceps
    T – Triceps
    S – Supinator
   Pl – Plantar

Musculoskeletal system (MSS)
 • Gait if abnormal
 • Muscle or soft-tissue changes
 • Swelling, colour, heat, tenderness
 • Deformities in the bones or joints
 • Limitation of range of movements (ROM) in any affected joint

Clinical diagnosis or impression
Record your conclusions and the most likely diagnoses in order
of probability.
In patients with multiple pathology make a problem list so the key
issues are seen immediately.

△ Diagnosis

21

Fig. 21.3 (Continued)

Plan

ECG performed on admission shows sinus rhythm and deep ST depression in leads II, III and aVF

Troponin at 12 hours
Repeat ECG in 1 hour
Chest X-ray
Full blood count
Urea and electrolytes, glucose

Oxygen and cardiac monitor
IV morphine and metoclopramide
Aspirin and clopidogrel
Low-molecular-weight heparin
Continue aspirin and diltiazem
Discuss beta-blocker with consultant in view of COPD
Advice to stop smoking

When stable
1 Review anti-anginal management
2 Referral for mammography and fine-needle aspiration of breast lump
3 Spirometry and assessment of inhaler technique

Information given
Diagnosis and treatment explained to patient and daughter
N.B. Breast lump not mentioned at this stage until discussed with senior staff

A. Doctor (signed)
A. DOCTOR   (Date and Time) capitals

Progress notes
3.8.13
1800 Ward Round – Dr Consultant

No further chest pain

O/E
P70 BP 100/70
JVP not elevated, °oedema
HS I + II and ESM as above
Chest clear
Breast lump noted

ECG at 4 hours – resolution of inferior ST changes

Impression

Acute coronary syndrome – no ST segment elevation

Plan
Await troponin
Continue LMW heparin
Check lipid profile
For echocardiography in view of murmur then consider ACE inhibitor
Spirometry and assessment of inhaler technique

Consultant to discuss finding of breast lump   A. Doctor (signed)
with patient and daughter   A. DOCTOR   (Date and Time) capitals

4

Fig. 21.3 (Continued)

Plan

List the investigations required. When a result is already available, e.g. an ECG, record it.

Record any immediate management instigated.

If uncertain about an investigation or treatment, precede with a '?' and discuss with a more senior member of staff.

Information given

Document what you have told the patient and any other family member. It is also important to document any diagnosis that you have not discussed.

If the patient voices any concerns or fears, document these too.

Progress notes

Follow the same structure with these additions:
• Changes in the patient's symptoms
• Examination findings
• Results of new investigations
• Clinical impression of the patient's progress
• Plans for further management, particularly drug changes.

Make progress notes regularly depending on the speed of change in the patient's condition; in an intensive therapy setting, this may be several times a day but, in a stable situation, daily or alternate days.

Date, note time and sign all entries.

Record any unexpected change in the patient's condition as well as routine progress notes.

ACE – angiotensin-converting enzyme
LMW – low-molecular-weight

21

Fig. 21.3 (Continued)

- **Background:** the information needed to make an assessment:
  - Relevant history: what were the key events leading up to the present situation?
  - Vital signs.
    - 'Mr Jackson had a sudden onset of severe headache after waking at about 07:00 this morning. The pain hasn't improved despite painkillers and he appears to be getting worse. He's hypertensive at 210/110 and vomiting.'
- **Assessment:** what is your assessment of the problem?
    - 'I'm concerned that Mr Jackson may be having an intracranial bleed.'
- **Recommendation/request:** what do you think should be done? What assistance are you asking for? Be clear about what you need and when you need it.
    - 'I'd like you to come and review the patient urgently please.'

If you are feeling out of your depth and need support from a senior colleague, be clear about that. It is better to endure the brief discomfort of having to admit that you need help than to put a patient's wellbeing in jeopardy.

SBAR can be applied as a standard framework to transfer important information in many situations. By using this method you are proactively giving the listener the information that they would be requesting anyway to assess the problem. You save time by assimilating and presenting information in a structured way.

Written communication

Conventionally, information was transferred between doctors by post, but increasingly communication is done electronically. Whatever the medium, the quality of written communication is crucial. Handwritten forms must be clear and legible. Doctors should write clear, well-structured referral, discharge or transfer letters (see Boxes 21.3 and 21.4). More and more, these letters are copied to, or read by, patients as well as other clinicians, so they must always contain appropriate language.

Clinical information is confidential and sensitive. It should never be transmitted by insecure electronic means. Nor should it be stored on, or copied to, equipment that could be stolen or lost, breaching confidentiality. Encryption should be used wherever possible to protect electronic records, and all clinical information should always be managed in accordance with local information governance regulations.

Index